Mosby's
Survival Guide to
MEDICAL
Abbreviations & Acronyms
Prefixes & Suffixes
Symbols
Greek Alphabet

Caution

Abbreviation and symbol usage can be extremely dangerous. One needs to decide if their convenience and space saving are worth the risk. For example, a physician wanted to order a prothrombin time (abbreviated PT) on a patient. A physical therapy routine (abbreviated PT) was ordered instead. An abbreviation should not be used to designate drugs or drug combinations because they are particularly dangerous. The abbreviation PBZ can mean phenoxybenzamine, phenylbutazone, or pyribenzamine. Also the form an abbreviation takes often varies from physician to physician, institution to institution, and specialty to specialty. With proper care and caution, abbreviations and symbols are a convenient and quick means of communication. However, THEY DO HAVE THEIR LIMITATIONS.

Mosby's
Survival Guide to
MEDICAL
Abbreviations & Acronyms
Prefixes & Suffixes
Symbols
Greek Alphabet

Joe Bill Campbell, PhD

June M. Campbell, MEd, MT(ASCP)

Edited by
C.O. Sennett, M.D.
President, SouthEastern Pathology
Rome, Georgia

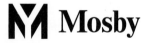 Mosby

An Affiliate of Elsevier Science

St. Louis   London   Philadelphia   Sydney   Toronto

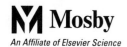
Mosby
An Affiliate of Elsevier Science

Editor: James Shanahan
Developmental Editors: Jennifer Roche, Anne J. Gleason
Editorial Assistant: Susan J. Eriksen
Project Manager: Peggy Fagen
Designer: Kay Kramer
Electronic Production Coordinator: Joan Herron
Manufacturing Supervisor: Linda Ierardi

Printed in the United States of America

Mosby, Inc.
11830 Westline Industrial Drive
St. Louis, MO 63146

ISBN 0-8151-1398-6

02 03 04 / 9 8 7 6 5 4 3

Preface

Abbreviations and symbols are used extensively in the medical community to speed communication among medical workers. They are a time and space saver. They are also a source of misinterpretation, confusion, and error. Their use is a great convenience. However, this is often achieved at the expense of safety and accuracy. This book is offered as a possible solution to some of these problems. It is meant to provide a single, comprehensive source of the abbreviations, symbols, prefixes, and suffixes used in medical communication.

Since abbreviations and symbols originate from various sources, many terms have more than one abbreviation or symbol. Also, many abbreviations and symbols have more than one meaning. The meaning given here may not even be the one intended in your source material. Great care should be exercised when interpreting abbrevations and symbols, since their use has led to delays in patient care and occasionally to patient harm.

No attempt has been made to state the best, most favored, or correct usage. Nor do the authors endorse the legitimacy of any inclusion, only that it has been used at one time or another in medical communication. All forms of the abbreviations and symbols have been given and all interpretations included. It is the responsibility of the person interpreting the abbreviations and symbols to assign the correct usage for that time and place.

It is recommended that everyone read the CAUTION notice at the beginning of this book and the introductory portion at the beginning of each section. The introduction sections give the format, style, and conventions used in this work.

Every effort has been made to see that the material presented here is accurate and many reference sources have been utilized. However, in a source of this magnitude, errors of both omission and commission are bound to occur. We ask your help in finding these areas. If you encounter an abbreviation, acronym, or symbol that is not included, please send it, along with its meaning and the situation in which it was used, to the authors at the address given below. An addendum has been added that includes entries found after the book went to press. This includes many entries relating to the Managed Health Care industry, as well as other new abbreviations and acronyms along with new meanings for some entries presently in the main list.

It is our sincere hope that the use of this work will make the task of good patient care easier, faster, and more reliable.

Joe Bill Campbell
June M. Campbell

P.O. Box 115
Cave Spring, Georgia 30124

Acknowledgments

Every effort has been made to see that these listings are accurate. To that end many sources have been used. We would like to acknowledge the efforts and expertise of the following people who have reviewed, corrected, and edited this material.

1. James H. Jordan, Teacher of Latin, Language Department, Darlington School, Rome, Georgia, for reviewing the Latin derivations and meanings.

2. Steven M. Sheeley, Ph.D., Associate Professor of Religion; Chair, The Mrs. Columbus Roberts Department of Religion and Philosophy, Shorter College, Rome, Georgia, for reviewing the Greek derivations and meanings.

3. Wilson Hall, Ph. D., Professor of Humanities, Shorter College, Rome, Georgia, for reviewing the German derivations and meanings.

4. Tom Moss III, Director of Research and Development, Peach State Laboratories, Rome, Georgia, for reviewing the chemical entries.

5. James E. Colbert, Ph.D., Assistant Professor of Chemistry, Shorter College, Rome, Georgia, for reviewing the biochemical entries.

6. Randa Mixon, Teacher of French, Language Department, Darlington School, Rome, Georgia, for reviewing the French derivations and meanings.

7. Alman Garrett, Pharm. D., M.B.A., R. Ph., Clinical Coordinator/Pharmacy Services, Redmond Regional Medical Center, Rome, Georgia, for reviewing the drug listings.

8. Gwynne D. Floyd, M.D., F.A.C.C., and Juanita Eury, C.M.A., Cardiology Department, Southeastern Cardiovascular Institute, Rome, Georgia, for reviewing the pacemaker codes.

Special thanks is given to Zaneta Arnold and Laura Falls, for their efforts in typing this difficult and tedious material, and to the many others who have contributed to this work.

Contents

Abbreviations & Acronyms

Abbreviations are shortened forms of words or phrases. Acronyms are words formed from the initial letters or groups of letters of the words in descriptive phases. Individuals or institutions have the prerogative to develop variations in the form of abbreviations so long as accurate and precise communication is maintained.

There are some considerations about the development of terms in modern medical nomenclature from Latin and Greek. The classical Latin alphabet consists of 23 letters. The "J", "U," and "W" were added during medieval times to give the 26 letters of the modern alphabet used in English. The letter "j" appears in the Latin roots given here, even though this is not proper in classical Latin. Since medical terminology developed from the more modern form of Latin, the prefixes and suffixes used in medical terms reflect this.

The process of transliterating Greek into English is a fairly smooth one. Dr. Steven Sheeley, whose work is acknowledged in the front matter of this book, gives two explanatory notes that relate to the development of terms from Greek origins. First, Greek does not contain the letter "h". Many words that begin with "r" or a vowel have aspirated first syllables indicated by a "rough" breathing mark. While this "h" sound would normally be transliterated by placing the "h" before the vowel or "r" (i.e., "hr"), English spelling of Greek words tends to reverse that order (i.e., "rh" as in "rheumatism"). A second note concerns the transliteration of the Greek letter upsilon ("v"). Where this letter would be transliterated with a "u," it shows up consistently in English spelling as a "y" (i.e., "hyper" rather than "huper").

The entries in this section are presented with the following conventions of format and style.

1. **CASE:** Upper and lower case letters are used in the manner in which they were found. Keep in mind that any given person may make his or her own refinements.

2. **PERIODS:** For consistency, periods are not used here with the abbreviations. Rules of classical grammar state that periods should follow abbreviations. However, in technical communication they are frequently not used; indeed, in some cases, rules of governing organizations prohibit the use of periods. For example, periods are not to be used with abbreviations of metric or SI units according to the Système-International. Individuals should consider whether or not to use periods in abbreviations in their communication.

3. **ALPHABETIZATION:** Entries are alphabetized by the letters in the abbreviations or acronyms. Spaces and punctuation are not considered. Numbers are considered when they are the only differences between entries. Entries that begin with a number are listed according to the first letter in the entry. The meanings for each abbreviation are listed in alphabetical order.

4. **OTHER ABBREVIATIONS:** Other abbreviations for the meanings of an entry are given following "also," after the meaning.

5. **PARENTHESES:** Parentheses have four uses in this work.
   a. When a meaning is used to modify or describe more than one term, the terms modified are given in parentheses and separated by commas.
   EXAMPLE: HBc hepatitis B core (antibody, antigen)
   b. Parentheses are used to contain explanatory material or to complete a term or phrase.
   EXAMPLE: H hydroxydaunomycin (doxorubicin)
        H Hoffmann (reflex)

c. Parentheses are used to provide a brief definition.
   EXAMPLE: H oersted (unit of magnetic field intensity)
d. Parentheses are used after foreign derivations if the meaning of the foreign word is different from the meaning of the abbreviation.
   EXAMPLE: H bacterial flagellar antigen [Ger. *Hauch* (breath)]

6. **BRACKETS:** Brackets following a meaning contain the foreign language derivations. Each derivation consists of the abbreviation of the language of origin (Fr., French; Gr., Greek; Ger., German; L., Latin;) with the foreign word or words in italics. If the meaning of the foreign word is different from the meaning of the abbreviation, the foreign word meaning is given in parentheses following the italicized words.

7. **GREEK LETTERS:** Entries beginning with a Greek letter are located at the beginning of each letter section.

8. **SYMBOLS:** Symbols that are composed of characters other than letters are listed in the Symbols Section.

A ALPHA, UPPER CASE, first letter of the Greek alphabet

α alpha, lower case, first letter of the Greek alphabet
alpha particle
angular acceleration
constituent of alpha plasma protein fraction
first in a series or group
heavy chain of immunoglobulin A
is proportional to
optical rotation (chemistry)
probability of type I error (statistics)
significance level
solubility coefficient (Bunsen's)

α₁AC alpha₁-anti-chymotrypsin

α-GLUC alpha-glucosidase

α-KG alpha-ketoglutarate

α-LP alpha-lipoprotein

α₂M alpha₂-macroglobulin; also AMG

α₁PI human alpha₁ proteinase inhibitor

γAbu gamma-aminobutyric acid

ε-Acp ε-aminocaproic acid

@c associated with

A abnormal; also AB, ABN, Abn, abn, abnor, abnorm
abortion; also AB, Ab, ab, ABO, Abor, abor
absolute temperature
absorbance; also *A,* abs
acceptor
accommodation; also a, ACC, Acc, acc, accom
acetum (vinegar)
acid; also a, AC
acidity; also a, AC
acidophil
acidophilic
actin
activity (radiation); also *A*
adenine; also Ade
adenoma
adenosine; also Ado
adenylic acid; also AA
admittance; also *A*
adrenalin; also Adr
adult
age [L. *aetas*]; also aet
akinetic
alanine (one-letter notation); also ALA, Ala
albumin (5%, followed by amount in mL)

albumin; also AL, ALB, Alb, alb
alive
allergic; also ALL, all
allergist
allergy; also ALL, all
alpha cell alternate
alveolar gas (subscript)
ambulatory; also AM, AMB, amb, ambul
ampere; also a, amp
amphetamine; also AMP, AMPH, AMT
ampicillin; also AM, AMP
anaphylaxis
androsterone; also ANDRO, Andro, Andros
anesthesia/anesthetic (start of)
angioplasty
angle; also ang
Angström; also Å
Angström unit; also Å, AU
anisotropic (band in striated muscle)
anodal; also a, AN, An
anode; also a, AN, An
anterior; also a, AN, ANT, ant
apical
aqueous
area; also *A,* a
argon; also Ar
arterial; also a, ART, art
artery; also a, ART, art
assessment; also asmt
atomic weight; also at wt, AW
atrium; also At
atropine; also AT, ATRO
auricle; also aur, auric
axial; also a, ax
axillary temperature; also (a)
blood group in the ABO system
ear [L. *auris*]; also a, aur
mass number; also *A*
subspinale (point A in cephalometrics)
systemic arterial blood (as subscript)
total acidity; also a
water [L. *aqua*]; also a, aq
year [L. *annus*]; also a

A absorbance; also A, abs
Actinomyces species
activity (radiation); also A
admittance; also A
Anopheles species
area; also A, a
disintegration rate
mass number; also A

A₁ aortic first heart sound

A₂ aortic second heart sound

°A degrees Absolute (replaced by °K, degrees Kelvin)

Å Angström; also A
Angström unit; also A, AU

Ã cumulated activity

AI angiotensin I; also AT I

AII angiotensin II

AIII angiotensin III

A250 5% albumin, 250 mL

A1000 5% albumin, 1000 mL

a absorptivity
acceleration; also *a*, Acc, acc, accel
accommodation; also A , ACC, Acc, acc, accom
acid; also A, AC
acidity; also A, AC
agar
alpha
ampere; also A, amp
annum
anodal; also A, AN, An
anode; also A, AN, An
anterior; also A, AN, ANT, ant
arabinose; also Ara, ara
are
area; also A, *A*
arterial; also A, ART, art
artery; also A, ART, art
arterial blood (subscript)
asymmetric; also AS, ASYM, asym
atto- (10⁻¹⁸)
axial; also A, ax
before [L. *ante*]; also ā, ante
ear [L. *auris*]; also A, aur
thermodynamic activity
total acidity; also A
water [L. *aqua*]; also A, aq
year [L. *annus*]; also A

a acceleration; also a, Acc, acc, accel
activity (of a chemical species)
specific absorptivity

ā before [L. *ante*]; also a, ante

(a) axillary temperature; also A

AA acetic acid; also AcOH
achievement age
active alcoholic
active-assistive (range of motion)
active avoidance
acupuncture analgesia
acute asthma

adenine arabinoside
adenylic acid; also A
adjuvant arthritis
adrenal androgen
adrenocortical autoantibody
aggregated albumin
agranulocytic angina
alcohol abuse
Alcoholics Anonymous
alopecia areata
alveolar-arterial (gradient); also A-a
aminoacetone
amino acid
aminoacyl
amyloid A
antiarrhythmic agent
anticipatory avoidance
antigen aerosol
aortic amplitude
aortic aneurysm
aortic arch
aplastic anemia
ARA-C and Adriamycin
arachidonic acid
arm to ankle (pulse ratio)
arteries [L. *arteriae];* also aa
ascaris antigen
ascending aorta; also AO, AS, Asc-A
ascorbic acid; also ASC
atomic absorption
audiologic assessment
Australia antigen; also AU, Au, Au(1), AuAg, Au Ag
authorized absence
autoanalyzer
automobile accident; also A/A
axonal arborization
of each [Gr. *ana* (so much of)]; also Ā Ā, aa, aā, ana

Ā Ā of each [Gr. *ana* (so much of)]; also AA, aa, āā, ana

A-A atlantoaxial

A/A automobile accident; also AA

A&A aid and attendance
arthroscopy and arthrotomy
awake and aware

A-a alveolar-arterial (gradient); also AA

aA abampere
azure A

a/A arterial to alveolar (oxygen ratio)

aa arteries [L. *arteriae*]; also AA
of each [Gr. *ana* (so much of)]; also AA, ĀĀ, āā, ana

āā of each [Gr. *ana* (so much of)]; also AA, ĀĀ, aa, ana

AAA abdominal aortic aneurysm
abdominal aortic aneurysmectomy
acquired aplastic anemia
acute anxiety attack
addiction, autoimmune diseases, and aging
amalgam; also aaa, AM, AMAL
American Academy of Allergy (now: AAAI, American Academy of Allergy and Immunology)
American Association of Anatomists
amino acid analysis
androgenic anabolic agent
aneurysm of ascending aorta
antiactin antibody
aromatic amino acid

aaa amalgam; also AAA, AM, AMAL

AAAA American Academy of Anesthesiologist's Assistants

AAAAA aphasia, agnosia, apraxia, agraphia, and alexia

AAAE amino acid-activating enzymes

AAAI American Academy of Allergy and Immunology

AAALAC American Association for Accreditation of Laboratory Animal Care

AA-AMP amino acid adenosine monophosphate

AAAS American Association for the Advancement of Science

AAATP Association for Anesthesiologist's Assistants Training Program

AAB action against burns
American Association of Bioanalysts
aminoazobenzene

AABB American Association of Blood Banks

AABCC alertness (consciousness), airway, breathing, circulation, and cervical spine

AAC antibiotic-associated colitis
antibiotic-associated pseudomembranous colitis; also AAPC, AAPMC
antimicrobial agent-induced colitis
antimicrobial agents and chemotherapy

AACA acylamino-cephalosporanic acid
American Association of Certified Allergists

AACAHPO American Association of Certified Allied Health Personnel in Ophthalmology (now: ATPO, Association of Technical Personnel in Ophthalmology)

AACC American Association for Clinical Chemistry

AACE American Association of Childbirth Education
antigen-antibody crossed electrophoresis

AACG acute angle closure glaucoma

AACIA American Association for Clinical Immunology and Allergy (now: ACAI, American College of Allergy and Immunology)

AACN American Association of Colleges of Nursing
American Association of Critical-Care Nurses

AACP American Academy for Cerebral Palsy (now: AACPDM, American Academy for Cerebral Palsy and Developmental Medicine)

AACPDM American Academy for Cerebral Palsy and Developmental Medicine

AACR American Association for Cancer Research

AACSH adrenal androgen corticotropic stimulating hormone

AAD acetoacetate decarboxylase
acid-ash diet
alloxazine adenine dinucleotide
alpha-1-antitrypsin deficiency
American Academy of Dermatology
antibiotic-associated diarrhea
aromatic-acid decarboxylase

AADC amino acid decarboxylase

AAdC anterior adductor of the coxa

(A-a)D$_{N2}$ difference in nitrogen tension between mixed alveolar gas and mixed arterial blood

(A-a)D$_{O2}$ difference in partial pressures of oxygen in mixed alveolar gas and mixed arterial blood

AADP American Academy of Denture Prosthetics

AADR American Academy of Dental Radiology (now: AAOMR, American Academy of Oral and Maxillofacial Radiology)

AADS American Association of Dental Schools

AAE active assistive exercise; also A/AEX
acute allergic encephalitis
American Association of Endodontists
annuloaortic ectasia

AAEE American Association of Electromyography and Electrodiagnosis (now: AAEM, American Association of Electrodiagnostic Medicine)

AAEM American Association of Electrodiagnostic Medicine

A/AEX active assistive exercise; also AAE

AAF 2-acetamidofluorene
acetic acid-alcohol-formalin (fixative)
2-acetylaminofluorene
ascorbic acid factor

AAFP American Academy of Family Physicians

AAG alpha$_1$-acid glycoprotein; also AGP

AaG alveolar arterial gradient

AAGP American Academy of General Practice (now: AAFP, American Academy of Family Physicians)

AAGS adult adrenogenital syndrome

A:AGT blood group A antiglobulin test

AAH adrenal androgenic hyperfunction

AAHA American Academy of Health Administration

AAHE Association for the Advancement of Health Education

AAHP American Association for Hospital Planning (now: Forum, The Forum for Health Care Planning)

AAHPER American Association for Health, Physical Education, and Recreation (now: AAHPERD, American Association for Health, Physical Education, Recreation and Dance)

AAHPERD American Association for Health, Physical Education, Recreation and Dance

AAI acute alveolar injury
American Association of Immunologists
arm-ankle indices
atrial demand inhibited (pacemaker code)

AAIA acquired artery immune augmentation

AAIB alpha$_1$-aminoisobutyrate

AAID American Academy of Implant Dentistry

AAIN acute allergic interstitial nephritis
American Association of Industrial Nurses (now: AAOHN, American Association of Occupational Health Nurses)

AAL anterior axillary line; also ant ax line

AALAS American Association for Laboratory Animal Science

AAM American Academy of Microbiology

AAMA American Association of Medical Assistants

AAMC American Association of Medical Clinics (now: AGPA, American Group Practice Association)
American Association of Medical Colleges

AAMD American Association on Mental Deficiency (now: AAMR, American Association on Mental Retardation)

AAME acetylarginine methyl ester

AAMI Association for the Advancement of Medical Instrumentation

AAMR American Association on Mental Retardation

AAMRL American Association of Medical Record Librarians (now: AMRA, American Medical Record Association)

AAMRS automated ambulatory medical record system

AAMS acute aseptic meningitis syndrome

AAMT American Association for Medical Transcription
American Association for Music Therapy

AAN alpha-amino acid nitrogen
American Academy of Neurology
American Academy of Nursing
amino acid nitrogen
analgesic abuse nephropathy
analgesic-associated nephropathy
attending's admission notes

AANA American Association of Nurse Anesthetists

AANN American Association of Neuroscience Nurses

AANP American Association of Neuropathologists

AAO American Academy of Ophthalmology
American Academy of Osteopathy
American Academy of Otolaryngology (now: AAO-HNS, American Academy of Otolaryngology–Head and Neck Surgery)
American Association of Orthodontists
amino acid oxidase
awake, alert, and oriented

(A-a)O$_2$ alveolar-arterial oxygen gradient

AAOx3 awake and oriented to time, place, and person

AAOHN American Association of Occupational Health Nurses

AAO-HNS American Academy of Otolaryngology–Head and Neck Surgery

AAOMR American Academy of Oral and Maxillofacial Radiology

AAOMS American Association of Oral and Maxillofacial Surgeons

AAOO American Academy of Ophthalmology and Otolaryngology (now: AAO, American Academy of Ophthalmology)

AAOP American Academy of Oral Pathology

AAOS American Academy of Orthopaedic Surgeons

AAP air at atmospheric pressure
alpha$_1$-antiprotease
Alzheimer's amyloid polypeptide
American Academy of Pediatrics
American Academy of Pedodontics (now: AAPD, American Academy of Pediatric Dentistry)
American Academy of Periodontology
American Association of Pathologists
assessment adjustment pass

AAPA American Academy of Physician Assistants
American Association of Pathologists' Assistants

AAPB American Association of Pathologists and Bacteriologists (now: AAP, American Association of Pathologists)

AAPC antibiotic-associated pseudomembranous colitis; also AAC, AAPMC

AAPD American Academy of Pediatric Dentistry

A-aP$_{CO2}$, (A-a)P$_{CO2}$ alveolar-arterial carbon dioxide difference

AAPF anti-arteriosclerosis polysaccharide factor

AAPHP American Association of Public Health Physicians

AAPMC antibiotic-associated pseudomembranous colitis; also AAC, AAPC

AAPMR American Academy of Physical Medicine and Rehabilitation

AAPS American Association of Physicians and Surgeons
American Association of Plastic Surgeons

AAR active avoidance reaction
acute articular rheumatism
antigen-antiglobulin reaction
Australia antigen radioimmunoassay

AARC American Association for Respiratory Care

AAROM active-assistive range of motion

AART American Association for Rehabilitation Therapy
American Association for Respiratory Therapy (now: AARC, American Association for Respiratory Care)

AAS acute abdominal series
aneurysm of atrial septum
anthrax antiserum
aortic arch syndrome
atlantoaxial subluxation
atomic absorption spectrometry
atomic absorption spectrophotometry
atomic absorption spectroscopy
atypical absence seizure

AASCRN amino acid screen

Aase asparaginase

AASH adrenal androgen stimulating hormone

AASP acute atrophic spinal paralysis
ascending aorta synchronized pulsation

AAT Aachen aphasia test
academic aptitude test
acute abdominal tympany
alanine aminotransferase; also ALAT, AlaAT, ALT
alkylating agent therapy
alpha-1-antitrypsin; also A1AT
aminoazotoluene
atrial demand triggered (pacemaker code)
auditory apperception test

A1AT alpha-1-antitrypsin; also AAT

AATA American Art Therapy Association

AATCC American Association of Textile Chemists and Colorists (bacteriostasis agar)

AATS American Association for Thoracic Surgery

AAU acute anterior uveitis

AAV adeno-associated virus
AIDS-associated virus

AAVV accumulated alveolar ventilatory volume

AAW anterior aortic wall

AB abdominal; also ABD, Abd, abd, ABDOM, Abdom, abdom
abnormal; also A, ABN, Abn, abn, abnor, abnorm
abortion; also A, Ab, ab, ABO, Abor, abor
Ace bandage
aid to the blind
air bleed
alcian blue

AB—cont'd
Alibert-Bazin (disease, syndrome)
antibiotic; also Anti bx, ATB
antibody; also Ab, ab
antigen binding
apex beat
asbestos body
asthmatic bronchitis
axiobuccal; also ab
Bachelor of Arts [L. *Artium Baccalaureus*]
blood group in the ABO system

A/B acid to base ratio
apnea and bradycardia; also A&B
apnea/bradycardia (moderate stimulation)

A&B apnea and bradycardia; also A/B

A>B air greater than bone (conduction)

Ab abortion; also A, AB, ab, ABO, Abor, abor
antibody; also AB, ab

aB azure B

ab abortion; also A, AB, Ab, ABO, Abor, abor
about; also abt
antibody; also AB, Ab
axiobuccal; also AB
from [L. *ab*]

ABA abscisic acid
allergic bronchopulmonary aspergillosis; also ABPA
American Board of Anesthesiology
antibacterial activity

ABAI American Board of Allergy and Immunology

AbAP antibody-against-panel (assay)

ABB Albright-Butler-Bloomberg (syndrome)
American Board of Bioanalysis

abbr abbreviated; also abbrev
abbreviation; also abbrev

abbrev abbreviated; also abbr
abbreviation; also abbr

ABC abbreviated blood count
absolute band count
absolute basophil count
absolute bone conduction
acalculous biliary colic
acid balance control
aconite-belladonna-chloroform
Adriamycin, BCNU, and cyclophosphamide
airway, breathing, and circulation
alternative birth center
American Blood Commission
aneurysmal bone cyst
antigen-binding capacity
apnea, bradycardia, and cyanosis

applesauce, bananas, and cereal (diet)
artificial beta cells
aspiration, biopsy, and cytology
atomic, biological, and chemical (warfare)
avidin-biotin peroxidase complex
axiobuccocervical

ABC and C&C airway, breathing, circulation, cervical spine, and consciousness level

ABCD Adriamycin, bleomycin, CCNU, and dacarbazine
asymmetry, border, color, and diameter (of melanoma)

ABCDE botulism toxin pentavalent

ABCIL antibody-mediated cell-dependent immunolympholysis

ABCM Adriamycin, bleomycin, cyclophosphamide, and mitomycin C

ABCP American Board of Cardiovascular Perfusion

ABCRS American Board of Colon and Rectal Surgery

ABCX Adriamycin, bleomycin, cisplatin, and radiation therapy

ABD abdomen; also Abd, abd, ABDOM, Abdom, abdom
abdominal; also AB, Abd, abd, ABDOM, Abdom, abdom
abduction; also Abd, abd, abduc
after bronchodilator
aged, blind, and disabled
aggressive behavioral disturbance
average body dose

ABd type of plain gauze dressing

Abd, abd abdomen; also ABD, ABDOM, Abdom, abdom
abdominal; also AB, ABD, ABDOM, Abdom, abdom
abduction; also ABD, abduc
abductor (muscle)

ABDCT atrial bolus dynamic computer tomography

Abd Hyst abdominal hysterectomy; also AH

ABDIC Adriamycin, bleomycin, dacarbazine, lomustine, and prednisone

ABDOM, Abdom, abdom abdomen; also ABD, Abd, abd
abdominal; also AB, ABD, Abd, abd

abd poll abductor pollicis (muscle)

abduc abduction; also ABD, Abd, abd

ABDV Adriamycin, bleomycin, dacarbazine, and vinblastine

ABE acute bacterial endocarditis
adult basic education
botulism equine trivalent antitoxin

ABEM American Board of Emergency
Medicine

ABEP auditory brainstem-evoked potentials

ABF aortobifemoral (bypass)

ABFP American Board of Family Practice

ABG aortoiliac bypass graft
arterial blood gas
axiobuccogingival

ABG's arterial blood gases

abg addictive behavior group

ABI ankle-brachial index
atherothrombotic brain infarction

ABIBN azobisisobutyronitrile

ABID antibody identification

ABIG absence of immunoglobulin G

ABIM American Board of Internal Medicine

ABK aphakic bullous keratopathy

ABL abetalipoproteinemia
African Burkitt lymphoma
Albright-Butler-Lightwood (syndrome)
allograft-bound lymphocyte
angioblastic lymphadenopathy
antigen-binding lymphocyte
axiobuccolingual

abl an oncogene involved in the Philadelphia
chromosome translocation in chronic granulocytic leukemia; found in the Abelson
strain of mouse leukemia virus

ABLB alternate binaural loudness balance

ABM adjusted body mass
alveolar basement membrane
autologous bone marrow

ABMO antibonding molecular orbital

ABMS Advisory Board for Medical Specialties
(now: American Board of Medical
Specialties)
American Board of Medical Specialties

A/B MS apnea/bradycardia mild stimulation

ABMT autologous bone marrow transplantation; also AuBMT

ABN, Abn, abn abnormal; also A, AB, abnor,
abnorm
abnormality; also abnor, abnorm

AbN antibody nitrogen

ABNC abnormal curve

ABNF Association of Black Nursing Faculty in
Higher Education

ABN F% abnormal forms percent (sperm
count)

ABNG AB negative (blood type)

ABNM American Board of Nuclear Medicine

abnor abnormal; also A, AB, ABN, Abn, abn,
abnorm
abnormality; also ABN, Abn, abn, abnorm

abnorm abnormal; also A, AB, ABN, Abn,
abn, abnor
abnormality; also ABN, Abn, abn, abnor

ABNS American Board of Neurological
Surgery

ABO abortion; also A, AB, Ab, ab, Abor, abor
absent bed occupancy
American Board of Otolaryngology
amethopterin, bleomycin, and Oncovin
antibodies
blood group system (groups A, AB, B, & O;
named for agglutinogens A, B, and O)

ABOG American Board of Obstetrics and
Gynecology

ABO-HD ABO hemolytic disease

Abor, abor abortion; also A, AB, Ab, ab, ABO

ABOS Adriamycin, bleomycin sulfate,
Oncovin, and streptozotocin
American Board of Orthopedic Surgery

ABP Adriamycin, bleomycin, and prednisone
American Board of Pathology
American Board of Pediatrics
androgen-binding protein
antigen-binding protein
arterial blood pressure

ABPA acute bronchopulmonary asthma; also ABA
allergic bronchopulmonary aspergillosis

ABPANC American Board of Post Anesthesia
Nursing Certification

ABPC antibody-producing cell

ABPE acute bovine pulmonary edema

ABPM ambulatory blood pressure monitoring
American Board of Preventive Medicine

ABPMR American Board of Physical
Medicine and Rehabilitation

ABPN American Board of Psychiatry and
Neurology

ABPS American Board of Plastic Surgery

ABR abortus-Bang reaction
abortus-Bang ring (test)
absolute bed rest
American Board of Radiology
auditory brainstem response

ABr agglutination for brucellosis (test)

Abr, abr abrasion(s); also Abras, abras

Abras, abras abrasion(s); also Abr, abr

ABS abdominal surgery
abnormal brainstem
absent; also abs
absorbed; also absorb
absorption; also Abs, abs, absorb
acrylonitrile-butadiene-styrene
acute brain syndrome
Adaptive Behavior Scale
admitting blood sugar
adult bovine serum
alkylbenzene sulfonate
aloin, belladonna, and strychnine (laxative)
American Board of Surgery
amniotic band sequence
anti-B serum
arterial blood sample
at bedside

1:5 ABS 1:5 Absorption-Reiter-Strain (cere-brospinal fluid test)

Abs absorption; also ABS, abs, absorb

abs absent; also ABS
absolute
absorbance; also A, *A*
absorption; also ABS, Abs, absorb

absc abscissa

abs config absolute configuration

ABSe ascending bladder septum

abs feb while fever is absent [L. *absente febre*]

absorb absorbed; also ABS
absorption; also ABS, Abs, abs

A/B ss apnea/bradycardia self-stimulation

abst abstract; also abstr

abstr abstract; also abst

ABT aminopyrine breath test
arteria basilaris thrombose

abt about; also ab

ABTS American Board of Thoracic Surgery
2,2-azine-di(3-ethylbenzthiazoline)-6-sulfonic acid

ABTX alpha-bungarotoxin

ABU American Board of Urology
aminobutyrate
asymptomatic bacteriuria

Abu alpha-aminobutyric acid

γ Abu gamma-aminobutyric acid

ABV actinomycin D, bleomycin, and vincristine

Adriamycin, bleomycin, and vinblastine
arthropod-borne virus

ABVD Adriamycin, bleomycin, vinblastine, and dacarbazine

ABW actual body weight

ABX, ABx, abx antibiotics

ABY acid bismuth yeast (medium/agar)

AC abdominal circumference
abdominal compression
absorption coefficient
absorptive cell
abuse case
acetate; also Ac
acetylcholine; also AcCh, ACH, ACh
acetylcysteine
acid; also A, a
acidified complement
acidity; also A, a
aconitine
acromioclavicular
activated charcoal
acupuncture clinic
acute; also ac
acute cholecystitis
adenocarcinoma; also ACA, adenoca
adenylate cyclase; also AdC
adherent cell
adrenal cortex; also AdC
adrenocorticoid
Adriamycin and carmustine
Adriamycin and cisplatin
Adriamycin and cyclophosphamide; also ACe
air changes
air conditioning
air conduction
all culture (broth)
alternating current
ambulatory care
ambulatory controls
anchored catheter
anesthesia circuit
anodal closure
antecubital
anterior chamber (of eye); also A/C
anterior column
anterior commissure
anterior cruciate
antibiotic concentrate
anticoagulant; also anticoag
anticomplement
anticomplementary
anti-inflammatory corticoid
antiphlogistic corticoid; also APC

aortic closure
aortocoronary
apophysitis calcanei
Arnold-Chiari (syndrome)
arterial capillary
ascending colon
atriocarotid; also A-C, a-c
auriculocarotid; also A-C, a-c
axiocervical

5-AC 5-azacytidine; also 5-AZA, 5-Aza

A-C adult-versus-child
Alberto Culver

A/C albumin to coagulin (ratio)
anterior chamber (of eye); also AC
assist/control
assisted control (ventilation); also ac

A2C apical two-chamber

Ac accelerator (globulin)
acetate; also AC
acetyl; also ac
actinium

aC abcoulomb
arabinosylcytosine (cytarabine); also ARA-C,
Ara-C, ara-C, araC
azure C

ac acetyl; also Ac
acute; also AC
assisted control (ventilation); also A/C
before meals [L. *ante cibum*]

A-C, a-c atriocarotid; also AC
auriculocarotid; also AC

ACA acute cerebellar ataxia
adenine-cytosine-adenine
adenocarcinoma; also AC, adenoca
adenylate cyclase activity
American College of Allergists (now: ACAI,
American College of Allergy and
Immunology)
American College of Anesthesiologists
American College of Angiology
American College of Apothecaries
aminocaproic acid
aminocephalosporanic acid
ammonia, copper, and arsenic
anomalous coronary artery
anterior cerebral artery
anterior communicating aneurysm
anterior communicating artery; also ACoA
anti-cardiolipin antibody
anti-centromere antibody
anti-collagen autoantibody
anticomplement activity
anti-cytoplasmic antibody

Automatic Clinical Analyzer

AC/A accommodation convergence to accommodation (ratio)

ACAC activated charcoal artificial cell

AcAcOH acetoacetic acid

acad academy

A-CAH autoimmune chronic active hepatitis

ACAI American College of Allergy and
Immunology

ACAN acanthocyte (acanthrocyte); also
ACANTH

ACANTH acanthocyte (acanthrocyte); also
ACAN

ACAO acylcoenzyme A oxidase

ACAT acylcholesterol acyltransferase
automatic computerized axial tomography

ACB alveolar-capillary block
antibody-coated bacteria
aortocoronary bypass
arterialized capillary blood
asymptomatic carotid bruit

AC&BC air conduction and bone conduction

AC/BC air conduction/bone conduction

ACBE air contrast barium enema

ACBG aortocoronary bypass graft

ACC accident; also Acc, acc, accid
accommodation; also A, a, Acc, acc, accom
acetylcoenzyme A carboxylase
acinar cell carcinoma
acute care center
adenoid cystic carcinoma; also Acc
administrative control center
adrenocortical carcinoma
alveolar cell carcinoma
ambulatory care center
American College of Cardiology
amylase creatinine clearance
anodal closure contraction; also AnCC
antitoxin-containing cell
aplastic cutis congenita
articular chondrocalcinosis
laboratory accident

Acc acceleration; also a, *a*, acc, accel
accident; also ACC, acc, accid
accommodation; also A, a, ACC, acc, accom
adenoid cystic carcinoma; also ACC

acc acceleration; also a, *a*, Acc, accel
accident; also ACC, Acc, accid
accommodation; also A, a, ACC, Acc, accom
according

accel acceleration; also a, *a*, Acc, acc

AcCh acetylcholine; also AC, ACH, ACh

AcChR acetylcholine receptor; also AChR

AcCHS acetylcholinesterase; also AChE

accid accident; also ACC, Acc, acc
accidental

ACCL, Accl anodal closure clonus

ACCME Accreditation Council for Continuing Medical Education

AcCoA acetylcoenzyme A; also acetyl-CoA

accom accommodation; also A, a, ACC, Acc, acc

ACCP American College of Chest Physicians

ACCR amylase creatinine clearance ratio

accum accumulated, accumulation

accur accurately, most carefully

ACD absolute cardiac dullness
absolute claudication
absolute claudication distance
actinomycin D (dactinomycin); also ACT, ACTD, Act-D, act-D, AMD
adult celiac disease
allergic contact dermatitis
alpha-chain disease
anterior chamber diameter
anterior chest diameter
anticonvulsant drug
area of cardiac disease
area of cardiac dullness
citric acid, trisodium citrate, dextrose (solution)

AcD alive with disease [L. *cum* (with)]

AC-DC alternating current or direct current; also AC/DC, ac/dc
bisexual (slang); also AC/DC, ac/dc

AC/DC, ac/dc alternating current or direct current; also AC-DC
bisexual (slang); also AC-DC

ACE acetonitrile
actinium emanation
acute coronary event
adrenocortical extract
Adriamycin, cyclophosphamide, and etoposide
aerobic chair exercises
alcohol, chloroform, and ether (mixture)
angiotensin converting enzyme

ACe Adriamycin and cyclophosphamide; also AC

Ace acetone

ace acentric

ACED anhydrotic congenital ectodermal dysplasia

ACEH acid cholesterol ester hydrolase

ACEI angiotensin-converting enzyme inhibitor

ACEP American College of Emergency Physicians

ACES automated clinical evaluation system

AcEst acetyl esterase

acetyl-CoA acetylcoenzyme A; also AcCoA

ACF accessory clinical findings
acute care facility
advanced communications function
area correction factor

ACFn additional cost of false negatives

ACFO American College of Foot Orthopedists

ACFp additional cost of false positives

ACFS American College of Foot Surgeons

ACFUCY actinomycin D, fluorouracil, and cyclophosphamide

ACG accelerator globulin (coagulation factor V); also AcG, AC-G, Ac-G, ac-G, ac-g
American College of Gastroenterology
angiocardiogram
angiocardiography
aortocoronary graft
apexcardiogram; also APCG

AcG, AC-G, Ac-G, ac-G, ac-g accelerator globulin (coagulation factor V); also ACG

ACGME Accreditation Council for Graduate Medical Education

ACGP American College of General Practice (now: ACM, American College of Medicine)

ACH acetylcholine; also AC, AcCh, ACh
achalasia
active chronic hepatitis
adrenocortical hormone
aerosolized aluminum chlorohydrate
aftercoming head
amyotrophic cerebellar hypoplasia
arm, chest, height
arm, chest, hip
arm girth, chest depth, and hip width (nutritional index)

ACh acetylcholine; also AC, AcCh, ACH

ACHA American College of Hospital Administrators (now: ACHE, American College of Healthcare Executives)

ACHCA American College of Health Care Administrators

ACHE American College of Healthcare Executives

AChE acetylcholinesterase; also AcCHS

ACHNE Association of Community Health Nurse Education

AChR acetylcholine receptor; also AcChR

AChRAb acetylcholine receptor antibody

AC&HS before meals and at bedtime [L. *ante cibum et hora somni*]

ACI acoustic comfort index
acute coronary infarction
acute coronary insufficiency
adenylate cyclase inhibitor
adrenocortical insufficiency
aftercare instructions
anti-clonus index
average cost of illness

ACID Arithmetic, Coding, Information, and Digit Span

acid phos acid phosphatase; also ACP, AcP, AC-PH, ac phos, acid PO_4, acid p'tase, AP

acid PO_4 acid phosphatase; also ACP, AcP, AC-PH, acid phos, ac phos, acid p'tase, AP

acid p'tase acid phosphatase; also ACP, AcP, AC-PH, acid phos, acid PO_4, ac phos, AP

ACIDS acquired cellular immunodeficiency syndrome

ACIF anticomplement immunofluorescence

ACIOC anterior chamber intraocular (lens)

ACIP acute canine idiopathic polyneuropathy
Advisory Committee on Immunization Practices

ACJ acromioclavicular joint

AcK actinium K

ACL anterior cruciate ligament

ACl aspiryl chloride

ACLA American Clinical Laboratory Association

ACLAM American College of Laboratory Animal Medicine

ACLC Assessment of Children's Language Comprehension

ACLR anterior cruciate ligament repair

ACLPS Academy of Clinical Laboratory Physicians and Scientists

ACLS advanced cardiac life support

ACM aclacinomycin (aclarubicin)
acute cerebrospinal meningitis
Adriamycin, cyclophosphamide, and methotrexate
albumin-calcium-magnesium
alveolar capillary membrane
American College of Medicine
anti-cardiac myosin
Arnold-Chiari malformation

ACME aphatic cystoid macular edema

ACMF arachnoid cyst of the middle fossa

ACMP alveolar-capillary membrane permeability

ACMT artificial circus movement tachycardia

ACMV assist-controlled mechanical ventilation

ACN acute conditioned neurosis
American College of Neuropsychiatrists

AcNeu *N*-acetylneuraminic acid

ACNHA American College of Nursing Home Administrators (now: ACHCA, American College of Health Care Administrators)

AcNHFln acetylaminofluorene

ACNM American College of Nuclear Medicine
American College of Nurse-Midwives

ACNP American College of Nuclear Physicians

AcNPV autographa californica nuclear polyhidrosis virus

ACO acute coronary occlusion
anodal closing odor

Ac_2O acetic anhydride

ACOA adult child of alcoholic

ACoA anterior communicating artery; also ACA

ACOAP Adriamycin, cyclophosphamide, Oncovin, Ara-C, and prednisone

ACOEM American College of Occupational and Environmental Medicine

AcOEt ethyl acetate

ACOG American College of Obstetricians and Gynecologists

AcOH acetic acid; also AA

ACOHA American College of Osteopathic Hospital Administrators (now: COHE, College of Osteopathic Healthcare Executives)

ACOI American College of Osteopathic Internists

A-comm anterior communicating (artery)

ACOOG American College of Osteopathic Obstetricians and Gynecologists

ACOP Adriamycin, cyclophosphamide, Oncovin, and prednisone
American College of Osteopathic Pediatricians

ACOPP Adriamycin, cyclophosphamide, Oncovin, prednisone, and procarbazine

ACOS American College of Osteopathic Surgeons

acous acoustic(s)

ACP accessory conduction pathway
acid phosphatase; also acid PO_4, acid phos, acid p'tase, AcP, AC-PH, ac phos, AP
acyl carrier protein
American College of Pathologists
American College of Physicians
Animal Care Panel (now: AALAS, American Association for Laboratory Animal Science)
anodal closing picture
aspirin-caffeine-phenacetin
Association of Clinical Pathologists (London, England)

AcP acid phosphatase; also acid PO_4, acid phos, acid p'tase, ACP, AC-PH, ac phos, AP

ϵ-Acp ϵ-aminocaproic acid

ACPA anti-cytoplasmic antibodies

AC-PH acid phosphatase; also acid PO_4, acid phos, acid p'tase, ACP, AcP, ac phos, AP

ac phos acid phosphatase; also acid PO_4, acid phos, acid p'tase, ACP, AcP, AC-PH, AP

ACPM American College of Preventive Medicine

ACPP adrenocortical polypeptide
adrenocorticopolypeptide

ACPP-PF acid phosphatase prostatic fluid

ACPS acrocephalopolysyndactyly

acq acquired
acquisition

ACR abnormally contracting regions
absolute catabolic rate
acriflavine; also Acr
adenomatosis of colon and rectum
American College of Radiology
American College of Rheumatology
anti-constipation regimen
axillary count rate

Acr acriflavine; also ACR
acrylic

ACRF ambulatory care research facility

ACRM American Congress of Rehabilitation Medicine

ACRP aminocarbonyl reaction product

ACS acetyl strophanthidin
acrocephalosyndactyly
acute confusional state
ambulatory care services
American Cancer Society
American Chemical Society
American College of Surgeons
anodal closing sound
antireticular cytotoxic serum
aperture current setting
arterial cannulation support
Association of Clinical Scientists

ACSM American College of Sports Medicine

ACSP Advisory Council on Scientific Policy

ACSV aortocoronary-saphenous vein (graft)

ACSVBG aortocoronary-saphenous vein bypass graft

ACT achievement through counseling and treatment
actinomycin
actinomycin D (dactinomycin); also ACD, ACTD, Act-D, act-D, AMD
activated clotting time
activated coagulation time
advanced coronary treatment
allergen challenge test
anodal closure tetanus; also ACTe
anti-chromotrypsin
anticoagulant therapy
antrocolic transposition
anxiety control training
asthma care training
atropine coma therapy

act active
activity; also activ

ACTA American Cardiology Technologists Association (now: NSCT/NSPT, National Society for Cardiovascular Technology/National Society for Pulmonary Technology)
American Corrective Therapy Association (now: AKA, American Kinesiotherapy Association)
automatic computerized transverse axial (scanner, scanning)

ACTC, Act-C, act-C actinomycin C

ACTD, Act-D, act-D actinomycin D (dactinomycin); also ACD, ACT, AMD

ACTe anodal closure tetanus; also ACT

Act Ex active exercise; also AE

ACTH adrenocorticotropic hormone (corticotropin)

ACTH-RF adrenocorticotropic hormone-releasing factor

activ activity; also act

ACTN adrenocorticotropin

ACTP adrenocorticotropic polypeptide

ACTSEB anterior chamber tube shunt encircling band

ACU acute care unit
ambulatory care unit

ACUTENS acupuncture and transcutaneous electrical nerve stimulation

ACV acyclovir
atrial/carotid/ventricular

ACVB aortocoronary venous bypass

ACVD acute cardiovascular disease

ACVM American College of Veterinary Microbiologists

ACVP American College of Veterinary Pathologists

ACVRD arteriosclerotic cardiovascular renal disease

AC/W acetone in water

acyl-CoA acylcoenzyme A

AD abdominal diameter
accident dispensary
acetate dialysis
achievement drive
active disease
acute dermatomyositis
Adair-Dighton (syndrome)
addict
addiction; also addict
adenoid degeneration (agent)
admitting diagnosis
Adriamycin; also ADM, ADR, Adr, ADRIA, Adria
aerosol deposition
after discharge
alcohol dehydrogenase; also ADH
Aleutian disease (of mink)
alveolar duct
Alzheimer's dementia
Alzheimer's disease
analgesic dose
anodal duration

anterior division
antigenic determinant
appropriate disability
arabinofuranosylcytosine (cytarabine) and daunomycin
arthritic dose
atopic dermatitis
attentional disturbance
autonomic dysreflexia
average day
average deviation
axiodistal; also ad
axis deviation
diphenylchlorarsine
right atrium [L. *atrium dextrum*]
right ear [L. *auris dextra*]; also ad

A/D analog-to-digital (converter); also A/O

A + D ARA-C and daunorubicin

A&D admission and discharge
alcohol and drugs
ascending and descending
vitamins A and D

Ad adipocyte
adrenal; also adr

A d anisotropic disk

ad add [L. *admove* (add)]; also admov
axiodistal; also AD
every other day [L. *alternis diebus*]; also alt dieb
let there be added [L. *addatur*]; also add
right ear [L. *auris dextra*]; also AD

ADA adenosine deaminase; also Adase, ADD
American Dental Association
American Dermatological Association
American Diabetes Association
American Dietetic Association
anterior descending artery
anti-deoxyribonucleic acid antibody

ADA # American Diabetes Association diet number

ADAA African Dental Assistants Association

ADAMHA Alcohol, Drug Abuse, and Mental Health Administration

ADase adenosine deaminase; also ADA, ADD

ADAU adolescent drug abuse unit

ADB accidental death benefit

ADBF azurophil-derived bactericidal factor

ADC affective disorders clinic
Aid to Dependent Children
albumin, dextrose, and catalase (medium)
ambulance design criteria
analog-to-digital converter
anodal duration contraction

ADC—cont'd
antral diverticulum of the colon
anxiety disorder clinic
average daily census
axiodistocervical

AdC adenylate cyclase; also AC
adrenal cortex; also AC

ADCC antibody-dependent cell-mediated
cytotoxicity
antibody-dependent cellular cytotoxicity
automated differential cell counter

ADCONFU Adriamycin, cyclophosphamide,
Oncovin, and fluorouracil

ADD adduction; also add
adenosine deaminase; also ADA, Adase
alcohol and drug dependency (unit)
attention deficit disorder
average daily dose

add adding
addition
adduction; also ADD
adductor
let there be added [L. *addatur*]; also ad

add c trit add with trituration [L. *adde cum
tritu*]

ad def an to the point of fainting [L. *ad
defectionem animi*]

ad deliq to fainting [L. *ad deliquium*]

addend to be added [L. *addendus*]

ADDH, ADD/H attention deficit disorder with
hyperactivity; also ADD-HA

ADD-HA attention deficit disorder with hyperactivity; also ADDH, ADD/H

addict addiction; also AD
addictive

add poll adductor pollicis (muscle)

ADDU alcohol and drug dependence unit

ADE acute disseminated encephalitis
antibody-dependent enhancement
apparent digestible energy

Ade adenine; also A

AdeCbl adenosyl cobalamine

ADEE age-dependent epileptic encephalopathy

ad effect until effective [L. *ad effectum*]

ADEK vitamins A, D, E, and K (the fat soluble
vitamins)

ADEM acute disseminated encephalomyelitis

adenoca adenocarcinoma; also AC, ACA

adeq adequate; also ADQ

ad feb fever being present [L. *adstante febre*]

ADFU agar diffusion for fungus

ADG atrial diastolic gallop
axiodistogingival

ad gr acid to an agreeable acidity or sourness
[L. *ad gratum aciditatem*]; also ad grat acid

ad grat acid to an agreeable acidity or sourness [L. *ad gratum aciditatem*]; also ad gr
acid

ad gr gust to an agreeable taste [L. *ad gratum
gustum*]

ADH adhesion
alcohol dehydrogenase; also AD
antidiuretic hormone

ADHA American Dental Hygienists'
Association

adhib to be administered [L. *adhibendus*]

ad hoc for this (purpose) [L. *ad hoc*]
temporary

ADI acceptable daily intake
allowable daily intake
American Drug Index
antral diverticulum of the ileum
autosomal-dominant ichthyosis
axiodistoincisal

ADIC Adriamycin and dacarbazine [(dimethyl-
triazenyl) imidazole-carboxamide]

ad int meanwhile [L. *ad interim*]

adj adjoining
adjunct

ADK adenosine kinase; also AK

ADKC atopic dermatitis with keratoconjunctivitis

ADL activities of daily living
adrenoleukodystrophy; also ALD

ADLC antibody-dependent lymphocyte-mediated cytotoxicity (test)

ad lib as desired [L. *ad libidinem* (at pleasure)]

ADL/DLS activities of daily living/daily living
skills

ADM administrative medicine
administrator
admission; also Adm, adm
Adriamycin; also AD, ADR, Ard, ADRIA,
Adria
apparent distribution mass

AdM adrenal medulla

Adm admission; also ADM, adm
admitted; also adm

adm administration; also Admin, admin
admission; also ADM, Adm

admitted; also Adm
apply [L. *admove*]

ad man med (to be delivered) into the hands of the (prescribing) physician [L. *ad manus medici*]

ADME absorption, distribution, metabolism, and excretion

Admin administration; also adm, admin

admin administer
administration; also adm, Admin

admov add [L. *admove*]; also ad
let there be applied or added [L. *admoveatur*]

ADN anti-deoxyribonuclease; also ADNase
aortic depressor nerve
Associate Degree in Nursing

ADNase anti-deoxyribonuclease; also ADN

ad naus to the point of producing nausea [L. *ad nauseam*]

ADN-B anti-deoxyribonuclease B

ad neut to neutralization [L. *ad neutralizandum*]

ADO adolescent medicine
axiodisto-occlusal

Ado adenosine; also A

ADOAP, Ad-OAP Adriamycin, Oncovin, ARA-C, and prednisone

AdoCbl adenosylcobalamin

ADOD arthrodentosteodysplasia

AdoDABA adenosyl-diaminobutyric acid

ADODM adult-onset diabetes mellitus; also AODM

AdoHcy *S*-adenosylhomocysteine; also AHCy

adol adolescent

AdoMet *S*-adenosylmethionine

Adox oxidized adenosine

ADP Academy of Denture Prosthetics
acute dermatomyositis and polymyositis
adenosine 5′-diphosphate
administrative psychiatry
advanced pancreatitis
ammonium dihydrogen phosphate
approved drug product
area diastolic pressure
arterial demand pacing
automatic data processing

ad part dolent to the painful parts [L. *ad partes dolentes*]

ADPase adenosine 5′-diphosphatase

ADPKD autosomal-dominant polycystic kidney disease

ADPL average daily patient load

ad pond om to the weight of the whole [L. *ad pondus omnium*]

ADPR adenosine diphosphate ribose

ADQ abductor digiti quinti (muscles)
adequate; also adeq

ADR acceptable dental remedies
acute dystonic reaction
Adriamycin; also AD, ADM, Adr, ADRIA, Adria
advanced diagnostic research
adverse drug reaction
airway dilation reflex

Adr adrenalin; also A
Adriamycin; also AD, ADM, ADR, ADRIA, Adria

adr adrenal; also Ad

Adrenex adrenalectomy

ADRIA, Adria Adriamycin; also AD, ADM, ADR, Adr

ADRS affective disorder rating scale

ADS acute diarrheal syndrome
adamantylsulphonyl
alternative delivery system
anatomical dead space
anonymous donor's sperm
anterior drawer sign
antibody deficiency syndrome
antidiuretic substance

ad sat to saturation [L. *ad saturandum*] ; also ad satur

ad satur to saturation [L. *ad saturandum*]; also ad sat

adst feb while fever is present [L. *adstante febre*]

ADT accepted dental therapeutics
adenosine triphosphate; also ATP
admission, discharge, transfer
agar-gel diffusion test
alternate day therapy
alternate day treatment
anodal duration tetanus; also ADTe, ANDTE, AnDTe
anticipate discharge tomorrow
any desired thing (placebo)
Auditory Discrimination Test
automated dithionite test

ADTA American Dance Therapy Association
American Dental Trade Association

ADTe anodal duration tetanus; also ADT, ANDTE, AnDTe

ad tert vic   three times [L. *ad tertiam vicem*]

ADTP   adolescent day treatment program
alcohol dependence treatment program

ADU   acute duodenal ulcer
arterial diagnostic unit

ad us   according to custom [L. *ad usum*]; also
AU

ad us ext   for external application or use [L. *ad usum externum*]; also ad us exter

ad us exter   for external application or use [L. *ad usum externum*]; also ad us ext

ADV   adenovirus; also Adv
adventitia; also Adv

Adv   adenovirus; also ADV
adventitia; also ADV
advisory
against [L. *adversum*]; also adv

A-DV   arterial–deep venous difference

A/DV   arterio/deep venous

adv   advice
advise
against [L. *adversum*]; also Adv

advert   advertisement
advertising

ad 2 vic   at two times [L. *ad duas vices*]
for two doses

ADVIRC   autosomal-dominant vitreo-retinochoroidopathy

A5D5W   alcohol 5% and dextrose 5%, in water

ADX   adrenalectomized (jargon)

AE   above elbow; also A-E
accident and emergency; also A&E
acrodermatitis enteropathica
activation energy
active exercise; also Act Ex
adrenal epinephrine
adult erythrocyte
after-effect
agarose electrophoresis
air embolism
air entry
alcoholic embryopathy
alveolar echinococcosis
anoxic encephalopathy
antitoxin unit [Ger. *Antitoxineinheit*];
   also AU
apoenzyme
aryepiglottic (fold)
energy of activation

A-E   above elbow; also AE

A&E   accident and emergency; also AE

A+E   analysis and evaluation

ae   of the age [L. *aetatis*]

AEA   above-elbow amputation
alcohol, ether, and acetone (solution)

AEB   acute erythroblastopenia
as evidenced by
avian erythroblastosis

AEC   ankyloblepharon, ectodermal defects, and
cleft lip (syndrome)
aortic ejection click
at earliest convenience
Atomic Energy Commission

AED   antiepileptic drug
automated external defibrillator

AEDP   automated external defibrillator pace-maker

AEEGS   American Electroencephalographic
Society

AEEU   admission, entrance, and evaluation unit

AEF   allogenic effect factor
amyloid enhancing factor
aryepiglottic fold

AEG   air encephalogram
air encephalography

Aeg, aeg   the patient [L. *aeger, aegra*]

AEI   atrial emptying index

AEL   acute erythroleukemia
after egg laying

AEM   ambulatory electrogram monitor
analytical electron microscope
analytical electron microscopy
avian encephalomyelitis

AEN   aseptic epiphyseal necrosis

AEP   acute edematous pancreatitis
appropriateness evaluation protocol
artificial endocrine pancreas
auditory evoked potential
average evoked potential

AEq   age equivalent

aeq   equal [L. *aequales*]

AER   acoustic evoked response
acute exertional rhabdomyolysis
agranular endoplasmic reticulum
aided equalization response
albumin excretion rate
aldosterone excretion rate
anion exchange resin
apical ectodermal ridge
auditory evoked response
average electroencephalic response
average evoked response

aer aerosol

AERA average evoked response audiometry

Aer m, AerM aerosol mask

Aero *Aerobacter* species

AERP atrial effective refractory period

Aer T, AerT aerosol tent

AES acetone-extracted serum
American Encephalographic Society
American Epidemiological Society
anti-embolic stockings
anti-eosinophilic sera
antral ethmoidal sphenoidectomy
Auger electron spectroscopy

AEST aeromedical evacuation support team

AET absorption-equivalent thickness
2-aminoethyl-isothiuronium bromide
atrial ectopic tachycardia

aet age [L. *aetas*]; also A

aetat aged, of the age [L. *aetatis*]

AEV avian erythroblastosis virus

AEVS automated eligibility verification system

AF abnormal frequency
acid-fast
aflatoxin; also AFT
albumose-free (tuberculin)
aldehyde fuchsin
alleged father
amaurosis fugax
aminophylline
amniotic fluid; also Amf
anchoring fibril
angiogenesis factor
anteflexed
anteflexion
anterior fontanel
anterofrontal
antibody forming
anti-fibrinogen
aortic flow
aortofemoral
arterial filter
artificially fed
ascitic fluid; also Ascit Fl
atrial fibrillation; also AFIB, AFib, A fib, At
Fib, at fib, ATR FIB, atr fib
atrial flutter; also AFL, AFl
atrial fusion
attenuation factor
attributable fraction
audiofrequency; also af
auricular fibrillation; also AUR FIB, aur fib

A-F ankle-foot (orthosis)
anti-fibrinogen

A/F air/fluid (level)

aF abfarad

af audiofrequency; also AF

AFA alcohol-formaldehyde-acetic (fixative or
solution)

AFAFP amniotic fluid alpha-fetoprotein

AFB acid-fast bacillus
acid-fast bacteria
aflatoxin B
aortofemoral bypass
aspirated foreign body

AFBG aortofemoral bypass graft

AFC adult foster care
air-filled cushions
antibody-forming cell

AFCI acute focal cerebral ischemia

AFCR American Federation for Clinical
Research

AFD accelerated freeze-drying

AFDC Aid to Families with Dependent
Children

AFE amniotic fluid embolization

AFEB, afeb afebrile

AFF atrial filling fraction

AF/F atrial fibrillation and/or flutter

aff afferent
having an affinity with but not identical with
[L. *affinis*]

AFG aflatoxin G
alpha fetal globulin
amniotic fluid glucose
auditory figure-ground

AFH anterior facial height

AFI amaurotic familial idiocy
amniotic fluid index

AFIB, Afib, A fib atrial fibrillation; also AF, At
Fib, at fib, ATR FIB, atr fib

AFID alkali flame ionization detectors

AFIP Armed Forces Institute of Pathology

AFL aflatoxicol
air/fluid level
anti-fatty liver (factor)
Aspergillus flavus
atrial flutter; also AF, AFl

AFl atrial flutter; also AF, AFL

AFLNH angiofollicular lymph node hyperplasia

AFLP acute fatty liver of pregnancy

AFM Adriamycin, fluorouracil, methotrexate, and leucovorin calcium
aflatoxin M

AFML Armed Forces Medical Library

AFN afunctional neutrophil

AFND acute febrile neutrophilic dermatosis

AFO ankle-foot orthosis

AFP alpha-fetoprotein; also aFP
anterior faucial pillar
atrial filling pressure
atypical facial pain

aFP alpha-fetoprotein; also AFP

AFPP acute fibrinopurulent pneumonia
acute fibropurulent pneumonia

AFQ aflatoxin Q

AFQT Armed Forces Qualification Test

AFR aqueous flare response
ascorbic free radical

AFRD acute febrile respiratory disease

AFRI acute febrile respiratory illness

AFS acid-fast smear
acquired Fanconi's syndrome
adult Fanconi's syndrome
American Fertility Society
anti-fibroblast serum

AFSP acute fibrinoserous pneumonia

AFT aflatoxin; also AF
agglutination-flocculation test

AFT₃ absolute free triiodothyronine

AFT₄ absolute free thyroxine

AFTC apparent free testosterone concentration

AFTN autonomously functioning thyroid nodule

AFV amniotic fluid volume

AFVSS afebrile, vital signs stable; also AVSS

AFX air-fluid exchange
atypical fibroxanthoma

AG abdominal girth
agarose
albumin to globulin (ratio); also A/G, A:G, ALB/GLOB
aminoglutethimide; also AGL
aminoglycoside; also AMG
analytical grade
anion gap
antigen; also Ag, ag, AGN
antiglobulin
antigravity; also anti-G
atrial gallop; also ag
attached gingiva

axiogingival
azurophilic granule

A/G albumin to globulin (ratio); also AG, A:G, ALB/GLOB

A:G albumin to globulin (ratio); also AG, A/G, ALB/GLOB

Ag antigen; also AG, ag, AGN
silver [L. *argentum*]; also arg

ag antigen; also AG, Ag, AGN
atrial gallop; also AG
attogram

AGA accelerated growth area
acetylglutamate
acute gonococcal arthritis
American Gastroenterological Association
American Genetic Association
anti-glomerular antibody
appropriate for gestational age
average for gestational age

Ag-Ab antigen-antibody (complex)

AGAG acidic glycosaminoglycans

AGAP antigen-against-panel

AGAS acetylglutamate synthetase
aerobiospheric genetic adaptation system

AGC absolute granulocyte count
automatic gain control

AGCT Army General Classification Test

AGD agar-gel diffusion (method)
agar-gel immunodiffusion (method)
agarose-gel diffusion (method)

AGDD agar-gel double diffusion (method)
agarose-gel double diffusion (method)

AGE acrylamide gel electrophoresis
acute gastroenteritis
agarose gel electrophoresis
angle of greatest extension

AGED automated general experimental device

AGEPC acetyl glyceryl ether phosphoryl choline

AGF angle of greatest flexion

ag feb while the fever increases or is coming on [L. *aggrediente febre*]; also aggred feb

AGG agammaglobulinemia

agg agglutinate; also aggl, agglut
agglutination; also aggl, agglut
aggravated
aggravation
aggregate; also aggreg
aggregation; also aggreg

aggl agglutinate; also agg, agglut
agglutination; also agg, agglut

agglut agglutinate; also agg, aggl
agglutination; also agg, aggl

aggred feb while the fever increases or is coming on [L. *aggrediente febre*]; also ag feb

aggreg aggregate; also agg
aggregation; also agg

AGGS anti-gas gangrene serum

agit shake [L. *agita*]

agit ante sum shake before taking [L. *agita ante sumendum*]

agit a us shake before using [L. *agita ante usum*]; also agit ante us

agit ante us shake before using [L. *agita ante usum*]; also agit a us

agit bene shake well [L. *agita bene*]

agit vas the vial being shaken [L. *agitato vase*]

AGL acute glomerular nephritis
acute granulocytic leukemia
aminoglutethimide; also AG

A-GLACTO-LK alpha-galactoside leukocytes

AGMK, AGMk African green monkey kidney (cell tissue culture)

AGML acute gastric mucosal lesion

AGN acute glomerulonephritis
agnosia; also agn
antigen; also AG, Ag, ag

agn agnosia; also AGN

AgNOR silver-staining nucleolar organizer region

AGOS American Gynecological and Obstetrical Society

AGP acid glycoprotein
agar-gel precipitation (test)
alpha$_1$-acid glycoprotein; also AAG

AGPA American Group Practice Association

AGPI agar-gel precipitin inhibition

AGPT agar-gel precipitation test

AGR aniridia, genitourinary abnormalities, and mental retardation
anticipatory goal response

AGS adrenal gland sympathogonioma
adrenogenital syndrome
American Geriatrics Society
American Gynecological Society (now: AGOS, American Gynecological and Obstetrical Society)
audiogenic seizure; also AS

AGT abnormal glucose tolerance
activity group therapy
acute generalized tuberculosis

adrenoglomerulotropin; also AGTr
antiglobulin test

agt agent

AGTH adrenoglomerulotropic hormone

AGTr adrenoglomerulotropin; also AGT

AGTT abnormal glucose tolerance test

AGU aspartylglycosaminuria

AGV aniline gentian violet

AH abdominal hysterectomy; also Abd Hyst
absorptive hypercalciuria
accidental hypothermia
acetohexamide
acid hydrolysis
acute hepatitis
Adie-Holmes (syndrome)
after-hyperpolarization (of a neuron); also AHP
alcoholic hepatitis
amenorrhea and hirsutism
amenorrhea and hyperprolactinemia; also A/H
aminohippurate
anterior hypothalamus
antihyaluronidase
arcuate hypothalamus
arterial hypertension
artificial heart
ascites hepatoma
astigmatic hypermetropia
autonomic hyperreflexia; also AHR
axillary hair
hypermetropic astigmatism; also ah, ASH, AsH
hyperopic astigmatism; also ah, ASH, AsH

A h ampere-hour; also A-h

A/H amenorrhea and hyperprolactinemia; also AH

A&H accident and health (insurance)

A-h ampere-hour; also A h

aH abhenry

ah hypermetropic astigmatism; also AH, ASH, AsH
hyperopic astigmatism; also AH, ASH, AsH

AHA acetohydroxamic acid
acquired hemolytic anemia
acute hemolytic anemia
American Heart Association
American Hospital Association
anterior hypothalamic area
anti-heart antibody
anti-histone antibody
area health authority
aspartylhydroxamic acid
autoimmune hemolytic anemia; also AIHA

AHB alpha-hydroxybutyric dehydrogenase

AHBC hepatitis B core antibody

AHC acute hemorrhagic conjunctivitis
acute hemorrhagic cystitis
Association of Academic Health Centers

AHCPR Agency for Health Care Policy and
Research

AHCy *S*-adenosylhomocysteine; also AdoHcy

AHD antihypertensive drug
arteriosclerotic heart disease; also ASHD
atherosclerotic heart disease; also ASHD
autoimmune hemolytic disease

AHDMS automated hospital data management
system

AHDP azacycloheptane diphosphonate

AHE acute hemorrhagic encephalomyelitis

AHEC area health education center

AHES artificial heart energy system

AHF acute heart failure
American Hospital Formulary
antihemophilic factor (coagulation factor
VIII)
Argentinian hemorrhagic fever

AHFS American Hospital Formulary Service

AHFS-DI American Hospital Formulary
Service–Drug Information

AHG aggregated human globulin
antihemophilic globulin (coagulation factor
VIII)
anti-human globulin

AHGG aggregated human gamma globulin
anti-human gamma globulin

AHGS acute herpetic gingival stomatitis

AHH alpha-hydrazine analog of histidine
anosmia and hypogonadotropic hypogonadism (syndrome)
arylhydrocarbon hydroxylase

AHI active hostility index
apnea-plus-hypopnea index

AHIP assisted health insurance plan

AHIS automated hospital information system

AHL apparent half-life

AHLE acute hemorrhagic leukoencephalitis

AHLG anti-human lymphocyte globulin

AHLS anti-human lymphocyte serum

AHM ambulatory Holter monitor
ambulatory Holter monitoring

AHMF American Holistic Medical Foundation

AHMI American Holistic Medical Institute
(now: AHMF, American Holistic Medical
Foundation)

AHN adenomatous hyperplastic nodule
Army head nurse
assistant head nurse

AHO Albright hereditary osteodystrophy

AHP acute hemorrhagic pancreatitis
after-hyperpolarization (of a neuron); also AH
air at high pressure
Assistant House Physician

AHPA American Health Planning Association

AHPAT Allied Health Practitioners
Aptitude/Admission Test

AHPO anterior hypothalamic preoptic (area)

AHR autonomic hyperreflexia; also AH

AHS adaptive hand skills
African horse sickness
alveolar hypoventilation syndrome
American Hearing Society (now: NAHSA,
National Association for Hearing and
Speech Action)
Assistant House Surgeon

AHSDF area health service development fund

AHT aggregation half-time
antihyaluronidase titer
augmented histamine test
autoantibodies to human thyroglobulin

AHTG anti-human thymocyte globulin; also
ATG
anti-human thymocytic globulin

AHTP anti-human thymocyte plasma

AHU acute hemolytic uremic (syndrome)
arginine, hypoxanthine, and uracil

AHuG aggregated human immunoglobulin G

AHV avian herpes virus

AI accidental injury
accidentally incurred
adiposity index
aggregation index
allergy and immunology; also A&I
allergy index
anaphylatoxin inhibitor
angiogenesis inhibitor
angiotensin I; also AT I
anxiety index
aortic incompetence
aortic insufficiency; also A Insuf
apical impulse
articulation index
artificial insemination; also art insem

artificial intelligence
atherogenic index
atrial insufficiency
autoimmune
axioincisal

A-I aortoiliac

A&I Allergy and Immunology (service); also AI

AIA allylisopropylacetamide
amylase inhibitor activity
anti-insulin antibody; also AI-Ab
aspirin-induced asthma
automated image analysis

AI-Ab anti-insulin antibody; also AIA

AIB aminoisobutyric acid; also AIBA
avian infectious bronchitis

AIBA aminoisobutyric acid; also AIB

AIBF anterior interbody fusion

AIBS American Institute of Biological Sciences

AIC aminoimidazole carboxamide
Association des Infirmières Canadiennes

AICA anterior inferior cerebellar artery
anterior inferior communicating artery

AICAR aminoimidazole carboxamide ribonucleotide

AICC anti-inhibitor coagulant complex

AICD automatic implantable cardioverter-defibrillator
automatic internal cardioverter-defibrillator

AICE angiotensin I-converting enzyme

AICF autoimmune complement fixation
autoimmune complement-fixing (antibody)

AID acquired immunodeficiency disease
acute infectious disease
acute ionization detector
Agency for International Development
American-Indian Dispensary
anti-inflammatory drug
argon ionization detector
artificial insemination donor
artificial insemination by donor (heterologous insemination)
autoimmune deficiency
autoimmune disease
automatic implantable defibrillator
average interocular difference

AIDH artificial insemination donor, husband

AIDS acquired immune deficiency syndrome
acquired immunodeficiency syndrome
acute infectious disease series
autoimmune deficiency syndrome

AIDS-KS acquired immunodeficiency syndrome with Kaposi's sarcoma

AIE acute inclusion body encephalitis
acute infectious encephalitis
acute infectious endocarditis

AIEP amount of insulin extractable from pancreas

AIF anemia-inducing factor
anti-inflammatory
anti-invasion factor
aortic-iliac-femoral

AIG anti-immunoglobulin

AIgA absence of immunoglobulin A

AIgM absence of immunoglobulin M

A-IGP activity-interview group psychotherapy

AIH American Institute of Homeopathy
artificial insemination by husband (homologous insemination)
artificial insemination, homologous

AIHA American Industrial Hygiene Association
autoimmune hemolytic anemia; also AHA

AIHD acquired immune hemolytic disease

AII angiotensin II

AIII angiotensin III

AIIS anterior inferior iliac spine

AIL acute infectious lymphocytosis
angiocentric immunoproliferative lesion
angioimmunoblastic lymphadenopathy

AILD alveolar-interstitial lung disease
angioimmunoblastic lymphadenopathy with dysproteinemia

AILT amiloride-inhibitable lithium transport

AIM Artificial Intelligence in Medicine

AIMD abnormal involuntary movement disorder

AIMS abnormal involuntary movement scale
arthritis impact measurement scale

AIN acute interstitial nephritis
anal intraepithelial neoplasia

AINS anti-inflammatory nonsteroidal (agent)

A Insuf aortic insufficiency; also AI

AIO amyloid of immunoglobulin origin

AION anterior ischemic optic neuropathy

AIP acute idiopathic pericarditis
acute infectious polyneuritis
acute inflammatory polyneuropathy
acute intermittent porphyria

AIP—cont'd
aldosterone-induced protein
annual implementation plan
arachidonate-insensitive platelet
automated immunoprecipitation
average intravascular pressure

AIR accelerated idioventricular rhythm;
also AIVR
aminoimidazole ribonucleotide
average impairment rating

AIRA anti-insulin receptor antibody

AIRF alteration in respiratory function

AIS Abbreviated Injury Score
alcohol intake sheet
androgen insensitivity syndrome
anterior interosseous nerve syndrome
anti-insulin serum

AISA acquired idiopathic sideroblastic a
nemia

AIS/ISS Abbreviated Injury Score/Injury
Severity Score

AIS/MR Alternative Intermediate Services for
the Mentally Retarded

AIT administrator-in-training

AITP autoimmune thrombocytopenia purpura;
also ATP

AITT arginine insulin tolerance test

AIU absolute iodine uptake
antigen-inducing unit

AIUM American Institute of Ultrasound in
Medicine

AIVR accelerated idioventricular rhythm;
also AIR

AIVV anterior internal vertebral vein

AJ ankle jerk; also A/J

A/J ankle jerk; also AJ

AJCC American Joint Committee on Cancer

AJCCS American Joint Committee for Cancer
Staging

AJR abnormal jugular reflex

AK above knee; also A/K, A-K
actinic keratosis
adenosine kinase; also ADK
adenylate kinase
artificial kidney

A/K above knee; also AK, A-K

A-K above knee; also AK, A/K

AKA above knee amputation; also AK amp
alcoholic ketoacidosis
all known allergies

alpha-allo-kainic acid
also known as; also aka
American Kinesiotherapy Association
anti-keratin antibody

aka also known as; also AKA

AK amp above knee amputation; also AKA

AKE acrokeratoelastoidosis

A/kg amperes per kilogram

AKP alkaline phosphatase; also ALK-P, alk
phos, Alk PO_4 tase, alk p'tase, ALP, AP,

AKS auditory and kinesthetic sensation

AL absolute latency
acinar lumina
active lipid
acute leukemia
adaptation level
Albright-Lightwood (syndrome)
albumin; also A, ALB, Alb, alb
alcoholism; also alc
alignment mark
amyloidosis
annoyance level
anti-human lymphocytic (globulin)
argininosuccinate lysate
argon laser
arterial line; also A-line
avian leukosis
axial length
axiolingual
left ear [L. *auris laeva*]; also al, AS, as
lethal antigen

Al allantoic
aluminum

al attoliter
left ear [L. *auris laeva*]; also AL, AS, as

ALA alanine; also A, Ala
American Laryngological Association
American Lung Association
aminolevulinic acid
anterior lip of the acetabulum
axiolabial; also ALa

ALa axiolabial; also ALA

Ala alanine; also A, ALA
alanyl

AlaAT alanine aminotransferase; also AAT,
ALAT, ALT

AL-Ab antilymphocyte antibody

ALAC antibiotic-loaded acrylic cement

ALAD abnormal left axis deviation
aminolevulinic acid dehydrase; also ALA-D

ALA-D aminolevulinic acid dehydrase; also ALAD

ALAG, ALaG axiolabiogingival

ALAL, ALaL axiolabiolingual

ALARA as low as reasonably achievable (radiation exposure)

ALAS aminolevulinic acid synthetase

ALAT alanine aminotransferase; also AAT, AlaAT, ALT
alanine transaminase; also ALT

ALAX apical long axis

ALB albumin; also A, AL, Alb, alb
avian lymphoblastosis

Alb albumin; also A, AL, ALB, alb

alb albumin; also A, AL, ALB, Alb
white [L. *albus*]

ALB/GLOB albumin to globulin (ratio); also AG, A/G, A:G

ALC absolute lymphocyte count
acute lethal catatonia
alcohol; also alc, alcoh
allogeneic lymphocyte cytotoxicity
alternate level of care
Alternative Lifestyle Checklist
approximate lethal concentration
avian leukosis complex
axiolinguocervical

alc alcohol; also ALC, alcoh
alcoholic; also alcoh
alcoholism; also AL
ethanol; also alcoh
ethyl alcohol; also alcoh

ALCA anomalous left coronary artery

ALCAPA anomalous origin of left coronary artery from pulmonary artery

alcoh alcohol; also ALC, alc
alcoholic; also alc
ethanol; also alc
ethyl alcohol; also alc

ALC R, ALCR, AlcR alcohol rub

AlCr aluminum crown

ALD adrenoleukodystrophy; also ADL
alcoholic liver disease
aldolase; also Ald
aldosterone; also Aldo, ALDOST
anterior latissimus dorsi
Appraisal of Language Disturbances
approximate lethal dose

Ald aldolase; also ALD

ALDH aldehyde dehydrogenase

Aldo aldosterone; also ALD, ALDOST

ALDOST aldosterone; also ALD, Aldo

ALE allowable limits of error

ALEC artificial lung-expanding compound

ALEP atypical lymphoepithelioid cell proliferation

ALF acute liver failure
anterior long fiber

ALFT abnormal liver function test

ALG Annapolis lymphoblast globulin
anti-lymphoblastic globulin
antilymphocyte globulin
antilymphocytic globulin
axiolinguogingival

ALGOL algorithm-oriented language
algorithmic oriented language

ALH anterior lobe hormone (of hypophysis)
anterior lobe of the hypophysis

ALI argon laser iridotomy

A-line arterial catheter
arterial line; also AL

ALIP abnormal localized immature myeloid precursor

ALK, alk alkaline
alkylating (agent)

ALK-P alkaline phosphatase; also AKP, alk phos, Alk PO$_4$ tase, alk p'tase, ALP, AP

alk phos alkaline phosphatase; also AKP, ALK-P, Alk PO$_4$ tase, alk p'tase, ALP, AP

Alk PO$_4$ tase alkaline phosphatase; also AKP, ALK-P, alk phos, alk p'tase, ALP, AP

alk p'tase alkaline phosphatase; also AKP, ALK-P, alk phos, Alk PO$_4$ tase, ALP, AP

ALL acute lymphatic leukemia
acute lymphoblastic leukemia
acute lymphocytic leukemia
allergic; also A, all
allergy; also A, all
anterior longitudinal ligament

all allergic; also A, ALL
allergy; also A, ALL
allose

ALLA acute lymphocytic leukemia antigen

ALLO atypical Legionella-like organism

ALM acral lentiginous melanoma
alveolar living material

ALME acetyl-lysine methyl ester

ALMI anterior lateral myocardial infarction

ALMV anterior leaflet of the mitral valve

ALN anterior lymph node

ALO average lymphocyte output
axiolinguo-occlusal

ALOMAD Adriamycin, Leukeran, Oncovin,
methotrexate, actinomycin D, and dacarbazine

ALOS average length of stay

ALP acute lupus pericarditis
alkaline phosphatase; also AKP, ALK-P, alk
phos, Alk PO$_4$ tase, alk p'tase, AP
Alupent
anterior lobe of pituitary
antilymphocyte plasma
antilymphocytic plasma
argon laser photocoagulation

ALPI alkaline phosphatase isoenzymes

ALPS angiolympho-proliferative syndrome
Aphasia Language Performance Scales

ALPZ alprazolam

ALRI anterolateral rotational instability

ALROS American Laryngological,
Rhinological and Otological Society

ALRR arthroscopic lateral retinacula release

ALS acute lateral sclerosis
advanced life support (system)
afferent loop syndrome
amyotrophic lateral sclerosis
angiotensin-like substance
anticipated life span
anti-lymphatic serum
antilymphocyte serum
antilymphocytic serum
antiviral lymphocyte serum

ALSD Alzheimer-like senile dementia

ALT alanine aminotransferase; also AAT,
ALAT, AlaAT
alanine transaminase; also ALAT
alternate; also Alt, alt
altitude; also Alt, alt
argon laser trabeculoplasty; also Alt, alt
avian laryngotracheitis

Alt, alt alternate; also ALT
altitude; also ALT
argon laser trabeculoplasty; also ALT

ALT/AST ratio of serum alanine aminotransferase to serum aspartate aminotransferase

ALTA apparent life-threatening agent

ALTB acute laryngotracheobronchitis

alt dieb every other day [L. *alternis diebus*];
also ad

ALTE apparent life threatening event

ALTEE acetyl-L-tyrosine ethyl ester

alt hor every other hour [L. *alternis horis*]

alt noc every other night [L. *alternis noctibus*];
also alt noct

alt noct every other night [L. *alternis
noctibus*]; also alt noc

ALU arithmetic and logic unit

ALV Abelson leukemia virus
adeno-like virus
alveolar; also Alv, alv
ascending lumbar vein
avian leukemia virus
avian leukosis virus

Alv, alv alveolar; also ALV
alveolus

ALVAD abdominal left ventricular assist device

alv adst when the bowels are constipated [L.
alvo adstricta]

alv deject discharge from the bowels [L. *alvi
dejectiones* (alvine dejections)]

ALVM alveolar mucosa; also AM

ALVT aortic and left ventricular tunnel

Alvx alveolectomy

ALW arch-loop-whorl (system)

ALWMI anterolateral wall myocardial infarct

AM acrylamide
actomyosin
acute myelofibrosis
adult male
adult monocyte
aerospace medicine
alveolar macrophage
alveolar mucosa; also ALVM
amacrine cell
amalgam; also AAA, aaa, AMAL
ambulate; also AMB, amb, ambul
ambulatory; also A, AMB, amb, ambul
amelanotic melanoma
amethopterin; also AMT
ametropia; also Am, am
ammeter
amperemeter
ampicillin; also A, AMP
amplitude modulation; also A-mode
anovular menstruation
antibodies to cardiac myosin
arithmetic mean
arousal mechanism
Austin-Moore (prosthesis)
aviation medicine; also AVM

aviation medicine; also AVM
axiomesial
before noon [L. *ante meridiem*]; also am
Master of Arts [L. *Artium Magister*]
meter-angle; also am
mixed astigmatism; also Am
myopic astigmatism; also am, ASM, AsM, As M

Am americium
ametropia; also AM, am
amnion
amyl
mixed astigmatism; also AM

a2M alpha-2 macroglobulin

A-m² ampere-square meter

A/m amperes per meter

am ametropia; also AM, Am
amplitude
attometer
before noon [L. *ante meridiem*]; also AM
meter-angle; also AM
myopic astigmatism; also AM, ASM, AsM,
As M

AMA actual mechanical advantage
Aerospace Medical Association
against medical advice
American Medical Association
anti-mitochondrial antibody
anti-myosin antibody
Australian Medical Association

AMAD morning admission

AMA-DE American Medical Association Drug
Evaluations

AMA-ERF American Medical Association -
Education and Research Foundation

AMAG adrenal medullary autograft

AMAL Aero-Medical Acceleration Laboratory
amalgam; also AAA, aaa, AM

AMAP as much as possible

AMAT amorphous material; also A-MAT
anti-malignant antibody test

A-MAT amorphous material; also AMAT

AMB ambulate; also AM, amb, ambul
ambulatory; also A, AM, amb, ambul
amphotericin B
anomalous bundle muscle
avian myeloblastosis

amb ambient
ambiguous; also ambig
ambulance
ambulate; also AM, AMB, ambul
ambulatory; also A, AM, AMB, ambul

ambig ambiguous; also amb

AMBL acute myeloblastic leukemia; also AML

ambul ambulate; also AM, AMB, amb
ambulatory; also A, AM, AMB, amb

AMC ammonium chloride (tablets)
antibody-mediated cytotoxicity
antimalaria campaign
arm muscle circumference
arthrogryposis multiplex congenita
automated mixture control
automatic mixture control
axiomesiocervical

AMCHA (aminomethyl)cyclohexanecarboxylic
acid

AMCN anteromedial caudate nucleus

AM/CR amylase to creatinine ratio

AMD acid maltase deficiency
acromandibular dysplasia
actinomycin D (dactinomycin); also ACD,
ACT, ACTD, Act-D, act-D
adrenomyelodystrophy
aeromedical data
age-related macular degeneration; also
ARMD
Aleutian mink disease
alpha-methyldopa
arthroscopic microdiskectomy
axiomesiodistal

AMDP Association for Methodology and
Documentation in Psychiatry (system)

AMDS Association of Military Dental
Surgeons

AME amphotericin B methyl ester
aseptic meningoencephalitis

AMEEGA American Medical
Electroencephalographic Association

AMEGL, AMegL acute megakaryoblastic
leukemia

AMEL Aero-Medical Equipment Laboratory

Amer American

Amerind American Indian sign language

Ameslan American sign language; also ASL

AMet adenosylmethionine (*S*-adenosylmethio-
nine)

AMF anti-muscle factor
autocrine motility factor

Amf amniotic fluid; also AF

AMG acoustic myography
alpha-1-microglobulin
alpha$_2$-macroglobulin; also α_2M

AMG—cont'd
  aminoglycoside; also AG
  amyloglucosidase
  amyloglucoside
  anti-macrophage globulin
  axiomesiogingival

AMH anti-muellerian hormone
  automated medical history

Amh mixed astigmatism with myopia predominating

AMHT automated multiphasic health testing

AMI acquired monosaccharide intolerance
  acute myocardial infarction
  amitriptyline; also AMT, AT
  anterior myocardial infarction
  Association of Medical Illustrators
  axiomesioincisal

AML acute monocytic leukemia; also AMOL
  acute myeloblastic leukemia; also AMBL
  acute myelocytic leukemia
  acute myelogenous leukemia
  acute myeloid leukemia
  anterior mitral leaflet

AMLB alternate monaural loudness balance
  (test)

AMLC adherent macrophage-like cell
  autologous mixed lymphocyte culture

AMLR autologous mixed lymphocyte reaction

AMLS anti-mouse lymphocyte serum

AMLSGA acute myeloblastic leukemia surface
  glycoprotein antigen

AMM agnogenic myeloid metaplasia
  ammonia; also ammon
  antibody to murine cardiac myosin

AMML acute myelomonocytic leukemia; also
  AMMOL, AMMoL

AMMOL, AMMoL acute myelomonocytic
  leukemia; also AMML
  acute myelomonoblastic leukemia
  acute myelomonoblastic lymphoma

ammon ammonia; also AMM

AMN adrenomyeloneuropathy
  alloxazine mononucleotide
  anterior median nucleus

amnio amniocentesis

AMN SC amniotic fluid scan

AMO acute mucocutaneous ocular (syndrome)
  Assistant Medical Officer
  axiomesio-occlusal

A-mode amplitude mode
  amplitude modulation; also AM

AMOL acute monoblastic leukemia
  acute monocytic leukemia; also AML

AMOR, amor amorphous; also AMORP,
  amorp, amorph

AMORP, amorp amorphous; also AMOR,
  amor, amorph

amorph amorphous; also AMOR, amor,
  AMORP, amorp

AMP accelerated mental processes
  acid mucopolysaccharide; also AMPS
  adenosine monophosphate (adenylic acid)
  2-amino-2-methyl-1-propanol
  amphetamine; also A, AMPH, AMT
  ampicillin; also A, AM
  ampule; also amp, ampul
  amputation; also amp
  Association for Methodology in Psychiatry
  (system)
  average mean pressure

amp ampere; also A, a
  amperage
  amplification
  ampule; also AMP, ampul
  amputation; also AMP
  amputated
  amputee

AMPA 2-(aminomethyl)phenylacetic acid

AMPase adenosine monophosphatase

AMP-c cyclic adenosine monophosphate; also
  cAMP, cAMP, cyclic AMP

AMPH amphetamine; also A, AMP, AMT

amph amphoric (respiratory sound)

amp-hr ampere-hour; also A h, A-h

ampl large [L. *amplus*]

A-M pr Austin-Moore prosthesis

AMPS abnormal mucopolysacchariduria
  acid mucopolysaccharide; also AMP

amps ampules

AMPT alpha-methyl-*p*-tyrosine

ampul ampule; also AMP, amp

AMR acoustic muscle reflex
  activity metabolic rate
  alternate motion rate
  alternating motion reflex

AMRA American Medical Record
  Association

AMRI anteromedial rotatory instability

AMRL Aerospace Medical Research
  Laboratories

AMRS automated medical record system

AMS accelerator mass spectrometry
    acute mountain sickness
    aggravated in military service
    altered mental status
    American Meteorological Society
    American Microscopical Society
    amylase; also AMY
    anti-macrophage serum
    Army Medical Service (British)
    Association of Military Surgeons
    atypical measles syndrome
    auditory memory span
    automated multiphasic screening
    automicrobic system

ams amount of a substance

AMSA American Medical Student Association
    amsacrine; also Amsa

Amsa amsacrine; also AMSA

AmSECT American Society of Extra-
    Corporeal Technology

AMSIT appearance, mood, sensorium, intelli-
    gence, and thought process (portion of
    mental status examination)

AMT acute miliary tuberculosis
    alpha-methyltyrosine
    American Medical Technologists
    amethopterin; also AM
    amitriptyline; also AMI, AT
    amphetamine; also A, AMP, AMPH

amt amount; also am't

am't amount; also amt

AMTP alpha-methyltryptophan

amu atomic mass unit

AmuLV Abelson murine leukemia virus

AMV assisted mechanical ventilation
    avian myeloblastosis virus

AMVI acute mesenteric vascular insufficiency

AMWA American Medical Women's
    Association
    American Medical Writers' Association

AMX amoxicillin

AMY amylase; also AMS

AMY-SP amylase urine spot (test)

AMZ anteromedial displacement osteotomy

AN acanthosis nigricans
    acne neonatorum
    acoustic neuroma
    administratively necessary
    adult normal
    aminonucleoside
    amyl nitrate

    aneurysm
    anisometropia; also An, anisometr
    anodal; also A, a, An
    anode; also A, a, An
    anorexia nervosa
    antenatal
    anterior; also A, a, ANT, ant
    anti-neuraminidase
    aseptic necrosis
    Aspergillus niger
    atrionodal
    autonomic neuropathy
    avascular necrosis; also AVN

A/N artery and/or nerve
    as needed

An actinon
    anatomy response
    anesthesia; also ANA, anes, anesth
    anesthesiology; also anes, anesth
    anesthetic; also ANA, anes, anesth
    aniridia
    anisometropia; also AN, anisometr
    anodal; also A, a, AN
    anode; also A, a, AN

A_n normal atmosphere

ANA acetylneuraminic acid
    American Neurological Association
    American Nurses Association
    anesthesia; also An, anes, anesth
    anesthetic; also An, anes, anesth
    antibody to nuclear antigens
    antinuclear antibody; also ANuA
    aspartyl naphthylamide

ana of each [Gr. *ana* (so much of)]; also AA,
    Ā Ā, aa, ā ā

ANAD anorexia nervosa and associated disorders
    anti-nicotinamide adenine dinucleotidase;
    also anti-NADase

ANA-FL antinuclear antibody fluid

anal analgesia
    analgesic
    analysis
    analyst
    analytic

ANAP agglutination negative, absorption posi-
    tive (reaction)

ANAS auditory nerve-activating substance

anast anastomosis

Anat, anat anatomical
    anatomist
    anatomy

ANC absolute neutrophil count

ANC—cont'd
  acid neutralization capacity
  antigen-neutralizing capacity
ANCA anti-neutrophil cytoplasmic antibodies
AnCC anodal closure contraction; also ACC
anch anchored
ANCOVA analysis of covariance
AND administratively necessary days
  algoneurodystrophy
  anterior nasal discharge
And androgen
ANDA Abbreviated New Drug Application
ANDRO, Andro androsterone; also A, Andros
Andros androsterone; also A, ANDRO, Andro
ANDTE, AnDTe anodal duration tetanus; also
  ADT, ADTe
anes anesthesia; also An, ANA, anesth
  anesthesiology; also An, anesth
  anesthetic; also An, ANA, anesth
ANESR apparent norepinephrine secretion rate
anesth anesthesia; also An, ANA, anes
  anesthesiology; also An, anes
  anesthetic; also An, ANA, anes
AnEx, an ex anodal excitation
  anode excitation
ANF alpha-naphthoflavone
  American Nurses' Foundation
  antineuritic factor
  antinuclear factor
  atrial natriuretic factor
ANG angiogram; also ang
  angiography; also ang, angio
ang angiogram; also ANG
  angiography; also ANG, angio
  angle; also A
  angular
Ang GR angiotensin generation rate
angio angiography; also ANG, ang
anh anhydrous; also anhydr
anhydr anhydrous; also anh
ANIS anisocytosis; also ANISO
ANISO anisocytosis; also ANIS
anisometr anisometropia; also AN, An
ANIT alpha-naphthyl-isothiocyanate
ank ankle
ANL acute non-lymphoblastic leukemia; also
  ANLL
  acute non-lymphocytic leukemia; also ANLL

ANLL acute non-lymphoblastic leukemia; also
  ANL
  acute non-lymphocytic leukemia; also ANL
ANM auxiliary nurse midwife
Ann annals; also Annls
  annual
Ann Justus Liebig's Annalen der Chemie
ann fib annulus fibrosus
Annls annals; also Ann
annot annotation
ANoA anti-nucleolar antibody
AnOC anodal opening contraction; also AOC
ANOVA analysis of variance; also ANOVAR
ANOVAR analysis of variance; also ANOVA
ANP acute necrotizing pancreatitis
  Adult Nurse Practitioner
  Advanced Nurse Practitioner
  A-norprogesterone
  atrial natriuretic peptide
A-NPP absorbed normal pooled plasma
ANRC American National Red Cross
ANRL antihypertensive neural renomedullary
  lipids
ANS anterior nasal spine
  anti-neutrophilic serum
  anti-rat neutrophil serum
  arterionephrosclerosis
  autonomic nervous system
ans answer
ANSA amino-naphthol-sulfonic acid
ANSCII American National Standard Code for
  Information Interchange
ANSI American National Standards Institute
ANT acoustic noise test
  aminoglycoside $2'$-o-nucleotidyltransferase
  2-amino-5-nitrothiazole (enpheptin)
  anterior; also A, a, AN, ant
  antimycin; also ant
ant antenna
  anterior; also A, a, AN, ANT
  antimycin; also ANT
AntA, Ant A antimycin A
antag antagonist
  antagonistic
ant ax line anterior axillary line; also AAL
ante before [L. *ante*]; also a,ā
Anthrop anthropology
anti antidote

ANTI A:AGT anti-blood group A antiglobulin test

Anti bx antibiotic; also AB, ATB

anticoag anticoagulant; also AC

anti-DNA anti-deoxyribonucleic acid

anti-G antigravity; also AG

anti-GBM anti-glomerular basement membrane

anti-HA anti-hepatitis antigen

anti-HAA antibody to hepatitis-associated antigen

anti-HAV antibody to hepatitis A virus

anti-HB$_c$ antibody to hepatitis B core antigen

anti-HB$_s$ antibody to hepatitis B surface antigen; also anit-HB$_s$Ag

anti-HB$_s$Ag antibody to hepatitis B surface antigen; also anit-HB$_s$

anti-HLTV III antibody to human lymphotrophic virus III

anti-IF anti-intrinsic factor

anti-LKM anti- liver and kidney microsomes

anti-log antilogarithm

anti-NADase anti-nicotinamide adenine dinucleotidase; also ANAD

anti-nRNP anti-nuclear ribonucleoprotein; also anti-RNP

anti-PNM Ab anti-peripheral nerve myelin antibody

anti-RANA anti-rheumatoid arthritis nuclear antigen

anti-RNP anti-nuclear ribonucleoprotein; also anti-nRNP

anti-S anti-sulfanilic acid

anti-SK anti-streptokinase; also ASK

anti-Sm anti-Smith (antibody)

anti-SM/RNP anti-Smith/anti-nuclear ribonucleoprotein

anti SS-A antibody to acidic nucleoprotein of human spleen extract

anti SS-B antibody to acidic nucleoprotein of rabbit thymus

anti-VCA anti-viral capsid antigen

ant jentac before breakfast [L. *ante jentaculum*]

Ant pit, ant pit anterior pituitary; also AP

ant prand before dinner [L. *ante prandium*]; also AP, ap

ANTR apparent net transfer rate

ant sag D anterior sagittal diameter; also ASD

ant sup anterior superior

ant sup sp anterior superior spine; also ant sup spine, ASS

ant sup spine anterior superior spine; also ant sup sp, ASS

ANTU alpha-naphthylthiourea

ANuA antinuclear antibody; also ANA

ANUG acute necrotizing ulcerative gingivitis

ANX, anx anxiety
anxious

anx neur anxiety neurosis

anx react anxiety reaction

AO abdominal aorta
achievement orientation
acid output
acridine orange (dye, test)
anodal opening
anterior oblique
aorta; also Ao
aortic opening
ascending aorta; also AA, AS, Asc-A
atomic orbital
atrioventricular valve opening
auriculoventricular valve opening
average optical density
avoidance of others
axio-occlusal

A-O acoustic-optic

A/O alert and oriented; also A&O
analog to digital (converter); also A/D

A&O alert and oriented; also A/O

A&Ox3 alert and oriented to person, place, and time

A&Ox4 alert and oriented to person, place, time, and date

Ao aorta; also AO

AOA abnormal oxygen affinity
Alpha Omega Alpha (honorary medical society)
American Optometric Association
American Orthopaedic Association
American Orthopsychiatric Association
American Osteopathic Association
average orifice area

AOAA amino-oxyacetic acid

AOAC Association of Official Analytical Chemists

AOAP as often as possible

AOB accessory olfactory bulb
alcohol on breath

AOBS acute organic brain syndrome

AOC abridged ocular chart
amyloxycarbonyl
anodal opening contraction; also AnOC
antacid of choice
aortic opening click
area of concern

AOCA American Osteopathic College of
Anesthesiologists

AOCD American Osteopathic College of
Dermatology
anemia of chronic disease

AOCl anodal opening clonus

AOCP American Osteopathic College of
Pathologists

AOCPr American Osteopathic College of
Proctology

AOCR American Osteopathic College of
Radiology

AOD adult-onset diabetes
alleged onset date
arterial occlusive disease
arterial oxygen desaturation
auriculo-osteodysplasia

AODA alcohol and other drug abuse

AODM adult-onset diabetes mellitus; also
ADODM

ao-il aorta-iliac

AOIVM angiographically occult intracranial
vascular malformation

AOL acro-osteolysis

AOM acute otitis media
atomic organic matter
azoxymethane
Master of Obstetric Art

AOMA American Occupational Medical
Association (now: ACOEM, American
College of Occupational and
Environmental Medicine)

AoMP aortic mean pressure

AONE American Organization of Nurse
Executives

AOO anodal opening odor
atrial asynchronous (pacemaker code)

AOP amino-oligopeptide
anodal opening picture
aortic pressure; also AP

AoP left ventricle to aorta pressure gradient

AOPA American Orthotic and Prosthetic
Association

AoPW aortic posterior wall

AOR auditory oculogyric reflex

AORN Association of Operating Room Nurses

aor regurg aortic regurgitation; also AR, aort
regurg

aort regurg aortic regurgitation; also AR, aor
regurg

aort sten aortic stenosis; also AS, A sten

AOS acridine orange staining
American Otological Society
anodal opening sound
anterior (o)esophageal sensor

AOSD adult-onset Still's disease

AOT accessory optic tract
anti-ovotransferrin
Association of Occupational Therapists

AOTA American Occupational Therapy
Association

AOTe anodal opening tetanus

AOU apparent oxygen utilization

AOV aortic valve; also AV

AP abdominoperineal (resection); also A-P
Academy of Periodontology
accessory pathway
acid phosphatase; also acid phos, acid PO_4,
acid p'tase, ACP, AcP, AC-PH, ac phos
acinar parenchyma
action potential
active pepsin
acute pancreatitis
acute phase
acute pneumonia
acute proliferative
adolescent psychiatry
Adriamycin and Platinol
after parturition
alkaline phosphatase; also AKP, ALK-P, alk
phos, Alk PO_4 tase, alk p'tase, ALP
alum-precipitated (vaccine)
aminopeptidase
aminopyrine
angina pectoris
antepartum
anterior pituitary; also Ant pit, ant pit
anteroposterior
antidromic potential
anti-parkinsonian; also APK
antipyrine
antral peristalsis

aortic pressure; also AOP
aortic pulmonary
apical pulse
apothecary; also ap, apoth
appendectomy; also Appy, appy
appendicitis
appendix; also APP, app, Appx
area postrema
arithmetic progression
arterial pressure
artificial pneumothorax
aspiration pneumonitis
assessment and plan(s); also A&P
association period
atherosclerotic plaque
atrial pacing
atrium pace
atrioventricular pathway
attending physician
axiopulpal
before dinner [L. *ante prandium*]; also ant
 prand, ap
before parturition [L. *ante partum*]
intra-abdominal voiding pressure

3-AP 3-acetylpyridine (nicotinic antagonist)

4-AP 4-aminopyridine

A-P abdominoperineal (resection); also AP
analytic-psychologic
anterior-posterior (radiologic projection)

A/P ascites to plasma (ratio)

A&P active and present
anatomy and physiology
anterior and posterior
assessment and plan(s); also AP
auscultation and palpation
auscultation and percussion

a&p abdominal and perineal

A$_2$P$_2$ aortic second sound, pulmonary second
sound

A$_2$>P$_2$ second aortic sound greater than second
pulmonary sound

A$_2$=P$_2$ second aortic sound equals second pulmonary sound

A$_2$<P$_2$ second aortic sound less than second
pulmonary sound

Ap apex

ap apothecary; also AP, apoth
before dinner [L. *ante prandium*]; also ant
 prand, AP
prior to [L. *a priori*]

APA acetyl-*para*-aminophenol; also APAP
aldosterone-producing adenoma

American Physiotherapy Association (now:
 APTA, American Physical Therapy
 Association)
American Psychiatric Association
American Psychological Association
aminopenicillanic acid
anti-parietal antibody
anti-pernicious anemia (factor)

6-APA 6-aminopenicillanic acid

APACHE Acute Physiology and Chronic
Health Evaluation (system)

APAD anterior-posterior abdominal diameter

APAF anti-pernicious anemia factor

APAP acetyl-*para*-aminophenol; also APA
Association of Physician Assistant Programs

APB abductor pollicis brevis (muscle)
atrial premature beat
auricular premature beat

APC acetylsalicylic acid, phenacetin, and caffeine
activated protein complex
acute pharyngoconjunctival (fever)
adenoidal-pharyngeal-conjunctival (agent or
 virus)
adenomatous polyposis coli
all-purpose capsule (jargon for aspirin-
 phenacetin-caffeine)
alternative patterns of complement
amsacrine, prednisone, and chlorambucil
antigen-presenting cell
anti-parietal cell
antiphlogistic corticoid; also AC
aperture current
apneustic center (of brain)
aspirin-phenacetin-caffeine
atrial premature contraction
atrial premature complex

APCA anti-parietal cell antibody

APCC, APC-C aspirin, phenacetin, and caffeine with codeine

APCD adult-onset polycystic kidney disease;
also APCKD, APKD

APCF acute pharyngoconjunctival fever

APCG apexcardiogram; also ACG

APCKD adult-onset polycystic kidney disease;
also APCD, APKD

APD action-potential duration
acute polycystic disease
adult polycystic disease
afferent pupillary defect
amino-hydroxypropylidene diphosphate
anteroposterior diameter; also A-PD

APD —cont'd
atrial premature depolarization
autoimmune progesterone dermatitis
automated peritoneal dialysis

A-PD anteroposterior diameter; also APD

APDC anxiety and panic disorder clinic

APDI adult personal data inventory

APE acetone powder extract
acute polioencephalitis
acute psychotic episode
acute pulmonary edema
Adriamycin, Platinol, and etoposide
airway pressure excursion
aminophylline, phenobarbital, and ephedrine
anterior pituitary extract
avian pneumoencephalitis

APECED autoimmune polyendocrinopathy-candidosis-ectodermal dystrophy

APF acidulated phosphofluoride
anabolism-promoting factor
animal protein factor (vitamin B_{12})
anti-perinuclear factor
arthritis pain formula

APG acid-precipitable globulin
acid-precipitated globulin
animal pituitary gonadotropin
Apgar (score)

APGAR adaptability, partnership, growth, affection, and resolve (family screening, not Apgar score of newborn physical status)

APGL alkaline phosphatase activity of granular leukocytes

APH adenohypophyseal hormone
adult psychiatric hospital
alcohol-positive history
antepartum hemorrhage
anterior pituitary hormone

aph aphasia

APHA American Protestant Hospital Association
American Public Health Association

APhA American Pharmaceutical Association

AP/HC accreditation program/hospice care

AP/HHC accreditation program/home health care

APHP anti-Pseudomonas human plasma

API alkaline protease inhibitor
analytical profile index
ankle-arm pressure index
atmospheric pressure ionization

APIC Association for Practitioners in Infection Control

APIE assessment plan, implementation, and evaluation

APIM Association Professionelle Internationale des Médecins

APIP additional personal injury protection

APIr atriopeptin-like immunoreactive (neurons)

APIVR artificial pacemaker-induced ventricular rhythm

APK anti-parkinsonian; also AP

APKD adult-onset polycystic kidney disease; also APCD, APCKD

APL abductor pollicis longus (muscle)
accelerated painless labor
acute promyelocytic leukemia; also AProL
animal placental lactogen
anterior pituitary-like (hormone)
trademark for a brand of chorionic gonadotropin

AP&L anteroposterior and lateral (radiologic view); also AP&Lat, A-P & Lat

AP&Lat anteroposterior and lateral (radiologic view); also AP&L, A-P & Lat

A-P & Lat anteroposterior and lateral (radiologic view); also AP&L, AP&Lat

AP/LTC accreditation program/long-term care

APM Academy of Physical Medicine
Academy of Psychosomatic Medicine
acid-precipitable material
alternating pressure mattress
aminopeptidase M
anterior papillary muscle
anteroposterior movement
aspartame

APMA 4-aminophenylmecuric acid
American Podiatric Medical Association

APMD automated percutaneous microdiskectomy

APMR Association for Physical and Mental Rehabilitation (now: AKA, American Kinesiotherapy Association)

APN acute pyelonephritis
average peak noise

APO adductor pollicis obliquus (muscle)
Adriamycin, prednisone, and Oncovin
adverse patient occurrences
aphoxide; also TEPA
apomorphine

Apo, apo apolipoprotein

ApoB, apoB, Apo B apolipoprotein B

Apo C apolipoprotein C

Apo D apolipoprotein D

Apo E apolipoprotein E

APORF acute postoperative renal failure

apoth apothecary; also AP, ap

APP acute phase protein
  alum-precipitated protein
  alum-precipitated pyridine
  amino-pyrazolopyrimidine
  antiplatelet plasma
  appendix; also AP, app, Appx
  aqueous procaine penicillin
  automated physiologic profile
  avian pancreatic polypeptide

app apparent; also appar
  appendix; also AP, APP, Appx
  applied; also appl
  approximate; also appr, approx

APPA American Psychopathological
  Association

appar apparatus
  apparent; also app

APPG aqueous procaine penicillin G

appl appliance
  applicable
  application
  applied; also app

applan flattened [L. *applanatus*]

applicand to be applied or administered [L.
  applicandus]

appoint appointment; also appt

APPR 4-amino-pyrazolopyrimidine ribonucle-
  oside

appr approximate; also app, approx
  approximately; also approx
  approximation; also approx

approx approximate; also app, appr
  approximately; also appr
  approximation; also appr

appt appointment; also appoint

Appx appendix; also AP, APP, app

Appy, appy appendectomy; also AP

APR abdominoperineal resection
  absolute proximal reabsorption
  accelerator-produced radiopharmaceuticals
  acute phase reactant
  amebic prevalence rate
  anatomic porous replacement

anterior pituitary reaction
auropalpebral reflex

aprax apraxia

APRL American Prosthetic Research
  Laboratory
  antihypertensive polar renomedullary lipid

APRO aprobarbital

AProL acute promyelocytic leukemia; also
  APL

APRP acidic proline-rich protein
  acute-phase reactant protein

APRT, aprt adenine phosphoribosyltransferase

APS Acute Pain Services
  acute physiology score
  adenosine phosphosulfate
  Adult Protective Services
  Adult Psychiatric Service
  American Pediatric Society
  American Physiological Society
  American Proctologic Society (now: ASCRS,
  American Society of Colon and Rectal
  Surgeons)
  American Psychosomatic Society
  aspirin, phenacetin, and salicylamide
  atrial pacing study

APsaA American Psychoanalytic Association

APSAC anisoylated plasminogen streptokinase
  activator complex (antistreplase)

APSD Alzheimer presenile dementia

APSGN acute post-streptococcal glomerulonephritis

APSQ Abbreviated Parent Symptom
  Questionnaire

APT alum-precipitated toxoid

APTA American Physical Therapy Association
  aneurysm of persistent trigeminal artery

APTD Aid to Permanently and Totally
  Disabled

APTT, aPTT activated partial thromboplastin
  time

APTX acute parathyroidectomy

APUD amine precursor uptake and decarboxy-
  lation (cell)

AVD aortic pulmonary valve

APVD anomalous pulmonary venous drainage

AQ accomplishment quotient
  achievement quotient
  any quantity
  cerebral aqueduct

aq aqueous; also aqu
  water [L. *aqua*]; also A, a

aq ad add water [L. *aquam ad*]

aq astr frozen water (ice) [L. *aqua astricta*]

aq bull boiling water [L. *aqua bulliens*]

aq cal hot water [L. *aqua calida*]; also aq ferv

aq com common water [L. *aqua communis*]; also aq comm

aq comm common water [L. *aqua communis*]; also aq com

aq dest distilled water [L. *aqua destillata*]

aq ferv hot water [L. *aqua fervens*]; also aq cal

aq fluv river water [L. *aqua fluvialis*]

aq font spring water [L. *aqua fontana*]

aq frig cold water [L. *aqua frigida*]

AQL acceptable quality limits

aq mar sea water [L. *aqua marina*]

aq niv snow water [L. *aqua nivalis*]

aq pluv rain water [L. *aqua pluvialis*]

aq pur pure water [L. *aqua pura*]

AQRS symbol for the mean manifest electrical axis of the QRS complex, measured in degrees and microvolt seconds (electrocardiography)

AQS additional qualifying symptoms

aq tep tepid water [L. *aqua tepida*]

aqu aqueous; also aq

AR abnormal record
achievement ratio
actinic reticuloid (syndrome)
active resistance
acute rejection
adherence ratio
adrenergic receptor
adverse reaction
airway resistance
alarm reaction
alcohol related
aldehyde reductase
allergic rhinitis
alloy restoration
amplitude ratio
anal retentive
analytical reagent
androgen receptor
anterior root
aortic regurgitation; also aor regurg, aort regurg
aortic root
apical-radial (pulse); also A-R, A/R
Argyll Robertson (pupil)
arsphenamine; also Ars

articulare (craniometric point); also Ar
artificial respiration
artificially ruptured
assisted respiration
atrial regurgitation
at risk
atrophic rhinitis
attack rate
aural rehabilitation
autoradiography
autorefractor
autosomal recessive

A-R apical-radial (pulse); also AR, A/R

A/R accounts receivable
apical/radial (pulse); also AR, A-R

A&R adenoidectomy with radium
advised and released

Ar argon; also A
articulare (craniometric point); also AR
aryl (group)

ARA acetylene reduction activity
American Rheumatism Association (now: ACR, American College of Rheumatology)
anti-reticulin antibody
aortic root angiogram

Ara, ara arabinose; also a
arabinosyl

ARA-A, Ara-A, ara-A, araA arabinosyladenine (vidarabine)

ARA-C, Ara-C, ara-C, araC arabinosylcytosine (cytarabine); also aC

araC-Hu arabinosylcytosine and hydroxyurea

ARAD abnormal right axis deviation

ARAS ascending reticular activating system

ARB adrenergic receptor binder
any reliable brand

arb arbitrary unit; also AU

ARBOR arthropod-borne (virus)

ARBOW artificial rupture of bag of waters

ARC accelerating rate calorimeter
accelerating rate calorimetry
acquired immunodeficiency syndrome-related complex
AIDS-related complex
active renin concentration
Addiction Research Center
alcohol rehabilitation center
American Red Cross
anomalous retinal correspondence
antigen-reactive cell
arcuate nuclei (of medulla oblongata)

average response computer

ARCA acquired red-cell aplasia
American Rehabilitation Counseling Association

ARCBS American Red Cross Blood Services

Arch archives

ARCI Addiction Research Center inventory

ARCO antigen-reactive cell opsonization

ArCO aromatic acyl radical

ARCS Associate of the Royal College of Science

ARD absolute reaction of degeneration
acute respiratory disease
acute respiratory distress
adult respiratory disease
adult respiratory distress
anorectal dressing
antibiotic removal device
antimicrobial removal device
aphakic retinal detachment
arthritis and rheumatic diseases
atopic respiratory disease

ARDS acute respiratory distress syndrome
adult respiratory distress syndrome

ARE active-resistive exercises

AREDYLD acrorenal field defect, ectodermal dysplasia, and lipoatrophic diabetes

ARF acute renal failure
acute respiratory failure
acute rheumatic fever
area resource file

ARFC active rosette-forming T cell

ARF/CRF acute renal failure and chronic renal failure

ARG, Arg arginine; also R
arginyl

arg silver [L. *argentum*]; also Ag

ARH adrenal regeneration hypertension

ARI acute respiratory infection
airway reactivity index
aldose reductase inhibitor

ARIA automated radioimmunoassay

ARIC Associate of the Royal Institute of Chemistry

ARK adrenergic receptor kinase

ARL average remaining lifetime

ARLD alcohol-related liver disease

ARM adrenergic receptor material
aerosol rebreathing method
allergy relief medicine

alternating rate of motion
anorectal manometry
anxiety reaction, mild
artificial rupture of membranes; also AROM
atomic resolution microscope
atomic resolution microscopy

Arm arm amputation

ARMD age-related macular degeneration; also AMD

ARMH Academy of Religion and Mental Health

ARMS amplification refractory mutation system

ARN acute renal necrosis
acute retinal necrosis
Association of Rehabilitation Nurses

ARNMD Association for Research in Nervous and Mental Disease

ARNP Advanced Registered Nurse Practitioner

ARO Association for Research in Ophthalmology (now: ARVO, Association for Research in Vision and Ophthalmology)

AROA autosomal recessive ocular albinism

AROM active range of motion
artificial rupture of membranes; also ARM

ARP absolute refractory period
Advanced Research Projects
alcohol rehabilitation program
American Registry of Pathology
asparagine-rich protein
assay reference plasma
assimilation regulatory protein
at-risk period
automaticity recovery phase

ARPT American Registry of Physical Therapists (defunct)

ARPES angular resolved photoelectron spectroscopy

ARROM active resistive range of motion

ARRS American Roentgen Ray Society

ARRT American Registered Respiratory Therapist
American Registry of Radiologic Technologists

Arry arrhythmia

ARS acquiescent response scale
adult recovery services
AIDS-related syndrome
alizarin red S (dye)
American Radium Society
American Rhinologic Society

ARS—cont'd
  antirabies serum
  autonomous replication sequence

Ars arsphenamine; also AR
  arylsulfatase

Ars-A arylsulfatase A; also ASA, AsA

Ars-B arylsulfatase B; also AsB

Ars-C arylsulfatase C; also AsC

ARSM acute respiratory system malfunction

ART absolute retention time
  Accredited Record Technician
  Achilles (tendon) reflex test
  acoustic reflex test
  acoustic reflex threshold(s)
  algebraic reconstruction technique
  anturane reinfarction trial
  arterial; also A, a, art
  artery; also A, a, art
  autologous reactive T cell
  automated reagin test (for syphilis)
  automaticity recovery time

art arterial; also A, a, ART
  artery; also A, a, ART
  articulated; also artic
  articulation; also artic
  artificial; also artif

arthr arthrotomy

arthro arthroscopy

ARTI acute respiratory tract illness

artic articulated; also art
  articulation; also art

artif artificial; also art

art insem artificial insemination; also AI

Art T art therapy

ARV AIDS-associated retrovirus
  AIDS-related virus
  anterior right ventricular (wall)

ARVD arrhythmogenic right ventricular dysplasia

ARVO Association for Research in Vision and Ophthalmology

ARW accredited rehabilitation worker

ARWY airway

AS above scale
  acetylstrophanthidin
  acidified serum
  acoustic stimulation
  active sarcoidosis
  active sleep
  acute salpingitis

  Adams-Stokes (disease, syndrome)
  adolescent suicide
  aerosol steroid
  affective style
  Alport syndrome
  alveolar sac
  alveolar space
  amyloid substance
  anal sphincter
  androsterone sulfate
  ankylosing spondylitis; also ASP
  annulospiral
  anomalous scattering
  anovulatory syndrome
  answering service
  antiserum
  antiserum to somatostatin
  antisocial
  antistreptolysin; also ASL
  antral spasm
  anxiety state
  aortic sac
  aortic stenosis; also aort sten, A sten
  aqueous solution
  aqueous suspension
  arteriosclerosis; also ASCL, ATS
  artificial sweetener
  ascending aorta; also AA, AO, Asc-A
  asthma astrocyte
  astigmatism; also As, AST, Ast, ASTIG, Astigm
  asymmetric; also a, ASYM, asym
  atherosclerosis; also ATS, Athsc
  atrial sense
  atrial septum
  atrial stenosis
  atropine sulfate
  audiogenic seizure; also AGS
  left ear [L. *auris sinistra*]; also AL, al, as
  sickle-cell trait (heterozygous genotype for sickle cell hemoglobin); also A/S

A-S Adam-Stokes (disease, syndrome)
  ascendance-submission

A/S sickle-cell trait (heterozygous genotype for sickle cell hemoglobin); also AS

As arsenic
  astigmatic
  astigmatism; also AS, AST, Ast, ASTIG, Astigm
  atmosphere, standard; also A_s, atm

A·s ampere-second; also A-s

A_s atmosphere, standard; also As, atm

A-s ampere-second; also A·s

A × s amperes per second

aS absiemens

as left ear [L. *auris sinistra*]; also AL, al, AS

ASA acetophenetidin, acetylsalicylic acid, and caffeine
acetylsalicylic acid (aspirin)
active systemic anaphylaxis
Adams-Stokes attack
American Society of Anesthesiologists
American Standards Association (now: ANSI, American National Standards Institute)
American Stomatological Association
American Surgical Association
antibody-to-surface antigen
anti-skin antibodies (test)
argininosuccinic acid
arylsulfatase A; also Ars-A, AsA
aspirin-sensitive asthma

ASA I-V American Society of Anesthesiologists patient classifications I to V, followed by "E" for emergency operations

ASA I healthy patient with localized pathologic process

ASA II patient with mild to moderate systemic disease

ASA III patient with severe systemic disease limiting activity but not incapacitating

ASA IV patient with incapacitating systemic disease

ASA V moribund patient not expected to live

AsA arylsulfatase A; also Ars-A, ASA

Asa arsenate
beta-carboxyaspartic acid

ASAA acquired severe aplastic anemia

ASAC acidified serum, acidified complement

ASACL American Society of Anesthesiologists classification

ASA-G guaiacolic acid ester of acetylsalicylic acid

ASAHP American Society of Allied Health Professions

ASAI aortic stenosis and aortic insufficiency (murmurs)

ASAIO American Society for Artificial Internal Organs

ASAL argininosuccinic acid lyase

ASAP as soon as possible

ASAS American Society of Abdominal Surgery
argininosuccinic acid synthetase

ASAT alanine-aspartate aminotransferase
aspartate aminotransferase; also AspAT, AST

ASB aloin, strychnine, and belladonna (pills)
American Society of Bacteriologists
anesthesia standby
asymptomatic bacteriuria

AsB arylsulfatase B; also Ars-B

ASBI aloin, strychnine, belladonna, and ipecac

ASBS arteriosclerotic brain syndrome

ASC *N*-acetylsulfanilyl chloride
adenosine-coupled spleen cell
altered state of consciousness
ambulatory surgery center
American Society of Cytology
anterior subcapsular cataract
antigen-sensitive cell
antimony-sulfur colloid
ascorbic acid; also AA

AsC arylsulfatase C; also Ars-C

Asc-A ascending aorta; also AA, AO, AS

ASCAD arteriosclerotic coronary artery disease
atherosclerotic coronary artery disease

ASCH American Society of Clinical Hypnosis

ASCI American Society for Clinical Investigation

ASCII American Standard Code for Information Interchange

ASCL arteriosclerosis; also AS, ATS

Ascit Fl ascitic fluid; also AF

ASCLT American Society of Clinical Laboratory Technicians (now: ASMT, American Society for Medical Technology)

ASCO American Society of Clinical Oncology
American Society of Contemporary Ophthalmology

ASCP American Society of Clinical Pathologists

ASCPC American Society of Clinical Pharmacology and Chemotherapy (now: ASCPT, American Society for Clinical Pharmacology and Therapeutics)

ASCPT American Society for Clinical Pharmacology and Therapeutics

ascr ascribed to [L. *ascriptum*]

ASCRS American Society of Colon and Rectal Surgeons

ASCT autologous stem-cell transplantation
American Society for Cytotechnology

ASCVD arteriosclerotic cardiovascular disease
atherosclerotic cardiovascular disease

ASD aldosterone secretion defect
Alzheimer senile dementia
anterior sagittal diameter; also ant sag D
anti-siphon device
arthritis syphilitica deformans
atrial septal defect

ASDC American Society of Dentistry for Children

ASDH acute subdural hematoma

ASE acute stress erosion
American Society of Echocardiography
axilla, shoulder, elbow (bandage)

ASEP American Society for Experimental Pathology (now: AAP, American Association of Pathologists)

ASES Adult Self-Expression Scale
American shoulder and elbow system

ASET American Society of Electroencephalographic Technologists (now: American Society of Electroneurodiagnostic Technologists)
American Society of Electroneurodiagnostic Technologists

ASF African swine fever
allergy-suppressing factor
aniline-sulfur-formaldehyde (resin)
asialofetium

ASFR age-specific fertility rate

ASG American Society for Genetics
advanced stage group

ASGE American Society for Gastrointestinal Endoscopy

AS/GP antiserum, guinea pig

ASH aldosterone-stimulating hormone
American Society of Hematology
ankylosing spinal hyperostosis
anti-streptococcal hyaluronidase
asymmetric septal hypertrophy
hypermetropic astigmatism; also ah, AH, AsH
hyperopic astigmatism; also ah, AH, AsH

AsH hypermetropic astigmatism; also ah, AH, ASH
hyperopic astigmatism; also ah, AH, ASH

ASHA American School Health Association
American Speech and Hearing Association (now: American Speech-Language-Hearing Association)
American Speech-Language-Hearing Association

ASHAP Adriamycin, cisplatin, ARA-C, methylprednisolone

ASHD arteriosclerotic heart disease; also AHD
atherosclerotic heart disease; also AHD
atrial septal heart disease

ASHN acute sclerosing hyaline necrosis

ASHI Association for the Study of Human Infertility

AS/Ho antiserum, horse

ASHP American Society of Hospital Pharmacists

ASI addiction severity index
Anxiety Status Inventory

ASIF Association for the Study of Internal Fixation

ASII American Science Information Institute

ASIM American Society of Internal Medicine

ASIS anterior superior iliac spine
aromatic solvent induced shift

ASK anti-streptokinase; also anti-SK

ASKA anti-skeletal antibody

ASL argininosuccinate lyase
American sign language; also Ameslan
ankylosing spondylitis, lung
antistreptolysin; also AS

ASLC acute self-limited colitis

ASLO, ASL-O antistreptolysin-O; also ASO, ASTO

ASLT antistreptolysin test

ASM airway smooth muscle
American Society for Microbiology
anterior scalenus muscle
myopic astigmatism; also AM, am, AsM, As M

AsM, As M myopic astigmatism; also AM, am, ASM

ASMA anti-smooth muscle antibody

ASMC aortic smooth muscle cells

ASMD atonic sclerotic musclar dystrophy

ASME Association for the Study of Medical Education

ASMI anteroseptal myocardial infarction

As/Mk antiserum, monkey

ASMR age-standardized mortality ratio

ASMRO Armed Services Medical Regulating Office

ASMT American Society for Medical Technology

asmt assessment; also A

ASN alkali-soluble nitrogen
arteriosclerotic nephritis

asparagine; also Asn, N

Asn asparagine; also ASN, N
asparaginyl; also Asx

ASNSA American Society for Nursing Service
Administrators (now: AONE, American
Organization of Nurse Executives)

ASO aldicarb sulfoxide
allele-specific oligonucleotide
American Society of Orthodontists (now:
AAO, American Association of
Orthodontists)
antistreptolysin-O; also ASLO, ASL-O,
ASTO
arteriosclerosis obliterans
automatic stop order

ASOR asialo-orosomucoid

ASOS American Society of Oral Surgeons
(now: AAOMS, American Association of
Oral and Maxillofacial Surgeons)

ASOT antistreptolysin-O titer

ASP acute suppurative parotitis
acute symmetric polyarthritis
African swine pox
aged substrate plasma
alkali-stable pepsin
American Society of Parasitologists
ankylosing spondylitis; also AS
antisocial personality
aortic systolic pressure
arachidonate-sensitive platelet
area systolic pressure
L-asparaginase; also Asp
aspartic acid (aspartate); also Asp, D
aspiration

Asp L-asparaginase; also ASP
aspartic acid (aspartate); also ASP, D

asp aspirate

ASPAN American Society of Post Anesthesia
Nurses

ASPAT anti-streptococcal polysaccharide A
test

AspAT aspartate aminotransferase; also ASAT,
AST
aspartate transaminase; also AST

ASPECT approach to systematic planning and
evaluation of clinical trials

Asper aspergillosis

ASPET American Society for Pharmacology
and Experimental Therapeutics

ASPG anti-spleen (cell) globulin

ASPH Association of Schools of Public Health

ASPVD arteriosclerotic peripheral vascular disease

ASQ abbreviated symptom questionnaire
anxiety scale questionnaire

ASR aldosterone secretion rate
atrial septal resection

AS/Rab antiserum, rabbit

ASRT American Society of Radiologic
Technologists

ASS acute serum sickness
anterior superior spine; also ant sup sp, ant
sup spine
argininosuccinate synthetase

ASSC acute splenic sequestration crisis

AS-SCORE assessing severity: age of patient,
systems involved, stage of disease, complications, response to therapy

assist assistive

Assn, assn association; also Assoc, assoc

Assoc, assoc associate
associated
association; also Assn, assn

assocd associated (with)

asst adult situational stress reaction
assist
assistant

AST angiotensin sensitivity test
anterior spinothalamic tract
antistreptokinase titer
antistreptolysin titer
aspartate aminotransferase; also ASAT,
AspAT
aspartate transaminase; also AspAT
Association of Surgical Technologists
astemizole
astigmatism; also AS, As, Ast, ASTIG,
Astigm
atrial overdrive stimulation rate
audiometry sweep test

Ast astigmatism; also AS, As, AST, ASTIG,
Astigm

ASTA anti-alpha-staphylolysin

ASTC Association of Science-Technology
Centers

ASTDN Association of State and Territorial
Directors of Nursing

A sten aortic stenosis; also aort sten, AS

Asth asthenopia

ASTHO Association of State and Territorial
Health Officials

ASTI anti-spasticity index

ASTIG astigmatism; also AS, As, AST, Ast, Astigm

Astigm astigmatism; also AS, As, AST, Ast, ASTIG

ASTM American Society for Testing and Materials

ASTMH American Society of Tropical Medicine and Hygiene

ASTO antistreptolysin O; also ASLO, ASL-O, ASO

AS TOL, as tol as tolerated

ASTR American Society for Therapeutic Radiologists (now: ASTRO, American Society for Therapeutic Radiology and Oncology)

ASTRO American Society for Therapeutic Radiology and Oncology

ASTZ anti-streptozyme (test)

ASU acute stroke unit
ambulatory surgical unit

ASUTS American Society of Ultrasound Technical Specialists (now: SDMS, Society of Diagnostic Medical Sonographers)

ASV, AS-V, A/SV anodic stripping voltammetry
anti-siphon valve
anti-snake venom
arterio-superficial venous (difference)
avian sarcoma virus

ASVD arteriosclerotic vascular disease

ASVG autologous saphenous vein graft

ASVIP atrial-synchronous ventricular-inhibited pacemaker

ASW artificial seawater

asw artificially sweetened

ASX asymptomatic; also Asx
symbol meaning "aspartic acid (Asp) or asparagine (Asn)" (to denote uncertainty between the two); also Asx, B

Asx asparaginyl; also Asn
aspartyl
asymptomatic; also ASX
symbol meaning "aspartic acid (Asp) or asparagine (Asn)" (to denote uncertainty between the two); also ASX, B

ASYM, asym asymmetric; also a, AS
asymmetry
asymmetrical

AT abdominal tympany

Achard-Thiers (syndrome)
achievement test
Achilles tendon
activity therapy
adaptive thermogenesis
adenine and thymine
adjunctive therapy
air temperature
air trapping
aminotransferase
aminotriazole (amitrole); also ATA
amitriptyline; also AMI, AMT
anaerobic threshold
anaphylotoxin
anionic trypsinogen
antithrombin
antitrypsin
antral transplantation
applanation tonometry
ataxia-telangiectasia; also A-T
atraumatic
atrial tachycardia
atropine; also A, ATRO
attenuated
attenuation
autoimmune thrombocytopenia
axonal terminal
old tuberculin [Ger. *altes Tuberkulin*]

A-T ataxia-telangiectasia; also AT

AT$_7$ hexachlorophene

AT-10 dihydrotachysterol; also AT$_{10}$

AT$_{10}$ dihydrotachysterol; also AT-10

AT I angiotensin I; also AI

AT III antithrombin III

AT III FUN antithrombin III functional

At astatine
atrial; also ATR
atrium; also A
symbol for the mean manifest direction and magnitude of repolarization of the myocardium determined algebraically and measured in degrees and microvolt seconds (electrocardiography)

at airtight
ampere turn
atom
atomic

ATA alimentary toxic aleukia
aminotriazole (amitrole); also AT
anti-thymic activity
anti-thyroglobulin antibody
antithyroid antibody

ATA—cont'd
anti-*Toxoplasma* antibody
atmosphere, absolute; also ata
aurintricarboxylic acid

ata atmosphere, absolute; also ATA

ATB antibiotic; also AB, Anti bx
atrial tachycardia with block
at the time of the bomb (A-bomb in Japan)
atypical tuberculosis

ATC activated cell
activated thymus cell
alcoholism therapy classes
around the clock

ATCC American Type Culture Collection

ATCS active trabecular calcification surface
anterior tibial compartment syndrome

ATD Alzheimer-type dementia
androstatrienedione
anthropomorphic test dummy
antithyroid drugs
asphyxiating thoracic dystrophy
autoimmune thyroid disease

ATE acute toxic encephalopathy
adipose tissue extract
autologous tumor extract

ATEE, ATEe *N*-acetyl-L-tyrosine ethyl ester

ATEM analytic transmission electron microscope

ATEN atenolol

Atetra P, A tetra P adenosine tetraphosphate

ATF ascites tumor fluid

ATFC alternative temporal forced choice

At Fib, at fib atrial fibrillation; also AF, AFIB, AFib, A fib, ATR FIB, atr fib

ATG adenine, thymine, and guanine
anti-human thymocyte globulin
anti-thrombocyte globulin
anti-thymocyte globulin; also AHTG
anti-thyroglobulin

ATGAM anti-thymocyte gamma-globulin

AT/GC adenine-thymine to guanine-cytosine (ratio)

ATH acetyltyrosine hydrazide

ATHC 3α-allotetrahydrocortisol

ATHR angina threshold heart rate

Athsc atherosclerosis; also AS, ATS

AT I angiotensin I; also AI

AT III antithrombin III

AT III FUN antithrombin III functional

ATL Achilles tendon lengthening
adult T-cell leukemia
adult T-cell lymphoma
anterior tricuspid leaflet
anti-tension line
atypical lymphocytes

ATLA adult T-cell leukemia (associated) antigen

ATLC adsorption thin-layer chromatography

ATLL adult T-cell leukemia/lymphoma

ATLS advanced trauma life support

ATLV adult T-cell leukemia virus

ATM abnormal tubular myelin
acute transverse myelitis
acute transverse myelopathy

atm atmosphere
atmospheric; also atmos
atmosphere, standard; also As, A_s

ATMA antithyroid plasma membrane antibody

At ma atrial milliampere

atmos atmospheric; also atm

ATN acute tubular necrosis
augmented transition network
tyrosinase-negative oculocutaneous albinism

ATNC atraumatic, normocephalic; also AT/NC

AT/NC atraumatic, normocephalic; also ATNC

aTNM at autopsy: tumor, nodes, and metastases (staging of cancer)

at no atomic number

ATNR asymmetric tonic neck reflex

ATP addiction treatment program
adenosine triphosphate; also ADT
ambient temperature and pressure
autoimmune thrombocytopenia purpura; also AITP

A-TP absorbed test plasma

ATPase adenosine triphosphatase

ATPD ambient temperature and pressure, dry

ATP-2Na adenosine triphosphate disodium

ATPO Association of Technical Personnel in Ophthalmology

ATPS ambient temperature and pressure, saturated (with water vapor)

ATPTX acute thyroparathyroidectomy

ATR Achilles tendon reflex
atrial; also At
attenuated total reflection (spectrum)

atr atrophy

ATR FIB, atr fib   atrial fibrillation; also AF, AFIB, AFib, A fib, At Fib, at fib

ATRO   atropine; also A, AT

ATS   Achard-Thiers syndrome
acid test solution
adjustable thigh anti-embolism stockings
American Thoracic Society
American Trudeau Society (medium)
anti-rat thymocyte serum
anti-tetanic serum (tetanus antitoxin)
anti-tetanus serum (tetanus antitoxin)
anti-thymocyte serum
anxiety tension state
arteriosclerosis; also AS, ASCL
atherosclerosis; also AS, Athsc

ATSDR   Agency for Toxic Substances and Diseases Registry

ATT   arginine tolerance test
aspirin tolerance time

att   attending

ATTR   attached report

ATU   alcohol treatment unit
allyl thiourea

ATV   avian tumor virus

AtV   arteriovenous; also AV, A-V
assisted ventilation; also AV
atrioventricular; also AV, A-V

at vol   atomic volume

at wt   atomic weight; also A, AW

ATZ   atypical transformation zone

AU   according to custom [L. *ad usum*] ;
also ad us
allergenic unit
Angström unit; also A, Å
antitoxin unit; also AE
arbitrary unit; also arb
atomic unit
Australia antigen; also AA, Au, Au(1), AuAg, Au Ag
azauridine; also AZU, AZUR, AzUr
both ears together [L. *aures unitas*]; also a u
each ear [L. *auris uterque*]; also a u

Au   Auberger blood group (antigen)
Australia antigen; also AA, AU, Au(1), AuAg, Au Ag
gold [L. *aurum*]; also aur

Au(1)   Australia antigen; also AA, AU, Au, AuAg, Au Ag

198Au   colloidal gold
gold 198, radioactive gold; halflife, 2.693 ± 0.005 days

a u   both ears together [L. *aures unitas*]; also AU
each ear [L. *auris uterque*]; also AU

AUA   American Urological Association

AuAg, Au Ag   Australia antigen; also AA, AU, Au, Au(1)

AUB   abnormal uterine bleeding

AuBMT   autologous bone marrow transplantation; also ABMT

AUC   area under the curve

auct   of authors [L. *auctorum*]

AUD, aud   arthritis of unknown diagnosis
auditory

aud-vis   audiovisual; also AV

AUFS   absorbance units, full scale

AUG   acute ulcerative gingivitis
adenine, uracil, guanine
adenine, uridine, guanosine

aug   increase [L. *augere*]

AUGIB   acute upper gastrointestinal bleeding

AUHAA   Australia hepatitis-associated antigen

AUI   alcohol use inventory

AUL   acute undifferentiated leukemia

AUM   asymmetric unit membrane

AUO   amyloid of unknown origin

AuP   Australia antigen protein

AUPHA   Association of University Programs in Health Administration

AUR   acute urinary retention

aur   auricle; also A, auric
auricular; also auric
ear [L. *auris*]; also A, a
gold [L. *aurum*]; also Au

auric   auricle; also A, aur
auricular; also aur

AUR FIB, aur fib   auricular fibrillation; also AF

AUS   acute urethral syndrome
auscultation; also aus, ausc, auscul

aus   auscultation; also AUS, ausc, auscul

ausc   auscultation; also AUS, aus, auscul

auscul   auscultation; also AUS, aus, ausc

AuSH, AuSh   Australia serum hepatitis (antigen)

AUTS   Adult Use of Tobacco Survey

aux   auxiliary

AV   Adriamycin and vincristine
alveolar (duct)

anteroventral
anteversion; also Av, av
anteverted; also Av, av
anticipatory vomiting
anti-virin
aortic valve; also AOV
arteriovenous; also AtV, A-V
artificial ventilation
assisted ventilation; also AtV
atrioventricular; also AtV, A-V
audiovisual; also aud-vis
auditory-visual
augmented vector
auriculoventricular; also A-V
average; also Av, av, avg
aviation (medicine)
avoirdupois; also Av, av, AVDP, avdp

A-V arteriovenous; also AtV, AV
atrioventricular; also AtV, AV
auriculoventricular; also AV

A/V amperes per volt
arterial/venous
atrial/ventricular
auricular/ventricular

A:V arterial to venous (ratio in fundi)

Av, av anteversion; also AV
anteverted; also AV
average; also AV, avg
avoirdupois; also AV, AVDP, avdp

aV abvolt
augmented voltage (unipolar limb lead)

AVA American Vocational Association
antiviral antibody
aortic valve area
aortic valve atresia
arteriovenous anastomosis
auditory vocal automatic (test)
availability

AV/AF anteverted, anteflexed

AVB atrioventricular block

AVBR automated ventricular brain ratio

AVC aberrant ventricular conduction
allantoin vaginal cream
associative visual cortex
atrioventricular canal
automatic volume control

AvCDO$_2$ arteriovenous oxygen content difference; also AVDO$_2$

AVCN anteroventral division of cochlear nucleus

AVCS atrioventricular conduction system

AVD aortic valve disease

apparent volume of distribution
arteriovenous difference
atrioventricular dissociation

AVDO$_2$ arteriovenous oxygen content difference; also AvCDO$_2$

AVDP, avdp asparaginase, vincristine, daunorubicin, and prednisone
avoirdupois; also AV, Av, av

AvDP average diastolic pressure

AVE all-valence-electron (method)
aortic valve echocardiogram
aortic valve electrocardiogram

AVEC-DIC Allen video-enhanced contrast - differential interference contrast (microscopy)

AVF antiviral factor
arteriovenous fistula

aVF augmented voltage unipolar left foot (lead) (electrocardiography)

AVG ambulatory visit groups (patient classification)

avg average; also AV, Av, av

AVH acute viral hepatitis

AVHB atrioventricular heart block

AVHD acquired valvular heart disease

AVI air velocity index

A-V IMA arteriovenous internal mammary (fistula)

AVJR atrioventricular junctional rhythm

AVJT atrioventricular junctional tachycardia

AVL anterior vein of the leg

aVL augmented voltage unipolar left (arm lead) (electrocardiography)

AVLINE audiovisuals on-line

AVM Adriamycin, vinblastine, and methotrexate
arteriovenous malformation
atrioventricular malformation
aviation medicine; also AM

AVMA American Veterinary Medical Association

AVN acute vasomotor nephropathy
arbitrary valve unit
arteriovenous nicking
atrioventricular nodal (conduction)
atrioventricular node
avascular necrosis; also AN

AVNFRP atrioventricular node functional refractory period

AVNR atrioventricular nodal re-entry

AVNRT atrioventricular nodal re-entry tachycardia

AVO atrioventricular opening

A-VO₂ arteriovenous oxygen difference

AVP actinomycin D, vincristine, and Platinol
Adriamycin, vincristine, and procarbazine
ambulatory venous pressure
antiviral protein
aqueous vasopressin
arginine vasopressin

AVPV anteroventral periventricular

AVR accelerated ventricular rhythm
aortic valve replacement

aVR augmented voltage unipolar right (arm lead) (electrocardiography)

AVr antiviral regulator

AVRB added viscous resistance to breathing

AVRI acute viral respiratory infection

AVRP atrioventricular refractory period

AVRT atrioventricular re-entrant tachycardia

AVS aneurysm of membranous ventricular septum
aortic valve stenosis
arteriovenous shunt
auditory vocal sequencing

AVCS aortic valve cusp separation

AVSD atrioventricular septal defect

AVSS afebrile, vital signs stable; AFVSS

AVSV aortic valve stroke volume

AVT Abelson virus transformed (cells)
Allen vision test
area ventralis of Tsai
arginine oxytocin
arginine vasotocin
atrioventricular tachycardia
atypical ventricular tachycardia

AVTB absolute volume of trabecular bone

Av3V anteroventral third ventricle

AVZ avascular zone

AW abdominal wall
abnormal wave
above waist
abrupt withdrawal
alcohol withdrawal
aluminum wafer
alveolar wall
alveolar wash
anterior wall
atomic warfare
atomic weight; also A, at wt

A/W able to work
in accordance with

A&W alive and well

A3W crystalline amino-acid solution

aw airways

AWA as well as
away without authorization

AWBM alveolar wall basement membrane

AWF adrenal weight factor

AWG American wire gage

AWI anterior wall infarction
authorized walk-in (patient)

AWMI anterior wall myocardial infarction

AWO airway obstruction

AWOL absent without leave

AWP airway pressure

AWRS anti-whole rabbit serum

AWRU active wrist rotation unit

AWS alcohol withdrawal syndrome

AWTA aniridia-Wilms tumor association

awu atomic weight unit

AX alloxan

Ax axilla; also ax
axillary; also ax
axis; also ax

ax axial; also A, a
axilla; also Ax
axillary; also Ax
axis; also Ax
axon

AXF advanced X-ray facility

axFem axillofemoral bypass

ax grad axial gradient

AXL axillary lymphoscintigraphy

AXM acetoxycyclohexamide

AXR abdominal X-ray

AXT alternating exotropia

AY aster yellow

AYA acute yellow atrophy (of liver)

AYF anti-yeast factor

AYP autolyzed yeast protein

AZ acetazolamide
Aschheim-Zondek (test)
azathioprine; also AZA

Az nitrogen [Fr. *azote*]

AZA azathioprine; also AZ

5-AZA, 5-Aza 5-azacytidine; also 5-AC

5-AZC azacitidine

AZG, azg azaguanine

AZO, azo indicates presence of the group -N:N-

AZQ aziridinylbenzoquinone

AZS automatic zero set

AZT Aschheim-Zondek test
azidothymidine (3′-azido-3′-deoxythymidine) (zidovudine)

AZU azauridine; also AU, AZUR, AzUr

AzU 6-azauracil; also 6-AzU

5-AzU 5-azauracil

6-AzU 6-azauracil; also AzU

AZUR azauridine; also AU, AZU, AzUr
6-azauridine; also AzUR, 6-AzUR

AzUR 6-azauridine; also AZUR, 6-AzUR

AzUr azauridine; also AU, AZU, AZUR

5-AzUR 5-azauridine

6-AzUR 6-azauridine; also AZUR, AzUR

B

B BETA, UPPER CASE, second letter of the Greek alphabet

B BETA, UPPER CASE, second letter of the Greek alphabet

β beta, lower case, second letter of the Greek alphabet
anomer of carbohydrate
beta chain of hemoglobin
buffer capacity
carbon separated from carboxyl by one other carbon in aliphatic compounds
constituent of plasma protein fraction
probability of type II error
second in a series or group
substituent group of steroid that projects above plane of ring

1-β power of statistical test

β₂m beta₂-microglobulin; also BMG

β-BuTX beta-bungarotoxin

ϱ beta, lower case, second letter of the Greek alphabet, medial or terminal

B aspartic acid (Asp) or asparagine (Asn) (one-letter notion, to denote uncertainty between the two); also ASX, Asx
bacillus; also Bac, bac
Bacillus species
bacitracin
bands (band neutrophils)
barometer; also BAR, bar
barometric; also BAR, bar
base (in chemistry); also b
base (in nucleic acid sequencing); also b
base (of a prism); also b
baseline
basophil; also ba, bas, baso
basophilic
bath; also b, BAL, bal
Baumé's (scale); also Be, Bè
behavior; also beh
bel
Benoist's scale
benzoate
beta
bicuspid
bilateral; also bi, BIL, bil, bilat
black; also Bl, blk
blood (whole blood); also bl, bld
bloody
blue; also bl
body
boils at; also b

Bolton's point; also bb, Bo, BP
bone marrow-derived (cell, lymphocyte)
born; also b
boron
both
bound; also BD
bovine
bregma; also Br
brother; also br, BRO, bro
buccal; also Buc, bucc
Bucky (film in cassette in Potter-Bucky diaphragm)
bursa cells
corticosterone (compound B)
gauss (unit of magnetic induction)
magnetic induction
supramentale (craniometric point); also b
tomogram with oscillating Bucky
twice [L. *bis*]; also b, BIS, bis

B *Brucella* species; also *Br,* Bruc
magnetic flux density

B✔ billing information posted

b barn (unit of area for atomic nuclei)
base (in chemistry); also B
base (in nucleic acid sequencing); also B
base (of a prism); also B
bath; also B, BAL, bal
boils at; also B
born; also B
brain; also BRA
supramentale (craniometric point); also B
twice [L. *bis*]; also B, BIS, bis

B4 before; also bef

B₀ constant magnetic field in nuclear magnetic resonance

B₁ radio-frequency magnetic field in nuclear magnetic resonance
thiamin

B₂ riboflavin

B₃ niacinamide

B₆ pyridoxine

B₇ biotin

B₈ adenosine phosphate

B₁₂ cyanocobalamin

BI Billroth I (operation)

BII Billroth II (operation)

BA Bachelor of Arts
Bacillus abortus
backache; also B/A

background activity
bacterial agglutination
basilar artery
basion; also Ba, ba
basket axon
benzanthracene; also BzAnth
benzyladenine
benzyl alcohol
benzylamine; also BZA
best amplitude
betamethasone acetate
bilateral asymmetric
bile acid
biliary atresia
biologic activity
blocking antibody
blood agar
blood alcohol
bone age
boric acid
Bourns' assist
bovine albumin
brachial artery
breathing apparatus
bronchial asthma
bronchoalveolar
buccoaxial
buffered acetone
butyric acid
sand bath [L. *balneum arenae*]; also bal are, bal arenae

B/A backache; also BA

B&A brisk and active

B>A bone greater than air (conduction); also BC>AC

B<A bone less than air (conduction); also BC<AC

Ba barium
basion; also BA, ba

ba basion; also BA, Ba
basophil; also B, bas, baso

BAA benzoyl arginine amide
branched-chain amino acid; also BCAA

BAB blood agar base

Bab Babinski (law, phenomenon, reflex, sign, syndrome, test)

BabK baboon kidney

BAC bacterial adherent colony
bacterial antigen complex
benzalkonium chloride
blood alcohol concentration
bronchoalveolar cells
buccoaxiocervical
butalbital, aspirin, and caffeine

Bac, bac bacillary
bacillus; also B

BACO bleomycin, Adriamycin, CCNU, and Oncovin

BACON bleomycin, Adriamycin, CCNU, Oncovin, and nitrogen mustard

BACOP bleomycin, Adriamycin, cyclophosphamide, Oncovin, and prednisone

BACT best available control technology
bischloroethylnitrosourea (BCNU), arabinosylcytosine, Cytoxan, and 6-thioguanine
bleomycin, Adriamycin, Cytoxan, and tamoxifen citrate

Bact, bact bacteria
bacterial
bacteriologist
bacteriology

BAD biologic aerosol detection
bipolar affective disorder

BAE bovine aortic endothelium
bronchial artery embolization

BaE barium enema; also BaEn, BE

BAEE benzoyl arginine ethyl ester
benzylarginine ethyl ester

BaEn barium enema; also BaE, BE

BAEP brainstem auditory evoked potential

BAER brainstem auditory evoked response; also BSAER

BAF B-cell activating factor

BAG buccoaxiogingival

BAGG buffered azide glucose glycerol (broth)

BAI basilar artery insufficiency

BAIB beta-aminoisobutyric (acid)

BAIF bile acid independent flow
bile acid independent fraction

BAIT bacterial automated identification technique

BAL balance; also bal
bath [L. *balneum*]; also B, b, bal
blood alcohol level
British anti-Lewisite (dimercaprol)
bronchoalveolar lavage

bal balance; also BAL
balsam; also bals
bath [L. *balneum*]; also B, b, BAL

bal are sand bath [L. *balneum arenae*]; also BA, bal arenae

bal arenae sand bath [L. *balneum arenae*]; also BA, bal are

BALB binaural alternate loudness balance (test)

bal cal hot bath [L. *balneum calidum*]

bal coen mud bath [L. *balneum coenosum*]

BALF bronchoalveolar lavage fluid

bal frig cold bath [L. *balneum frigidum*]

B ALL, B-ALL B-cell acute lymphoblastic leukemia

bal lact milk bath [L. *balneum lacteum*]

bal mar salt-water or sea-water bath [L. *balneum maris*]; also BM, bm

bal pneu air bath [L. *balneum pneumaticum*]

BALS bile acid-losing syndrome

bals balsam; also bal

BALT binaural alternate loudness balance test
bronchus-associated lymphoid tissue

bal tep warm bath [L. *balneum tepidum*]

bal vap steam or vapor bath [L. *balneum vaporis*]; also BV, bv

BAM basophil-associated mononuclear
bronchoalveolar macrophage

BAm mean brachial artery (pressure)

BaM barium meal

Bam benzamide

BAME benzoyl arginine methyl ester

BAMON bleomycin, Adriamycin, methotrexate, Oncovin, and nitrogen mustard

BAN British Approved Name

BAND band neutrophil (stab); also BD

B and M 693 Sulfapyridine

BANF bilateral acoustic neurofibromatosis

BANS back, arm, neck, and scalp

BAO Bachelor of the Art of Obstetrics
basal acid output
brachial artery output

BAO/MAO ratio of basal acid output to maximal acid output

BAP bacterial alkaline phosphatase
basic adaptive process
Behavior Activity Profile
bleomycin, Adriamycin, and prednisone
blood agar plate
bovine albumin in phosphate buffer
brachial artery pressure; also BrAP

BaP benzo[*a*]pyrene

BAPI barley alkaline protease inhibitor

BAPN beta-aminopropionitrile fumarate

BAPP bleomycin, Adriamycin, Platinol, and prednisone

BAPS bovine albumin phosphate saline

BAPTA 1,2-bis(*o*-aminophenoxy)ethane-*N,N,N′,N′*-tetraacetic acid

BAPV bovine alimentary papilloma virus

BAQ brain-age quotient

BAQD 10 1,1′-decamethylene-bis[4-aminoquinaldinium chloride] (dequalinium chloride)

BAR, bar bariatrics
barometer; also B
barometric; also B

Barb, barb barbiturate

BARN bilateral acute retinal necrosis

BART blood-activated recalcification time

BAS ballon atrial septostomy
benzyl analogue of serotonin
benzyl antiserotonin
bioanalytical systems
biologically active substance
boric acid solution
British Anatomical Society

BaS barium swallow; also BS

bas basilar
basophil; also B, ba, baso

BASCA brain-associated small cell lung cancer antigen

BASH body acceleration given synchronously with heart rate

BASK basket cell; also BC

baso basophil; also B, ba, bas

basos basophils

BASO STIP basophilic stippling (on differential); also BSTP

BAT Basic Aid Training
basic assurance test
benzilic acid 3α-tropanyl ester
best available technology
brown adipose tissue

batt battery

BAV bicuspid aortic valve

BAVFO bradycardia after arteriovenous fistula occlusion

BAVIP bleomycin, Adriamycin, vinblastine, imidazole carboxamide, and prednisone

BAVP balloon aortic valvuloplasty

BAW bronchoalveolar washing

BB baby boy
backboard
bad breath
bath blanket
bed bath

bed board
Besnier-Boeck (disease)
beta blockade
beta-blocker
BioBreeding (rat)
blanket bath
blood bank; also BLBK
blood buffer (base)
blow bottle
blue bloaters (emphysema)
body belts
Bogdän-Buday (disease)
both bones (fractures)
bowel and bladder; also B&B
breakthrough bleeding; also BTB
breast biopsy; also B Bx, br bx
brush border
buffer base
bundle branch
Busse-Buschke (disease)
isoenzyme of creatine kinase that contains
     two B subunits

B/B backward bending

B&B bowel and bladder; also BB

bb Bolton's point; also B, Bo, BP

BBA born before arrival

BBB blood-brain barrier
     blood buffer base
     bundle branch block

BBBB bilateral bundle branch block

BBC bromobenzyl cyanide

BBD before bronchodilator
     benign breast disease

BBE *Bacteroides* bile esculin (agar)

BBEP brush border endopeptidase

BBF bronchial blood flow

BBG big big gastrin

BBI Bowman-Birk soybean inhibitor
     Bowman-Birk trypsin inhibitor

BBM banked breast milk
     Berneimer's basal medium
     brush border membrane

BBMV brush border membrane vesicle

BBN broad band noise

BBOT 2,5-bis-2-(5-*t*-butylbenzoxazol-2-yl)thio-
     phene

BBOW bulging bag of water

BBP butylbenzyl phthalate

BBPRL big big prolactin

BBS bashful bladder syndrome
     benign breast syndrome

bilateral breath sounds
bombesin

BBSO black braided silk out (removed)

BBS black braided silk

BBSS black braided silk suture

BBT basal body temperature

BB to MM belly button to medial malleolus

BB/W BioBreeding/Worcester (rat)

B Bx breast biopsy; also BB, br bx

BC Bachelor of Surgery [L. *Chirurgiae
     Baccalaureus*]; also BCh, BS, CB, ChB
     back care; also bc
     backcross
     background counts
     bactericidal concentration
     basal cell
     basket cell; also BASK
     battle casualty
     bed and chair; also B&C
     bicarbonate; also Bicarb, bicarb
     biliary colic
     biotin carboxylase
     bipolar cell
     birth control
     blastic crisis
     blood cardioplegia
     blood center
     blood culture; also BlC, BL CULT, bl cult
     Blue Cross; also BX
     board certified
     bone conduction
     Bourns' control
     Bowman's capsule
     brachiocephalic
     bronchial carcinoma
     buccal cartilage
     buccocervical
     Budd-Chiari (syndrome)
     buffy coat
     bulbus chordae

B/C because
     blood urea nitrogen to creatinine (ratio)

B&C bed and chair; also BC
     biopsy and curettage
     board and care
     breathed and cried

bc back care; also BC

b/c benefit to cost (ratio)

BCA balloon catheter angioplasty
     basal-cell atypia
     blood color analyzer
     Blue Cross Association

BCA—cont'd
brachiocephalic artery
branchial cleft anomaly
breast cancer antigen

BCAA branched chain amino acid; also BAA

BC>AC bone conduction greater than air conduction; also B>A

BC<AC bone conduction less than air conduction; also B<A

BCAC Breast Cancer Advisory Center

BCAF basophil chemotaxis augmentation factor

B-CAVE, B-CAVe bleomycin, CCNU, Adriamycin, and Velban

BCB brilliant cresyl blue (stain)

BCBR bilateral carotid body resection

BC/BS Blue Cross/Blue Shield; also BX/BS, BX BS

BCC basal cell carcinoma; also BCCa
biliary cholesterol concentration
birth control clinic

bcc body-centered-cubic

BCCa basal cell carcinoma; also BCC

BCCG British Cooperative Clinical Group

BCCP biotin carboxyl carrier protein

BCD basal cell dysplasia
binary-coded decimal
bleomycin, cyclophosphamide, and dactinomycin

BCDDP Breast Cancer Detection Demonstration Project

BCDF B-cell differentiation factor

BCDSP Boston Collaborative Drug Surveillance Program

BCE basal cell epithelioma
B-cell enriched
bubble chamber equipment

BCECF 2′,7′-bis(carboxyethyl)-5,6-carboxyfluorescein

B cell bone marrow derived cell
bursa of Fabricius derived cell

BCF basophil chemotactic factor
bioconcentration factor
breast cyst fluid

BCFP breast cyst fluid protein

BCG Bacillus of Calmette-Guérin (TB vaccine) [Fr. *Bacille bilié de Calmette-Guérin*]
ballistocardiogram
ballistocardiograph
ballistocardiography
bicolor guaiac (test); also BG

bilateral cystogram
bromcresol green

BCGF B-cell growth factor

BCH basal-cell hyperplasia
basal-cell hypoplasia

BCh Bachelor of Surgery [L. *Chirurgiae Baccalaureus*]; also BC, BS, CB, ChB

BChD Bachelor of Dental Surgery [*L. Baccalaureus Chirurgiae Dentalis*]; also BDS

bChl, Bchl bacterial chlorophyll

BCHS Bureau of Community Health Services

BCIC Birth Control Investigation Committee

BCKA branched-chain keto acids

BCL basic cycle length

BCLL, B-CLL B-cell chronic lymphocytic leukemia

BCLP bilateral cleft of lip and palate

BCLS Basic Cardiac Life Support (system)

BCM birth control medication
body cell mass

BCME bis(chloromethyl) ether

BCNP board-certified nuclear pharmacist

BCNS basal cell nevus syndrome

BCNU 1,3-bis(2-chloroethyl)-1-nitrosourea (carmustine); also BiCNU

BCO biliary cholesterol output

BCOC bowel care of choice

BCOP BCNU, cyclophosphamide, Oncovin, and prednisone

BCP BCNU (carmustine), cyclophosphamide, and prednisone
biochemical profile
birth control pill
blood cell profile
Blue Cross Plan
bromcresol purple
5-butyl-1-cyclohexyl-2,4,6(1H,3H,5H)-pyrimidinenetrione (bucolome)

BCP-D bromocresol purple desoxycholate (agar)

BCPS battery-charging power supply

BCPV bovine cutaneous papilloma virus

BCR B-cell reactivity
bromocriptine; also BRO
bulbocavernosus reflex

bcr breakpoint cluster region

BCRC Baltimore Cancer Research Center

BCS battered child syndrome
biopolymer crosslinking system

blood cell separator
Budd-Chiari syndrome
BCSI breast cancer screening indicator
BCT brachiocephalic trunk
BCTF Breast Cancer Task Force
BCtg bovine chymotrypsinogen
BCtr bovine chymotrypsin
BCU burn care unit
BCW biologic and chemical warfare
BCVP BCNU, cyclophosphamide, vincristine, and prednisone
BCVPP BCNU, cyclophosphamide, vinblastine, prednisone, and procarbazine
BCYE buffered charcoal yeast extract
BD band neutrophil (stab); also BAND
barbital-dependent
barbiturate dependence
base deficit
base of prism down
basophilic degeneration
Batten's disease
beclomethasone dipropionate; also BDP
Becton-Dickinson
behavior disorder
Behçet's disease
belladonna
below diaphragm
benzidine; also Benz
benzodiazepine; also BDZ, BZ, bz, BZD, BZDZ
bicarbonate dialysis
bile duct
binocular deprivation
birth date
birth defect
black death
Blackfan-Diamond (syndrome)
block design (test)
blood donor
blue diaper (syndrome)
board; also Bd
borderline dull
bound; also B
brain dead
bronchial drainage
bronchodilator
buccodistal
twice a day [L. *bis die*]; also bd, BID, bid
Bd board; also BD
bd twice a day [L. *bis die*]; also BD, BID, bid
B&D bondage and discipline

BDA British Dental Association
BDAC Bureau of Drug Abuse Control
BDAE Boston Diagnostic Aphasia Examination
BDB bis-diazotized-benzidine
BDBS Bonnet-Dechaume-Blanc syndrome
BDC burn-dressing change
BDE bile duct examination
bile duct exploration
BDF black divorced female
BDG bilirubin diglucuronide
buccal developmental groove
buffered desoxycholate glucose (broth)
BDI Beck Depression Index
burn depth indicator
BDIBS Boston Diagnostic Inventory of Basic Skills
BDID bystander dominates initial dominant (psychology)
BDI SF Beck Depression Index–Short Form
BDL below detectable limits
bile duct ligation
BDLS Brachmann-de Lange syndrome
BDM benzphetamine demethylase
black divorced male
border detection method
BDMP Birth Defects Monitoring Program
B-DOPA bleomycin, dacarbazine, Oncovin, prednisone, and Adriamycin
BDP beclomethasone dipropionate; also BD
bilateral diaphragm paralysis
BDPE 1-(2-bromo-1,2-diphenylethenyl)-4-ethylbenzene (broparoestrol)
BDR background diabetic retinopathy
BDS Bachelor of Dental Surgery; also BChD
biological detection system
British Dental Society
bds to be taken twice a day [L. *bis in die sumendus*]
BDSc Bachelor of Dental Science
BDTA 3,3′,4,4′-benzophenone tetracarboxylic dianhydride
BDTVMI Beery Development Test of Visual-Motor Integration
BDUR bromodeoxyuridine
BDW buffered distilled water
BDZ benzodiazepine; also BD, BZ, bz, BZD, BZDZ
BE bacillary emulsion (tuberculin)
bacterial endocarditis; also BEC

BE—cont'd
 barium enema; also BaE, BaEn
 Barrett esophagus
 base excess; also Bex
 below-elbow; also B/E
 bile esculin (test)
 board eligible
 bovine enteritis
 brain edema
 brain encephalitogen
 bread equivalent
 breast examination
 bronchoenterology
 bronchoesophagology

B/E below-elbow; also BE

Be Baumé's (scale); also B, Bé
 beryllium

Bé Baumé's (scale); also B, Be

B&E brisk and equal

B↑E both upper extremities; also BUE

B↓E both lower extremities; also BLE

BEA below-elbow amputation
 bromoethylamine

BEAM BCNU, etoposide, Ara-C, and melphalan
 brain electrical activity mapping
 brain electrical activity monitoring

BEAR Biologic Effects of Atomic Radiation (Committee)

BEC bacterial endocarditis; also BE
 blood ethanol concentration
 blood ethanol content
 bromoergocryptine
 buffer exchange column

BECF blood extracellular fluid

BEE basal energy expenditure

BEEP both end-expiratory pressures

BEF bronchoesophageal fistula

bef before; also B4

beg begin
 beginning

beh behavior; also B
 behavioral

Beh Sp behavioral specialist

BEI back-scattered electron imaging
 butanol-extractable iodine

Beilstein *Beilsteins Handbuch der Organischen Chemie* (a comprehensive German encyclopedia of organic chemistry [Springer-Verlag])

BEIR biologic effects of ionizing radiation

BEK bovine embryonic kidney (cell)

BEL blood ethanol level
 bovine embryonic lung

ben well [L. *bene*]

Benz benzidine; also BD

BEP bleomycin, etoposide, and Platinol
 brainstem evoked potential; also BSEP

BEPI beta-endorphin immunoreactivity

bepti bionomics, environment, *Plasmodium*, treatment, and immunity (malaria epidemiology)

BER basic electrical rhythm

Ber *Chemische Berichte* [Ger. *Berichte der Deutschen Chemischen Gesellschaft* (Reports of the German Chemical Society)]

BERA brainstem electric response audiometry

BES balanced electrolyte solution

BESM bovine embryo skeletal muscle

BESP bovine embryonic spleen (cells)

BET benign epithelial tumor
 Brunauer-Emmet-Teller (method)

bet between; also bi

Beta HCG beta subunit human chorionic gonadotropin

BETS benign epileptiform transients of sleep

BEV baboon endogenous virus
 billion electron volts; also BeV, Bev, bev
 bleeding esophageal varices

BeV, Bev, bev billion electron volts; also BEV

Bex base excess; also BE

BF bentonite flocculation (test)
 bile flow
 black female; also B/F
 blastogenic factor
 blister fluid
 blocking factor
 blood flow
 body fat
 Bolivian hemorrhagic fever; also BHF
 bone fragment
 bouillon filtrate (tuberculin) [Fr. *bouillon filtre*]; also bf
 boyfriend
 breakfast fed
 breast fed
 buccofacial
 buffered
 burning feet (syndrome)
 butter fat

B/F black female; also BF
 bound to free (antigen ratio)
bf bouillon filtrate (tuberculin) [Fr. *bouillon filtre*]; also BF
BFA baby for adoption
 bifemoral arteriogram
b'fast breakfast; also bkf, bkfst, bkft, Brkf, brkf
BFB biologic feedback
BFC benign febrile convulsion
BFD bias flow down
BFDI bronchodilation following deep inspiration
BFDT Békésy Functionality Detection Test
BFDU brain function diagnostic unit
BFE 60 befunolol hydrochloride
bFGF basic fibroblast growth factor
BFH benign familial hematuria
BFL bird fancier's lung
 breast firm and lactating
BFLS Börjeson-Forssman-Lehmann syndrome
BFM bendroflumethiazide
BFO balanced forearm orthesis
 ball-bearing forearm orthesis
 blood-forming organ
 buccofacial obturator
BFP basic fetoprotein
 biologically false positivity
 biologic false-positive (reaction)
BFPR biologic false-positive reaction; also BFR
BFR biologic false-positive reaction; also BFPR
 biologic false-positive reactor
 biologic false reaction
 blood filtration rate
 blood flow rate
 bone formation rate
 buffered Ringer (solution)
BFR sol buffered Ringer solution
BFS blood fasting sugar
BfS rate of occurrence [Ger. *Befindlichkeitsskala*]
BFSW buffered filtered seawater
BFT bentonite flocculation test
 biofeedback training
 bladder flap tube
BFU burst-forming unit
BFU-E burst-forming unit(s), erythroid
BG baby girl

background; also Bkg
Barré-Guillain (syndrome)
basal ganglion
basic gastrin
Bertolotti-Garcin (syndrome)
beta-galactosidase; also B-GALACTO
beta-glucuronidase
Beurmann-Gougerot (disease)
bicolor guaiac (test); also BCG
big gastrin
blood glucose; also BGlu
bone graft
Bordet-Gengou (agar, bacillus, phenomenon); also B-G
brilliant green
Brock-Graham (syndrome)
buccogingival
Buerger-Grütz (disease)
B-G Bender's gestalt (test)
 Bordet-Gengou (agar, bacillus, phenomenon); also BG
BGA blue-green algae
BGAg blood group antigen
B-GALACTO beta-galactosidase; also BG
BGAV blue-green algae virus
BGC basal-ganglion calcification
 blood group class
BGCA bronchogenic carcinoma
BG-corr background corrected
BGD blood group degrading (enzyme)
BGDC Bartholin gland duct cyst
BGE butyl glycidyl ether
BGG bovine gamma-globulin
BGH, bGH bovine growth hormone
Bg^J beige (mouse)
BGL blood glucose level
BGLB brilliant green lactose broth
BGlu blood glucose; also BG
BGM blood glucose monitor
BGP beta-glycerophosphatase
BGRS blood glucose reagent strip
BGS blood group substance
BGSA blood granulocyte-specific activity
BGT basophil granulation test
 Bender's gestalt test
 bungarotoxin; also BuTX
BGTT borderline glucose tolerance test
BH base hospital

BH—cont'd
  benzalkonium and heparin
  Bernard-Horner (syndrome)
  bill of health
  Board of Health; also BOH
  Bolton-Hunter (reagent)
  borderline hypertensive
  both hands
  brain hormone
  Braxton-Hicks (contraction)
  breath holding
  bronchial hyperactivity
  bronchial hyper-reactivity
  Bryan high titer
  bundle of His; also BOH

BH$_4$ tetrahydrobiopterin

BHA benign hilar adenopathy
  bilateral hilar adenopathy
  bound hepatitis antibody
  butylated hydroxyanisole

BH-AC behenoylcytosine arabinoside (enoc-itabine)

BHAT beta-blocker heart attack trail

BHB beta-hydroxybutyrate; also BOH
  l-[1-*p*-*n*-butoxybenzyl (hyoscyaminium) bro-mide (butropium bromide)]

BHb, bHb bovine hemoglobin

BHBA beta-hydroxybutyric acid; also BOHB

BHBAD beta-hydroxybutyric acid dehydro-genase

BHC benzene hexachloride

BHCDA Bureau of Health Care Delivery and Assistance

BHD BCNU, hydroxyurea, and dacarbazine

BHD-V BCNU, hydroxyurea, dacarbazine, and vincristine

BHE Bolton-Hunter (reagent-labeled) eledoisin

B-HEXOS-A-LK beta-hexosaminidase A leukocytes

BHF Bolivian hemorrhagic fever; also BF

BHI beef heart infusion (broth)
  biosynthetic human insulin
  brain-heart infusion (broth)
  Bureau of Health Insurance

BHIA brain-heart infusion agar

BHI-ac brain-heart infusion broth with acetone

BHIB beef heart infusion broth
  brain-heart infusion broth

BHIBA brain-heart infusion blood agar

BHIRS brain-heart infusion and rabbit serum

BHIS beef heart infusion supplemented (broth)

BHK baby hamster kidney (cells)
  type B Hong Kong (influenza virus)

BHL bilateral hilar lymphadenopathy
  biological half-life

BHM Bureau of Health Manpower

BHN bephenium hydroxynaphthoate
  bridging hepatic necrosis
  Brinell hardness number

BHP basic health profile
  Bureau of Health Professions; also BHPR

BHPR Bureau of Health Professions; also BHP

BHR basal heart rate

BHRD Bureau of Health Resources Development

BHS beta-hemolytic streptococcal (infection)
  beta-hemolytic streptococcus
  breath-holding spell

BHSK Bolton-Hunter reagent-labeled sub-stance K

BHSP Bolton-Hunter reagent-labeled substance P

BHT beta-hydroxytheophylline
  breath hydrogen test
  butylated hydroxytoluene

BHU basic health unit

BHV bovine herpes virus

BH/VH body hematocrit to venous hematocrit (ratio)

BI background interval
  bacterial index
  bactericidal index
  bacteriologic index
  bacteriological index
  base of prism in
  basilar impression
  bifocal; also BIF, bif
  Billroth I (operation)
  biologic indicator
  biological indicator
  bodily injury
  bone injury
  bowel impaction
  brain injured
  brain injury
  burn index

Bi bismuth

bi between; also bet
  bilateral; also B, BIL, bil, bilat

BIB, bib brought in by
  drink [L. *bibe*]; also Bib

Bib drink [L. *bibe*]; also BIB, bib

biblio bibliography

BIC blood isotope clearance
brain injury center

Bic biceps

Bicarb, bicarb bicarbonate; also BC

BiCNU 1,3-bis(2-chloroethyl)-L-nitrosourea
(carmustine); also BCNU

BICROS bilateral contralateral routing of
signals

BID bibliographic information and documentation
brought in dead
twice a day [L. *bis in die*]; also BD, bd, bid

bid twice a day [L. *bis in die*]; also BD, bd,
BID

BIDLB block in posteroinferior division of left
branch

BIDS bedtime insulin, daytime sulfonylurea
(therapy)
brittle hair, impaired intelligence, decreased
fertility, and short stature

BIER biological indicator evaluator resistome-
ter

BIF, bif bifocal; also BI

BIGGY bismuth glycine glucose yeast (agar)

BIH benign intracranial hypertension
bilateral inguinal hernia

bihor during two hours [L. *bihorium*]

BII Billroth II (operation)

Bi Isch, bi isch between ischial tuberosities

BIL, bil basal insulin level
bilateral; also B, bi, bilat
bilirubin; also Bil, bili, bilirub, BR, Bu
brother-in-law

Bil bilirubin; also BIL, bil, bili, bilirub, BR, Bu

BIL/ALB bilirubin to albumin (ratio)

bilat bilateral; also B, bi, BIL, bil

BILAT SLC bilateral short-leg cane

BILAT SXO, bilat sxo bilateral salpingo-
oophorectomy; also BSO

bili bilirubin; also BIL, Bil, bil, bilirub, BR,
Bu

bili-c conjugated bilirubin

bilirub bilirubin; also BIL, Bil, bil, bili, BR,
Bu

BIMA bilateral internal mammary arteries

BIN benign intradermal nerves
twice a night [L. *bis in nocte*]; also bin

bin twice a night [L. *bis in nocte*]; also BIN

biochem biochemistry
biochemical

BIOETHICSLINE Bioethical Information On-
Line

BIOF biofeedback

biol biologic
biological
biology

biophys biophysical
biophysics

BIOS British Intelligence Objectives
Subcommittee

BIOSIS BioScience Information Service

BIP Background Interference Procedure
bacterial intravenous protein
biparietal (diameter)
bismuth iodoform paraffin
bismuth iodoform paste
Blue Cross interim payment
brief infertile period

BiP immunoglobulin-binding protein

BiPD biparietal diameter (fetal skull)

BIPLED bilateral, independent, periodic, lateralized epileptiform discharge

BIPM International Bureau of Weights and
Measures [Fr. *Bureau International des
Poids et Mesures*]

BIPP bismuth iodoform paraffin paste
bismuth iodoform petrolatum paste

BIR backward internal rotation
basic incidence rate

BIS, bis Brain Information Service
sodium bicarbonate in invert sugar
twice [L. *bis*]; also B, b

BISP, BiSP between ischial spines

Bisp, bisp bispinous or interspinous diameter

BIT, BiT between great trochanters

BIU barrier isolation unit

BIW, biw, bi wk biweekly (twice a week)

BIZ-PLT bizarre platelets

BJ Bence Jones (protein, proteinuria)
biceps jerk
Bielschowsky-Jansky (disease)
bones and joints; also B&J

B&J bones and joints; also BJ

BJE bone and joint examination

BJM bones, joints, and muscles

BJP Bence Jones protein
Bence Jones proteinuria

BK Bassen-Kornzweig (syndrome)
  bekanamycin
  below-knee; also B-K, B/K
  bovine kidney (cells)
  bradykinin
  bullous keratopathy

B-K below-knee; also BK, B/K
  initials of two patients after whom a multiple
    cutaneous nevus (mole) was named

B/K below-knee; also BK, B-K

Bk berkelium

bk back

BKA below-knee amputation

BK-A basophil kallikrein of anaphylaxis

BKC blepharokerato-conjunctivitis

bkf breakfast; also b'fast, bkfst, bkft, Brkf, brkf

bkfst breakfast; also b'fast, bkf, bkft, Brkf, brkf

bkft breakfast; also b'fast, bkf, bkfst, Brkf, brkf

Bkg background; also BG

bkly back lying

BKS beekeeper serum

BKTT below-knee to toe (cast)

BKV BK virus

BKWC below-knee walking cast

BKWP below-knee walking plaster (cast)

BL bacterial levan
  baralyme
  Barré-Liéou (syndrome)
  basal lamina
  baseline (fetal heart rate)
  Bessey-Lowry (method, unit)
  black light
  bland; also bl
  blast (cells)
  bleeding; also bl, bldg
  bleomycin; also BLEO, bleo, BLM
  blind loop
  blood level
  blood loss
  bone marrow lymphocyte
  borderline lepromatous
  bronchial lavage
  buccolingual
  Burkitt's lymphoma
  butyrolactone
  complaint list [Ger. *Beschwerdenliste*]

B-L bursa-equivalent lymphocyte

Bl black; also B, blk

bl bland; also BL
  bleeding; also BL, bldg

  blood (whole blood); also B, bld
  blue; also B

BLa buccolabial

BLAD borderline left axis deviation

blad bladder

BLB Bessey-Lowry-Brock (method, unit)
  Boothby-Lovelace-Bulbulian (oxygen mask)

BLBK blood bank; also BB

BL=BS bilateral equal breath sounds

BLC beef liver catalase

BlC blood culture; also BC, BL CULT, bl cult

BLCL Burkitt's lymphoma cell line

BL CULT, bl cult blood culture; also BC, BlC

BLD basal-cell liquefactive degeneration
  benign lymphoepithelial disease
  beryllium lung disease

bld blood (whole blood); also B, bl

bldg bleeding; also BL, bl

bld tm bleeding time; also BT

BLE Basal level enhancer
  bilateral lower extremity
  both lower extremities; also B↓E

BLEO, bleo bleomycin; also BL, BLM

BLEO-MOPP bleomycin, mechlorethamine,
  Oncovin, procarbazine, and prednisone

BLEP Breast Lesion Evaluation Project

bleph blepharoplasty

BLESS bath, laxative, enema, shampoo, and
  shower

BLF bovine lactoferrin

BLFD buccolinguofacial dyskinesia

BLFG bilateral firm hand grips

BL-FST blood-fasting

BLG beta-lactoglobulin

BLI bombesin-like immunoreactivity

BLIPS Biometrics Laboratory Information
  Processing System

blk black; also B, Bl

BLL below lower limit
  bilateral lower lobe
  brows, lids, and lashes

BLLS bilateral leg strength

BLM basolateral membrane
  bilayer lipid membrane
  bimolecular liquid membrane
  black lipid membrane
  bleomycin; also BL, BLEO, bleo

BLN bronchial lymph node

BLOBS bladder obstruction

BLP beta-lipoprotein
bombesin-like peptide

BlP blood pressure; also BL PR, bl pr, BP, B/P

BLPO beta-lactamase-producing organism

BL PR, bl pr blood pressure; also BlP, BP, B/P

BLQ both lower quadrants

BLRA beta-lactamase-resistant antimicrobial

BLROA British Laryngological, Rhinological, and Otological Association

BLS basic life support
blind loop syndrome
blood and lymphatic system
blood sugar
Bloom's syndrome; also BS

BlS blood sugar; also BS

BLSD bovine lumpy skin disease

BLST Bankson Language Screening Test

BLT, BlT blood-clot lysis time
blood test
blood type; also BT
blood typing; also BT

BLU Bessey-Lowry unit

BLV blood volume; also BV
bovine leukemia virus

BM Bachelor of Medicine
Bamberger-Marie (disease)
basal medium
basal metabolism
basement membrane
basilar membrane
Batten-Mayou (disease)
Bergersen medium
betamethasone; also BMS
Bingold's myorenal (syndrome)
biomedical
black male; also B/M
blood monocyte
body mass
Boehringer Mannheim
Bohr's magneton
bone marrow
bone mass
bowel movement
Brailsford-Morquio (disease)
breast milk; also BrM
buccal mass
buccomesial
salt-water or sea-water bath [L. *balneum maris*]; also bal mar, bm

B/M black male; also BM

bm salt-water or sea-water bath [L. *balneum maris*]; also bal mar, BM

BMA bone marrow arrest
bone marrow aspirate
British Medical Association

BmA *Brugia malayi* adult antigen

BMAP basement membrane associated protein
bone marrow acid phosphatase

BMB biomedical belt
bone marrow biopsy

BMBL benign monoclonal B-cell lympho-cytosis

BMC blood mononuclear cell
bone marrow cells
bone mineral content

BMD Becker's muscular dystrophy
Boehringer Mannheim Diagnostics
bone marrow depression
bone mineral density
bovine mucosal disease
Bureau of Medical Devices

BMDC Biomedical Documentation Center

BME biundulant meningoencephalitis
brief maximal effort
Eagle's basal medium

BMET biomedical equipment technician

BMF black married female

BMG benign monoclonal gammopathy
beta$_2$-microglobulin; also β_2m

BMI bicuculline methiodide
body mass index

BMJ bones, muscles, joints
British Medical Journal

BMK, bmk birthmark

BML bone marrow lymphocytosis

BMLM basement membrane-like material

BMLS billowing mitral leaflet syndrome

BMM black married male

BMMP benign mucous membrane pemphigus

BMN bone marrow necrosis

BMNR bone marrow neutrophil reserve

BmNPV bombyx mori nuclear polyhidrosis virus

BMO bonding molecular orbital

BMOC Brinster medium for ovum culture

Bmod, B-mod behavior modification

B-mode brightness modulation

BMP BCNU, methotrexate, and procarbazine
  behavior management plan
  bleomycin, methotrexate, and Platinol
  bone marrow pressure
  bone morphogenetic protein
BMPI bronchial mucous proteinase inhibitor
BMR basal metabolic rate
  best motor response
BMS Bachelor of Medical Science
  betamethasone; also BM
  biomedical monitoring system
  bleomycin sulfate
BMST Bruce maximal stress test
BMT bacterial mutagenicity test (Ames test)
  basement membrane thickness
  benign mesenchymal tumor
  bilateral myringotomy and tubes
  bone marrow transplant
  bone marrow transplantation
BMTU bone marrow transplant unit
BMU basic multicellular unit
BMV Brome mosaic virus
  Bromegrass mosaic virus
BMZ basement membrane zone
BN Babinski-Nageotte (syndrome)
  bladder neck
  brachial neuritis
  bronchial nodes
  brown Norway (rat)
  bucconasal
BNA Basle Nomina Anatomica
BNB blood-nerve barrier
BNC bladder neck contracture
BNCT boron neutron capture therapy
BNDD Bureau of Narcotics and Dangerous
  Drugs
bne but not exceeding
BNEG B negative (blood type)
BNF British National Formulary
BNG bromonaphthyl-β-galactoside
BNGase bromonaphthyl-β-galactosidase
BNGF beta-nerve growth factor
BNIST National Bureau of Scientific
  Information [Fr. *Bureau National
  d'Information Scientifique*]
BNL breast needle location
BNMSE Brief Neuropsychologic Mental Status
  Examination
BNO bladder neck obstruction
  bowels not open

BNPA binasal pharyngeal airway
BNR bladder neck resection
BNS benign nephrosclerosis
BNT brain neurotransmitter
BO base of prism out
  behavior objective
  belladonna and opium; also B&O
  body odor
  bowel; also bo
  bowel obstruction
  bowels open
  bucco-occlusal
B/O because of
B&O belladonna and opium; also BO
Bo bohemium
  Bolton's point; also B, bb, BP
bo bowel; also BO
BOA behavioral observation audiometry
  born on arrival
  born out of asepsis
  British Orthopaedic Association
BOB ball on back
BOBA beta-oxybutyric acid
BOC blood oxygen capacity
  t-butoxycarbonyl (former abbreviation, pre-
  sent usage is Boc); also *t*BOC, Boc
***t*BOC** *t*-butoxycarbonyl (former abbreviation,
  present usage is Boc); also BOC, Boc
Boc *t*-butoxycarbonyl; also BOC, *t*BOC
BOCG Brudzinski, Oppenheim, Chaddock, and
  Guilland (reflexes, signs)
BOD bilateral orbital decompression
  biochemical oxygen demand
  biologic oxygen demand
  borderline; also BORD
  Bureau of Drugs
Bod units Bodansky units
BOE bilateral otitis externa
BOEA ethyl biscoumacetate
BOFA beta-oncofetal antigen
BOH beta-hydroxybutyrate; also BHB
  Board of Health; also BH
  bundle of His; also BH
Bol, bol a large pill [L. *bolus* (pill)]
BOHB beta-hydroxybutyric acid; also BHBA
BOLD bleomycin, Oncovin, lomustine, and
  dacarbazine

BOM bilateral otitis media

BOMA bilateral otitis media, acute

BOO bladder outlet obstruction

BOOP bronchiolitis obliterans with organizing pneumonia

BOP bleomycin, Oncovin, and prednisone
bromo-oxyprogesterone
Buffalo orphan prototype (virus)

BOPAM bleomycin, Oncovin, prednisone, Adriamycin, and methotrexate

BOPP bleomycin, Oncovin, procarbazine, and prednisone

BOR basal optic root
before time of operation
bowels open regularly
branchio-otorenal (syndrome)

BORD borderline; also BOD

BORR blood oxygen release rate

BOS behavioral observation scale (for autism)

B-O$_2$S blood oxygen saturation

BOT base of tongue; also BT
botulinum toxin

bot botany
bottle

BOW bag of waters

BOWI bag of waters intact

BP back pressure
Bard-Pic (syndrome)
barometric pressure
base pair; also bp
basic protein
bathroom privileges; also BRP, brp
bedpan
before present
behavior pattern
Bell's palsy
benzopyrene
benzoyl peroxide
benzpyrene
bioequivalance problem
biotic potential
biparietal
biphenyl
bipolar
birthplace
blood pressure; also BlP, BL PR, bl pr, B/P
body part
body plethysmography
boiling point; also bp
Bolton's point; also B, bb, Bo
borderline personality

British Pharmacopoeia; also BPh, B Ph
bronchopleural
bronchopulmonary
buccopulpal
bullous pemphigoid
bullous pemphigus
bypass

B/P blood pressure; also BlP, BL PR, bl pr, BP

bp base pair; also BP
boiling point; also BP

BPA Bauhinia purpura agglutinin
blood pressure assembly
bovine plasma albumin
breast, pubic and axillary hair (in Tanner staging)
British Paediatric Association
bronchopulmonary aspergillosis
burst-promoting activity

BPAA (1,1′-biphenyl)-4-acetic acid (felbinac)

BPAS benzoylpas, sodium salt of

BPB bromphenol blue

BPC Behavior Problem Checklist
bile phospholipid concentration
British Pharmaceutical Codex
bronchial provocation challenge

B-P$_{CO2}$ blood partial pressure of carbon dioxide

BPD biparietal diameter
blood pressure decreased
borderline personality disorder
bronchopulmonary dysplasia

BPd diastolic blood pressure

BPE bacterial phosphatidylethanolamine
bovine pancreatic enzyme

BPEAOA Bureau of Professional Education of the American Osteopathic Association

BPEC bipolar electrocoagulation

BPF bradykinin-potentiating factor
bronchopleural fistula
burst-promoting factor

BPG blood pressure gauge
bypass graft

BPH benign prostatic hyperplasia
benign prostatic hypertrophy

BPh, B Ph British Pharmacopoeia; also BP
buccopharyngeal

B-pH blood pH

Bph bacteriopheophytin

BPI Basic Personality Inventory
beef-pork insulin

BPI—cont'd
  bipolar affective disorder, type 1
  blood pressure increased

BPIG bacterial polysaccharide immune globulin

BPL benign proliferative lesion
  benzylpenicilloyl polylysine
  beta-propiolactone
  bone phosphate of lime

BP lar blood pressure, left arm

BPLN bilateral pelvic lymph nodes

BPLND bilateral pelvic lymph node dissection

BPM, bpm beats per minute
  bipiperidyl mustard
  births per minute
  breaths per minute
  brompheniramine maleate

BPMG *N,N*-bis(phosphonomethyl)glycine

BPMS blood plasma measuring system

BPN bacitracin, polymyxin B, and neomycin sulfate
  brachial plexus neuropathy

BPO basal pepsin output
  bilateral partial oophorectomy
  bile phospholipid output

BPP biophysical profile
  bovine pancreatic polypeptide
  bradykinin potentiating peptide
  breast parenchymal pattern

BPPN benign paroxysmal positioning nystagmus

BPPP bilateral pedal pulses present

BP,P,R,T blood pressure, pulse, respiration, and temperature

BPPS 2-(*p-tert*-butylphenoxy)cyclohexyl propargyl sulfite (propagite)

BPPV benign paroxysmal positional vertigo
  bovine paragenital papilloma virus

BPR bilirubin production rate
  blood per rectum
  blood pressure recorder
  blood production rate

BP rar blood pressure, right arm

BPRS brief psychiatric rating scale

BPS Baseline Prevalence Survey
  beats per second
  bilateral partial salpingectomy
  bovine papular stomatitis
  brain protein solvent
  breaths per second

BPs blood pressure, systolic

BPSD bronchopulmonary segmental drainage

BPT benign paroxysmal torticollis

BPTI basic pancreatic trypsin inhibitor
  basic polyvalent trypsin inhibitor

BPV benign paroxysmal vertigo
  benign positional vertigo
  bioprosthetic valve
  bovine papilloma virus

BP(VET) British Pharmacopoeia (Veterinary)

Bq becquerel (SI unit of radionuclide activity)

BQA Bureau of Quality Assurance

BQC sol 2,6-dibromoquinone-4-chlorimide solution

BR bacteriorhodopsin
  barrier-reared (experimental animals)
  baseline recovery
  bathroom
  bedrest
  bedside rounds
  Benzing retrograde
  benzodiazepine receptor
  bilirubin; also BIL, Bil, bil, bili, bilirub, Bu
  biologic response
  Birmingham Revision (of Basle Nomina Anatomica terminology)
  blink reflex
  bowel rest
  brachialis
  breathing rate
  British Revision (of Basle Nomica Anatomica terminology)
  bronchitis; also Br
  brown; also Br, br

Br breech
  bregma; also B
  bridge
  bromide
  bromine
  bronchitis; also BR
  brown; also BR, br

Br *Brucella* species; also *B,* Bruc

br boiling range
  brachial; also Brach
  branch
  breath; also brth
  broiled
  bromo
  brother; also B, BRO, bro
  brown; also BR, Br

BRA beta-resorcylic acid
  bilateral renal agenesis

brain; also b

BRAC basic rest-activity cycle

Brach brachial; also br

BRADY bradycardia

BRAO branch retinal artery occlusion; also BR RAO

BRAP burst of rapid atrial pacing

BrAP brachial artery pressure; also BAP

BRAT bananas, rice (or rice cereal), applesauce, and toast (diet)

BRATT bananas, rice (or rice cereal), applesauce, tea, and toast (diet)

BRB blood-retinal barrier
bright red blood

BRBC bovine red blood cell
burro red blood cell

BRBNS blue rubber bleb nevus syndrome

BRBPR bright red blood per rectum; also BRBR

BRBR bright red blood per rectum; also BRBPR

br bx breast biopsy; also BB, B Bx

BRCM below right costal margin

BRD bladder retraining drill

BRDU, BrDu, BrdU 5-bromodeoxyuridine; also BrdUrd

BrdUrd 5-bromodeoxyuridine; also BRDU, BrDu, BrdU

BRET bretylium tosylate

BRFSS Behavioral Risk Factor Surveillance System

BRH benign recurrent hematuria
Bureau of Radiological Health

BRI Bio-Research Index

BRIC benign recurrent intrahepatic cholestasis

Brit Britain
British

Brit pat British patent

BRJ brachial radialis jerk

Brkf, brkf breakfast; also b'fast, bkf, bkfst, bkft

BRM biologic response modifier(s)
biuret-reactive material

BrM breast milk; also BM

BRMP Biologic Response Modification Program

BRN Board of Registered Nursing

BRO bilirubin oxidase

bromocriptine; also BCR
bronchoscope; also bronch
bronchoscopy; also bronch
brother; also B, br, bro

bro brother; also B, br, BRO

Bron bronchi
bronchial

bronch bronchoscope; also BRO
bronchoscopy; also BRO

BRP bathroom privileges; also BP, brp
bilirubin production

brp bathroom privileges; also BP, BRP

Brph bronchophony

BRR baroreceptor reflex response

BR RAO branch retinal artery occlusion; also BRAO

BR RVO branch retinal vein occlusion; also BRVO

BRS breath sounds; also BS, bs
British Roentgen Society

brth breath; also br

BRU bromide urine

BrU bromouracil; also BU

Bruc Brucella; also *B, BR*

BRVO branch retinal vein occlusion; also BR RVO

BS Bachelor of Science; also BSc
Bachelor of Surgery; also BC, BCh, CB, ChB
Bacillus subtilis
Baehr-Schiffrin (disease)
barium swallow; also BaS
Bartter's syndrome
bedside
before sleep
Behçet's syndrome
Bennett seal
bilateral symmetric
bile salt
bismuth subgallate
bismuth subsalicylate; also BSS
Bloch-Sulzberger (syndrome)
blood sugar; also BlS
Bloom's syndrome; also BLS
Blue Shield
borderline schizophrenia
bowel sounds; also bs
Boyd-Stearns (syndrome)
breaking strength
breath sounds; also BRS, bs
Brill-Symmers (disease, syndrome)
British Standard

BS—cont'd
  Brown-Séquard (disease, syndrome)
  Brown-Symmers (disease)
  Bureau of Standards

B-S Björk-Shiley (valve prosthesis)
  Binet-Simon (test)

B&S Bartholin and Skene's (glands)

bs bowel sounds; also BS
  breath sounds; also BRS, BS

BSA beef serum albumin
  benzenesulfonic acid
  bismuth-sulfite agar
  bistrimethysilylacetamide
  Blue Shield association
  body surface area; also bsa
  bovine serum albumin; also bsa
  bowel sounds active

bsa body surface area; also BSA
  bovine serum albumin; also BSA

BSAB Balthazar Scales of Adaptive Behavior

BSAER brain-stem auditory evoked response;
    also BAER

BSAG Bristol Social Adjustment Guides

BSAP brief short-action potential
  brief, small, abundant potentials

BSB bedside bag
  body surface burned

BSBC buffer-soluble binding component

BSC bedside care
  bedside commode
  bench scale calorimeter
  bile salt concentration
  Biological Stain Commission
  burn scar contracture

BSc Bachelor of Science; also BS

BSCIF bile salt independent canalicular fraction

BSCP bovine spinal cord protein

BSD baby soft diet
  bedside drainage

BSDLB block in anterosuperior division of left
    branch

BSE bacillus species enzyme
  bilateral, symmetrical, and equal
  breast self-examination

BSEP brainstem evoked potential; also BEP

BSepF black separated female

BSepM black separated male

BSER brainstem evoked response (audiometry)

BSF backscatter factor
  basal skull fracture
  black single female
  busulfan; also BUS, bus

BSF-2 B-cell stimulatory factor 2

BSG branchioskeletogenital (syndrome)

BSGA beta-hemolytic streptococcus group A

BSI body substance isolation
  borderline syndrome index
  bound serum iron
  brainstem injury

BSID Bayley Scales of Infant Development

BSIF bile salt independent fraction

BSL benign symmetric lipomatosis
  blood sugar level

BS L base breath sounds diminished, left base

BSM bile salt metabolism
  black single male

BSN Bachelor of Science in Nursing
  bowel sounds normal

BSNA bowel sounds normal and active

BSNT breast soft and non-tender

BSO bilateral sagittal osteotomy
  bilateral salpingo-oophorectomy; also BILAT
    SXO, bilat sxo
  bilateral serous otitis
  buthionine sulphoximine

BSOM bilateral serous otitis media

BSP body segment parameter
  bromsulfophthalein
  bromsulphalein
  sulphobromophthalein sodium

BSp bronchospasm

BSPA bowel sounds present and active

BSPM body surface potential mapping

BSQ Behavior Style Questionnaire

BSR basal skin resistance
  blood sedimentation rate
  bowel sounds regular
  brain stimulation reinforcement

BSRI Bem Sex Role Inventory

BSS balanced salt solution
  bedside scale
  Bernard-Soulier syndrome; also B-SS
  bismuth subsalicylate; also BS
  black silk suture
  buffered saline solution
  buffered salt solution
  buffered single substrate

B-SS Bernard-Soulier syndrome; also BSS

BSSE bile salt-stimulated esterase

BSSG sitogluside

BSSI Basic School Skills Inventory

BSSL bile salt-stimulated lipase

BSSS benign sporadic sleep spikes

BST Bacteriuria Screening Test
bedside testing
biceps semitendinosus
blood serologic test
bovine somatotropin
breast stimulation test
brief stimulus therapy

BSTFA bis-trimethylsilyl-trifluoroacetamide

BSTP basophilic stippling (on differential);
also BASO STIP

BSU Bartholin, Skene, and urethral (glands)
British Standard Unit

BSV Batten-Spielmeyer-Vogt (syndrome)

BSVM bovine seminal vesical microsomal
(preparation)

BT *Bacillus thuringiensis*
base of tongue; also BOT
bedtime
Behçet-Touraine (syndrome)
bitemporal (diameter of fetal head)
bituberous
bladder tumor
bleeding time; also bld tm
blood transfusion
blood type; also BLT, B1T
blood typing; also BLT, B1T
blue tetrazolium
blue tongue
body temperature
borderline tuberculoid
bovine turbinate (cells)
brain tumor
breast tumor
bulbotruncal

BTA *N*-benzoyl-L-tyrosine amide
brief tone audiometry

BTB breakthrough bleeding; also BB
bromthymol blue

BTBC Boehm Test of Basic Concepts

BTBL bromothymol blue lactose

BTBV beat-to-beat variability

BTC basal temperature chart
bilateral tubal coagulation
bladder tumor check
by the clock

BTE Baltimore Therapeutic Equipment Work
Simulator
behind-the-ear (hearing aid)
bovine thymus extract

BTEA Boston Test for Examining Aphasia

BTF blenderized tube feeding

BTFS breast tumor frozen section

BTG beta-thromboglobulin

BTg bovine trypsinogen

BThU British thermal unit; also BTU, Btu

BTL bilateral tubal ligation

BTLS basic trauma life support

BTM benign tertian malaria
bilateral tympanic membranes

BTMD Botten-Turner muscular dystrophy

BTMSA bis-trimethylsilylacetylene

BTP biliary tract pain

BTPD body temperature, pressure, dry

BTPS body temperature, ambient pressure, saturated (gas volume expressed as if it were
saturated with water vapor at body temperature and at the ambient barometric pressure)

BTR Bezold-type reflex
bladder tumor recheck
blood transfusion recipient
bovine trypsin; also BTr

BTr bovine trypsin; also BTR

BTS bioptic telescopic spectacle
bithional sulfoxide
blood transfusion service
bradycardia-tachycardia syndrome

BTSG Brain Tumor Study Group

BTSH, bTSH beef thyroid-stimulating hormone
bovine thyroid-stimulating hormone

BTU, Btu British thermal unit; also BThU

BTV blue tongue virus

BTX batrachotoxin
benzene, toluene, and xylene

BTX-B brevetoxin-B

BU base of prism up
below the umbilicus
blood urea
Bodansky unit
Bonnevie-Ullrich (syndrome)
bromouracil; also BrU
burn unit

Bu bilirubin; also BIL, Bil, bil, bili, bilirub, BR
butyl

BUA blood uric acid

Buc, bucc buccal; also B

BUD budesonide

BUDS bilateral upper dorsal sympathectomy

BUE bilateral upper extremity
both upper extremities ; also B ↑ E
built-up edge

BUF Buffalo (rat)

BUFA baby up for adoption

BUG buccal ganglion

BUI brain uptake index

BULL buccal or upper lingual of lower

Bull, bull bulletin
let it boil [L. *bulliat*]

BUMP Behavioral Regression or Upset in Hospitalized Medical Patients (scale)

BUN blood urea nitrogen
bunion

BUO bilateral ureteral occlusion
bilirubin of undetermined origin
bleeding of undetermined origin
bruising of undetermined origin

BUPA British United Provident Association

BUR back-up rate (ventilator)

Bur bureau

Burd Burdick (suction)

BUS Bartholin, urethral, and Skene's (glands)
busulfan; also BSF, Bus

Bus busulfan; also BSF, BUS

BUSEG Bartholin, urethral, and Skene's glands, and external genitalia

BUT break-up time

But, but alpha-aminobutyric acid (butyrine)
butter
butyrate
butyric

BuTX bungarotoxin, also BGT

BV bacitracin V
bacterial vaginitis
Bacto V factor (differentiation disks)
billion volts
biological value
blood vessel
blood volume; also BLV
bronchovesicular
buccoversion
bulboventricular
steam or vapor bath [L. *balneum vaporis*];
also bal vap, bv

bv steam or vapor bath [L. *balneum vaporis*];
also bal vap, BV

BVAD biventricular assist device

BVAP BCNU, vincristine, Adriamycin, and prednisone

BVAT Binocular Visual Acuity Test
blood-stage variant antigen type

BVC British Veterinary Codex

BVD BCNU, vincristine, and dacarbazine
bovine viral diarrhea

BVDT Brief Vestibular Disorientation Test

BVDU 5-(2-bromovinyl)-2′-deoxyuridine

BVE binocular visual efficiency
biventricular enlargement
blood vessel endothelium
blood volume expander
blood volume expansion

BVH biventricular hypertrophy

BVI Better Vision Institute
blood vessel invasion

BVL bilateral vas ligation

BVM bronchovascular markings
Bureau of Veterinary Medicine

BVMGT Bender Visual-Motor Gestalt Test

BVO branch vein occlusion
brominated vegetable oil

BVP blood vessel prosthesis
blood volume pulse
Bonhoeffer van der Pol
burst of ventricular pacing

BVR baboon virus replication
Bureau of Vocational Rehabilitation

BVRT-R Benton Visual Retention Test, Revised

BVS blanked ventricular sense

BVU bromoisovaleryl urea (bromisovalum)

BVV bovine vaginitis virus

BVX Bacto V factor and X factor (differentiation disks)

BW bacteriologic warfare
below waist
biologic warfare
biologic weapon
birth weight; also BWt
bite-wing (radiograph)
bladder washout
blood Wassermann
body water
body weight; also bw

B&W black and white (milk of magnesia and cascara extract)

bw body weight; also BW

BWA bed wetter admission

BWC body weight change

BWCS bagged white-cell study

BWD bacillary white diarrhea

BWFI bacteriostatic water for injection

BWG Bland-White-Garland (syndrome)

BWidF black widowed female

BWidM black widowed male

BWS battered woman syndrome
Beckwith-Wiedemann syndrome

BWST black widow spider toxin

BWSV black widow spider venom

BWt birth weight; also BW

BX bacitracin X
Bacto X factor (differentiation disks)
biopsy; also Bx, bx
Blue Cross; also BC

Bx, bx biopsy; also BX

BX/BS, BX BS Blue Cross/Blue Shield; also BC/BS

BXM B-cell cross-match

BYE Barile-Yaguchi-Eveland (medium)

BZ, bz benzodiazepine; also BD, BDZ, BZD, BZDZ
benzoyl; also Bz
benzyl; also Bzl, bzl

Bz benzoyl; also BZ, bz

BZA benzylamine; also BA

Bza benzimidazole
benzimidazolyl

BzAnth benzanthracene; also BA

BZD benzodiazepine; also BD, BDZ, BZ, bz, BZDZ

BZDZ benzodiazepine; also BD, BDZ, BZ, bz, BZD

BzH benzaldehyde

Bzl, bzl benzyl; also BZ, bz

BzOH benzoic acid

Bz-TY-PABA *N*-benzoyl-L-tyrosyl-*p*-aminobenzoic acid (test)

BZQ benzquinamide

C

X CHI, UPPER CASE twenty-second letter of the Greek alphabet

χ chi, lower case, twenty-second letter of the Greek alphabet

χ^2 chi-square (distribution test)

χ_e electric susceptibility

χ_m magnetic susceptibility

C ascorbic acid
bruised [L. *contusus*]; also cont, contus
calcitonin-forming (cell)
calculus
canine (tooth); also c
capacitance; also *C*
carbohydrate; also CARB, carb, carbo, CHO, COH
carbon
cardiovascular (disease)
carrier
cathodal; also CA, Ca
cathode; also CA, Ca, Cath, cath
Catholic
Caucasian; also Cau, Cauc, cauc
Celsius; also CEL, Cel, Cels
centigrade; also CENT, cent
central; also cen, CENT, cent
central electrode placement in electroencephalography
centromeric or constitutive heterochromatic chromosome (banding)
cerebrospinal (fluid)
certified; also Cert, cert, CRT
cervical (collar, spine, vertebra)
cesarean (section)
chest (precordial lead in electrocardiography)
chloramphenicol; also CAP, CHL, chloro, CMC, CP
cholesterol; also CH, Ch, CHO, CHOL, Chol, chol
clear; also Cl, cl, cler
clearance; also *C*, Cx
clearance rate (renal)
clonus, also Cl
closure; also Cl, cl
clubbing
coarse (bacterial colonies)
cocaine
coefficient; also coef, coeff
colored (guinea pig)
color sense
communicating (pacemaker code)
complement; also C′
compliance
component
compound; also cmp'd, CO, co, comp, compd, CP, CPD, cpd
concentration; also c, conc, concn, concentr
conditioned; also cond
conditioning
condyle
constant; also const
contact; also c
content
contraction; also contr, contrx, CTX, CTXN, Cx
contracture
control; also CO
conventionally reared (experimental animal)
cornea
correct
cortex; also cort
coulomb; also coul
creatinine; also CR, Cr, Cre, CREAT, creat
crit (hematocrit); also Crit, crit, Hc, H'crit, HCT, Hct, hemat, HMT
cubic; also c, cu
cup; also c
curie; also c, Ci, CU, cu
cuspid (secondary dentition)
cuticular
cyanosis
cylinder; also cyl
cylindrical lens; also cyl
cysteine (one-letter notation); also Cys, cys
cytidine; also Cyd
cytochrome; also CYT
cytosine; also Cyt
gallon [L. *congius*]; also cong
hundred [L. *centum*]; also c
large calorie (kilocalorie); also Cal
molar heat capacity
rib [L. *costa*]
speed of light
with [L. *cum*]; also c, c̄

C capacitance; also C
clearance; also C, Cx
Clostridium species; also Cl, *Cl*, Clostr
Cryptococcus species

ℂ complex number

C′ complement; also C

°C degree Celsius
degree centigrade

© confidential (patient may be unaware)
copyright

C§ cesarean section; also CS, C/S, C sect, C-section

C-I – C-V DEA (Drug Enforcement Administration) controlled substances, schedules I through V

CI – CXII, C_I – C_{XII} cranial nerves I through XII; also CNI – CNXII

C1 – C7, C_1 – C_7 cervical vertebrae 1 through 7

C1 – C8, C_1 – C_8 cervical nerves 1 through 8

C1 – C9, C_1 – C_9 components of complement 1 through 9

C-1 – C-9 activated components of complement 1 through 9

C_1 – C_{12} first through twelfth ribs [L. *costa*]

C_3 Collin's solution

C-6 hexamethonium

C-10 decamethonium

C14, ^{14}C carbon-14, radioactive carbon: halflife 5,730 years

^{137}C Cesium 137, radioactive cesium: halflife' 9.0 hours

C23O catechol 2,3-dioxygenase

c about, approximately [L. *circa*]; also ca
candle; also ca
canine (tooth); also C
capacity; also cap
capillary blood (subscript)
carat
centi- (10^{-2})
concentration; also C, conc, concn, concentr
concentration by volume (after optical rotations only)
contact; also C
cubic; also C, cu
cup; also C
curie; also C, Ci, CU, cu
cuspid (primary dentition)
cycle; also cyc
cyclic
hundred [L. *centum*]; also C
meal [L. *cibus*]
small calorie; also cal
specific heat capacity; also *c*
with [L. *cum*]; also C, c̄

c molar concentration
specific heat capacity; also c

speed of light in a vacuum

c̄ with [L. *cum*]; also C, c

c′ coefficient of partage
pulmonary end-capillary (blood phase)

CA anterior commissure [L. *commissura anterior*]
calcium antagonist
California (rabbit)
cancer; also Ca, ca, Can
cancer antigen
caproic acid
carbohydrate antigen
carbonic anhydrase
carcinoma; also Ca
cardiac-apnea (monitor)
cardiac arrest
cardiac arrhythmia
carotid artery
catecholamine; also CAT
catecholaminergic
cathodal; also C, Ca
cathode; also C, Ca, Cath, cath
celiac artery
cellulose acetate
cerebellopontine angle (syndrome)
cerebral aqueduct
cervicoaxial; also CO
Chemical Abstracts (service)
chemotactic activity; also CTA
chloroamphetamine
cholic acid
chronic anovulation
chronological age
citric acid
clotting assay
coagglutination (test)
coarctation of the aorta; also CoA, C of A
Cocaine Anonymous
coefficient of absorption
cold agglutinin; also COLD A, cold agg
collagen antigen
collagenolytic activity
colloid antigen
commissural associated
common antigen
community acquired
compressed air
conceptional age
conditioned abstinence
conditioned air
condylomata acuminata
coronary angioplasty
coronary arrest
coronary artery

CA—cont'd
corpora allata
corpora amylacea
cortisone acetate
cricoid arch
croup-associated (virus)
cyclophosphamide and Adriamycin
cytosine arabinoside
cytotoxic antibody

CA (#) cancer antigen (#)
carbohydrate antigen (#)

C/A, c/a Clinitest/Acetest; also C&A

C&A Clinitest and Acetest; also C/A, c/a
conscious and alert

Ca calcium; also CAL, Calc
cancer; also CA, ca, Can
Cancer – A Cancer Journal for Clinicians
carcinoma; also CA
carmustine
carpal
carpal amputation
cathodal; also C, CA
cathode; also C, CA, Cath, cath
NIOSH (National Institute for Occupational
Safety and Health) recommends that the
substance be treated as a potential human
carcinogen

⁴⁵Ca calcium 45, radioactive calcium: halflife,
165 days

ca about, approximately [L. *circa*]; also c
cancer; also CA, Ca, Can
candle; also c

CAA carotid audiofrequency analysis
chloroacetaldehyde
computer-aided assessment
computer-assisted assessment
constitutional aplastic anemia
crystalline amino acids

CAAH carbobenzoxy-L-arginine amidehydro-
lase

CAAT computer-assisted axial tomography

CAB captive air bubble
catheter-associated bacteriuria
cellulose acetate butyrate
coronary artery bypass

CABG coronary artery bypass graft

CABGS coronary artery bypass graft surgery

CaBI calcium bone index

CABO cisplatin, Amethopterin, bleomycin, and
Oncovin

CABOP, CA-BOP cyclophosphamide,
Adriamycin, bleomycin, Oncovin, and
prednisone

CaBP calcium-binding protein; also CBP

CABS coronary artery bypass surgery

CAC cancer cell
cardiac-accelerator center
cardiac arrest code
carotid artery canal
circulating anticoagulant
comprehensive ambulatory care

CACB calcium carbonate

CACC, CaCC cathodal closure contraction;
also CCC

CACE counteracting chromatographic electrophoresis

CACI computer-assisted continuous infusion

CACMS Committee on Accreditation of
Canadian Medical Schools

CACP *cis*-diamminedichloroplatinum (cisplatin); also CDDP, cis-DDP, *cis*-DDP

CaCV *Calicivirus*

CACX cancer of cervix

CAD cadaver; also Cad
cold agglutinin disease
compressed air disease
computer-assisted design
computer-assisted diagnosis
coronary artery disease
cyclophosphamide, Adriamycin, and dacarbazine
cytosine arabinoside and daunorubicin

Cad cadaver; also CAD

CADI computer-assisted diabetic instruction

CADIC cyclophosphamide, Adriamycin, and
DIC (dacarbazine); also CyADIC

CADL Communicative Abilities in Daily
Living

CADS calcium-dependent cell adhesion system

CaDTe cathodal duration tetanus

CAE caprine arthritis-encephalitis
cellulose acetate electrophoresis
contingent aftereffects
coronary artery embolization
cyclophosphamide, Adriamycin, and etoposide

CaE calcium excretion

CAEC cardiac arrhythmia evaluation center

CaEDTA, CaEdTA calcium disodium ethyl-
enediaminetetraacetate

CAER caerulein

CAEV caprine arthritis-encephalitis virus

CAF cell adhesion factor
citric acid fermenters
continuous atrial fibrillation
continuous atrial flutter
contract administration fees
cyclophosphamide, Adriamycin, and 5-fluorouracil

CaF correction of area factor

Caf caffeine

CAFP cyclophosphamide, Adriamycin, fluorouracil, and prednisone

CAFT cisplatin, Adriamycin, fluorouracil, and teniposide
Clinitron air fluidized therapy

CAFVP cyclophosphamide, Adriamycin, fluorouracil, vincristine, and prednisone

CAG cholangiogram
chronic atrophic gastritis
continuous ambulatory gamma-globulin (infusion)
coronary angiogram
coronary angiography

CaG calcium gluconate; also CG

CaGP calcium glycerophosphate

CAH central alveolar hypoventilation
chronic active hepatitis
chronic aggressive hepatitis
combined atrial hypertrophy
congenital adrenal hyperplasia
congenital adrenogenital hyperplasia
cyanacetic acid hydrazide

CaHA calcium hydroxyapatite

CAHC chronic active hepatitis with cirrhosis

CAHD coronary arteriosclerotic heart disease; also CASHD
coronary atherosclerotic heart disease; also CASHD

CAHEA Committee on Allied Health Education and Accreditation

CAI complete androgen insensitivity
computer-assisted instruction
confused artificial insemination

CAIS complete androgen insensitivity syndrome

CAL calcium; also Ca, Calc
calculated average life
callus
calories
chronic airflow limitation
computer-assisted learning

Cal large calorie (kilocalorie); also C

cal caliber
small calorie; also c

C$_{alb}$ albumin clearance

Calc calcium; also Ca, CAL

calc calculate
calculated; also calcd

calcd calculated; also calc

cal ct calorie count

CALD chronic active liver disease

CALEF, calef make warm [L. *calefacio*]
warmed [L. *calefactus*]

CALGB cancer and leukemia group B

calib calibrated

cALL common null cell acute lymphocytic leukemia

CALLA, cALLA, cALLa common acute lymphoblastic leukemia antigen
common acute lymphocytic leukemia antigen

CAM calf aortic microsome
carminomycin
Caucasian adult male
cell adhesion molecule
cell-associating molecule
chorioallantoic membrane
computer-aided myelography
computer-assisted myelography
contralateral axillary metastasis
cyclophosphamide, Adriamycin, and methotrexate

CaM calmodulin

C$_{am}$ amylase clearance

CAMAC computer-automated measurement and control

CAMB cyclophosphamide, Adriamycin, methotrexate, and bleomycin

CAMEO cyclophosphamide, Adriamycin, methotrexate, etoposide, and Oncovin

CAMF cyclophosphamide, Adriamycin, methotrexate, and fluorouracil

CAMP Christie-Atkins-Munch-Peterson (test)
computer-assisted menu planning
concentration of adenosine monophosphate
cyclophosphamide, Adriamycin, methotrexate, and procarbazine

cAMP, *c*AMP cyclic adenosine monophosphate; also AMP-c, cyclic AMP

c amplum heaping spoonful [L. *cochleare amplum*]; also cochl amp

CAMPPDE 3′,5′-cyclic adenosine monophosphate phosphodiesterase

CAMS computer-assisted monitoring system

CAMU cardiac ambulatory monitoring unit
coronary arrhythmia monitoring unit

CaMV cauliflower mosaic virus; also CLMV

CAN umbilical cord around neck

CA/N child abuse and neglect

(CA)n contain

Can cancer; also CA, Ca, ca

can cannabis

CANC, canc cancelled

CANCERLIT Cancer Literature (an electronic database including citations relating to oncology)

CancerProj Cancer Research Projects

CANP calcium-activated neutral protease

Can pat Canadian patent

CANS central auditory nervous system

CAO chronic airway obstruction
coronary artery obstruction
coronary artery occlusion

Ca$_{O2}$ arterial oxygen concentration

CaOC cathodal opening contraction; also COC

CaOCl cathodal opening clonus; also COC, COCL, COCl

CAOD coronary artery occlusive disease

CAOM chronic adhesive otitis media

Ca ox calcium oxalate (crystal)

CAP cancer of prostrate
capsule; also cap, caps, capsul
captopril
cardioacceleratory peptide
catabolite activator protein
cell attachment protein
cellular acetate propionate
cellulose acetate phthalate
central apical portion
chloramphenicol; also C, CHL, chloro, CMC, CP
chloroacetophenone
cholesteric analysis profile
chronic alcoholic pancreatitis
College of American Pathologists
community-acquired pneumonia
complement-activated plasma
compound action potential
computerized automated psycho-physiologic (device)
coupled atrial pacing

cyclic AMP-binding protein
cyclophosphamide, Adriamycin, and Platinol
cyclophosphamide, Adriamycin, and prednisone
cystine aminopeptidase

Ca/P calcium to phosphorus ratio

Cap let him take [L. *capiat*]; also cap

cap capacity; also c
capillary
capsule; also CAP, caps, capsul
let him take [L. *capiat*]; also Cap

CAPA caffeine, alcohol, pepper and aspirin (diet free of)
cancer-associated polypeptide antigen

CAPB central auditory processing battery

CAPD chronic ambulatory peritoneal dialysis
continuous ambulatory peritoneal dialysis

CAPERS Computer-assisted Psychiatric Evaluation and Review System

capiend to be taken [L. *capiendus*]

cap moll soft capsule [L. *capsula mollis*]

CAPP cell-associated peplomer

CAPPS Current and Past Psychopathology Scales

cap quant vult let him take as much as he wants [L. *capiat quantum vult*]

CAPRCA chronic, acquired, pure red cell aplasia

CAPRI Cardiopulmonary Research Institute

CAPS caffeine, alcohol, pepper, and spicy foods (diet free of)
Community Adjustment Profile System

caps capsule; also CAP, cap, capsul

capsul capsule; also CAP, cap, caps

CAPYA child and adolescent psychoanalysis

CAR Canadian Association of Radiologists
cardiac ambulation routine
chronic articular rheumatism
cis-acting antirepression (sequence)
computer-assisted research
conditioned avoidance response

car carotid

CARB carbohydrate; also C, carb, carbo, CHO, COH

carb carbohydrate; also C, CARB, carbo, CHO, COH
carbonate

CARBAM carbamazepine; also CBZ

carbo carbohydrate; also C, CARB, carb, CHO, COH

CARD, Card cardiology; also Cardiol

Cardiol cardiology; also CARD, Card

CARE Coronary Atherosclerosis Risk Evaluations

CARF Commission on Accreditation of Rehabilitation Facilities

CAROT carotene

CARS childhood autism rating scale
Children's Affective Rating Scale

CART computer-assisted real time transcription

CARTOS computer-assisted reconstruction by tracing of serial sections

CAS calcarine sulcus
calcified aortic stenosis
Cancer Attitude Survey
carbohydrate-active steroid
cardiac adjustment scale
cardiac surgery
carotid artery stenosis
casein
Celite-activated normal serum
Center for Alcohol Studies
cerebral arteriosclerosis
Chemical Abstracts Service
chronic anovulation syndrome
cold agglutinin syndrome
Community Adaptation Schedule
congenital alcoholic syndrome
congenital asplenia syndrome
control adjustment strap
coronary artery spasm
Council of Academic Societies

Cas casualty

cas castrated
castration

CASA computer-assisted self-assessment

CASH Commission for Administrative Services in Hospitals

CASHD coronary arteriosclerotic heart disease; also CAHD
coronary atherosclerotic heart disease; also CAHD

CASMD congenital atonic sclerotic muscular dystrophy

CA-SP calcium urine spot (test)

CAS-REGN Chemical Abstracts Service Registry Number

CASRT corrected adjusted sinus node recovery time

CASS computer-aided sleep system

Coronary Artery Surgery Study

CAST cardiac arrhythmia suppression trial
Children of Alcoholism Screening Test
color allergy screening test

C-AST cytoplasmic aspartate aminotransferase

CASTNO cast number (urinalysis)

CAT capillary agglutination test
catalase; also CAT'ase
cataract; also cat
catecholamine; also CA
cellular atypia
Children's Apperception Test
chloramphenicol acetyltransferase
chlormerodrin accumulation test
choline acetyltransferase; also ChAc, ChAct, CHAT, ChaT
chronic abdominal tympany
classified anaphylatoxin
computed abdominal tomography
computed axial tomography
computer-assisted tomography
computerized axial tomography
computer of average transients
cytosine arabinoside, Adriamycin, and thioguanine

cat catalyst
cataract; also CAT

CAT-A-KIT Catecholamine Radioenzymatic Assay Kit

CAT'ase catalase; also CAT

CAT-CAM contoured adducted trochanteric-controlled alignment method

CATCH Community Actions to Control High Blood Pressure

cat c̄ IL cataract with intraocular lens

Cath, cath cathartic
catheter
catheterization
catheterize
cathode; also C, CA, Ca

CATLINE Catalog On-Line

CAT-MET catecholamine and metabolites

CATS combined abdominal transsacral resection technique

CAT-S Children's Apperception Test, Supplemental

Catt, CATT calcium tolerance test

Cau Caucasian; also C, Cauc, cauc

Cauc, cauc Caucasian; also C, Cau

caud caudal; also CD, Cd, cd

caute cautiously [L. *cautē*]

CAV computer-assisted ventilation
congenital absence of vagina
congenital adrenal virilism
constant angular velocity
croup-associated virus
cyclophosphamide, Adriamycin, and vincristine

cav cavity

CAVB complete atrioventricular block

CAVC common arterioventricular canal

CAVD complete atrioventricular dissociation
completion, arithmetic problems, vocabulary, following directions (battery)

C(a-VDO₂) arteriovenous oxygen difference

CAVE CCNU (lomustine), Adriamycin, and vinblastine

CAVH continuous arteriovenous hemofiltration

CAVHD continuous arteriovenous hemodialysis
continuous arteriovenous hemofiltration with dialysis

CAVmP cyclophosphamide, Adriamycin, Vumon (teniposide), and prednisone

CAVO common atrioventricular orifice

CAVP CCNU (lomustine), Alkeran, VP-16-213 (etoposide), and prednisone
cyclophosphamide, Adriamycin, vincristine, and prednisone

CAV-P-VP cyclophosphamide, Adriamycin, vincristine, Platinol, and VP-16-213 (etoposide)

CAW central airways

C$_{aw}$ airway conductance

CAWO closing abductory wedge osteotomy

CAZ ceftazidime

CB Bachelor of Surgery [L. *Chirurgiae Baccalaureus*]; also BC, BCh, BS, ChB
carbenicillin; also CBC, CBCN
carbobenzoxy; also Cbo, CBZ, CBz, Cbz
carbonated beverage
carotid body
catheterized bladder
ceased breathing
cesarean birth
chair and bed; also C&B
chest-back; also C-B, C/B
chlorambucil; also CHL, Chl, CLB
chocolate blood (agar)
chronic bronchitis
circumflex branch
code blue

color blind
compensated base
conjugated bilirubin; also CBIL
contrast baths
Cruveilhier-Baumgarten (syndrome)
cytochalasin B

C-B chest-back; also CB, C/B

C/B chest-back; also CB, C-B

C&B chair and bed; also CB
crown and bridge

CB$_{11}$ phenadoxone hydrochloride

Cb columbium (old name for niobium)

cb cardboard or plastic film holder without intensifying screens

CBA carcinoma-bearing animal
chronic bronchitis with asthma
competitive-binding assay
cost-benefit analysis

CBAB complement-binding antibody

CBAT Coulter battery

CBB Coomassie brilliant blue R-250 (stain)

CBBB complete bundle branch block

CBC carbenicillin; also CB, CBCN
cerebrobuccal connective
child behavior characteristics
complete blood count; also cbc

cbc complete blood count; also CBC

CBCL Child Behavior Checklist

CBCME computer-based continuing medical education

CBCN carbenicillin; also CB, CBC

CBD cannabidiol
carotid body denervation
closed bladder drainage
common bile duct
community based distribution

CBDC chronic bullous disease of childhood

CBDE common bile duct exploration

CBDL chronic bile duct ligation

CBDS Carcinogenesis Bioassay Data System

CBE Council of Biology Editors

CBF capillary blood flow
carcino-breaking factor
cerebral blood flow
ciliary beat frequency
coronary blood flow
cortical blood flow

CBFS cerebral blood flow studies

CBFV cerebral blood flow velocity

CBG capillary blood gases; also CPG
  capillary blood glucose
  centromeric banding
  coronary bypass graft
  corticosteroid-binding globulin
  cortisol-binding globulin

CBG$_V$ corticosteroid-binding globulin variant

CBH chronic benign hepatitis
  cutaneous basophilic hypersensitivity

CBI Children's Behavior Inventory
  continuous bladder irrigation

CBIL conjugated bilirubin; also CB

CBL circulating blood lymphocytes
  umbilical cord blood leukocytes

Cbl cobalamin

cbl chronic blood loss

CBM capillary basement membrane

CBMMP chronic benign mucous membrane
    pemphigus

CBMT capillary basement membrane thickness

CBMW capillary basement membrane width

CBN cannabinol
  central benign neoplasm
  chronic benign neutropenia
  Commission on Biological Nomenclature

CBOC completion bed occupancy care

Cbo carbobenzoxy; also CB, CBZ, CBz, Cbz

CBP calcium-binding protein; also CaBP
  carbohydrate-binding protein
  chlorobiphenyl(s)
  cobalamin-binding protein

CBPP contagious bovine pleuropneumonia

CBPPA cyclophosphamide, bleomycin, procar-
    bazine, prednisone, and Adriamycin

CBPS coronary bypass surgery

CBR carotid bodies resected
  chemical, bacteriological, and radiological
    (warfare)
  chemical, biological and radiological
  chemically bound residue
  chronic bed rest
  complete bed rest
  crude birth rate

C$_{BR}$ bilirubin clearance

CBS Central Bureau voor Schimmelcultures
  chronic brain syndrome; also ChrBrSyn
  conjugated bile salts
  Cruveilhier-Baumgarten syndrome
  Curschmann-Batten-Steinert (syndrome)

CBT carotid body tumor

cognitive behavior therapy
  computed body tomography

CBV capillary blood flow velocity
  central blood volume
  cerebral blood volume
  circulating blood volume
  corrected blood volume
  Coxsackie B virus
  cyclophosphamide, BCNU (carmustine), and
    Vepesid (etoposide)

CBVD cerebrovascular disease; also CVD

CBW chemical and biological warfare
  critical bandwidth (range of frequencies)

CBX computer-based examination

CBZ carbamazepine; also CARBAM
  carbobenzoxy; also CB, Cbo, CBz, Cbz

CBz carbobenzoxy; also CB, Cbo, CBZ, Cbz

Cbz carbobenzoxy; also CB, Cbo, CBZ, CBz

CC calcaneo-cuboid
  calcium cyclamate
  cardiac catheterization
  cardiac cycle
  cardio-vascular clinic
  carotid-cavernous
  case coordinator
  caval catheterization
  cell culture
  cellular compartment
  central compartment
  cerebral commissure
  cerebral concussion
  cervical collar
  Céstan-Chenais (syndrome)
  chest circumference; also cc
  chief complaint; also C/C
  cholecalciferol
  chondrocalcinosis
  choriocarcinoma; also CCA
  chronic complainer
  ciliated cell
  circulatory collapse
  classical conditioning
  clean catch (urine)
  clinical course
  closing capacity
  coefficient of correlation
  colony count
  colorectal cancer
  column chromatography
  commission-certified (stain)
  complications and comorbidities
  compound cathartic
  computer calculated

CC—cont'd
concave; also Cc, cc
continuing care
contractile component
coracoclavicular
cord compression
coronary collateral
corpus callosum
costo-chondral
Coulter counter
creatinine clearance; also Ccr, ccr, C_{cr}, CrCl
critical care
critical condition
crus cerebri
crus communis
cubic centimeter; also cc, cm^3, c cm, cu cm
culture collection
cup cell
current complaint(s)
cytochrome C
with correction (with glasses) [L. *cum* (with)]

C/C chief complaint; also CC
cholecystectomy and operative cholangiogram
complete upper and lower dentures

C&C cold and clammy
confirmed and compatible

Cc concave; also CC, cc

cc chest circumference; also CC
concave; also CC, Cc
condylocephalic
corrected; also cor, corr
cubic centimeter; also CC, cm^3, c cm, cu cm

c̄ c with meals [L. *cum cibo*]

CCA Career College Association
cephalin cholesterol antigen
chenodeoxycholic acid; also CDA, CDCA
chick-cell agglutination (unit)
chimpanzee coryza agent (respiratory syncytial virus)
choriocarcinoma; also CC
chromated copper arsenic
circumflex coronary artery
colitis colon antigen
common carotid artery
concentrated care area
congenital contractual arachnodactyly
constitutional chromosome abnormality

CCABA cold, cough, allergy, bronchodilator
and antiasthmatic

CCAP capsule cartilage articular preservation
Culture Collection of Algae and Protozoa
(United Kingdom)

CCAT conglutinating complement absorption
test

CCB calcium channel blocker

CCBV central circulating blood volume

CCC calcium cyanamide citrated (carbimide)
Cancer Care Center
care-cure coordination
cathodal closure contraction; also CACC,
CaCC
central counteradaptive changes
child care clinic
chronic calculous cholecystitis
citrated calcium carbimide
Commission on Clinical Chemistry
comprehensive cancer center
comprehensive care clinic
consecutive case conference
continuing community care
covalently closed circular (DNA)
critical care complex

CC&C colony count and culture

CCCC centrifugal counter-current chromatography

CCCL, CCCl cathodal closure clonus

CCCP carbonyl cyanide *m*-chlorophenyl-
hydrazone

CCCR closed-chest cardiac resuscitation
closed-chest cardiopulmonary resuscitation

CCCS condom catheter collecting system

CCCT closed craniocerebral trauma

CCCU comprehensive cardiovascular care unit

CCD calibration curve data
charge-coupled device
childhood celiac disease
cortical collecting duct
countercurrent distribution
cumulative cardiotoxic dose

CCDC Canadian Communicable Disease
Center

CCDN Central Council for District Nursing

CCDPHP Center for Chronic Disease
Prevention and Health Promotion

CCE carboline-carboxylic acid ester
chamois contagious ecthyma
clubbing, cyanosis, and edema
countercurrent electrophoresis; also CEP

CCEI Crown-Crisp Experimental Index

CCF carotid-cavernous fistula
centrifuged culture fluid
cephalin-cholesterol flocculation
compound comminuted fracture

congestive cardiac failure
crystal-induced chemotactic factor

CCFA cycloserine-cefoxitin-fructose agar

CCFE cyclophosphamide, cisplatin, fluorouracil, and estramustine

CCG cholecystogram; also CG

CCGC capillary column gas chromatography

CCGG cytosine-cytosine-guanine-guanine

CCH chronic cholestatic hepatitis

CCh carbamylcholine

CCHD cyanotic congenital heart disease

CCHE Central Council for Health Education

CCHP Consumer Choice Health Plan

CCHS congenital central hypoventilation syndrome

CCI chronic coronary insufficiency
corrected count increment; also CI

CCJ costochondral junction

CCK cholecystokinin; also CK

CCK-8 cholecystokinin octapeptide; also CCK-OP

CCK-GB cholecystokinin-gallbladder (cholecystogram)

CCKLI cholecystokinin-like immunoreactivity

CCK-OP cholecystokinin octapeptide; also CCK-8

CCK-PZ cholecystokinin-pancreozymin; also CK-PZ

CCL carcinoma cell line
cardiac catheterization laboratory
certified cell line
critical carbohydrate level
critical condition list

CCLC chemically crosslinked collagen

CCLI composite clinical and laboratory index

CCM cerebrocostomandibular (syndrome)
congestive cardiomyopathy
contralateral competing message
craniocervical malformation
critical care medicine
cyclophosphamide, CCNU (lomustine), and methotrexate

c cm cubic centimeter; also CC, cc, cm³, cu cm

CCME Coordinating Council on Medical Education

CCMS clean catch midstream (urine)
clinical care management system

CCMSU clean-catch midstream urine

CCMSUA clean-catch midstream urinalysis

CCMT catechol-o-methyltransferase; also CMT, COMT

CCMU critical care medicine unit

CCN caudal central nucleus
coronary care nursing
critical care nursing

CCNS cell-cycle nonspecific (agent)

CCNSC Cancer Chemotherapy National Service Center

CCNU, Ccnu N-(2-chloroethyl)-N'-cyclohexyl-N-nitrosourea (lomustine)

CCNU-OP CCNU, Oncovin, and prednisone

CcO$_2$ pulmonary end-capillary blood oxygen concentration

CCOF chromosomally competent ovarian failure

CCOP CCNU, Oncovin, and prednisone

CCP calcitonin cleavage product
chronic calcifying pancreatitis
ciliocytophthoria
Crippled Children's Program
cytidine cyclic phosphate

CCPD continuous cyclical peritoneal dialysis
continuous cycling peritoneal dialysis
crystalline calcium pyrophosphate dihydrate

CCPDS Centralized Cancer Patient Data System

CCPR crypt cell production rate

CCR cardiac catheterization recovery
complete continuous remission
continuous complete remission

Ccr, ccr, C$_{cr}$ creatinine clearance; also CC, CrCl

CCRC continuing care residential community

CCRN Critical Care Registered Nurse

CCRS carotid chemoreceptor stimulation

CCRU critical care recovery unit

CCS casualty clearing station
cell cycle specific (agent)
cholecystosonography
cloudy cornea syndrome
concentration camp syndrome
costoclavicular syndrome
Crippled Children's Services
Critical Care Services
Cronkhite-Canada syndrome

CC&S cornea, conjuctiva, and sclera

CCSA central chemosensitive area

CCSCS central cervical spinal cord syndrome

CCSG Children's Cancer Study Group

CCT calcitriol
carotid compression tomography
central conduction time
chocolate-coated tablet
closed cerebral trauma
coated compressed tablet
combined cortical thickness
composite cyclic therapy
congenitally corrected transposition (of the great vessels)
controlled cord traction
coronary care team
cranial computed tomography
crude coal tar
cyclocarbothiamine

cct circuit; also cir

CCTe cathodal closure tetanus

CCTGA congenitally corrected transposition of the great arteries

CCT in PET crude coal tar in petroleum

CCTP Coronary Care Training Project

CCTV closed circuit television

CCU cardiac care unit
cardiovascular care unit
Cherry-Crandall unit
community care unit
coronary care unit
critical care unit

CCUA clean catch urinalysis

CCUP colpocystourethropexy

CCV canine coronavirus
CCNU (lomustine), cyclophosphamide, and vincristine
channel catfish virus
conductivity cell volume

CCVB CCNU (lomustine), cyclophosphamide, vincristine, and bleomycin

CCVD chronic cerebrovascular disease

CCVPP CCNU (lomustine), cyclophosphamide, vinblastine, procarbazine, and prednisone

CCW childcare worker
counterclockwise

Ccw chest wall compliance

CCX complications(s); also CM, cm, COMP, compl, complic, Cx

CD cadaver donor
canine distemper
carbohydrate dehydratase
carbon dioxide; also CO_2
cardiac disease

cardiac dullness
cardiac dysrhythmia
cardiovascular deconditioning
cardiovascular disease; also CVD
Carrel-Dakin (fluid)
cat dander (test)
caudad
caudal; also caud, Cd, cd
cefaloridin
celiac disease
cell dissociation
central deposition
cesarean delivered
cesarean delivery
channel down
character disorder
chemical dependency
chemotactic difference
childhood disease(s); also CHD
circular dichroism
civil defense
Clostridium difficile
cluster designation
colloid droplet
combination drug
common duct
communicable disease; also commun dis
communication deviance
communication disorder(s)
compact optical disk
completely denatured
complicated delivery
conduct disorder
conjugate diameter
consanguineous donor
contact dermatitis
contagious disease
continuous drainage
control diet
convulsive disorder
convulsive dose
copying drawings
corneal dystrophy
covert dyskinesia
Crohn's disease
crossed diagonal
curative dose
current diagnosis
cutdown
cystic duct
cytarabine and daunorubicin
Czapek-Dox (agar, solution)
diagonal conjugate diameter of the pelvic inlet [L. *conjugata diagonalis*]
with the right hand [L. *cum dextra*]

C/D cigarettes per day
cup-to-disc ratio

C&D curettage and desiccation
cystoscopy and dilatation

CD$_{50}$ median curative dose

Cd cadmium
caudal; also caud, CD, cd
coccygeal; also cd, COC, Coc, coc
color denial
condylion

^{115}Cd cadmium 115, radioactive cadmium;
halflife, 53.5 hours

cd candela
caudal; also caud, CD, Cd
coccygeal; also Cd, COC, Coc, coc
cord

CDA Certified Dental Assistant
chenodeoxycholic acid; also CCA, CDCA
ciliary dyskinesia activity
complement-dependent antibody
completely denatured alcohol
congenital dyserythropoietic anemia

CDAA chlorodiallylacetamide

CDAI Crohn Disease Activity Index

CDAK Cordis Dow Artificial Kidney

CDAO caudal portion of the dorsal accessory
olive

CDB cough and deep breath; also C&DB

C&DB cough and deep breath; also CDB

CDC calculated date of confinement
cancer detection center
capillary diffusion capacity
carboplatin, doxorubicin, and cyclophosphamide
cardiac diagnostic center
cell division cycle
Centers for Disease Control
chenodeoxycholic (acid)
child development clinic
Communicable Disease Center
complement-dependent cytotoxicity
Crohn's disease of the colon

CD-C controlled drinker-control

CDCA chenodeoxycholic acid; also CCA, CDA

CDC/AIDS Centers for Disease Control definition of acquired immunodeficiency syndrome

CDCF *Clostridium difficile* culture filtrate

CDD certificate of disability for discharge
chronic degenerative disease
chronic disabling dermatosis

critical degree of deformation

CDDP *cis*-diamminedichloroplatinum (cisplatin); also CACP, cis-DDP, *cis*-DDP

CDE antigens in the Rh blood group system
(antigens C, D, and E)
canine distemper encephalitis
Certified Diabetes Educator
chlordiazepoxide; also CDP, CDX, CDZ
common duct exploration

CD-E controlled drinker-experimental

CDF chondrodystrophia fetalis
ciliary dyskinesia factor

cdf cumulative distribution function

CDFR cumulative duration of the first remission

CDG central developmental groove

CDGD constitutional delay in growth and
development

CDGF cartilage-derived growth factor

CDGP constitutional delay of growth and
puberty

CDH ceramide dihexoside
chronic daily headache
chronic disease hospital
congenital diaphragmatic hernia
congenital dislocation of the hip
congenital dysplasia of the hip

CDI cell diabetes insipidus
cell-directed inhibitor
central diabetes insipidus
Children's Depression Inventory
chronic diabetes insipidus
Cotrel-Dubousset instrumentation

CDILD chronic diffuse interstitial lung disease

CDK climatic droplet keratopathy

CDL chlorodeoxylincomycin
Copying Drawings with Landmarks

CDLE chronic discoid lupus erythematosus

CDLS Cornelia de Lange's syndrome

CDM chemically defined medium
clinical decision making

cDNA complementary deoxyribonucleic acid
copy deoxyribonucleic acid

CDP chlordiazepoxide; also CDE, CDX, CDZ
chronic destructive periodontitis
collagenase-digestible protein
constant distending pressure
continuous distending pressure
Coronary Drug Project
cystic disease protein
cytidine diphosphate

CDPC cytidine diphosphate choline
CDPS common duct pigment stones
CDQ corrected development quotient
CDR calcium-dependent regulator
chronologic drinking record
complementarity determining region (of a
protein)
computed digital radiography
continuing disability review
correct delayed reaction
CDRH Center for Devices and Radiological
Health (of the United States Food and Drug
Administration)
CDR(H) cup-to-disc ratio, horizontal
CDRS-R Children's Depression Rating Scale -
Revised
CDR(V) cup-to-disc ratio, vertical
CDS caudal dysplasia syndrome
Chemical Data System
clonidine-displacing substance
cul-de-sac
cumulative duration of survival
cyclodextrine sulphate
cd-sr candela-steradian
CDSS clinical decision support system
CDT carbon dioxide therapy
Certified Dental Technician
combined diphtheria tetanus
CDTe cathode duration tetanus
CDU chemical dependency unit
cumulative dose unit
CDV canine distemper virus
Carr's disease virus
CDX chlordiazepoxide; also CDE, CDP, CDZ
CDYN, Cdyn, cdyn, C$_{dyn}$ dynamic compliance (of lung in pulmonary function test)
CDZ chlordiazepoxide; also CDE, CDP, CDX
CE California encephalitis
Camurati-Engelmann (disease)
cardiac emergency
cardiac enlargement
cardioesophageal (junction); also CEJ
cataract extraction
cell extract
central episiotomy
Charcot-Erb (disease)
chemical energy
chick embryo
chloroform-ether; also C-E
cholera exotoxin
cholesterol ester(s); also CHE, ChE, chol est

cholinesterase; also CEA, CHE, ChE, CHS
chromatoelectrophoresis
clinical emphysema
columnar epithelium
community education
conjugated estrogens
constant error
constant estrus
continuing education
contractile element
contrast echocardiology
converting enzyme
crude extract
cytopathic effect; also CPE
C-E chloroform-ether; also CE
C&E consultation and examination
cough and exercise
curettage and electrodesiccation
Ce cerium
CEA carcinoembryonic antigen
carotid endarterectomy
cholesterol-esterifying activity
cholinesterase; also CE, CHE, ChE, CHS
cost-effectiveness analysis
crystalline egg albumin
CeA central nucleus of the amygdala
CEARP Continuing Education Approval and
Recognition Program
CEB cotton elastic bandage
CEBD controlled extrahepatic biliary drainage
CEBV chronic Epstein-Barr virus
CEC ciliated epithelial cell
contractile electrical complex
CECT contrast enhancement computed tomog-
raphy
CED chondroectodermal dysplasia
chronic enthusiasm disorder
cultural/ethnic diversity
CEE chick embryo extract
CEEC calf esophagus epithelial cell
CEEG computer-analyzed EEG
CEEV Central European encephalitis virus
CEF centrifugation extractable fluid
chick embryo fibroblast; also CHF
constant electric field
CEG chronic erosive gastritis
CEH cholesterol ester hydrolase
CEHC calf embryonic heart cell
CEI character education inquiry
continuous extravascular infusion

converting enzyme inhibitor
corneal epithelial involvement

CEID crossed electroimmunodiffusion

CEJ cardioesophageal junction
cement-enamel junction

CEK chick embryo kidney

CEL cardiac exercise laboratory
Celsius; also C, Cel, Cels

Cel Celsius; also C, CEL, Cels

Cels Celsius; also C, CEL, Cel

Cell celluloid

CELO chicken-embryo-lethal-orphan (virus)

CELOV chick embryonal lethal orphan virus

CEM CCNU (lomustine), etoposide, and
methotrexate
conventional transmission electron microscope

cemf counterelectromotive force

CEN Certificate for Emergency Nursing
Certified Emergency Nurse

cen central; also C, CENT, cent
centromere

CENP centromere protein

CENT, cent centigrade; also C
centimeter; also cm
central; also C, cen

CEO chick embryo origin
chloroethylene oxide

CEOT calcifying epithelial odontogenic tumor

CEP CCNU (lomustine), etoposide, and pred-
nimustine
chronic eosinophilic pneumonia
chronic erythropoietic porphyria
cognitive evoked potential
congenital erythropoietic porphyria
continuing education program
cortical evoked potential
countercurrent electrophoresis
counterelectrophoresis; also CCE
counterimmunoelectrophoresis; also CIE, CIEP

CEPA chloroethane phosphoric acid
couple electron pair approximation

CEPB Carpentier-Edwards porcine bioprostheses

CEPH, ceph cephalic
cephalin
cephalosporin

CEPH FLOC, ceph-floc cephalin flocculation
(test)

CEPT cyclophosphamide, Efudex (fluorouracil), prednisone, and tamoxifen

CEQ Council on Environmental Quality

CER capital expenditure review
ceramide; also Cer
ceruloplasmin; also CERULO, CP, Cp
conditioned emotional response
conditioned escape response
control electrical rhythm
cortical evoked response

CE&R central episiotomy and repair

Cer ceramide; also CER

CERA cardiac evoked response audiometry

cerat wax ointment [L. *ceratum*]

CERD chronic end-stage renal disease

CERP Continuing Education Recognition
Program

Cert, cert certificate; also CTF
certified; also C, CRT

CERULO ceruloplasmin; also CER, CP, Cp

CERV, cerv cervical
cervix; also CX, Cx

CES cat's-eye syndrome
central excitatory state; also ces
chronic electrophysiological study
cognitive environmental stimulation

ces central excitatory state; also CES

CESD cholesterol ester storage disease

CES-D Center for Epidemiologic Studies
depression scale

CET capital expenditure threshold
cephalothin; also CF
congenital eyelid tetrad
controlled environment treatment

CETE Central European tick-borne encephalitis

CETP cholesteryl ester transfer protein

CEU congenital ectropion uvea
continuing education unit

CEV citrus exocortis viroid
cyclophosphamide, etoposide, and vincristine

CEVD CCNU (lomustine), etoposide, vindesine, and dexamethasone

CEZ cefazolin; also CZ

CF antibody titer (complement fixation)
calf blood flow
calibration factor
cancer-free
carbol-fuchsin (stain)
carboxyfluorescein
cardiac failure
carotid foramen

CF—cont'd
carrier-free
cascade filtration
case file
Caucasian female
cephalothin; also CET
characteristic frequency
chemotactic factor
chest and left leg (foot) (lead in electrocardiography)
Chiari-Frommel (syndrome)
chick fibroblast
choroid fissure
Christmas factor
cisplatin and fluorouracil
citrovorum factor (calcium leucovorin)
clastogenic factor
climbing fiber
clotting factor
colicin factor
collected fluid
colonization factor
colony-forming
color and form
column of fornix
compare [L. *confer* (compare, bring together)]; also cf, *cf*, comp, cp
complement fixation; also CMP-FX, com fix
complement fixing; also C′F
completely follicular
constant frequency
contractile force
coronary flow
cough frequency
count fingers (visual acuity test); also C/F, cf
coupling factor
crystal field
cycling fibroblast
cystic fibrosis; also C/F
cytolytic factor

C′F complement fixing; also CF

C/F colored female
count fingers (visual acuity test); also CF, cf
cystic fibrosis; also CF

C&F cell and flare
curettage and fulguration

CFII Cohn fraction II

Cf californium
carrier of iron [L. *ferrum* (iron)]

cf bring together [L. *confer* (compare, bring together)]; also CF, *cf*, cp
centrifugal force

compare [L. *confer* (compare, bring together)]; also CF, *cf*, comp, cp
count fingers (visual acuity test); also CF, C/F

cf compare [L. *confer* (compare, bring together)]; also CF, cf, comp, cp

CFA clofibric acid
colonization factor antigen
colony-forming assay
common femoral artery
complement-fixing antibody
complete Freund's adjuvant
cryptogenic fibrosing alveolitis

CFAC complement-fixing antibody consumption

C-factor cleverness factor

CFB central fibrous body

CFC capillary filtration coefficient
chlorofluorocarbon(s)
colony-forming capacity
colony-forming cells
continuous flow centrifugation

CFCL continuous flow centrifugation leukapheresis

CFC-S colony-forming cells–spleen

CFD cephalofacial deformity
craniofacial dysostosis

CFE carrageenan-induced foot edema

CFF critical flicker frequency
critical flicker fusion; also cff
critical fusion frequency; also cff
cystic fibrosis factor
Cystic Fibrosis Foundation

cff critical flicker fusion; also CFF
critical fusion frequency; also CFF

CFFA cystic fibrosis factor activity

Cf-Fe carrier-bound iron (ferrum)

CFH Council on Family Health

CFI cardiac function index
chemotactic-factor inactivator
complement fixation inhibition
confrontation fields intact

CFL cisplatin, fluorouracil, and leucovorin calcium

CFM chlorofluoromethane
close-fitting mask
craniofacial microsomia
cyclophosphamide, fluorouracil, and mitoxantrone

cfm cubic feet per minute

CFMG Commission on Foreign Medical Graduates

CFNS chills, fever, and night sweats

CFO chief financial officer

CFP chronic false positive
Clinical Fellowship Program
cyclophosphamide, fluorouracil, and prednisone
cystic fibrosis of pancreas
cystic fibrosis patients
cystic fibrosis protein

CFPD critical frequency of photic driving

CFPMV cyclophosphamide, fluorouracil, prednisone, methotrexate, and vincristine

CFPT cyclophosphamide, fluorouracil, prednisone, and tamoxifen

CFR case-fatality ratio
citrovorum-factor rescue
Code of Federal Regulations
complement-fixation reaction
correct fast reaction
cyclic flow reduction

CFS call for service
cancer family syndrome
chronic fatigue syndrome
contoured femoral stem
craniofaciostenosis
crush fracture syndrome
Cystic Fibrosis Society

cfs cubic feet per second

CFSE crystal field stabilization energy

CFSTI Clearinghouse for Federal Scientific and Technical Information

CFT cardiolipin flocculation test
clinical full-time
complement fixation test
complement-fixing titer

CFU colony-forming unit

CFU-C colony-forming unit – culture

CFU-E colony-forming unit – erythroid

CFU$_{EOS}$ colony-forming unit – eosinophil

CFU-F colony-forming unit – fibroblastoid

CFU$_{GM}$ colony-forming unit – granulocyte macrophage

CFU$_L$ colony-forming unit – lymphoid

CFU$_M$ colony-forming unit – megakaryocyte; also CFU$_{MEG}$

CFU$_{MEG}$ colony-forming unit – megakaryocyte; also CFU$_M$

CFU/mL colony-forming units/mL

CFU$_{NM}$ colony-forming unit – neutrophil-monocyte

CFU-S, CFU$_S$ colony-forming unit – spleen
colony-forming unit – stem (cell)

CFW cancer-free white (mouse)
Carworth farm (mouse), Webster strain

CFWM cancer-free white mouse

CFX cefoxitin
circumflex (coronary artery); also Cx

CFZ capillary-free zone

CFZC continuous-flow zonal centrifugation

CG calcium gluconate; also CaG
cardio-green
Ceelen-Gellerstedt (syndrome)
center of gravity; also cg
central gray
choking gas (phosgene)
cholecystogram; also CCG
cholecystography
choriogenic gynecomastia
chorionic gonadotropin; also CGT
chronic glomerulonephritis; also CGN, Ch Gn
cingulate gyrus
colloidal gold
contact guarding
control group
cryoglobulin; also cryo
cystine guanine

cg center of gravity; also CG
centigram; also cgm
chemoglobulin

CGA catabolite gene activator
chromogranin-A

CGAS Children's Global Assessment Scale

CGB chronic gastrointestinal bleeding

CGC Certified Gastrointestinal Clinician

CGD chromosomal gonadal dysgenesis
chronic granulomatous disease

CGDE contact glow discharge electrolysis

CGFH congenital fibrous histiocytoma

CGFNS Commission on Graduates of Foreign Nursing Schools

CGH chorionic gonadotropic hormone

CGI chronic granulomatous inflammation
Clinical Global Impression (Scale); also cgi

cgi Clinical Global Impression (Scale); also CGI

CGL chronic granulocytic leukemia
correction with glasses; also c gl

c gl correction with glasses; also CGL

CGM central gray matter (spinal cord)

cgm centigram; also cg

CGMMV cucumber green mottle mosaic virus

cGMP cyclic guanosine monophosphate; also cyclic GMP

CGN chronic glomerulonephritis; also CG, Ch Gn
Convalescent Growing Nursery

CGNA Canadian Gerontological Nursing Association

CGNB composite ganglioneuroblastoma

CG/OQ cerebral glucose-oxygen quotient

CGP choline glycerophosphatide
chorionic growth hormone prolactin
circulating granulocyte pool
N-carbobenzoyl-glycyl-L-phenylalanine

CGPM General Conference on Weights and Measures [Fr. *Conférence Générale des Poids et Mesures*]

CGPF cell-growth potentiating factor

CGRP calcitonin gene-related peptide

CGS cardiogenic shock; also CS
catgut suture
centimeter-gram-second (system); also cgs

cgs centimeter-gram-second (system); also CGS

CGT chorionic gonadotropin; also CG
cyclodextrin glucanotransferase
cyclodextrin glycosyltransferase
N-carbobenzoyl-α-glutamyl-L-tryosine

CGTT cortisol glucose tolerance test
cortisone glucose tolerance test

cGy centigray

CH case history
casein hydrolysate
Chang liver (cell culture)
Chédiak-Higashi (syndrome)
child; also Ch, ch
children; also Ch, ch
Chinese hamster
chloral hydrate
cholesterol; also C, Ch, CHO, CHOL, Chol, chol
Christchurch chromosome; also Ch¹, ch¹
chronic hepatitis
chronic hypertension
Clarke-Hadfield (syndrome)
cluster headache
common hepatic (duct)
communicating hydrocele
Community Health
Community Hospital

complete healing
congenital hypothyroidism
Conradi-Hünermann (syndrome)
continuous heparinization
convalescent hospital; also CONV HOSP
crown-heel (length of fetus)
cycloheximide
hemolytic complement
wheelchair

C$_H$ constant region of an immunoglobulin H (heavy) chain

C&H cocaine and heroin

CH50, CH$_{50}$ total serum hemolytic complement

Ch chapter
chest; also ch
Chido (antibody)
chief; also ch
child; also CH, ch
children; also CH, ch
cholesterol; also C, CH, CHO, CHOL, Chol, chol
choline; also ch
chromosome; also chr
surgery [L. *chirurgiae*]

Ch¹, ch¹ Christchurch chromosome; also CH

cH hydrogen ion concentration

ch chest; also Ch
chief; also Ch
child; also CH, Ch
children; also CH, Ch
choline; also Ch
chronic; also chr, chron

CHA Catholic Hospital Association (now: Catholic Health Association of the United States)
chronic hemolytic anemia
common hepatic artery
congenital hypoplastic anemia
continuous heated aerosols
cyclohexyladenosine
cyclohexylamine

ChA choline acetylase

CHAC cyclophosphamide, hexamethylmelamine, Adriamycin, and carboplatin

ChAc choline acetyltransferase; also CAT, ChAct, CHAT, ChaT

ChAct choline acetyltransferase; also CAT, ChAc, CHAT, ChaT

CHAD cyclophosphamide, hexamethymelamine, Adriamycin, and *cis*-diamminedichloroplatinum (cisplatin)

CHAI continuous hepatic artery infusion

CHAID chi-square automatic interaction detection

CHAL chromic haloperidol

CHAMOCA, CHAM-OCA cyclophosphamide, hydroxyurea, actinomycin D, methotrexate, Oncovin, citrovorum factor (calcium leucovorin), and Adriamycin

CHAMPUS Civilian Health and Medical Program of Uniformed Services

CHAMPVA Civilian Health and Medical Program of Veterans Administration

Chang C Chang conjunctiva cells

Chang L Chang liver cells

CHAP Certified Hospital Admission Program
Child Health Assessment Program
cyclophosphamide, hexamethylmelamine, Adriamycin, and Platinol

CHAP-5 cyclophosphamide, hexamethylmelamine, Adriamycin, Platinol and 5-fluorouracil

CHARGE coloboma, heart disease, atresia choanae, retarded growth and retarded development and/or CNS anomalies, genital hypoplasia, and ear anomalies and/or deafness (syndrome)

chart paper [L. *charta*]

chart cerat waxed paper, parchment paper [L. *charta cerata*]

CHAS Center for Health Administration Studies

CHAT, ChaT choline acetyltransferase; also CAT, ChAc, ChAct

CHB complete heart block
congenital heart block

ChB Bachelor of Surgery [L. *Chirurgiae Baccalaureus*]; also BC, BCh, BS, CB

CHBHA congenital Heinz body hemolytic anemia

CHC community health center
community health council

CHCP correctional health care program

CHD center hemodialysis
Chédiak-Higashi disease
childhood disease(s); also CD
chronic hemodialysis
common hepatic duct
congenital heart disease
congenital hip disease
congenital hip dysplasia

congestive heart disease
constitutional hepatic dysfunction
coordinate home care
coronary heart disease
cyanotic heart disease
cyclophosphamide, hexamethylmelamine, and *cis*-diamminedichloroplatinum (cisplatin)

ChD Doctor of Surgery [L. *Chirurgiae Doctor*]; also Chir Doct

CHE, ChE cholesterol ester(s); also CE, chol est
cholinesterase; also CE, CEA, CHS

CHEC Community Hypertension Evaluation Clinic

CHEF Chinese hamster embryo fibroblast

Chem chemical; also chem
chemistry; also chem
chemotherapy; also chemo, ChemoRx, CT

chem chemical; also Chem
chemistry; also Chem

CHEMLINE Chemical Dictionary On-Line

chemo chemotherapy; also Chem, ChemoRx, CT

ChemoRx chemotherapy; also Chem, chemo, CT

CHEP Cuban/Haitian Entrant Program

CHERSS continuous high-amplitude electroencephalogram rhythmical synchronous slowing

CHEST Chick Embryotoxicity Screening Test

CHF chick embryo fibroblast; also CEF
chronic heart failure
congenital hepatic fibrosis
congestive heart failure
Crimean hemorrhagic fever
cyclophosphamide, hexamethylmelamine, and 5-fluorouracil

CHFV combined high-frequency ventilation

CHG, chg change
changed

Ch Gn chronic glomerulonephritis; also CG, CGN

CHH cartilage-hair hypoplasia

CHI chalcone isomerase
closed head injury
creatinine-height index

CHILD congenital hemidysplasia with ichthyosiform erythroderma and limb defects (syndrome)

CHINA chronic infectious neuropathic agent
chronic infectious neurotropic agent

CHINS child in need of service (petition)

CHIP comprehensive health insurance plan
comprehensive hospital infections project

Chir Doct Doctor of Surgery [L. *Chirurgiae Doctor*]; also ChD

chirurg surgical [L. *chirurgicalis*]

Chix chickenpox; also CHPX, chpx, Cp

CHL Chinese hamster lung
chlorambucil; also CB, Chl, CLB
chloramphenicol; also C, CAP, chloro, CMC, CP

Chl chlorambucil; also CB, CHL, CLB
chloroform; also chl, chlor

chl chloroform; also Chl, chlor

CHLA cyclohexyllinoleic acid

Chlb chlorobutanol

CHLD chronic hypoxic lung disease

chlor chloride; also Cl, CR
chloroform; also Chl, chl

chloro chloramphenicol; also C, CAP, CHL, CMC, CP

ChlVPP chlorambucil, vinblastine, procarbazine, and prednisone; also C1VPP

ChM Master of Surgery [L. *Chirurgiae Magister*]; also CM

CHMD clinical hyaline membrane disease

CHN carbon, hydrogen, and nitrogen
central hemorrhagic necrosis
Certified Hemodialysis Nurse
Child Neurology
Chinese (hamster)
community health network

CHO carbohydrate; also C, CARB, carb, carbo, COH
Chinese hamster ovary
cholesterol; also C, CH, Ch, CHOL, Chol, chol
chorea
cyclophosphamide, hydroxydaunomycin, and Oncovin

C_{H2O} water clearance

Cho choline

CHOB cyclophosphamide, hydroxydaunomycin, Oncovin, and bleomycin

choc chocolate

CHOI considered characteristic of osteogenesis imperfecta

CHOL, Chol, chol cholesterol; also C, CH, Ch, CHO

c̄hold withhold

Chole cholecystectomy

chol est cholesterol ester(s); also CE, CHE, ChE

CHOP cyclophosphamide, hydroxydaunomycin, Oncovin, and prednisone

CHOP-B cyclophosphamide, hydroxydaunomycin, Oncovin, prednisone, and bleomycin; also CHOP-BLEO

CHOP-BLEO cyclophosphamide, hydroxydaunomycin, Oncovin, prednisone, and bleomycin; also CHOP-B

CHOR cyclophosphamide, hydroxydaunomycin, Oncovin, and radiation

chord chirurg surgical "catgut" [L. *chorda chirurgicalis*]

CHP capillary hydrostatic pressure
charcoal hemoperfusion
child psychiatry; also CP
comprehensive health planning
coordinating hospital physician
cutaneous hepatic porphyria

ChP chest physician

CHPX, chpx chickenpox; also Chix, Cp

CHQ chlorquinol

CHR Cercarien-Hüllen-Reaktion (test) [Ger. *Reaktion* (reaction)]

Chr *Chromobacterium* species

chr chromosome; also Ch
chronic; also ch, chron

c hr candle hour

c-hr curie-hour; also Ci-hr, ci-hr

ChRBC chicken red blood cell; also CRBC

ChrBrSyn chronic brain syndrome; also CBS

CHRIS Cancer Hazards Ranking and Information System

chron chronic; also ch, chr
chronological

CHRS cerebrohepatorenal syndrome (Zellweger syndrome)
congenital hereditary retinoschisis

CHS central hypoventilation syndrome
Chédiak-Higashi syndrome
cholinesterase; also CE, CEA, CHE, ChE
chondroitin sulfate; also CS
chondroitin sulfuric acid
compression hip screw
contact hypersensitivity

CHSD Children's Health Services Division

CHSS cooperative health statistics system

CHT closed head trauma

contralateral head turning

ChTg chymotrypsinogen; also CTG

ChTK chicken thymidine kinase

CHU closed head unit

CHV canine herpes virus

CI cardiac index
cardiac insufficiency
cell immunity
cell inhibition
cellular immunity
cephalic index
cerebral infarction
cesium implant
chain initiating
chemical ionization
chemotactic index
chemotherapeutic index
chromatid interchange
chronically infected
clinical impression
clinical investigation
clinical investigator
clomipramine
clonus index
closure index
cochlear implant
coefficient of intelligence
colloidal iron
colony inhibition
color index
Colour Index (British)
complete iridectomy
compliance index
confidence interval
configuration interaction
contamination index
continuous infusion
coronary insufficiency
corrected count increment; also CCI
crystalline insulin
cytotoxic index

C-I - C-V DEA (Drug Enforcement
Administration) controlled substances,
schedules I through V

CI – CXII, C$_I$ – C$_{XII}$ cranial nerves I through
XII; also CNI – CNXII

Ci curie; also C, c, CU, cu

CIA canine inherited ataxia
chronic idiopathic anhidrosis
chymotrypsin inhibitor activity
colony-inhibiting activity

CIAA competitive insulin autoantibodies

CIAED collagen-induced autoimmune ear disease

CIB crying-induced bronchospasm; also cib
Current Intelligence Bulletin
cytomegalic inclusion bodies; also CMB
food [L. *cibus*]; also Cib, cib

Cib food [L. *cibus*]; also CIB, cib

cib crying-induced bronchospasm; also CIB
food [L. *cibus*]; also CIB, Cib

CIBD chronic inflammatory bowel disease

CIBHA congenital inclusion-body hemolytic
anemia

CIBP chronic intractable benign pain

CIC cardioinhibitor center
Certified Infection Control
circulating immune complex
constant initial concentration
coronary intensive care

CICA cervical internal carotid artery

CICC circulating immune complex content

CICE combined intracapsular cataract extraction

CICU cardiac intensive care unit
cardiovascular inpatient care unit
coronary intensive care unit

CID Central Institute for the Deaf
central integrative deficit
cervical immobilization device
chick infective dose
combined immunodeficiency disease
cytomegalic inclusion disease; also CMID

CIDEP chemically induced dynamic electron
polarization

CIDNP chemically induced dynamic nuclear
polarization

CIDP chronic inflammatory demyelinating
polyradioneuropathy

CIDS cellular immunodeficiency syndrome
continuous insulin delivery system

CIE countercurrent immunoelectrophoresis
counterimmunoelectrophoresis; also CEP,
CIEP
crossed immunoelectrophoresis; also CIEP

CIEA continuous infusion epidural analgesia

CIEBM Committee on the Interplay of
Engineering with Biology and Medicine

CIE-C counterimmunoelectrophoresis–colorimetric

CIE-D counterimmunoelectrophoresis–densito-
metric

CIEP counterimmunoelectrophoresis; also CEP, CIE
crossed immunoelectrophoresis; also CIE

CIF cartilage induction factor
claims inquiry form
cloning inhibitory factor; also CLIF

CIFC Council for the Investigation of Fertility Control

CIG cigarettes; also cig, cigs
cold-insoluble globulin

CIg intracytoplasmic immunoglobulin

cig cigarettes; also CIG, cigs

cigs cigarettes; also CIG, cig

cIgM cytoplasmic immunoglobulin M

CIH carbohydrate-induced hyperglyceridemia
Certificate in Industrial Health
children in hospital

CIHD chronic ischemic heart disease

Ci-hr, ci-hr curie-hour; also c-hr

CII Carnegie Interest Inventory

CIIA common internal iliac artery

CIIPS chronic idiopathic intestinal pseudo-obstruction syndrome

CIIS Cattell's Infant Intelligence Scale

CIL Center for Independent Living

CIM cimetidine
cortical induction of movement
cortically induced movement
Cumulated Index Medicus

Ci/mL curies per milliliter

CIMS chemical ionization mass spectrometry
clinical information scale
Conflict in Marriage Scale

CIN cefsulodin-irgasan-novobiocin (agar)
cerebriform intradermal nevus
cervical intraepithelial neoplasia
chronic interstitial nephritis
cinoxacin

C_{IN}, C_{in} inulin clearance

CIN 1 cervical intraepithelial neoplasia, grade 1; also CIN I

CIN 2 cervical intraepithelial neoplasia, grade 2; also CIN II

CIN 3 cervical intraepithelial neoplasia, grade 3; also CIN III

CINE chemotherapy-induced nausea and emesis
cineangiogram

C1 INH C1 esterase inhibitor

CIN I cervical intraepithelial neoplasia, grade 1; also CIN 1

CIN II cervical intraepithelial neoplasia, grade 2; also CIN 2

CIN III cervical intraepithelial neoplasia, grade 3; also CIN 3

CIOMS Council for International Organizations of Medical Sciences

CIOP chromosomally incompetent ovarian failure

CIP Carcinogen Information Program
Cardiac Injury Panel
cellular immunocompetence profile
chronic idiopathic polyradiculoneuropathy
chronic inflammatory polyneuropathy; also CIPN

CIPD chronic inflammatory polyradiculoneuropathy, demyelinating
chronic intermittent peritoneal dialysis

CIPF clinical illness promotion factor

CIPN chronic inflammatory polyneuropathy; also CIP

cir circuit; also cct
circular
circumference; also Circ, circ

Circ, circ circulation
circumcision; also circum
circumference; also cir

circ & sen circulation and sensation

circum circumcision; also Circ, circ

CIRR cirrhosis

CIS carcinoma in situ
catheter-induced spasm
central inhibitory state
Chemical Information Service
clinical information system

CI-S calculus index, simplified

CiS cingulate sulcus

CISCA cisplatin, cyclophosphamide, and Adriamycin

cis-DDP, *cis*-DDP *cis*-diamminedichloro-platinum (cisplatin); also CACP, CDDP

CIT citrate; also cit
combined intermittent therapy
conjugated-immunoglobulin technique
conventional immunosuppressive therapy
conventional insulin therapy

cit citrate; also CIT

cit disp let it be dispensed quickly [L. *cito dispensetur*]; also cito disp

cito quickly [L. *cito*]

cito disp let it be dispensed quickly [L. *cito dispensetur*]; also cit disp

CIU chronic idiopathic urticaria

CIV Chilo iridescent virus
common iliac vein
continuous intravenous (infusion)

CIVII continuous intravenous insulin infusion

CIXU constant infusion excretory urogram

CJ Creutzfeldt-Jakob (disease)

CJD Creutzfeldt-Jakob disease

CJR centric jaw relationship

CJS Creutzfeldt-Jakob syndrome

CK calf kidney
check; also ck
checked; also ck
chicken kidney
cholecystokinin; also CCK
choline kinase
contralateral knee; also ck
creatine kinase
cyanogen chloride

CK₁, CK₂, CK₃ isoenzymes of creatine kinase

ck check; also CK
checked; also CK
contralateral knee; also CK

CK-BB creatine kinase BB band (isoenzyme of creatine kinase with brain subunits)

CKC cold-knife conization

CKG cardiokymograph
cardiokymography

C/kg coulombs per kilogram

CK-ISO creatine kinase isoenzyme

CK-MB creatine kinase MB band (isoenzyme of creatine kinase with muscle and brain subunits)

CK-MM creatine kinase MM band (isoenzyme of creatine kinase with muscle subunits)

CK-PZ cholecystokinin-pancreozymin; also CCK-PZ

CKW clockwise; also CW, cw

CL capacity of the lung
capillary lumen
cardinal ligament
cardiolipin
ceiling level
cell line
center line
centralis lateralis
chemiluminescence

chest and left arm (lead in electrocardiography)
cholelithiasis
cholesterol-lecithin
chronic leukemia
cirrhosis of liver
clamp lamp
clear liquid; also cl liq
cleft lip
clinical laboratory
cloudy; also cl, cldy
complex loading
compliance of the lungs; also C_L
composite lymphoma
confidence level
contact lenses
continence line
corpus luteum; also cl
cricoid lamina
criterion level
critical list
current liabilities
cutis laxa
cycle length
cytotoxic lymphocyte

CL1 - CL5 Papanicolaou classes 1 through 5

C-L consultation-liaison (psychiatry)

C_L compliance of the lungs; also CL
constant region of an immunoglobulin L (light) chain

Cl chloride; also chlor, CR
chlorine
clavicle; also cl, CLAV, clav
clear; also C, cl, cler
clinic; also cl, Clin, clin
clonus; also C
Clostridium; also *C, Cl*, Clostr
closure; also C, cl
colistin; also CS

Cl *Clostridium* species; also *C*, Cl, Clostr

cL centiliter; also cl

cl centiliter; also cL
clavicle; also Cl, CLAV, clav
clear; also C, Cl, cler
cleft
clinic; also Cl, Clin, clin
closure; also C, Cl
cloudy; also CL, cldy
corpus luteum; also CL

CLA Certified Laboratory Assistant
cervicolinguoaxial
common leukocyte antigen
community living arrangements

CLA—cont'd
  contralateral local anesthesia
  cyclic lysine anhydride
CLAH congenital lipoid adrenal hyperplasia
C lam cervical laminectomy
CLAS congenital localized absence of skin
class classification
CLAV, clav clavicle; also Cl, cl
CLB chlorambucil; also CB, CHL, Chl
  curvilinear body
CLBBB complete left bundle branch block
CLC Charcot-Leyden crystal
  cork, leather, and celastic (orthotic)
CL/CP cleft lip and cleft palate
CLD central language disorder
  chronic liver disease
  chronic lung disease
  congenital limb deficiency
  crystal ligand field
cld cleared
  colored; also COL, Col, col
CLDH choline dehydrogenase
CLDM clindamycin
cldy cloudy; also CL, cl
CLE centrilobular emphysema
  continuous lumbar epidural (anesthesia)
CLEC chiral ligand exchange chromatography
CLED cystine lactose-electrolyte-deficient
  (agar)
cler clear; also C, Cl, cl
CLF cardiolipin fluorescence (antibody)
  cholesterol-lecithin flocculation
CLH chronic lobular hepatitis
  cutaneous lymphoid hyperplasia
ClHgBzO chloromercuribenzoate; also CMB
CLI corpus luteum insufficiency
CLIA Clinical Laboratories Improvement Act
CLIF cloning inhibitory factor; also CIF
  Crithidia luciliae immunofluorescence
Clin, clin clinic; also Cl, cl
  clinical
Clin Path clinical pathology; also CIP, CP
Clin Proc clinical procedure(s)
CLINPROT Clinical Cancer Protocols
CLIP cerebral lipidosis (without visceral
  involvement and with onset of disease past
  infancy)
  corticotropin-like intermediate lobe peptide

CLL cholesterol-lowering lipid
  chronic lymphatic leukemia
  chronic lymphocytic leukemia
  cow lung lavage
CLLE columnar-lined lower esophagus
cl liq clear liquid; also CL
CLMA Clinical Laboratory Management
  Association
CLML Current List of Medical Literature
CLMN complete lower motor neuron (lesion)
clmp clumped
CLMV cauliflower mosaic virus; also CaMV
CLN cervical lymph node
  computer liaison nurse
CLO cod liver oil
CLOF clofibrate
C-loop anatomical position (shape) of duode-
  num
Clostr Clostridium; also *C*, Cl, *Cl*
CLOT R clot retraction; also CR
CLP chymotrypsin-like protein
  cleft lip with cleft palate; also CL&P
  cycle length, paced
CL&P cleft lip and palate; also CLP
ClP clinical pathology; also CP, Clin Path
Clpal cleft palate; also CP
CLQ cognitive laterality quotient
CLR cerebellar ataxia
CLRO community leave for reorientation
CLS Clinical Laboratory Scientist
  confused language syndrome
CLSH corpus luteum stimulating hormone
CLSL chronic lymphosarcoma cell leukemia
CLSP clinical laboratory specialist
CLT Certified Laboratory Technician
  chronic lymphocytic thyroiditis
  Clinical Laboratory Technician
  Clinical Laboratory Technologist
  clot lysis time
  clotting time
ClT total plasma clearance
CLV constant linear velocity
CL VOID clean voided specimen (urine); also
  CVS
ClVPP chlorambucil, vinblastine, procarbazine,
  and prednisone; also Ch1VPP
CLX cloxacillin; also CX
clysis hypodermoclysis

CM California mastitis (test)
  calmodulin
  capreomycin
  carboxymethyl (cellulose)
  cardiac monitor
  cardiac muscle
  cardiomyopathy; also CMP
  Caucasian male
  cell membrane
  center of mass
  centrum medianum
  cerebral mantle
  cervical mucus
  chemotactic migration
  Chick-Martin (coefficient)
  chloroquine-mepacrine
  chondromalacia
  chopped meat (medium)
  chylomicron
  circular muscle
  circulating monocyte
  clinical medicine
  coccidioidal meningitis
  cochlear microphonic(s)
  common migraine
  community meeting
  competing message
  complete medium
  complication(s); also CCX, cm, COMP,
    compl, complic, Cx
  conditioned medium
  congenital malformation
  congestive myocardiopathy
  continuous murmur
  contrast medium
  copulatory mechanism
  costal margin; also cm
  cow's milk
  culture medium
  cystic mesothelioma
  cytometry
  cytoplasmic membrane
  Master of Surgery [L. *Chirurgiae Magister*];
    also ChM
  narrow-diameter endosseous screw implant
    [Fr. *crête manche*]
  tomorrow morning [L. *cras mane*]; also cm

C/M counts per minute; also CPM, cpm

C&M cocaine and morphine

Cm curium
  maximal clearance; also C_m

C_m maximal clearance; also Cm

cM centimorgan; also cMO, cMo

cm centimeter; also CENT, cent
  complication(s); also CCX, CM, COMP,
    compl, complic, Cx
  costal margin; also CM
  tomorrow morning [L. *cras mane*]; also CM

cm^2 square centimeter

cm^3 cubic centimeter; also CC, cc, c cm, cu cm

CMA California Medical Association
  Canadian Medical Association
  Candida metabolic antigen
  Certified Medical Assistant
  Chemical Manufacturers Association
  Chinese Medical Association
  chronic metabolic acidosis
  compound myopic astigmatism
  cow's milk allergy
  cultured macrophages

CMAF centrifuged microaggregate filter

c magnum tablespoonful [L. *cochleare magnum*]; also cochl mag

CMAJ Canadian Medical Association Journal

CMAmg corticomedial amygdaloid (nucleus)

CMAP compound motor action potential
  compound muscle action potential

CMB carbolic methylene blue
  Central Midwives' Board
  chloromercuribenzoate; also C1HgBzO
  cytomegalic inclusion bodies; also CIB

p-CMB *para*-chloromercuribenzoate

CMBBT cervical mucous basal body temperature

CMC carboxymethylcellulose
  care management continuity
  carpometacarpal
  cell-mediated cytolysis
  cell-mediated cytotoxicity
  chloramphenicol; also C, CAP, CHL, chloro, CP
  Chloromycetin
  chronic mucocutaneous candidiasis; also CMCC
  critical micellar concentration; also cmc
  cyclophosphamide, methotrexate, and CCNU (lomustine)

cmc critical micellar concentration; also CMC

CMCC chronic mucocutaneous candidiasis; also CMC

CMCt care management continuity (across settings)

CMD cerebromacular degeneration
  childhood muscular dystrophy

CMD —cont'd
  congenital muscular dystrophy
  count median diameter (of particles)
  Current Medical Dialog
  cytomegalic disease
CMDS Christian Medical & Dental Society
CME cervical mediastinal exploration
  cervical mucous extract
  continuing medical education
  Council on Medical Education
  crude marijuana extract
  cystic macular edema
  cystoid macular edema
CMER current medical evidence of record
CMF calcium-magnesium free
  catabolite modular factor
  chondromyxoid fibroma
  cortical magnification factor
  craniomandibulofacial
  cyclophosphamide, methotrexate, and
    fluorouracil
CMFE calcium and magnesium free plus
    ethylenediaminetetraacetic acid (EDTA)
CMFH cyclophosphamide, methotrexate,
    fluorouracil, and hydroxyurea
CMFP cyclophosphamide, methotrexate,
    fluorouracil, and prednisone
CMF-TAM cyclophosphamide, methotrexate,
    fluorouracil, and tamoxifen
CMFV cyclophosphamide, methotrexate,
    fluorouracil, and vincristine
CMFVP cyclophosphamide, methotrexate,
    fluorouracil, vincristine, and prednisone
CMG canine myasthenia gravis
  chopped meat glucose (medium)
  compressed medical gas
  congenital myasthenia gravis
  cyanmethemoglobin
  cystometrogram
  cystometrography
CMGN chronic membranous glomerulo-
    nephritis
CMGS chopped meat-glucose-starch (medium)
CMGT chromosome-mediated gene transfer
CMH congenital malformation of the heart
CMHC Community Mental Health Center
CMHN Community Mental Health Nurse
cmH₂O centimeters of water (cuff pressure)

cmH_2O centimeters of water (cuff pressure)
CMI carbohydrate metabolism index
  care management integration
  cell-mediated immunity

cell multiplication inhibition
  chronically mentally ill
  chronic mesenteric ischemia
  circulating microemboli index
  Commonwealth Mycological Institute
  computerized medical information
  computer-managed instruction
  Cornell Medical Index
CMI-CC Culture Collection of the
    Commonwealth Mycological Institute
CMID cytomegalic inclusion disease; also CID
c/min cycles per minute; also cpm
CMIR cell-mediated immune response
CMIT Current Medical Information and
    Terminology
CMJ carpometacarpal joint
CMK chloromethyl ketone
  congenital multicystic kidney
CML cell-mediated lymphocytotoxicity
  cell-mediated lympholysis
  cell-mediated lysis
  chronic myelocytic leukemia
  chronic myelogenous leukemia
  chronic myeloid leukemia
  count median length
  cross midline
CML-BC chronic myeloid leukemia in blast
    crisis
CMM cell-mediated mutagenesis
  cutaneous malignant melanoma
cmm, c mm cubic millimeter; also cu mm,
    mm^3
cm/m² centimeters per square meter
CMME chloromethyl methyl ether
CMML chronic myelomonocytic leukemia
CMN caudal mediastinal node
  cystic medial necrosis
CMN-AA cystic medial necrosis of the ascend-
    ing aorta
CMO calculated mean organism
  canonical molecular orbital (method)
  cardiac minute output
  card made out
  Chief Medical Officer
  comfort measures only
  corticosterone methyl oxidase
cMO, cMo centimorgan; also cM
CMoL chronic monoblastic leukemia
  chronic monocytic leukemia
CMOMC cell meeting our morphologic
    criteria

C-MOPP cyclophosphamide, mechlorethamine, Oncovin, procarbazine, and prednisone

CMOR craniomandibular orthopedic repositioning device

CMOS complementary metal-oxide semiconductor (logic)

CMP cardiomyopathy; also CM
cervical mucus penetration
chondromalacia patellae
competitive medical plan
comprehensive medical plan
cytidine monophosphate (cytidylic acid)

cmp'd compound; also C, CO, co, comp, compd, CP, CPD, cpd

CMP-FX complement fixation; also CF, com fix

CMPGN chronic membranoproliferative glomerulonephritis

CMPT cervical mucus penetration test

CMR cerebral metabolic rate
Certified Medical Representative
common mode rejection
crude mortality ratio

CMRG cerebral metabolic rate of glucose

CMRL cerebral metabolic rate of lactate

CMRNG chromosomally mediated resistant *Neisseria gonorrhoeae*

CMRO cerebral metabolic rate of oxygen; also CMRO$_2$

CMRO$_2$ cerebral metabolic rate of oxygen; also CMRO

CMRR common mode rejection ratio (of amplifiers)

CMS cardiomediastinal silhouette
central material section
central material supply
cervical mucous solution
Christian Medical Society (now: CMDS, Christian Medical & Dental Society)
chromosome modification site
chronic myelodysplastic syndrome
circulation, motion sensation
circulation, muscle sensation
clean, midstream (urine)
click murmur syndrome
clofibrate-induced muscular syndrome
Clyde Mood Scale
council of medical staffs
to be taken tomorrow morning [L. *cras mane sumendus*]; also cms

cms to be taken tomorrow morning [L. *cras mane sumendus*]; also CMS

cm/s centimeters per second

CMSS circulation, motor (ability), sensation, and swelling
Council of Medical Specialty Societies

CMSUA clean, midstream urinalysis

CMT California mastitis test
cancer multistep therapy
catechol-*o*-methyltransferase; also CCMT, COMT
Certified Medical Transcriptionist
Charcot-Marie-Tooth (disease, syndrome)
chronic motor tic
circus movement tachycardia
continuous memory test
culture mutant Tübingen
Current Medical Terminology

CMTD Charcot-Marie-Tooth disease

CMU cardiac monitoring unit
chlorophenyldimethylurea
complex motor unit

CMUA continuous motor unit activity

CMV cisplatin, methotrexate, and vinblastine
continuous mechanical ventilation
controlled mechanical ventilation
conventional mechanical ventilation
cool mist vaporizer
cucumber mosaic virus
cytomegalic inclusion virus
cytomegalovirus; also CYTOMG

CMVIG cytomegalovirus immune globulin

CMV-IGIV cytomegalovirus immune globulin, intravenous

CMVS culture mid-void specimen

CN caudate nucleus
cellulose nitrate
charge nurse
child nutrition
clinical nursing
cochlear nucleus
congenital nephrosis
congenital nystagmus
cranial nerve(s)
Crigler-Najjar (syndrome)
cyanide; also Cn, CYN
cyanogen; also CY, Cy
cyanosis neonatorum
tomorrow night [L. *cras nocte*]; also cn

CN⁻, -CN cyanide radical

C/N carbon to nitrogen (ratio)
carrier to noise (ratio)
contrast to noise (ratio)

Cn color naming
cyanide; also CN, CYN

cn tomorrow night [L. *cras nocte*]; also CN

CNA calcium nutrient agar
Canadian Nurses' Association
chart not available

CNAG chronic narrow angle glaucoma

CNAP cochlear nucleus action potential

CNB cutting needle biopsy

CNBr cyanogen bromide

CNC clear, no creamy (layer)
Clinical Nursing Conference

CNCbl, CN-Cbl cyanocobalamin

CNCM Collection Nationale de Cultures des
Microorganismes

CND canned
cannot determine

CNDC chronic nonspecific diarrhea of childhood

CNDO complete neglect of differential overlap

CNE chronic nervous exhaustion
concentric needle electrode
could not establish

CNEMG concentric needle electromyography

CNF cancer normalizing factor
chronic nodular fibrositis
congenital nephrotic (syndrome), Finnish
cyclophosphamide, Novantrone, and
fluorouracil

CNH central neurogenic hyperpnea
central neurogenic hyperventilation
community nursing home

CNHD congenital nonspherocytic hemolytic
disease

CNHI Committee for National Health
Insurance

CNI–CNXII cranial nerves I through XII; also
CI–CXII, C_I–C_{XII}

CNK cortical necrosis of the kidneys

CNL cardiolipin natural lecithin

CNM Certified Nurse-Midwife
computerized nuclear morphometry

CNMT Certified Nuclear Medicine
Technologist

CNN congenital nevocytic nevus

CNOH cyanic acid

CNOR Certified Nurse, Operating Room

CNP community nurse practitioner
continuous negative pressure (breathing)
cranial nerve palsy
cyclic nucleotide phosphodiesterase

CNPase cyclic nucleotide phosphohydrolase

CNPV continuous negative pressure ventilation

CNRN Certified Neurosurgical Registered
Nurse

CNRR Chinese National Relief and
Rehabilitation Administration

CNRS citrated normal rabbit serum

CNS central nervous system
clinical nurse specialist
computerized notation system
cyanide sulfonate (sulfocyanate)

cns to be taken tomorrow night [L. *cras nocte
sumendus*]

CNSD chronic nonspecific diarrhea

CNSHA congenital nonspherocytic hemolytic
anemia

CNS-L central nervous system leukemia

CNSN Certified Nutrition Support Nurse

CNT could not test
current night terrors

CNV choroidal neovascularization
colistin sulfate, nystatin, and vancomycin
(antimicrobic disk)
conative negative variation
contingent negative variation
cutaneous necrotizing vasculitis

CNVT colistin sulfate, nystatin, vancomycin,
and trimethoprim lactate (antimicrobic
disk)

CO candidal onychomycosis
carbon monoxide
cardiac output
castor oil
casualty officer
centric occlusion
cervical orthosis
cervicoaxial; also CA
choline oxidase
coenzyme; also Co
community organization
compound; also C, cmp'd, co, comp, compd,
CP, CPD, cpd
control; also C
corneal opacity
crossover

C/O, c/o check out

complains of
complaint(s); also comp, Cx
in care of

CO₂ carbon dioxide; also CD

Co cobalt
coenzyme; also CO

Co I coenzyme I (nicotinamide adenine dinucleotide)

Co II coenzyme II (nicotinamide adenine dinucleotide phosphate)

Co 57, ⁵⁷Co cobalt 57, radioactive cobalt: halflife, 270 days

Co 58, ⁵⁸Co cobalt 58, radioactive cobalt: halflife, 71.3 days

Co 60, ⁶⁰Co cobalt 60, radioactive cobalt: halflife, 5.26 years

co compound; also C, cmp'd, CO, comp, compd, CP, CPD, cpd
compounded; also comp, compd
cutoff

COA calculated opening area
Canadian Orthopaedic Association
cervico-oculoacusticus (syndrome)

CoA coarctation of the aorta; also CA, C of A
coenzyme A

COAD chronic obstructive airway disease
chronic obstructive arterial disease

COAG, coag chronic open angle glaucoma
coagulated
coagulation

COAG PD coagulation profile–diagnosis

COAG PP coagulation profile–presurgery

COAGSC coagulation screen

COAP cyclophosphamide, Oncovin, ARA-C, and prednisone

coarc coarctation (of the aorta)

CoASH reduced coenzyme A; also CoA-SH

CoA-SH reduced coenzyme A; also CoASH

CoA-SPC coenzyme A–synthesizing protein complex

COB chronic obstructive bronchitis
cisplatin, Oncovin, and bleomycin
coordination of benefits

COBMAM cyclophosphamide, Oncovin, bleomycin, methotrexate, Adriamycin, and methyl-CCNU (semustine)

COBOL common business-oriented language

COBRA Consolidated Omnibus Budget Reconciliation Act (of 1985)

COBS cesarean-obtained barrier-sustained (animals)
chronic organic brain syndrome

COBT chronic obstruction of biliary tract

COC calcifying odontogenic cyst
cathodal opening clonus; also CaOCl, COCL, COCl
cathodal opening contraction; also CaOC
coccygeal; also Cd, cd, Coc, coc
combination oral contraceptive

Coc, coc coccygeal; also Cd, cd, COC

Cocci coccidioidomycosis

coch spoonful [L. *cochleare*]; also cochl

cochl spoonful [L. *cochleare*]; also coch

cochl amp heaping spoonful [L. *cochleare amplum*]; also c amplum

cochl mag tablespoonful [L. *cochleare magnum*]; also c magnum

cochl med dessertspoonful [L. *cochleare medium*]; also cochl mod

cochl mod dessertspoonful [L. *cochleare modicum*]; also cochl med

cochl parv teaspoonful [L. *cochleare parvum*]; also c parvum

COCI Consortium on Chemical Information

COCL, COCl cathodal opening clonus; also CaOCl, COC

Coct, coct boiling [L. *coctio*]

COD cause of death
chemical oxygen demand
codeine; also cod
condition on discharge

cod codeine; also COD

CODATA Committee on Data for Science and Technology

COD-MD cerebro-oculardysplasia–muscular dystrophy

COE court-ordered examination

COEAMRA Council on Education of the American Medical Record Association

coef coefficient; also C, coeff

coeff coefficient; also C, coef

COEPS cortical originating extrapyramidal system

COF cut-off frequency

CoF cobra venom factor; also CoVF, CVF
cofactor

C of A coarctation of the aorta; also CA, CoA

COFS cerebro-oculofacial-skeletal (syndrome)

COG Central Oncology Group
　clinical obstetrics and gynecology
　cognitive (function tests)

COGN cognition

COGTT cortisone-primed oral glucose tolerance test

COH carbohydrate; also C, CARB, carb, carbo, CHO

CoH coefficient of haze

COHB, COHb, CoHb carboxyhemoglobin

COHE College of Osteopathic Healthcare Executives

COHSE Confederation of Health Service Employees

COI Central Obesity Index

COL colicin; also Col
　colony; also Col, col
　color; also Col, col
　colored; also cld, Col, col
　column; also Col, col
　cost of living; also Col, col
　strain [L. *cola*]; also Col, col

Col colicin; also COL
　colicinogenic
　colony; also COL, col
　color; also COL, col
　colored; also cld, COL, col
　column; also COL, col
　cost of living; also COL, col
　strain [L. *cola*]; also COL, col

col colony; also COL, Col
　color; also COL, Col
　colored; also cld, COL, Col
　column; also COL, Col
　cost of living; also COL, Col
　strain [L. *cola*]; also COL, Col

COLAT, colat strained [L. *colatus*]

COLD chronic obstructive lung disease

COLD A cold agglutinin; also CA, cold agg

cold agg cold agglutinin; also CA, COLD A

colet let it be strained [L. *coletur*]

COLL, coll collect
　collection
　collective
　college
　colloidal
　eyewash [L. *collyrium*]; also COLLYR, Collyr, collyr

collat collateral

collun nose wash [L. *collunarium*]

COLLUT, collut mouthwash [L. *collutorium*]

coll vol collective volume

COLLYR, Collyr, collyr eyewash [L. *collyrium*]; also COLL, coll

col/mL colonies per milliliter

color colorimetry (including spectrophotometry and photometry)
　let it be colored [L. *coloretur*]

colp colporrhaphy; also colpo
　colposcopy; also colpo

colpo colporrhaphy; also colp
　colposcopy; also colp

COM chronic otitis media
　College of Osteopathic Medicine
　computer output on microfilm
　cyclophosphamide, Oncovin, and methotrexate
　cyclophosphamide, Oncovin, and methyl-CCNU (semustine)

com commitment

COMA cyclophosphamide, Oncovin, methotrexate, and ARA-C

COMB cyclophosphamide, Oncovin, methyl-CCNU (semustine), and bleomycin

comb combination
　combine

COMF comfortable; also comf
　cyclophosphamide, Oncovin, methotrexate, and fluorouracil

comf comfortable; also COMF

com fix complement fixation; also CF, CMP-FX

COMLA cyclophosphamide, Oncovin, methotrexate, leucovorin calcium, and ARA-C

comm commission; also commn
　commissioner; also commn
　committee
　communicable; also commun

commn commission; comm
　commissioner; also comm

commun communicable; also comm

commun dis communicable disease; also CD

COMP complication(s); also CCX, CM, cm, compl, complic, Cx
　cyclophosphamide, Oncovin, methotrexate, and prednisone

comp comparable
　comparative
　compare; also CF, cf, *cf*, cp

compensated
compensation
complaint(s); also C/O, c/o, Cx
composition; also compn
compound; also C, cmp'd, CO, co, compd,
    CP, CPD, cpd
compounded; also co, compd
compress
compression
computer

compd compound; also C, cmp'd, CO, co,
    comp, CP, CPD, cpd
compounded; also co, comp

compet competition

compl complete; also cpl
completed; also cpl
completion; also cpl
complicated; also complic
complication(s); also CCX, CM, cm, COMP,
    complic, Cx

complic complicated; also compl
complicating
complication(s); also CCX, CM, cm, COMP,
    compl, Cx

compn composition; also comp

COMS chronic organic mental syndrome

COMT catechol-*o*-methyltransferase; also
    CCMT, CMT

COMTRAC computer-based (case) tracing

CON certificate of need

Con concanavalin

con against [L. *contra*]; also cont

ConA, Con A concanavalin A

Con A-HRP concanavalin A–horseradish per-
    oxidase

conc concentrated; also concd, concentr
concentration; also C, c, concn, concentr

concd concentrated; also conc, concentr

concn concentration; also C, c, conc, concentr

concentr concentrated; also conc, concd
concentration; also C, c, conc, concn

concis cut [L. *concisus*]

cond condensation
condensed
condition
conditional
conditioned; also C
conductivity

cond ref conditioned reflex; also CR

cond resp conditioned response; also CR

cone conization (of cervix); also coniz

conf confection
conference

config configuration

cong congenital; also congen
congress
gallon [L. *congius*]; also C

congen congenital; also cong

congr congruent

coniz conization (of cervix); also cone

conj conjunctiva
conjunctival

conjug conjugated
conjugation

CONPADRI I cyclophosphamide, Oncovin,
    L-phenylalanine mustard, and Adriamycin

CONPADRI II CONPADRI I plus high dose
    methotrexate

CONPADRI III CONPADRI I plus intensi-
    fied doxorubicin

CONS consultant; also cons
consultation; also cons

cons conservation
conservative
conserve
consultant; also CONS
consultation; also CONS
keep [L. *conserva*]

consperg dust, sprinkle [L. *consperge*]

const constant; also C

constit constituent

cont against [L. *contra*]; also con
bruised [L. *contusus*]; also C, contus
containing; also contg
contains
contents
continuation
continue
continuously
contusions

contag contagion
contagious

conter rub together [L. *contere*]

contd continued

contg containing; also cont

contin let it be continued [L. *continuetur*]

contr contraction; also C, contrx, CTX,
    CTXN, Cx

contra contraindicated

contralat contralateral

cont rem let the medicine be continued [L. *continuetur remedium*]

contrib contributory

contrit broken down [L. *contritus*]

contrx contraction; also C, contr, CTX, CTXN, Cx

contus bruised [L. *contusus*]; also C, cont

conv convalescence; also CS
convalescent; also CS
convalescing
conventional (rat)
convergence
convergent

CONV HOSP convalescent hospital; also CH

conv strab convergent strabismus

COOD chronic obstructive outflow disease

coord coordinated
coordination

COP capillary osmotic pressure
change of plaster
cicatricial ocular pemphigoid
cicumoval precipitin
coefficient of performance
colloid oncotic pressure
colloid osmotic pressure
cyclophosphamide, Oncovin, and prednisone

COPB cyclophosphamide, Oncovin, prednisone, and bleomycin

COP-BLAM cyclophosphamide, Oncovin, prednisone, and bleomycin, Adriamycin, and Matulane

COPC community-oriented primary care

COPD chronic obstructive pulmonary disease

COPE chronic obstructive pulmonary emphysema
Committee on Political Education

COPI California Occupational Preference Inventory

COP$_i$ colloid osmotic pressure in interstitial fluid

COPP cyclophosphamide, Oncovin, procarbazine, and prednisone

COP$_p$ colloid osmotic pressure in plasma

COPRO coproporphyria; also CP
coproporphyrin; also CP

CoQ coenzyme Q (ubiquinone)

coq boil [L. *coque*]

coq in s a boil in sufficient water [L. *coque in sufficiente aqua*]

coq s a boil properly [L. *coque secunda arte*]

coq simul boil together [L. *coque simul*]

COR body [L. *corpus*]
cardiac output recorder
comprehensive outpatient rehabilitation (facility)
conditioned orientation reflex (audiometry)
coroner
corrosion
corrosive
cortisone
heart [L. *cor*]

Cor Congo red; also CR

cor coronary
corrected; also cc, corr
correction; also corr

CORA conditioned orientation reflex audiometry

CORD chronic obstructive respiratory disease
Commissioned Officer Residency Deferment

corr corrected; also cc, cor
correction; also cor
correspondence

corresp corresponding

CORT Certified Operating Room Technician

cort cortex; also C
cortical

CORTIS cortisol

COS Canadian Ophthalmological Society
Chief of Staff
clinically observed seizure
Clinical Orthopaedic Society

cos change of shift
cosine

COSMIS Computer System for Medical Information Systems

COSTAR Computer-stored Ambulatory Record

COSTEP Commissioned Officer Student Training and Extern Program

COSY correlation spectroscopy

COT colony overlay test
content of thought
continuous oxygen therapy
contralateral optic tectum
critical off-time

CO$_2$T total carbon dioxide content

COTA Certified Occupational Therapy Assistant

COTD cardiac output by thermodilution

COTe cathodal opening tetanus

COTH Council of Teaching Hospitals

COTRANS Coordinated Transfer Application System

COTX cast off, to x-ray

COU cardiac observation unit

coul coulomb; also C

COV crossover value

CoVF cobra venom factor; also CoF, CVF

COWAT Controlled Oral Word Association Test

COWS cold to opposite and warm to same side (Hallpike caloric stimulation response)

COX coxsackie virus

CP candle-power; also cp
capillary pressure
carbamoyl phosphate
cardiac pacing
cardiac performance
cardiac pool
cardiopulmonary; also C/P
cardiopulmonary performance
carotid pressure
caudate putamen; also CPU
caudatus putamen; also CPU
cell passage
central pit
centric position
cerebellopontine
cerebral palsy
certified prosthetist
ceruloplasmin; also CER, CERULO, Cp
cervical probe
chemically pure; also cp
chest pain; also C/P
child psychiatry; also CHP
child psychology
chloramphenicol; also C, CAP, CHL, chloro, CMC
chloropurine
chloroquine and primaquine (combination tablets)
chondrodysplasia punctata
chondromalacia patellae
chronic pain
chronic pancreatitis
chronic pyelonephritis, also CPN
cicatricial pemphoid
circular polarization
cisplatin
cleft palate; also Clpal
clinical pathology; also Clin Path, CIP
closing pressure
clottable protein
cochlear potential

code of practice
cold pressor
color perception
combination product
combining power
complete physical
compound; also C, cmp'd, CO, co, comp, compd, CPD, cpd
compressed
congenital phosphoruria
constant pressure
coproporphyria; also COPRO
coproporphyrin; also COPRO
coracoid process
cor pulmonale
cortical plate
Corynebacterium parvum
costal plaque
C peptide
creatine phosphate; also CrP
creatine phosphokinase; also CPK
cross-linked protein
crude protein
current practice
cyclophosphamide; also CPA, CPM, CY, Cy, CYC, Cyc, CYCLO, CyClo, Cyclo
cyclophosphamide and Platinol
cyclophosphamide and prednisone
cystosarcoma phyllodes
cytosol protein

C/P cardiopulmonary; also CP
chest pain; also CP
cholesterol – phospholipid ratio

C&P compensation and pension
complete and pain-free (range of motion)
cystoscopy and pyelography

Cp ceruloplasmin; also CER, CERULO, CP
chickenpox; also Chix, CHPX, chpx
peak concentration
phosphate clearance; also C_p

C_p heat capacity (constant pressure); also C_p, C_p
phosphate clearance; also Cp

C_p, C_p heat capacity (constant pressure); also C_p

cP centipoise; also cp

cp candle-power; also CP
centipoise; also cP
chemically pure; also CP
compare; also CF, cf, *cf*, comp

CPA carboxypeptidase A
cardiophrenic angle
cardiopulmonary arrest

CPA—cont'd
carotid phonoangiograph
carotid phonoangiography
cerebellar pontine angle
chlorophenylalanine
chronic pyrophosphate arthropathy
circulating platelet aggregate
costophrenic angle
cyclophosphamide; also CP, CPM, CY, Cy,
CYC, Cyc, CYCLO, CyClo, Cyclo
cyproterone acetate; also CTA

C3PA complement 3 proactivator (convertase)

CPAF chlorpropamide-alcohol flushing

Cpah, C$_{pah}$ *para*-aminohippuric acid clearance

CPAI central principal axis of inertia

CPAN Certified Post-Anesthesia Nurse

CPA/OPG carotid phonoangiography/oculo-
plethysmography

CPAP continuous positive airway pressure
(breathing)

c parvum teaspoonful [L. *cochleare parvum*];
also cochl parv

C3PAse C3 proactivator convertase

CPB cardiopulmonary bypass
competitive protein binding

CPBA competitive protein-binding analysis
competitive protein-binding assay

CPBS cardiopulmonary bypass surgery
Colorado potato beetle spiroplasma

CPBV cardiopulmonary blood volume

CPC capillary packed column
cerebellar Purkinje cell
cerebral palsy clinic
cetylpyridinium chloride
chronic passive congestion
circumferential pneumatic compression
Clinical Pathology Conference
clinicopathological conference
coil planet centrifuge (method, tube)
committed progenitor cell
cresolphthalein complexone

CPCL congenital pulmonary cystic lymphangiectasia

CPCN capitated primary care network

CPCP chronic progressive coccidioidal pneumonitis

CPCR cardiopulmonary-cerebral resuscitation

CPCS circumferential pneumatic compression
suit
clinical pharmaco-kinetics consulting service

CPD calcium pyrophosphate deposition
calcium pyrophosphate dihydrate; also CPPD
cephalopelvic disproportion
childhood polycystic disease
chorioretinopathy and pituitary dysfunction
chronic peritoneal dialysis
citrate-phosphate-dextrose (blood preservative)
compound; also C, cmp'd, CO, co, comp,
compd, CP, cpd
contact potential difference
contagious pustular dermatitis
critical point drying
cyclopentadiene

cpd compound; also C, cmp'd, CO, co, comp,
compd, CP, CPD

CPDA citrate-phosphate-dextrose-adenine; also
CPD-A, CPDA-1

CPD-A citrate-phosphate-dextrose-adenine;
also CPDA, CPDA-1

CPDA-1 citrate-phosphate-dextrose-adenine;
also CPDA, CPD-A

CPDD calcium pyrophosphate deposition disease
cis-platinum diamminedichloride (cisplatin)

CPDL cumulative population doubling level

CPE cardiac pulmonary edema
cardiogenic pulmonary edema
chronic pulmonary emphysema
compensation, pension, and education
complete physical examination; also CPX
complex partial epilepsy
corona-penetrating enzyme
cytopathic effect; also CE
cytopathogenic effect

C Ped Certified Pedorthist

CPEHS Consumer Protection and
Environmental Health Service

CPEO chronic progressive external ophthalmoplegia

CPF clot-promoting factor
contraction peak force

CPFV cucumber pale fruit viroid

CP&FD cephalopelvic disproportion and fetal
distress

CPG capillary blood gases; also CBG
carotid phonoangiogram

CPGN chronic progressive glomerulonephritis
chronic proliferative glomerulonephritis

CPH centrophenoxine
Certificate in Public Health

chronic paroxysmal hemicrania
chronic persistent hepatitis

CPHA Commission on Professional and Hospital Activities

CPI California Personality Inventory
Cancer Potential Index
congenital palatopharyngeal incompetence
constitutional psychopathic inferiority
consumer price index
coronary prognostic index
cysteine proteinase inhibitor

CP\I chest pain or indigestion

CPIB chlorophenoxyisobutyrate

CPID chronic pelvic inflammatory disease

CPIP chronic pulmonary insufficiency of prematurity
common peak developed isovolumetric pressure

CPK Corey-Paulin-Koltun (molecular model)
creatine phosphokinase; also CP

CPKD childhood polycystic kidney disease

CPKI creatine phosphokinase isoenzyme(s); also CPKISO

CPKISO creatine phosphokinase isoenzyme(s); also CPKI

CPL caprine placental lactogen
conditioned pitch level
congenital pulmonary lymphangiectasia

C/PL cholesterol to phospholipid ratio

cpl complete; also compl
completed; also compl
completion; also compl

CPLM cysteine-peptone-liver infusion medium

CPM CCNU (lomustine), procarbazine, and methotrexate
central pontine myelinosis
chlorpheniramine maleate
Clinical Practice Model
cognitive-perceptual-motor
Colored Progressive Matrices
continue present management
continuous passive motion (device)
counts per minute; also C/M, cpm
cyclophosphamide; also CP, CPA, CY, Cy, CYC, Cyc, CYCLO, CyClo, Cyclo

cpm counts per minute; also C/M, CPM
cycles per minute; also c/min

CPmax peak (maximum) serum concentration

CPMDI computerized pharmacokinetic model-driven drug infusion

CPMG Carr-Purcell-Meiboom-Gill (spin-echo technique)

CPMI central principal moments of inertia

CPmin trough (minimum) serum concentration

CPMM constant passive motion machine

CPMP computer-patient management problems

CPMS chronic progressive multiple sclerosis

CPMV cowpox mosaic virus

CPN carboxypeptidase N
chronic polyneuropathy
chronic pyelonephritis; also CP

CPNA Certified Pediatric Nurses Association

CPNM corrected perinatal mortality

CPNP Certified Pediatric Nurse Practioner

CPNP/A Certified Pediatric Nurse Practitioner/Associate

CPOB cyclophosphamide, prednisone, Oncovin, and bleomycin

CPOC ethyl 2-[5-(4-chlorophenyl)pentyl]-oxirane-2-carboxylate

CPP cancer proneness phenotype
canine pancreatic polypeptide
cerebral perfusion pressure
cryoprecipitate; also cryo
cyclopentenophenanthrene

CPPB continuous positive-pressure breathing

CPPD calcium pyrophosphate dihydrate; also CPD
calcium pyrophosphate dihydrate disease
chest percussion and postural drainage; also CP&PD

CP&PD chest percussion and postural drainage; also CPPD

CPPT coronary primary prevention trial

CPPV continuous positive-pressure ventilation

CPR cardiac and pulmonary rehabilitation
cardiac pulmonary reserve
cardiopulmonary resuscitation
carrageenan pleural reaction
centripetal rub
cerebral cortex perfusion rate
chlorophenyl red
cochleopalpebral reflex
cortisol production rate
cumulative potency rate
customary, prevailing, and reasonable

CPRAM controlled partial rebreathing anesthesia method

CPRS Children's Psychiatric Rating Scale
Comprehensive Psychiatric Rating Scale

CPRS—cont'd
Comprehensive Psychopathological Rating Scale

CPS carbamoyl phosphate synthetase
cardioplegic perfusion solution
cardiopulmonary support
Center for Preventive Services
characters per second; also cps
Child Personality Scale
Child Protective Services
chloroquine, pyrimethamine, and sulfisoxazole
clinical performance score
clinical pharmacokinetic service
coagulase-positive staphylococci
Compendium of Pharmaceuticals and Specialties
complex partial seizure
constitutional psychopathic state
contagious pustular stomatitis
C-polysaccharide
cumulative probability of success
current population survey

cps characters per second; also CPS
counts per second
cycles per second; also c/s

CPSC Consumer Product Safety Commission

CPSI carbamoyl phosphate synthetase I

CPS-I Cancer Prevention Study I

CPSII carbamoyl phosphate synthetase II

CPS-II Cancer Prevention Study II

CPT carnitine palmityltransferase
carotid pulse tracing
chest physiotherapy
child protection team
choline phosphotransferase
ciliary particle transport
clinical pharmacokinetics team
cold pressor test
combining power test
continuous performance task
continuous performance test
Current Procedural Terminology

CPTH chronic post-traumatic headache
C-terminal parathyroid hormone

CPU caudate putamen; also CP
caudatus putamen; also CP
central processing unit (in a computer)

CPUE chest pain of unknown etiology

CPV canine parvovirus
cytoplasmic polyhidrosis virus

CPVD congenital polyvalvular disease

CPX complete physical examination; also CPE

CPZ cefoperazone
chlorpromazine
Compazine (prochlorperazine dimaleate)

CQ carboquone
chloroquine
chloroquine-quinine
circadian quotient
conceptual quotient

CQA concurrent quality assurance

CQM chloroquine mustard

CQUCC Commission on Quantities and Units in Clinical Chemistry

CR Cacchi-Ricci (disease)
calcification rate
calculus removal
calculus removed
calorie restricted
cardiac rehabilitation
cardiorespiratory
caries resistant
cartilage residue
case report
cathode ray
central ray
centric relation
chest and right arm (lead in electrocardiography)
chest roentgenogram
chest roentgenography
chief resident
child-resistant (closure, container)
chloride; also chlor, Cl
choice reaction
chromium; also Cr
chronic rejection
clinical record
clinical research
closed reduction
clot retraction; also CLOT R
coefficient of fat retention
cold recombinant
colon resection
colony-reared (animal)
colorectal
complement receptor
complete remission
complete response
complete responders
conditioned reflex; also cond ref
conditioned response; also cond resp
congenital rubella
Congo red; also Cor

contact record
continuous reinforcement; also CRF
controlled release
controlled respiration
controlled response
conversion rate
cooling rate
correct response
corticoresistant
cranial; also Cr, cran
cranium; also Cr, cran
creamed
creatinine; also C, Cr, Cre, CREAT, creat
cresyl red
critical ratio (response)
crown-rump (length) (fetal measurement)

C&R cardiac and respiratory
convalescence and rehabilitation
cystoscopy and retrograde

CR₁ first cranial nerve

CR₂ second cranial nerve

Cr chromium; also CR
cranial; also CR, cran
cranium; also CR, cran
creatinine; also C, CR, Cre, CREAT, creat
crown

Cr 51, ⁵¹Cr chromium 51, radioactive
chromium: halflife, 27.8 days

cr tomorrow [L. *cras*]

CRA central retinal artery
chronic rheumatoid arthritis
colorectal anastomosis
cytochrome *c* reductase

CRABP cellular retinoic acid-binding protein
cytoplasmic retinoic acid-binding protein

CRAG cerebral radionuclide angiography

CRAMS circulation, respiration, abdomen,
motor, and speech

cran cranial; also CR, Cr
cranium; also CR, Cr

CRAO central retinal artery occlusion

crast for tomorrow [L. *crastinus*]

CRBBB complete right bundle-branch block

CRBC chicken red blood cell; also ChRBC

CRBP cellular retinol-binding protein

CRC cardiovascular reflex conditioning
child-resistant container
clinical research center
colorectal carcinoma
concentrated red blood cells
Crisis Resolution Center

cross-reacting cannabinoids

CR&C closed reduction and cast

CrCl creatinine clearance; also CC, Ccr, C_{cr},
ccr

CRCS Canadian Red Cross Society
cardiovascular reflex conditioning system

CRD childhood rheumatic disease
child-restraint device
chorioretinal degeneration
chronic renal disease
chronic respiratory disease
completely randomized design
complete reaction of degeneration
cone-rod dystrophy
congenital rubella deafness
crown-rump distance (fetal measurement)

CRE cumulative radiation effect

Cre creatinine; also C, CR, Cr, CREAT, creat

CREAT, creat creatinine; also C, CR, Cr, Cre

CREA-S creatinine urine spot (test)

CREG cross-reactive group (of HLA antigens)

C region constant region

CRENA crenated (red blood cells)

crep crepitation

CREST calcinosis cutis, Raynaud's phenomenon, esophageal motility disorder(s), sclerodactyly, and telangiectasia (syndrome)

CRF case report form
chronic renal failure
chronic respiratory failure
citrovorum rescue factor
continuous-reacting factor
continuous reinforcement; also CR
corticotropin-releasing factor

CRFK Crandell feline kidney cells

CRG cardiorespirogram

CRH corticotropin-releasing hormone

CRHL Collaborative Radiological Health
Laboratory

CRHV cottontail rabbit herpes virus

CRI Cardiac Risk Index
catheter-related infection
chronic renal insufficiency
Composite Risk Index
concentrated rust inhibitor
congenital rubella infection
cross-reactive idiotype

CRIE crossed radioimmunoelectrophoresis

CRIS controlled release infusion syndrome

Crit, crit critical

Crit, crit —cont'd
hematocrit; also C, Hc, H'crit, HCT, Hct, hemat, HMT

CRITOE capitellum, radial head, internal condyle, trochlea, olecranon, external condyle (ossification sequence in elbow)

crit press critical pressure

crit temp critical temperature

CRL cell repository line
Certified Record Librarian
complement receptor location
complement receptor lymphocyte
crown-rump length (fetal measurement)

CRM certified raw milk
Certified Reference Materials
contralateral remote masking
cross-reacting material
crown-rump measurement (fetal measurement)

CRN complement-requiring neutralizing (antibody)

Crn corrin

CRNA Certified Registered Nurse Anesthetist

cRNA chromosomal ribonucleic acid

CRNF chronic rheumatoid nodular fibrositis

cr nn cranial nerves; also cr ns, crns

CRNP Certified Registered Nurse Practitioner

cr ns, crns cranial nerves; also cr nn

CRO cathode ray oscillograph
cathode ray oscilloscope
centric relation occlusion

CROP cyclophosphamide, Rubidazone, Oncovin, and prednisone

CROS contralateral routing of signal(s)

CRP carbon-reactive protein (C-reactive protein)
chronic relapsing pancreatitis
confluent, reticulate papillomatosis
corneal-retinal potential
coronary rehabilitation program
cyclic adenosine monophosphate receptor protein

CrP creatine phosphate; also CP

CRPA C-reactive protein antiserum

CRPD chronic restrictive pulmonary disease

CRPF chloroquine-resistant *Plasmodium falciparum*
contralateral renal plasma flow

CRS catheter-related sepsis
caudal regression syndrome
central supply room
Chinese restaurant syndrome
cis-acting repression (effect)
colon-rectal surgery
colorectal surgery
compliance of the respiratory system
congenital rubella syndrome

CRSP comprehensive renal scintillation procedure

CrSp craniospinal

CRST calcinosis cutis, Raynaud's phenomenon, sclerodactyly, and telangiectasia (syndrome)

CRT cadaver renal transplant
cardiac resuscitation team
cathode ray tube
central reaction time
certified; also C, Cert, cert
Certified Record Technique
choice reaction time
chromium release time
complex reaction time
computed renal tomography
controlled release time
copper reduction test
corrected retention time
cortisone resistant thymocyte
cranial radiation therapy

CRTP Consciousness Research and Training Project

CrTr crutch training; also CT

CRTT Certified Respiratory Therapy Technician

CRTX cast removed, take x-ray

CRU cardiac rehabilitation unit
Clinical Research Unit

CRV central retinal vein

cr vesp tomorrow evening [L. *cras vespere*]; also CV, cv

CRVF congestive right ventricular failure

CRVO central retinal vein occlusion

CRY-AB cryptococcal antibody

CRY-AG cryptococcal antigen

cryo cryoglobulin; also CG
cryoprecipitate; also CPP
cryosurgery
cryotherapy

Crys, crys crystal(s); also cryst
crystalline; also cryst
crystallinized; also cryst

CRYST crystal examination screen

cryst crystal(s); also Crys, crys
crystalline; also Crys, crys
crystallinized; also Crys, crys
crystallization; also crystn

crystn crystallization; also cryst

CS calf serum
carcinoid syndrome
cardiogenic shock; also CGS
caries susceptible
carotid sheath
carotid sinus
cat scratch (disease)
celiac sprue
Central Service
central supply
cerebrospinal
cervical spine; also C-S, C-spine, C/spine
cervical stimulation
cesarean section; also C§, C/S, C-sect,
C-section
chemical sympathectomy
chest strap
cholesterol stone
chondroitin sulfate; also CHS
chorionic somatomammotropin
chronic schizophrenia
cigarette smoke (solution)
cigarette smoker
circumsporozoite
citrate synthetase
clinical (laboratory) scientist
clinical specialist
clinical stage
clinical state
close supervision
Cockayne's syndrome
colistin; also Cl
Collet-Sicard (syndrome)
colorimetric solution
completed stroke
completed suicide
concentrated strength (of solution)
conditioned stimulus
congenital syphilis
conjunctival secretion
conjunctiva-sclera
conscious; also Cs, cs
consciousness; also Cs, cs
constant spring
consultation service
contact sensitivity
continue same (treatment)
continuing smoker
continuous stripping

control serum
convalescence; also conv
convalescent; also conv
convalescent status
coronary sclerosis
coronary sinus
corpus striatum
cortical spoking
corticoid sensitive
corticosteroid; also CTS
crush syndrome
Curschmann-Steinert (syndrome)
current smoker
current strength
Cushing's syndrome
cycloserine
cyclosporin; also CSP
with the left hand [L. *cum sinistra*]

C-S cervical spine; also CS, C-spine, C/spine

C/S cesarean section; also C§, CS, C sect,
C-section
Cost-Stirling (antibody)
culture and sensitivity; also C&S

C&S conjunctiva and sclera
cough and sneeze
culture and sensitivity; also C/S
culture and susceptibility

C4S chondroitin 4-sulfate

C$_S$ concentration of the standard
standard clearance; also Cs
static compliance (lung); also CST, Cst, C$_{st}$,
C$_{stat}$

Cs case; also cs
cell surface (antigen)
cesium
conscious; also CS, cs
consciousness; also CS, cs
standard clearance; also C$_S$

cS centistoke; also cSt

cs case; also Cs
conscious; also CS, Cs
consciousness; also CS, Cs

c/s cycles per second; also cps

CSA canavaninosuccinic acid
chemical shift anisotropy
chondroitin sulfate A
colon-specific antigen
colony-stimulating activity
compressed spectral assay
controlled substance analog
cross-sectional area
cyclosporin A; also CsA, CyA

CsA cyclosporin A; also CSA, CyA

CSAA Child Study Association of America
CSAD cysteine sulfinic acid decarboxylase
CSAP colon-specific antigen protein
CSAT cell-substrate attachment (antigen)
CSB caffeine sodium benzoate
Cheyne-Stokes breathing
contaminated small bowel
CSB I&II Chemistry Screening Batteries I and II
CSBF coronary sinus blood flow
CSBO complete small bowel obstruction
CSC administration of small doses of drugs at short intervals [Fr. *coup sur coup* (blow on blow)]
central serous choroidopathy
cigarette smoke condensate
collagen sponge contraceptive
cornea, sclera, and conjunctiva
corticostriatocerebellar
cryogenic storage container
C/S & CC culture, sensitivity and colony count
CSCD Center for Sickle Cell Disease
CSCI continuous subcutaneous infusion
CSCT comprehensive support care team
CSD carotid sinus denervation
cat scratch disease
colloidal silicon dioxide
combined system disease
conditionally streptomycin dependent
conduction system disease
cortically spreading depression
craniospinal defect
critical stimulus duration
CS&D cleaned, sutured, and dressed
CSE clinical-symptom/self-evaluation (questionnaire)
control standard exotoxin
cross-sectional echocardiography
C sect cesarean section; also C§, CS, C/S, C-section
C-section cesarean section; also C§, CS, C/S, C sect
CSER cortical somatosensory evoked response
CSF cerebrospinal fluid
circumferential shortening fraction
colony-stimulating factor
coronary sinus flow
CSF-1 macrophage colony-stimulating factor
CSFH cerebrospinal fluid hypotension
CSFN cell surface fibronectin

CSFP cerebrospinal fluid pressure
CSFV cerebrospinal fluid volume
CSF-WR cerebrospinal fluid–Wassermann reaction
CSGBI Cardiac Society of Great Britain and Ireland
CSGBM collagenase-soluble glomerular basement membrane
CSH carotid sinus hypersensitivity
chronic subdural hematoma
cortical stromal hyperplasia
C-Sh chair shower
CSI calculus surface index
cancer serum index
cavernous sinus infiltration
cholesterol saturation index
CSICU cardiac surgery intensive care unit
CSII continuous subcutaneous insulin infusion
CSIIP continuous subcutaneous insulin infusion pump
CSIN Chemical Substances Information Network
CSIS clinical supplies and inventory system
CSL cardiolipin synthetic lecithin
CSLM confocal scanning laser microscopy
CSLU chronic stasis leg ulcer
CSM carotid sinus massage
cerebrospinal meningitis
circulation, sensation, movement
Committee on Safety of Medicines
Consolidated Standards Manual
cornmeal, soybean, and milk
CSMA chronic spinal muscular atrophy
CSMB Center for Study of Multiple Births
CSME cotton-spot macular edema
CSMMG Chartered Society of Massage and Medical Gymnastics (British)
CSMP chloramphenicol-sensitive microsomal protein
CSN cardiac sympathetic nerve
carotid sinus nerve
CS(NCA) Clinical Laboratory Scientist, certified by the National Certification Agency (for Medical Laboratory Personnel)
CSNRT, cSNRT corrected sinus node recovery time; also CSRT
CSNS carotid sinus nerve stimulation
CSO common source outbreak
copied standing orders

CSOM chronic serous otitis media
chronic suppurative otitis media

CSP carotid sinus pressure
cavum septi pellucidi
cell surface protein
cellulose sodium phosphate
chemistry screening profile
circumsporozite precipitation
circumsporozoite precipitin
Cooperative Statistical Program
criminal sexual psychopath
cyclosporin; also CS

CSPG chondroitin sulfate proteoglycan

C-spine cervical spine; also CS, C-S, C/spine

C/spine cervical spine; also CS, C-S, C-spine

CSR Central Supply Room
Cheyne-Stokes respiration
continued stay review
corrected sedimentation rate
corrected survival rate
corrective septorhinoplasty
cortisol secretion rate
cumulative survival rate

CSRT corrected sinus node recovery time; also
CSNRT, cSNRT

CSS Cancer Surveillance System
carotid sinus stimulation
carotid sinus syndrome
Central Sterile Supply
chewing, sucking, and swallowing
chronic subclinical scurvy
Churg-Strauss syndrome
coronary sinus stimulation
cranial sector scan
subclinical scurvy syndrome

CSSD central sterile supply department

CST cardiac stress test
cavernous sinus thrombosis
Certified Surgical Technician
Christ-Siemens-Touraine (syndrome)
Compton scatter tomography
contraction stress test
convulsive shock therapy
cosyntropin stimulation test
static compliance (lung); also C_S, Cst, C_{st},
C_{stat}

Cst, C_{st} static compliance (lung); also C_S, CST,
C_{stat}

C_{stat} static compliance (lung); also C_S, CST,
Cst, C_{st}

cSt centistoke; also cS

CSTI Clearinghouse for Scientific and
Technical Information

CSU cardiac surgery unit
cardiac surveillance unit
cardiovascular surgery unit
casualty staging unit
catheter specimen of urine
Central Statistical Unit (of Venereal Disease
Research Laboratory)
clinical specialty unit
cryosurgical unit

CSUF continuous slow ultrafiltration

CSV chick syncytial virus
chrysanthemum stunt viroid

CSW Certified Social Worker
current sleepwalker

CT calcitonin; also CTN
calcitonin-sensitive (cell)
calf testis
cardiac tamponade
cardiothoracic (ratio)
Cardiovascular Technologist
carotid tracing
carpal tunnel
catastrophe theory
cationic trypsinogen
cell therapy
center thickness
cerebral thrombosis
cerebral tumor
cervical traction; also CXTX
chemotaxis; also CTX
chemotherapy; also Chem, chemo, ChemoRx
chest tube
chloramine T
chlorothiazide; also CTZ
cholera toxin
chordae tendineae
chronic thyroiditis
chymotrypsin
circulation time
classic technique
clotting time
coagulation time
coated tablet
cobra toxin
cognitive therapy
coil test
collecting tubule
combined tumor
compressed tablet
computed tomography
computerized tomography
connective tissue

CT—cont'd
continue treatment
continuous-flow tub
contraction time
controlled temperature
Coombs test
corneal thickness
corneal transplant
coronary thrombosis
corrected transposition
corrective therapy
cortical thickness
cough threshold
counseling and testing
Courvoisier-Terrier (syndrome)
crest time
crutch training; also CrTr
cystine-tellurite (medium)
cytolytic thymus (derived lymphocyte)
cytotechnologist
cytotoxic therapy

C/T compression to traction ratio
cross-match to transfusion ratio

Ct carboxy terminal; also C-terminal

C$_{T-1824}$ T-1824 (Evans blue) clearance

CTA Canadian Tuberculosis Association
chemotactic activity; also CA
chromotropic acid
clear to auscultation
Committee on Thrombolytic Agents (units)
computed tomoangiography
conditioned taste aversion
congenital trigeminal anesthesia
cyproterone acetate; also CPA
cystine trypticase agar
cytoplasmic tubular aggregate
cytotoxic assay
menses [L. *catamenia*]; also Cta

Cta menses [L. *catamenia*]; also CTA

CTAB cetyltrimethylammonium bromide
(cetrimonium bromide); also CTBM

C-TAB cyanide tablet

CTAC Cancer Treatment Advisory Committee
Carrow Test for Auditory Comprehension
cetyltrimethylammonium chloride

CTAL cortical thick ascending limb

c tant, ctant with the same amount [L. *cum tanto]*

CTAP computed tomography during arterial
portography
connective tissue activating peptide

CT(ASCP) Cytotechnologist (American
Society of Clinical Pathologists)

CTAT computerized transaxial tomography

CTB ceased to breath

CTBM cetyltrimethylammonium bromide
(cetrimonium bromide); also CTAB

CTC chlortetracycline
clinical trial certificate
computer-assisted tomographic cisternography
cultured T cell

CTCL cutaneous T-cell leukemia
cutaneous T-cell lymphoma

ctCO$_2$ concentration of total carbon dioxide

CTD carpal tunnel decompression
chest tube drainage
congenital thymic dysplasia
connective tissue disease
Corrective Therapy Department

CT&DB cough, turn, and deep breathe

CTDI computed tomography dose index

CTDW continues to do well

CTE calf thymus extract
clinical trial exemption; also CTX
cultured thymic epithelium

CTEM conventional transmission electron
microscopy

C-terminal carboxyl terminal; also Ct

CTF cancer therapy facility
certificate; also Cert, cert
Colorado tick fever
cytotoxic factor

CTFA The Cosmetic, Toiletry, and Fragrance
Association

CTFE chlorotrifluoroethylene

CTG cardiotocography
chymotrypsinogen; also ChTg

C/TG cholesterol to triglyceride (ratio)

CTGA complete transposition of great arteries

CTH ceramide trihexoside
clot to hold

CTI certification of terminal illness

CTIU cardiac-thoracic intensive care unit

CTL cervical, thoracic, and lumbar
cytotoxic T-lymphocyte (cytotoxic thymus-
derived lymphocyte)

ctl contact lens

CTLD chlorthalidone

CTLL cytotoxic T-lymphocyte line

CTLp cytotoxic T-lymphocyte precursor

CTLSO cervicothoracolumbosacral orthosis

CTM calibration and test material
cardiotachometer
Chlamydia transport media
Chlor-Trimeton
continuous tone masking
cricothyroid muscle

CTMM computed tomographic metrizamide
myelography

CT/MPR computed tomography with multiplanar reconstructions

CTN calcitonin; also CT
Certified Transcultural Nurse
computed tomography number
continuous noise condition

C&TN BLE color and temperature normal,
both lower extremities

CTND computed tomography nominal dose

CTNE calf thymus nuclear extract

cTNM tumors, nodes, and metastases (clinical
staging of tumors as determined by nonin-
vasive examination)

cTOX cerebral toxoplasmosis

CTP comprehensive treatment plan
cytidine triphosphate
cytosine triphosphate

CTP-³H cytidine triphosphate, tritium-labeled

C-TPN cyclic total parenteral nutrition

CTPP cerebral tissue perfusion pressure

CTPV coal tar pitch volatiles

CTPVO chronic thrombotic pulmonary
vascular obstruction

CTR cardiothoracic ratio
carpal tunnel release

ctr center

CTS carpal tunnel syndrome
composite treatment score
computed tomographic scanner
contralateral threshold shift
corticosteroid; also CS

CT scan computed tomography scan

CTSP called to see patient

CTT cefotetan
central tegmental tract
compressed tablet triturate
computed transaxial tomography
critical tracking task

CTTT carotid-thyroid transit time

CTU cardiac-thoracic unit
centigrade thermal unit
constitutive transcription unit

CTUWSD chest tube underwater seal drainage

CTV cervical and thoracic vertebrae

CTW central terminal of Wilson
combined testicular weight

CTX cefotaxime
cerebrotendinous xanthomatosis
charybdotoxin
chemotaxis; also CT
chemotoxins
clinical trial exemption; also CTE
contraction; also C, contr, contrx, CTXN,
Cx
Cytoxan (cyclophosphamide); also CY, CYT

CTx cardiac transplantation

CTXN contraction; also C, contr, contrx, CTX,
Cx

CTZ chemoreceptor trigger zone
chlorothiazide; also CT

CU cardiac unit
casein unit
cause unknown
chymotrypsin unit
clinical unit
color unit
contact urticaria
control unit
convalescent unit
curie; also C, c, Ci, cu

Cu copper [L. *cuprum*]

Cu-7 Copper-7 (intrauterine contraceptive
device)

C_U, C_u concentration of the unknown
urea clearance

⁶¹Cu Copper 61, radioactive copper: halflife,
3.41 hours

⁶⁴Cu Copper 64, radioactive copper: halflife,
12.9 hours

cu cubic; also C, c
curie; also C, c, Ci, CU
curved; also cvd

CuB copper band

CUC chronic ulcerative colitis

cu cm cubic centimeter; also CC, cc, c cm, cm³

CUD cause undetermined
congenital urinary (tract) deformities

CUE cumulative urinary excretion

cu ft cubic feet

CUG cytidine, uridine, and guanidine
cystourethrogram
cystourethrography

CuHVL copper half-value layer

cu in cubic inch

Cuj, cuj of which [L. *cujus*]

cuj lib of whatever you please [L. *cujus libet*]

cult culture ; also CX, Cx

CUM cumulative report

cum cubic micrometer; also μm^3

cu m cubic meter; also m^3

CUMITECH Cumulative Techniques and
Procedures in Clinical Microbiology

cu mm cubic millimeter; also cmm, c mm,
mm^3

CUP carcinoma of unknown primary (site)

CUPS carcinoma of unknown primary site

CUR curettage

cur curative
cure
current

curat dressing [L. *curatio*]

CURN Conduct and Utilization of Research in
Nursing

CUS chronic undifferentiated schizophrenia
contact urticaria syndrome

CUSA Cavitron ultrasonic surgical aspirator

cusp cuspid

CUT chronic undifferentiated type (schizophrenia)

CuTS cubital tunnel syndrome

cu yd cubic yard

CV cardiovascular
carotenoid vesicle
cell volume
central venous
cerebrovascular
cervical vertebra
chikungunya virus
cisplatin and Vepesid (etoposide)
closed vitrectomy
closing volume
coefficient of variation
color vision
concentrated volume
conducting vein
conduction velocity
consonant vowel (syllable)
contrast ventriculography; also CVG

conventional ventilation
conversational voice
corpuscular volume
Coxsackie virus; also Cvirus, C virus
cresyl violet
critical value
crystal violet
curriculum vitae
cutaneous vasculitis
cyclophosphamide and vincristine
tomorrow evening [L. *cras vespere*]; also cr
vesp, cv
true conjugate diameter of pelvic inlet [L.
conjugata vera]

C/V coulombs per volt

Cv, C$_v$, *C$_v$* heat capacity (constant volume)

cv tomorrow evening [L. *cras vespere*]; also cr
vesp, CV

CVA cardiovascular accident
cerebrovascular accident
cervicovaginal antibody
chronic villous arthritis
costovertebral angle
cresyl violet acetate
cyclophosphamide, vincristine, and
Adriamycin

CVA-BMP cyclophosphamide, vincristine,
Adriamycin, and BCNU (carmustine),
methotrexate, and procarbazine

CVAH congenital virilizing adrenal hyperplasia

C-Vasc cerebral vascular (profile study)

CVAT costovertebral angle tenderness; also
CVT

CVB CCNU (lomustine), vinblastine, and
bleomycin
chorionic villi biopsy

CVC central venous catheter
consonant vowel consonant (syllable)

CVCT cardiovascular computed tomography

CVD cardiovascular disease; also CD
cerebrovascular disease; also CBVD
cerebrovascular disorder
collagen vascular disease
color vision deviant
color vision deviate

cvd curved; also cu

CVE cerebrovascular evaluation

CVEB cisplatin, vinblastine, etoposide, and
bleomycin

CVF cardiovascular failure
central visual field

cervicovaginal fluid
cobra venom factor; also CoF, CoVF
cyclophosphamide, vincristine, and
   fluorouracil

CVG contrast ventriculography; also CV

CVH cervicovaginal hood
combined ventricular hypertrophy
common variable hypogammaglobulinemia

CVHD chronic valvular heart disease

CVI cardiovascular insufficiency
cerebrovascular insufficiency
common variable immunodeficiency; also
   CVID
continuous venous infusion
Cox Uphoff International (tissue expander)

CVID common variable immunodeficiency;
also CVI

Cvirus, C virus Coxsackie virus; also CV

CVL clinical vascular laboratory

CVM cardiovascular monitor
cyclophosphamide, vincristine, and
   methotrexate

CVN central venous nutrient

CVO central vein occlusion
central venous oxygen
Chief Veterinary Officer
circumventricular organs
obstetric conjugate diameter of pelvic inlet
   [L. *conjugata vera obstetrica*]

C$_v$O$_2$ mixed venous oxygen content

CVOD cerebrovascular obstructive disease

CVOR cardiovascular operating room

CVP cardiac valve procedure
cardioventricular pacing
cell volume profile
central venous pressure
cerebrovascular profile
cyclophosphamide, vincristine, and prednisone

CVP lab cardiovascular-pulmonary laboratory

CVPP CCNU (lomustine), vinblastine, procarbazine, and prednisone
cyclophosphamide, vincristine, prednisone,
and procarbazine

CVR cardiovascular-renal (disease)
cardiovascular resistance
cardiovascular-respiratory
cardiovascular review
cephalic vasomotor response
cerebrovascular resistance

contraceptive vaginal ring

CVRD cardiovascular-renal disease

CVRI cardiovascular resistance index

CVRR cardiovascular recovery room

CVS cardiovascular surgery
cardiovascular system
challenge virus strain
chorionic villi sampling
clean voided specimen (urine); also CL VOID

CVSF conduction velocity of slower fibers

CVSU cardiovascular specialty unit

CVT central venous temperature
congenital vertical talus
costovertebral angle tenderness; also CVAT

CVT-ICU cardiovascular-thoracic–intensive
care unit

CVTP-ICU cardiovascular-thoracic-pul-
monary–intensive care unit

CVTR charcoal viral transport medium

CVTS cardiovascular-thoracic surgery

CVUG cysto-void-urethrogram

CVV calf venous volume

CW cardiac work
careful watch
case work
case worker
Cavare-Westphal (syndrome)
cell wall
chemical warfare
chemical weapon
chest wall
children's ward
Christian-Weber (disease)
clockwise; also CKW, cw
compare with
continuous wave; also cw
cotton-wool (spots); also C-W
crutch walking; also c/w

C-W cotton-wool (spots); also CW

C/W compatible with; also c/w
consistent with; also c/w

cw clockwise; also CKW, CW
continuous wave; also CW

c/w compatible with; also C/W
consistent with; also C/W
crutch walking; also CW

CWB Charcot-Weiss-Baker (syndrome)

CWBTS capillary whole blood true sugar

CWD cell wall defective
continuous-wave Doppler

CWDF cell wall-deficient form (bacteria)

CWE cotton-wool exudates

CWF Cornell Word Form

CWI cardiac work index

CWL cutaneous water loss

CWMS color, warmth, movement, and sensation

CWOP childbirth without pain; also CWP

CWP childbirth without pain; also CWOP
coal workers' pneumoconiosis

CWS cell wall skeleton
chest wall stimulation
Child Welfare Service
cold water soluble
comfortable walking speed
cotton-wool spots

CWT cold water treatment

Cwt, cwt hundredweight

CX cancel; also Cx
cerebral cortex
cervix; also cerv, Cx
chest x-ray; also Cx, CXR, CxR
cloxacillin; also CLX
critical experiment
culture; also cult, Cx
cylinder axis

Cx cancel; also CX
cervix; also cerv, CX
circumflex (coronary artery); also CFX
chest x-ray; also CX, CXR, CxR
clearance; also C, *C*
complaint(s); also C/O, c/o, comp
complex
complication(s); also CCX, CM, cm, COMP,
compl, complic
contraction; also C, contr, contrx, CTX,
CTXN
convex
culture; also cult, CX

CXM cefuroxime
cyclohexamide

CxMT cervical motion tenderness

CXR, CxR chest x-ray; also CX, Cx

CXTX cervical traction; also CT

CY calendar year
cyanogen; also CN, Cy
cyclophosphamide; also CP, CPA, CPM, Cy,
CYC, Cyc, CYCLO, CyClo, Cyclo
Cytoxan (cyclophosphamide); also CTX,
CYT

Cy cyanogen; also CN, CY
cyclonium

cyclophosphamide; also CP, CPA, CPM, CY,
CYC, Cyc, CYCLO, CyClo, Cyclo
cyst
cytarabine

cy copy

CyA cyclosporin A; also CSA, CsA

CyADIC cyclophosphamide, Adriamycin, and
DIC (dacarbazine); also CADIC

cyath a glassful [L. *cyathus*]

cyath vin a wineglassful [L. *cyathus vinarius*]

CYC, Cyc cyclophosphamide; also CP, CPA,
CPM, CY, Cy, CYCLO, CyClo, Cyclo

cyc cyclazocine
cycle; also c
cyclotron

cyclic AMP cyclic adenosine monophosphate;
also AMP-c, cAMP, *c*AMP

cyclic GMP cyclic guanosine monophosphate;
also cGMP

CYCLO, CyClo cyclophosphamide; also CP,
CPA, CPM, CY, Cy, CYC, Cyc, Cyclo

Cyclo cyclophosphamide; also CP, CPA, CPM,
CY, Cy, CYC, Cyc, CYCLO, CyClo
cyclopropane

Cyclo C cyclocytidine hydrochloride

Cyd cytidine; also C

CYE charcoal yeast extract (medium)

CYL casein yeast lactate (medium)

cyl cylinder; also C
cylindrical lens; also C

CYN cyanide; also CN, Cn

CYNAP cytotoxicity negative, absorption positive

CYP cyproheptadine

CYPIA Cytochrome P-450 induction assay

CYS cystoscopy; also CYSTO, cysto

Cys cyclosporin
cysteine; also C, cys

Cys-Cys cystine

cys cysteine; also C, Cys

CYSTO, cysto cystogram
cystoscopic examination
cystoscopy; also CYS

CYT Cytoxan (cyclophosphamide); also CTX,
CY
cytochrome; also C

Cyt cytosine; also C

cyt cytologic; also cytol
cytology; also cytol

cytoplasm
cytoplasmic

Cy/TBI cyclophosphamide and total body irradiation

cytol cytologic; also cyt
cytology; also cyt

CYTOMG cytomegalovirus; also CMV

Cyt ox cytochrome oxidase

cyt sys cytochrome system

CYVADIC, CyVADIC, CY-VA-DIC cyclophosphamide, vincristine, Adriamycin, and DIC (dacarbazine)

CZ cefazolin; also CEZ

Cz central midline placement of electrodes in electroencephalography

CZD cefazedone

CZI crystalline zinc insulin (regular insulin)

CZP clonazepam

D

Δ DELTA, UPPER CASE, fourth letter of the Greek alphabet
absence of heat in a reaction
change in a component of a physical system
delta gap
diagnosis; also D, DG, Dg, Diag, diag, DX, Dx, dx
difference (mathematics)
double bond
increment

ΔEF ejection fraction response

Δ9 THC delta-9-tetrahydrocannabinol

δ delta, lower case, fourth letter of the Greek alphabet
fourth in a series or group
heavy chain of immunoglobulin D
the delta chain of hemoglobin
thickness in a biological system, as of a layer of fluid

δALA delta-aminolevulinic acid; also DALA

D aspartic acid (one-letter notation); also ASP, Asp
cholecalciferol
coefficient of diffusion
dacryon; also dac
dalton; also Da
date; also d
daughter; also da, dau
daunorubicin; also DAUNO, DNR, Dnr, DRB
day(s); also d, da
dead; also d
dead air space; also DS
Debye
decease; also d, DEC, dec
deceased; also d, DEC, dec, dec'd, decd
deciduous; also DEC, dec
decimal reduction time; also D value
decrease; also d, DC, D/C, DEC, dec, DECR, decr
decreased; also d, DC, D/C, DEC, dec, DECR, decr
degree; also d, DEG, Deg, deg
density; also d, *d*
dental; also Dent, dent
dermatologic; also DERM, Derm, derm
dermatologist; also DERM, Derm, derm, DM
dermatology; also DERM, Derm, derm, DM
detail response
deuterium; also d
deuteron; also d
develop; also dev

development; also dev, devel
developmental; also dev, devel
deviant; also DEV, dev
deviate; also DEV, dev
deviation; also DEV, dev
dextro- (to the right, clockwise); also d-, *d*-
dextrorotary (rotated to the right or clockwise); also d-, *d*-
dextrose
diagnosis; also Δ, DG, Dg, Diag, diag, DX, Dx, dx
diagonal; also Diag, diag
diameter; also d, *d,* Dia, dia, diam
diarrhea; also d
diastole; also dias
diastolic; also dias
diathermy; also Dia, dia, diath
didymium (praseodymium); also Di
died; also d
difference; also DIFF, Diff, diff
different; also DIFF, Diff, diff
diffusing; also DIFF, Diff, diff
diffusing capacity
diffusion; also DIFF, Diff, diff
dihydrouridine
diopter; also d
diplomate; also Dip
disease; also dis, DZ, Dz, dz
distal; also d, dist
diuresis
diurnal; also d
diverticulum
divorced; also d, div
dominance; also DOM, dom
dominant; also DOM, dom
donor
dorsal; also d, Dors
dosage; also d, dos
dose; also d, dos
drive
drug
dual
duodenal; also duod
duodenum; also duod
duration; also d, DUR, dur
dwarf (colony)
electric displacement
give [L. *da* (give), *dare* (to give)]; also d, DA
let it be given [L. *detur*]; also d, det
right [L. *dexter*]; also d, dex
vitamin D unit

D̄ mean dose

D dilution factor

D- sterically related to D-glyceraldehyde

D1–D12 first through twelfth dorsal vertebra;
also D_1–D_{12}

D_1–D_{12} first through twelfth dorsal nerve
first through twelfth dorsal vertebra; also
D1–D12

D/3 distal third; also distal/3

D5, D_5 dextrose 5% in water; also D5W, D_5W,
D5/W, D5&W

1-D one-dimensional

2-D two-dimensional

2,4-D (2,4-dichlorophenoxy)acetic acid

3-D delayed double diffusion (test)
three-dimensional

D (as subscript) dead space gas

d 24 hours [L. *diem*]
atomic orbital with angular momentum quantum number 2
date; also D
day(s); also D, da
dead; also D
death
decease; also D, DEC, dec
deceased; also D, DEC, dec, dec'd, decd
deci- (10^{-1})
decrease; also D, DC, D/C, DEC, dec, DECR,
decr
decreased; also D, DC, D/C, DEC, dec,
DECR, decr
degree; also D, DEG, Deg, deg
density; also D, *d*
deoxy
deoxyribose; also DR, dRib
deuterium; also D
deuteron; also D
diameter; also D, *d*, Dia, dia, diam
diarrhea; also D
died; also D
diopter; also D
distal; also D, dist
diurnal; also D
divorced; also D, div
dorsal; also D, Dors
dosage; also D, dos
dose; also D, dos
doubtful
duration; also D, DUR, dur
dyne; also dyn
give [L. *da* (give), *dare* (to give)]; also D, DA
let it be given [L. *detur*]; also D, det
relative to rotation of a bean of polarized light
right [L. *dexter*]; also D, dex

1/d daily; also DD, dd
one per day

2/d twice a day

d- dextro- (to the right, clockwise); also D, *d*-
dextrorotary (rotated to the right or clockwise); also D, *d*-

d density; also D, d
diameter; also D, d, Dia, dia, diam

d- dextro- (to the right, clockwise); also D, d-
dextrorotary (rotated to the right or clockwise); also D, d-

DA dark agouti (rat)
daunomycin and arabinofuranosylcytosine
(cytarabine)
decubitus angina
degenerative arthritis
delayed action
delivery awareness
Dental Assistant
developmental age
diabetic acidosis
diagnostic arthroscopy
dietetic assistant
differentiation antigen
diphenylchlorarsine
direct admission
direct agglutination
disability assistance
disaggregated
dispense as directed; also DAD
dopamine; also DM, DPM
drug addict
drug addiction
drug aerosol
ductus arteriosus
give [L. *da* (give), *dare* (to give)]; also D, d

D-A donor-acceptor

D/A date of admission; also DOA
digital-to-analog (converter)
discharge and advise

Da dalton; also D

dA deoxyadenosine; also dAdo

da daughter; also D, dau
day(s); also D, d
deca- (10^1)

/da per day

DAA dehydroacetic acid; also DHA

DA/A drug/alcohol addiction

DAAO D-amino acid oxidase

DAB days after birth
3'3-diaminobenzidine

DAB—cont'd
diaminobutyric acid
dimethylaminoazobenzene; also DMAB
dysrhythmic aggressive behavior
German Medications Book (Ger. *Deutsches Arzneibuch*)

DABA 2,4-diaminobutyric acid

DABCO diazabicyclooctane

DAC diazacholesterol
digital-to-analog converter
disabled adult child
disaster assistance center
Division of Ambulatory Care

dac dacryon; also D

DACA dissecting aneurysm of the coronary artery
Drug Abuse Control Amendments

DACL Depression Adjective Check List

DACT, Dact dactinomycin (actinomycin D)

DAD delayed after-depolarization
diffuse alveolar damage
dispense as directed; also DA
drug administration device

DADA dichloroacetic acid diisopropylammonium salt

DADDS diacetyldiaminodiphenyl sulfone

dAdo deoxyadenosine; also dA

dADP deoxyadenosine diphosphate

DAE diphenylanthracene endoperoxide
diving air embolism

DAF decay-accelerating factor
delayed auditory feedback
differentiation-activating factor

DAFT Draw-A-Family test

DAG diacylglycerol

dag decagram; also dkg

DAGT direct antiglobulin test (Coombs test); also DAT

DAH disordered action of the heart

DAHEA Department of Allied Health Education and Accreditation

DAHM Division of Allied Health Manpower

DAI diffuse axonal injury

DAL defect anion level
drug analysis laboratory

daL, dal decaliter; also dkL, dkl

DALA delta-aminolevulinic acid; also δALA

DALE Drug Abuse Law Enforcement

DALU-SMUSPG domestic animal luteolytic uterine smooth muscle prostaglandin

DAM degraded amyloid
diacetylmonoxime
diacetylmorphine
discriminant analytic model

dam decameter; also dkm

dam² square decameter

dam³ cubic decameter

DAMA discharged against medical advice

dAMP deoxyadenosine monophosphate
deoxyadenosine-5'-phosphate
deoxyadenylic acid

DANA drug-induced antinuclear antibodies

dand to be given [L. *dandus*]

D and C dilatation and curettage: also DC, D&C
dilation and curettage; also DC, D&C

DANS dansyl chloride [5-(dimethylamino)-1-naphthalenesulfonyl chloride]

DAO diamine oxidase
duly authorized officer

DAP data acquisition processor
delayer after polarization
depolarizing afterpotential
diabetes-associated peptide
diaminopimelic acid; also DAPA
dihydrogalactital, Adriamycin, and Platinol
dihydroxyacetone phosphate; also DHAP, DHP
dipeptidyl amino peptidase
direct latex agglutination pregnancy (test)
Draw-A-Person (test)
dynamic aortic patch

DAPA diaminopimelic acid; also DAP

DAPI diaminophenylindole

DAPRU Drug Abuse Prevention Resource Unit

DAPST Denver Auditory Phoneme Sequencing Test

DAPT diaminophenylthiazole
direct latex agglutination pregnancy test

Dapt Daptazole

DAR daily affective rhythm
dual asthmatic reaction

DARF direct antiglobulin rosette-forming

DARP drug abuse rehabilitation program

DARTS Drug and Alcohol Rehabilitation Testing System

DAS death anxiety scale
delayed anovulatory syndrome

developmental apraxia of speech
dextroamphetamine sulfate
died at scene

DASE Denver Articulation Screening
Examination

DASH Distress Alarm for the Severely
Handicapped

DASI Developmental Activities Screening
Inventory

DASP double antibody solid phase

DAT daunorubicin, ARA-C, and thioguanine
delayed-action tablet
dementia of the Alzheimer type
Dental Admission Test
Dental Aptitude Test
diet as tolerated
differential agglutination test
differential agglutination titer
Differential Aptitude Test
diphtheria antitoxin
direct agglutination test; also dAT
direct antiglobulin test (Coombs test); also
DAGT
Disaster Action Team (Red Cross)

dAT direct agglutination test; also DAT

DATE dental auxiliary teacher education

dATP deoxyadenosine triphosphate

DAU 3-deazauridine
Dental Auxiliary Utilization

dau daughter; also D, da

DAUNO daunorubicin; also D, DNR, Dnr, DRB

DAV duck adenovirus

DAVP deamino-arginine vasopressin

DAW dispense as written

DB Baudelocque's diameter
database
date of birth; also D/B, DOB
deep breath
dense body
dextran blue
diabetic; also DIA, Dia, dia, diab
diagonal band
Diamond-Blackfan (syndrome)
diet beverage
direct bilirubin; also DBIL, D bili, DBR
disability; also dis, DSBL
distobuccal
Dollinger-Bielschowsky (syndrome)
double-blind (study)
dry bulb
duodenal bulb

Dutch belted (rabbit)

D/B date of birth; also DB, DOB

dB, db decibel

db diabetes; also DIA, Dia, dia, diab

DBA dibenzanthracene
Dolichos biflorus agglutinin

dBA decibel, weighted according to the A scale

DBAE dihydroxyborylaminoethyl

DBC dibencozide
dye-binding capacity

DB&C deep breathing and coughing

DBCL dilute blood clot lysis (method)

DBCP dibromochloropropane

DBD definite brain damage
dibromodulcitol (milolactol)

DBDG distobuccal developmental groove

DBE deep breathing exercise
dibromoethane

DBED dibenzylethylenediamine dipenicillin G
(penicillin G benzathine)

DBF disturbed bowel function

DBG dextrose, barbital, gelatin

DBH dacarbazine, BCNU (carmustine), and
hydroxyurea
dopamine beta-hydroxylase

DBI development-at-birth index
diazepam-binding inhibitor ("anxiety
peptide")

DBIL direct bilirubin; also DB, D bili, DBR

D bili direct bilirubin; also DB, DBIL, DBR

DBIOC database input/output control

DBIP Discrimination by Identification of
Pictures

dBk decibels above 1 kilowatt

dbl double

DBM database management
decarboxylase base Moeller
demineralized bone matrix
diabetic management
dibromomannitol
dobutamine; also DOB

dBm decibels above 1 milliwatt

DBMC dystrophica bullosa Mendes da Costa

DBMS database management systems

DBO distobucco-occlusal

db/ob diabetic obese (mouse)

DBP demineralized bone powder
diastolic blood pressure; also DIAS BP

DBP—cont'd
dibutyl phthalate
distobuccopulpal
di-*tert*-butyl peroxide; also DTBP
Döhle body panmyelopathy
vitamin D-binding protein

DBPPEE diisobutylphenoxypolyethoxyethanol

DBQ debrisoquin(e)

DBR direct bilirubin; also DB, DBIL, D bili
disordered breathing rate

DBS deep brain stimulation
Denis Browne splint
despeciated bovine serum
dibromosalicil
diminished breath sounds
direct bonding system
Division of Biological Standards

DBT disordered breathing time
dry bulb temperature

DBV dacarbazine, BCNU (carmustine), vincristine

DBW desirable body weight

dBW decibels above 1 watt

DBZ dibenzamine

DC daily census
data communication
daunorubicin and cytarabine
decarboxylase
decrease; also D, d, D/C, DEC, dec, DECR, decr
decreased; also D, d, D/C, DEC, dec, DECR, decr
deep compartment
degenerating cell
Deiters' cell
dendritic cell(s)
Dental Corps
deoxycholate; also DOC
descending colon
dextran charcoal
diagonal conjugate (diameter)
diagnostic center
diagnostic code
diarrhea/constipation; also D/C
differentiated cell
diffuse cortical
digit copying
dilatation and curettage; also D and C, D&C
dilation and curettage; also D and C, D&C
dilation catheter
diphenylarsine cyanide
diphenylcyanarsine
direct and consensual; also D&C

direct Coombs (test)
direct current; also dc
Direction Circular
discharge; also D/C, d/c, disch
discontinue; also D/C, d/c, dc, disc
distal colon
distocervical
Doctor of Chiropractic
donor cells
dorsal column
duodenal cap
dyskeratosis congenita

DC65 Darvon compound 65

D/C decrease; also D, d, DC, DEC, dec, DECR, decr
decreased; also D, d, DC, DEC, dec, DECR, decr
diarrhea/constipation; also DC
discharge; also DC, d/c, disch
discontinue; also DC, d/c, dc, disc
discontinued; also D/c'd, DXD, Dxd

D&C dilatation and curettage; also D and C, DC
dilation and curettage; also D and C, DC
direct and consensual; also DC
drug and cosmetic (dyes)

dC deoxycytidine

dc direct current; also DC
discontinue; also DC, D/C, d/c, disc

d/c discharge; also DC, D/C, disch
discontinue; also DC, D/C, dc, disc

DCA deoxycholate-citrate agar
deoxycholic acid
desoxycorticosterone acetate
dicarboxylic acid
dichloroacetate

DCAG double coronary artery graft

DCB dichlorobenzidine
dilutional cardiopulmonary bypass

DC&B dilation, curettage, and biopsy

DCBE double contrast barium enema

DCBF dynamic cardiac blood flow

DCC day care center
dextran-coated charcoal
dicyclohexylcarbodiimide; also DCCD
Disaster Control Center
dorsal cell column
double concave; also DCc, DDc

DCc double concave; also DCC, DDc

DCCD dicyclohexylcarbodiimide; also DCC

DCCF dural carotid-cavernous fistula

DCCMP daunomycin, cyclocytidine, mercaptopurine, and prednisolone

DC$_{CO2}$ diffusing capacity for carbon dioxide

DCD Dennis Test of Child Development

D/c'd discontinued; also D/C, DXD, Dxd

DCDA deuterium with cesium dihydrogen arsenate

dCDP deoxycytidine diphosphate

DCE delayed contrast enhancement
designated compensable event
desmosterol-to-cholesterol enzyme

DCF data collection form
deoxycoformycin
direct centrifugal flotation
dopachrome conversion factor
French approved non-proprietary name [Fr. *Dénomination Commune Française*]

DCFM Doppler color flow mapping

DCG deoxycorticosterone glucoside; also DOCG
disodium cromoglycate; also DSC, DSCG
dynamic electrocardiogram

DCH delayed cutaneous hypersensitivity
Diploma in Child Health

DCh Doctor of Surgery [L. *Doctor Chirurgiae*]

DCHA dicyclohexylamine

DCHFB dichlorohexafluorobutane

DCHN dicyclohexylamine nitrate
dicyclohexylamine nitrite

DCI dichloroisoprenaline
dichloroisoproterenol
International approved non-proprietary name [Fr. *Dénomination Commune Internationale*]

DCIS ductal carcinoma in situ

DCL dicloxacillin; also diclox, DX
diffuse cutaneous leishmaniasis
digital counter/locator
disseminated cutaneous leishmaniasis

DCLS deoxycholate citrate lactose saccharose (agar)

DCM dichloromethane
dichloromethotrexate; also DCMXT
dilated cardiomyopathy
Doctor of Comparative Medicine
dyssynergia cerebellaris myoclonica

DCMHQ Denver community mental health questionnaire

DCML dorsal column medical lemniscal

DCMO dihydrocarboxanilidomethyloxathiin

DCMP daunorubicin, cytarabine, mercaptopurine, and prednisone

dCMP deoxycytidine monophosphate
deoxycytidine-5′-phosphate
deoxycytidylic acid

dCMV disseminated cytomegalovirus (infection)

DCMX dichloro-*meta*-xylenol

DCMXT dichloromethotrexate; also DCM

DCN Data Collection Network (medical records)
delayed conditional necrosis
delayed conditioned necrosis
dorsal column nucleus
dorsal cutaneous nerve

DCNU chloroethyl-nitrosoglucosyl urea (chlorozotocin)

D$_{CO}$ diffusing capacity for carbon monoxide

DCOG Diploma of the College of Obstetricians and Gynaecologists (British)

DCP dicalcium phosphate
dichlorophen(e)
discharge planner
District Community Physician
dynamic compression plate

DCPC dichlorodiphenylmethyl carbinol; also DMC

DCPM daunorubicin, cytarabine, prednisolone, and mercaptopurine

DCPN direction-changing positional nystagmus

DCPU dorsal caudate putamen

DCR dacryocystorhinostomy
delayed cutaneous reaction
direct cortical response

DCS decompression sickness
Deleage-Curschmann-Steinert (syndrome)
dense canalicular system
diffuse cerebral sclerosis
diffuse cortical sclerosis
disease control serum
dorsal column stimulation
dorsal column stimulator

DCSA double-contrast shoulder arthrography

DCT daunorubicin, cytarabine, and thioguanine
deep chest therapy
direct Coombs' test
distal convoluted tubule
diurnal cortisol test
dynamic computed tomography

DCTM delay computer tomographic myelography

DCTMA desoxycorticosterone trimethylacetate

dCTP deoxycytidine triphosphate

DCTPA desoxycorticosterone triphenylacetate

DCU dichloral urea

DCV dacarbazine, CCNU (lomustine), and vincristine

DCX double-charge exchange

DCx double convex

DD daily [L. *de die*]; also dd
dangerous drug
day of delivery
degenerative disease
delusional disorder
dependent drainage
detrusor
developmental disability
developmentally disabled
dialysis dementia
diaper dermatitis
died of the disease; also DOD
differential diagnosis; also D/D, DDX, DDx, DIAGNO, diff diag
digestive disease
Di Guglielmo's disease
discharged dead
discharge diagnosis
disk diameter
Distortion of Dots
dog dander (test)
double density (disk)
double diffusion (test)
double dose
down drain
drug dependence
dry dressing; also dd
Duchenne's dystrophy
Dupuytren's disease
dyssynergia
let it be given to [L. *detur ad*]; also dd

DD-8 dodecahedral

D/D differential diagnosis; also DD, DDX, DDx, DIAGNO, diff diag

D-D discharge to duty

D&D diarrhea and dehydration

Dd unusual detail response

dD confabulated detail response

dd daily [L. *de die*]; also DD
dideoxynucleoside
dry dressing; also DD
let it be given to [L. *detur ad*]; also DD

DDA Dangerous Drugs Act
dideoxyadenosine
digital differential analyzer
digital display alarm

DDAVP, dDAVP 1-deamino-8-D-arginine vasopressin (desmopressin acetate)

DDBJ DNA Database of Japan

DDC dangerous drug cabinet
dideoxycytidine (zalcitabine); also ddC
diethyldithiocarbamate; also DDTC
dihydrocollidine
direct display console
diverticular disease of colon

DDc double concave; also DCC, DCc

ddC dideoxycytidine (zalcitabine); also DDC

DDD defined daily dose
degenerative disk disease
dense deposit disease
Denver dialysis disease
dichlorodiphenyldichloroethane
dihydroxydinaphthyl disulfide
drug distribution data
universal (pacemaker code)

o,p-DDD 2,4'-dichlorodiphenyldichloroethane (mitotane)

DDE dichlorodiphenyldichloroethylene
direct data entry

DDFS distant-disease-free survival

DDG deoxy-D-glucose

DDGB double-dose gallbladder (cholecystogram)

DDH Division of Dental Health

DDHT double dissociated hypertropia

DDI atrioventricular sequential (pacemaker code); also DVI
dideoxyinosine; also ddI
dressing dry and intact

ddI dideoxyinosine; also DDI

DDIB Disease Detection Information Bureau

dd in d from day to day [L. *de die in diem*]; also de d in d

DDM Doctor of Dental Medicine; also DMD

DDMS degenerative dense microsphere

dDNA denatured deoxyribonucleic acid

DDP *cis*-diamminedichloroplatinum (cisplatin); also Ddp
density-dependent phosphoprotein
difficult-denture patient
distributed data processing

Ddp *cis*-diamminedichloroplatinum (cisplatin); also DDP

DDR diastolic descent rate
discharged during referral

DDS damaged disk syndrome
Demon Dropout Scale
dendrodendritic synaptosome
dental distress syndrome
depressed deoxyribonucleic acid synthesis
dialysis disequilibrium syndrome
diaminodiphenylsulfone (dapsone); also DDSO
directional Doppler sonography
Director of Dental Services
disease disability scale
Doctor of Dental Surgery
dodecyl sulfate
double decidual sac
dystrophia-dystocia syndrome

Dds detail response to small white space

DDSc Doctor of Dental Science

DDSO diaminodiphenyl-sulfone (dapsone);
also DDS
diaminodiphenyl sulfoxide

DDST Denver Developmental Screening Test

DDT Degos-Delort-Tricot (syndrome)
dichlorodiphenyltrichloroethane (chloro-phenothane)
ductus deferens tumor

DDTC diethyldithiocarbamate; also DDC

DDTP drug dependence treatment program

ddTTP dideoxythymidine triphosphate

DDVP dimethyldichlorovinyl phosphate (dichlorvos)

DDW distilled deionized water
double distilled water

DdW detail response elaborating the whole

DDX, DDx differential diagnosis; also DD
D/D, DIAGNO, diff diag

DE dendritic expansion
deprived eye
diagnostic error
digestive energy
dose equivalent
dream elements
drug evaluation
Duchenne-Erb (syndrome)
duodenal exclusion
duration of ejection

-DE -dimensional echocardiography (eg, two-DE)

D₅E₄₈ 5% dextrose and electrolyte #48 (solution)

2DE two-dimensional echocardiography

D&E diet and elimination
dilatation and evacuation
dilation and evacuation

de edge detail

DEA dehydroepiandrosterone; also DHA,
DHE, DHEA
diethanolamine
diethylamine
Drug Enforcement Administration

DEA# Drug Enforcement Administration number (physician's federal narcotic number)

DEA-D diethylaminoethyldextran; also
DEAE-D

DEAE diethlaminoethanol
diethylaminoethyl (cellulose)

DEAE-D diethylaminoethyldextran; also
DEA-D

dearg pil let the pills be silverized [L. *deargentur pilulae*]

deaur pil let the pills be gilded [L. *deaurentur pilulae*]

DEB diepoxybutane
diethylbutanediol
dystrophic epidermolysis bullosa

deb debridement

DEBA diethylbarbituric acid

debil debility

DEBS dominant epidermolysis bullosa simplex

deb spis of proper consistency [L. *debita spissutudine*]

DEC decant, pour off [L. *decanta*]; also Dec, dec
decease; also D, d, dec
deceased; also D, d, dec, dec'd, decd
deciduous; also D, dec
decimal
decimeter; also dm
decrease; also D, d, DC, D/C, dec, DECR, decr
decreased; also D, d, DC, D/C, dec, DECR, decr
deoxycholate citrate
diethylcarbamazine
dynamic environmental conditioning (cycle)

Dec decant, pour off [L. *decanta*]; also DEC, dec

dec decant, pour off [L. *decanta*]; also DEC, Dec

decease; also D, d, DEC

deceased; also D, d, DEC, dec'd, decd

deciduous; also D, DEC

decompose; also decomp

decomposition; also decomp, decompn

decrease; also D, d, DC, D/C, DEC, DECR, decr

decreased; also D, d, DC, D/C, DEC, DECR, decr

deca- ten (10^1); also deka-

decd, dec'd deceased; also D, d, DEC, dec

DECEL, decel deceleration

deci- a tenth (10^{-1})

DECO decreasing consumption of oxygen

decoct a decoction

decomp decompose; also dec

decomposition; also dec, decompn

decompn decomposition; also dec, decomp

decon decontamination

dec(R) decrease, relative

DECR, decr decrease; also D, d, DC, D/C, DEC, dec

decreased; also D, d, DC, D/C, DEC, dec

DECUB, decub lying down [L. *decubitus*]

DED date of expected delivery

defined exposure dose

delayed erythema dose

diabetic eye disease

de d in d from day to day [L. *de die in diem*]; also dd in d

DEEG depth electroencephalogram

depth electroencephalography

depth electrography

DEET diethyltoluamide

DEF decayed, extracted, and/or filled; also def

defecation; also def

deficiency; also def, defic

duck embryo fibroblast

def decayed, extracted, and/or filled; also DEF

defecation; also DEF

deficiency; also DEF, defic

deficient; also defic

definite

definition

defib defibrillate

defibrillation

defic deficiency; also DEF, def

deficient; also def

deform deformed

deformity

DEG, Deg, deg degeneration; also degen

degenerative; also degen

degree; also D, d

degen degeneration; also DEG, Deg, deg

degenerative; also DEG, Deg, deg

deglut let it be swallowed [L. *deglutiatur*]

DEH dysplasia epiphysealis hemimelica

DEHFT developmental hand function test

DEHP di(2-ethylhexyl)phthalate

DEHS Division of Emergency Health Services

dehyd dehydrated

dehydration

DEJ, dej dentoenamel junction

deka- ten (10^1); also deca-

del deletion

delivery

delusion

deliq deliquescence

deliquescent; also deliquesc

deliquesc deliquescent; also deliq

DEM, Dem Demerol (meperidine)

DEN dengue

device experience network

diethylnitrosamine

denat denatured

denom denominator

DENT Dental Exposure Normalization Technique

Dent, dent dental; also D

dentist

dentistry

dentition

dent tal dos let such doses be given [L. *dentur tales doses*]

DEP diethylpropanediol

diethyl pyrocarbonate; also DEPC

dilution end point

dep dependent

deposit

purified [L. *depuratus*]

DEPA diethylenephosphoramide

DEPC diethyl pyrocarbonate; also DEP

depr depressed

depression

DEPS distal effective potassium secretion

DEP ST SEG depressed ST segment

Dept, dept department; also DPT

DER disulfiram-ethanol reaction
DeR reaction of degeneration
der derivative of chromosome
derive
deriv derivative
derived
DERM, Derm, derm dermatologic; also D
dermatologist; also D, DM
dermatology; also D, DM
DES dermal-epidermal separation
dialysis encephalopathy syndrome
diethylstilbestrol; also Des
diffuse esophageal spasm
disequilibrium syndrome
Doctor's Emergency Service
Des diethylstilbestrol; also DES
DESAT, desat desaturated
desc descent
descendant
descending
DESI drug efficacy study implementation
DEST dichotic environmental sounds test
dest distill [L. *destilla*]; also destil, dist
distilled [L. *destillatus*]; also destil, dist
destil distill [L. *destilla*]; also dest, dist
distilled [L. *destillatus*]; also dest, dist
DET diethyltryptamine
det determine
let it be given [L. *detur*]; also D, d
Det-6 detroid-6 (human sternum marrow cells)
determ determination; also determin, determn
determined; also determin
determin determination; also determ, determn
determined; also determ
determn determination; also determ, determin
det in dup let twice as much be given
[L. *detur in duplo*]; also det in 2 plo
det in 2 plo let twice as much be given
[L. *detur in duplo*]; also det in dup
detn detention
detox detoxification; also DTX
d et s let it be given and labeled [L. *detur et signetur*]
DEUC direct electronic urethrocystometry
DEV deviant; also D, dev
deviate; also D, dev
deviation; also D, dev
duck embryo rabies vaccine
duck embryo rabies virus

dev develop; also D
development; also D, devel
developmental; also D, devel
deviant; also D, DEV
deviate; also D, DEV
deviation; also D, DEV
devel development; also D, dev
developmental; also D, dev
DevPd developmental pediatrics
DEVR dominant exudative vitreoretinopathy
DEX, dex dexamethasone
dex right [L. *dexter*]; also D, d
DEXA dual energy x-ray absorptiometry
DF Daae-Finsen (disease)
Debré-Fibiger (syndrome)
decapacitation factor (sperm)
decayed and filled (permanent teeth)
decontamination factor
deferoxamine
deficiency factor
defined flora (animal)
degrees of freedom; also df
dengue fever
desferrioxamine; also DFX
diabetic father; also df
diaphragmatic function
diastolic filling
dietary fiber
differentiation factor
digital fluoroscopy
discriminant function
disseminated foci; also dF
distribution factor
dome fragment
dorsiflexion; also df
drug free
dry gas fractional (concentration)
dye free
dysgonic fermenter
Df duodenal fluid
dF disseminated foci; also DF
df decayed and filled (deciduous teeth)
degrees of freedom; also DF
diabetic father; also DF
dorsiflexion; also DF
DFA diet for age
difficulty falling asleep
direct fluorescence antibody (test)
direct fluorescent antibody (test)
dorsiflexion assist
DFB dinitrofluorobenzene (Sanger's reagent);
also DNFB
dysfunctional uterine bleeding; also DUB

DFC deletion of final consonants
dry-filled capsule

DFD defined formula diets
degenerative facet disease
diisopropylphosphorofluoridate; also DIPF

DFDD difluorodiphenyldichloroethane

DFDNB 1,5-difluoro-2,4-dinitrobenzene

DFDT difluorodiphenyltrichloroethane

DFE diffuse fasciitis with eosinophilia
distal femoral epiphysis

DFECT dense fibroelastic connective tissue

DFG direct forward gaze

DFI disease-free interval(s)

DFM decreased fetal movement

DFMC daily fetal movement count

DFMD difluoromethylDOPA

DFMO difluoromethylornithine

DFMR daily fetal movement record

DFO deferoxamine; also DFOM

DFOM deferoxamine; also DFO

DFP diastolic filling period
diisopropyl fluorophosphonate; also DIFP

DF^{32}P radiolabeled diisopropyl fluorophosphonate

DFR diabetic floor routine
dialysate filtration rate

DFRC deglycerolized frozen red cells

DFS disease-free survival
dynamic flow study

DFSP dermatofibrosarcoma protuberans

DFT defibrillation threshold
discrete Fourier transform

DFT$_4$ dialyzable free thyroxine

DFU dead fetus in utero
dideoxyfluorouridine

DFV diarrhea with fever and vomiting

DFX desferrioxamine; also DF

DG dark ground
dentate gyrus
deoxyglucose; also 2DG
diagnosis; also Δ, D, Dg, Diag, diag, DX, Dx,
dx
diastolic gallop
diglyceride
distogingival
Duchenne-Griesinger (disease)

Dg diagnosis; also Δ, D, DG, Diag, diag, DX,
Dx, dx

D$_g$ sterically related to D-glyceraldehyde (Used
to denote that carbohydrate nomenclature is
being used. The subscript refers to the standard substance 'glyceraldehyde'.)

dG deoxyguanosine

dg decigram; also dgm

2DG 2-deoxy-D-glucose; also DG

DGAVP desglycinamide vasopressin

DGBG dimethylglyoxal-bis(guanylhydrazone)

DGCI delayed gamma camera image

dGDP deoxyguanosine diphosphate

DGE delayed gastric emptying
density gradient electrophoresis

DGF digoxin-like factor; also DLF

DGGE denaturing gradient gel electrophoresis

DGI disseminated gonococcal infection

DGL deglycyrrhizined liquorice

DGM ductal glandular mastectomy

dgm decigram; also dg

dGMP deoxyguanosine monophosphate
deoxyguanosine-5′-phosphate
deoxyguanylic acid

DGMS Division of General Medical Services

DGN diffuse glomerulonephritis

DGP deoxyglucose phosphate

DGR Degranol (mannomustine)

DGS diabetic glomerulosclerosis

dGTP 2-deoxyguanosine-5′-triphosphate

DGV dextrose-gelatin-Veronal (buffer)

DGVB dextrose-gelatin-Veronal buffer

DH daily habits
day hospital
dehydrocholic acid
dehydrogenase
delayed hypersensitivity
dental habits
dental hygiene
dental hygienist
dermatitis herpetiformis
developmental history
diaphragmatic hernia
diffuse histiocytic (lymphoma)
disseminated histoplasmosis
dominant hand
dorsal horn
ductal hyperplasia
Dunkin-Hartley (guinea pig)

D/H deuterium to hydrogen (ratio)

DHA dehydroacetic acid; also DAA
dehydroascorbic acid
dehydroepiandrosterone; also DEA, DHE, DHEA
dihydroxyacetone
district health authority

Dha dihydroalanine

DHAD dihydroxy-bis(hydroxyethyl)ami-noethylamino-anthraquinone dihydrooride (mitoxantrone hydrochloride)

DHAP dexamethasone, ARA-C, and Platinol
dihydroxyacetone phosphate; also DAP, DHP

DHAS dehydroepiandrosterone sulfate; also DHEAS, DS

DHB dihydroxybenzoic acid

Dhb dehydrobutyrine

DHBS dihydrobiopterin synthetase

DHBV duck hepatitis B virus

DHC dehydrocholate
dehydrocholesterol

DHCA deep hypothermia and circulatory arrest

DHCC dihydroxycholecalciferol

DHD district health department

DHE dehydroepiandrosterone; also DEA, DHA, DHEA
dihydroergocryptine; also DHEC, DHK
dihydroergotamine; also DHE-45

DHE-45 dihydroergotamine; also DHE

DHEA dehydroepiandrosterone; also DEA, DHA, DHE

DHEAS dehydroepiandrosterone sulfate; also DHAS, DS

DHEC dihydroergocryptine; also DHE, DHK

DHES Division of Health Examination Statistics

DHEW Department of Health, Education, and Welfare (now; DHHS, Department of Health and Human Services)

DHF dengue hemorrhagic fever
dorsihyperflexion

DHFR dihydrofolate reductase

DHFS dengue hemorrhagic fever shock (syndrome)

DHg Doctor of Hygiene; also DHy, DHyg, DrHyg

DHGG deaggregated human gamma-globulin

DHHS Department of Health and Human Services

DHI Dental Health International

dihydroisocodeine; also DHIC
dihydroxyindole

DHIA dehydroisoandrosterone

DHIC dihydroisocodeine; also DHI

DHJ doing his job

DHK dihydroergocryptine; also DHE, DHEC

DHL diffuse histiocytic lymphoma

DHM dihydromorphine

DHMA 3,4-dihydroxymandelic acid

DHN Department of Hospital Nursing

DHO deuterium hydrogen oxide
dihydroergocornine; also DHO 180
Dhori orthomyxovirus

DHO 180 dihydroergocornine; also DHO

DHODH dihydroorotate dehydrogenase

DHP dehydrogenated polymer
dihydroprogesterone
dihydropyridine
dihydroxyacetone phosphate; also DAP, DHAP

DHPc dorsal hippocampus

DHPG dihydroxyphenylethylene glycol
dihydroxyphenylglycol; also DOPEG
dihydroxyproproxymethylguanine (ganciclovir)

DHPR dihydropteridine reductase

dhPRL decidual human prolactin

DHR delayed hypersensitivity reaction

DHS delayed hypersensitivity (reaction)
dihydrostreptomycin; also DHSM, DS, DSM, DST
duration of hospital stay
dynamic hip screw

D-5-HS dextrose 5% in Harman solution

DHSM dihydrostreptomycin; also DHS, DS, DSM, DST

DHSS dihydrostreptomycin sulfate

DHST delayed hypersensitivity test

DHT dihydroergotoxine
dihydrotachysterol
dihydrotestosterone
dihydrothymine
dihydroxypropyltheophylline
dissociated hypertropia

DHTP dihydrotestosterone propionate

DHy Doctor of Hygiene; also DHg, DHyg, DrHyg

DHyg Doctor of Hygiene; also DHg, DHy, DrHyg

DHZ dihydralazine

DI (Beck) Depression Inventory
date of injury; also DOI
Debris Index
defective interfering (particle)
degradation index
dentinogenesis imperfecta
deoxyribonucleic acid index
desorption ionization
deterioration index
detrusor instability
diabetes insipidus
diagnostic imaging
diaphragm; also diaph, DPH
diaphragmatic; also diaph, DPH
disability insurance
dispensing information
distal intestine
distoincisal
dorsal interosseous
dorsoiliacus
double indemnity
drug information
drug interactions
dyskaryosis index
dyspnea index

D&I debridement and irrigation
dry and intact

D$_I$ insulin dialysance

Di didymium (praseodymium); also D
Diego blood group

di inside detail

DIA depolarization-induced automaticity
diabetes; also db, Dia, dia, diab
diabetic; also DB, Dia, dia, diab
Diego blood group antigen; also DiA, Di^a
differentiation inhibitory activity

DiA Diego blood group antigen; also DIA, Di^a

Dia, dia diabetes; also db, DIA, diab
diabetic; also DB, DIA, diab
diathermy; also D, diath
diameter; also D, d, *d,* diam

Di^a Diego blood group antigen; also DIA, DiA

diab diabetes; also db, DIA, Dia, dia
diabetic; also DB, DIA, Dia, dia

DIAC diiodothyroacetic acid

Diag, diag diagnosis; also Δ, D, DG, Dg, DX,
Dx, dx
diagnostic
diagonal; also D
diagram

DIAGNO differential diagnosis; also DD, D/D,
DDX, DDx, diff diag

diam diameter; also D, d, *d,* Dia, dia

diaph diaphragm; also DI, DPH
diaphragmatic; also DI, DPH

DIAR dextran-induced anaphylactoid reaction

dias diastole; also D
diastolic; also D

DIAS BP diastolic blood pressure; also DBP

diath diathermy; also D, Dia, dia

DIATH SW diathermy short wave

DIAZ diazepam; also DZ, DZP

DIB Diagnostic Interview for Borderlines
disability insurance benefits
dot immunobinding

DIC differential interference contrast
(microscopy)
diffuse intravascular coagulation
dimethyltriazenylimidazole carboxamide
(dacarbazine); also DTIC
disseminated intravascular coagulation;
also DIVC
disseminated intravascular coagulopathy
drug information center

dic dicentric

DICD dispersion-induced circular dichroism

diclox dicloxacillin; also DCL, DX

DID dead of intercurrent disease
delayed ischemia deficit
double immunodiffusion (technique)
dystonia-improvement-dystonia

DIDD dense intramembranous deposit disease

DIDMOAD diabetes insipidus, diabetes mellitus, optic atrophy, and deafness (syndrome); also DIMOAD

DIE died in Emergency Room

dieb alt on alternate days [L. *diebus alternis*]

dieb secund every second day [L. *diebus
secundis*]

dieb tert every third day [L. *diebus tertiis*]

DIEDA diethyliminodiacetic acid

Diet Tech Dietetic Technician; also DT

DIF differentiation-inducing factor
diffuse interstitial fibrosis
diflunisal
direct immunofluorescence
dose increase factor

dif differential blood count; also DIFF, Diff, diff

DIFF, Diff, diff difference; also D
different; also D
differential
differential blood count; also dif
diffusing; also D

diffusion; also D

diff diag differential diagnosis; also DD, D/D, DDX, DDx, DIAGNO

DIFP diffuse interstitial fibrosing pneumonitis diisopropyl fluorophosphonate; also DFP

DIG digitalis; also dig
digitoxin; also DT
digoxin; also Dig, DO

Dig digoxin; also DIG, DO

dig digitalis; also DIG
let it be digested [L. *digeretur*]

dig tox digitalis toxicity

DIH died in hospital

DIHPPA diiodohydroxyphenylpyruvic acid

DIJOA dominantly inherited juvenile optic atrophy

DIL dilute; also dil, dilut
diluted; also dil, dilut
dilution; also dil, dilut, diln
drug-induced lupus; also dil
drug information log; also dil

Dil Dilantin
dilation; also dil

dil dilation; also Dil
dilute; also DIL, dilut
diluted; also DIL, dilut
dilution; also DIL, dilut, diln
dissolve [L. *dilue*]; also diss, dslv
drug-induced lupus; also DIL
drug information log; also DIL

dilat dilatation

DILD diffuse infiltrative lung disease
diffuse interstitial lung disease

DILE drug-induced lupus erythematosus

diln dilution; also, DIL, dil, dilut

Diluc, diluc at daybreak [L. *diluculo*]

dilut dilute; also DIL, dil
diluted; also DIL, dil
dilution; also DIL, dil, diln

DIM digital imaging microscopy
diminish; also dim
diminished; also dim
divalent ion metabolism

dim diminish; also DIM
diminished; also DIM
one-half [L. *dimidius*]

DIME Division of International Medical Education

DIMOAD diabetes insipidus, diabetes mellitus, optic atrophy, and deafness (syndrome); also DIDMOAD

dIMP deoxyinosine monophosphate (deoxy-inosinate)

DIMS disorders of initiating and maintaining sleep

DIMSA disseminated intravascular multiple systems activation

DIN drug identification number

d in dup give twice as much [L. *detur in duplo*]

d in p aeq divide into equal parts [L. *divide in partes aequales*]; also div in par aeq

diopt diopter

DIP desquamative interstitial pneumonia
desquamative interstitial pneumonitis
dichlorophenolindophenol
diisopropyl phosphate
distal interphalangeal (joint)
drip-infusion pyelogram
drug-induced parkinsonism
dual-in-line package (integrated circuits)

Dip diplomate; also D

dip diploid

DIPA diisopropylamine

DIPC diffuse interstitial pulmonary calcification

DIPF diisopropylphosphorofluoridate; also DFD

diph diphtheria

diph-tox diphtheria toxoid; also DT

diph-tox AP alum-precipitated diphtheria toxoid

DIPJ distal interphalangeal joint

DIR director; also Dir, dir
double isomorphous replacement

Dir, dir direct
direction
directions
director; also DIR

DIRD drug-induced renal disease

dir prop with proper direction [L. *directione propria*]; also DP, dp

DIS Diagnostic Interview Schedule
dislocated; also dis, disloc
dislocation; also dis, disl, disloc

DI-S Debris Index-Simplified

dis disability; also DSBL
disabled; also DSBL
disease; also D, DZ, Dz, dz
dislocated; also DIS, disloc
dislocation; also DIS, disl, disloc
distance; also dist

dis—cont'd
distribute; also dist
distribution; also dist

disc discontinue; also DC, D/C, dc, d/c

disch discharge; also DC, D/C, d/c
discharged

DISH diffuse idiopathic skeletal hyperostosis
disseminated idiopathic skeletal hyperostosis

DISI dorsiflexed intercalated segment
instability

DISIDA diisopropyliminodiacetic acid

disinfect disinfection

disl dislocation; also DIS, dis, disloc

disloc dislocated; also DIS, dis
dislocation; also DIS, dis, disl

disod disodium

D₅ISOM dextrose 5% in Isolyte M

disp dispensary
dispense
to dispense [L. *dispensare*]

dispo disposition

DISS diameter index safety system

diss dissolve; also dil, dslv
dissolved

dissem disseminated
dissemination

dist distal; also D, d
distance; also dis
distill; also dest, destil
distillation; also distill, distln
distilled; also dest, destil
distribute; also dis
distribution; also dis
district

distal/3 distal third; also D/3

dist fr distinguished from

distill distillation; also dist, distln

distln distillation; also dist, distill

DIT diet-induced thermogenesis
diiodotyrosine
drug-induced thrombocytopenia

dITP deoxyinosine triphosphate

DIV double-inlet ventricle

div divergence
divergent
divide
divided
division
divorced; also D, d
to divide [L. *dividere*]

DIVA digital intravenous angiography

DIVBC disseminated intravascular blood
coagulation

DIVC disseminated intravascular coagulation;
also DIC

DIVD decentralized in vitro diagnostic

div in par aeq divide into equal parts [L.
divide in partes aequales]; also d in p aeq

DJ Dubin-Johnson (syndrome)

DJD degenerative joint disease

DJS Dubin-Johnson syndrome

DK dark; also dk
decay
degeneration of keratinocytes
Déjérine-Klumpke (syndrome)
diabetic ketoacidosis; also DKA
diet kitchen
diseased kidney
dog kidney (cells)

dk dark; also DK
deka- (10¹)

DKA diabetic ketoacidosis; also DK
didn't keep appointment

DKB deep knee bends
dideoxykanamycin B

DKDP deuterium with potassium dihydrogen
phosphate [L. *kalium* (potassium)]

dkg dekagram; also dag

dkL, dkl dekaliter; also daL, dal

dkm dekameter; also dam

DKP dibasic potassium phosphate
[L. *kalium* (potassium)]
dikalium phosphate
diketopiperazine

DKTC dog kidney tissue culture

DKV deer kidney virus

DL danger list
dansyl lysine
deep lobe
developmental level
diagnostic laparoscopy
difference limen (test, threshold)
diffuse lymphoma
diffusing capacity of the lungs; also D_L
directed listening
direct laryngoscopy
disabled list
distolingual
Donath-Landsteiner (antibody, test); also D-L
doxorubicin and lomustine
drug level

Duchenne-Leyden (syndrome)
Dunning leukemia
lethal dose [L. *dosis letalis*]
racemic (optically inactive, containing equal
quantities of D- and L- enantiomorphs; also
DL-, DL-

DL-, DL- racemic (optically inactive, containing
equal quantities of D- and L- enantiomorphs; also DL

D-L Donath-Landsteiner (antibody, test); also DL

D_L diffusing capacity of the lungs; also DL

dL, dl deciliter

dl-, *dl*- racemic (optically inactive, containing
equal quantities of dextrorotary and levorotary enantiomorphs)

DLA, DLa distolabial

D-L Ab Donath-Landsteiner antibody

DLAI, DLaI distolabioincisal

DLAP, DLaP distolabiopulpal

DLB diffuse and lymphoblastic
direct laryngoscopy and bronchoscopy

DLC differential leukocyte count
double-lumen catheter

DLCO, DL$_{CO}$, D$_{LCO}$ carbon monoxide diffusing capacity of the lungs

DLCO$_2$, DL$_{CO2}$, D$_{LCO2}$ carbon dioxide diffusing capacity of the lungs

D$_{LCO}$RB, D$_{LCO}$^{RB} diffusing capacity of the
lungs, rebreathing methods

D$_{LCO}$SB, D$_{LCO}$^{SB} diffusing capacity of the
lungs, single breath

D$_{LCO}$SS, D$_{LCO}$^{SS} diffusing capacity of the
lungs, steady-state

DLE delayed light emission
dialyzable leukocyte extract
discoid lupus erythematosus
disseminated lupus erythematosus

D$_1$LE diagonal 1 lower extremity

D$_2$LE diagonal 2 lower extremity

DLF digitalis-like factor
digoxin-like factor; also DGF
dorsolateral funiculus

DLG distolingual groove

DLI distolinguoincisal
double label index

DLIF digoxin-like immunoreactive factors

DLIS digoxin-like immunoreactive substance

DLL dihomo-gammalinoleic acid

DLLI dulcitol lysine lactose iron (agar)

DLMP date of last menstrual period

DLNMP date of last normal menstrual period

DLO distolinguo-occlusal
drug license opportunity

D$_L$O$_2$, D$_{LO2}$ diffusing capacity of lungs for
oxygen

DLP delipidized serum protein
developmental learning problems
direct linear plotting
dislocation of patella
distolinguopulpal
dysharmonic luteal phase

D$_5$LR dextrose 5% in lactated Ringer's
(solution)

DLS daily living skills

DLT dehydroepiandrosterone loading test

DLU disposable loading unit

DLV defective leukemia virus

DLWD diffuse lymphocytic, well differentiated

DM dermatologist; also D, DERM, Derm,
derm
dermatology; also D, DERM, Derm, derm
dermatomyositis; also DMS
Descemet's membrane
dextromaltose
dextromethorphan
diabetes mellitus
diabetic mother
diastolic murmur
diffuse mixed (histiocytic-lymphocytic lymphoma)
diphenylamine-arsine chloride
diphenylaminechlorarsine
distant metastases
Doctor of Medicine [L. *Doctor Medicinae*]
dopamine; DA, DPM
dorsomedial
dose modification
double membrane
double minute (chromosome)
drug monograph
dry matter
duodenal mucosa
membrane diffusing capacity

D$_M$ membrane component of diffusion

dM decimorgan

dm decimeter; also DEC

dm^2 square decimeter

dm^3 cubic decimeter

DMA dimethoxyamphetamine
dimethyladenosine
dimethylamine
dimethylaniline
dimethylarginine

DMA—cont'd
  direct memory access (computers)
  direct memory address (computers)
DMAARD delayed-mechanism-of-action antirheumatic drug
DMAB dimethylaminoazobenzene; also DAB
  dimethylaminobenzaldehyde (Ehrlich's reagent); also DMABA
DMABA dimethylaminobenzaldehyde (Ehrlich's reagent); also DMAB
DMAC *N,N*-dimethylacetamide
DMAD disease-modifying antirheumatic drug; also DMARD
DMAE dimethylaminoethanol
DMARD disease-modifying antirheumatic drug; also DMAD
DMAS dimethylamine sulfate
DMAT Disaster Medical Assistance Team
DMBA 7,12-dimethylbenz[*a*]anthracene
DMC dactinomycin, methotrexate, and cyclophosphamide
  demeclocycline
  dichlorodiphenylmethyl carbinol; also DCPC
  dimethylcysteine
  direct microscopic count
DMCC direct microscopic clump count
DMCT demethylchlortetracycline (demeclocycline); also DMCTC
DMCTC demethylchlortetracycline (demeclocycline); also DMCT
DMD desmethyldiazepam; also DMDZ
  disease-modifying drug
  Doctor of Dental Medicine; also DDM
  Duchenne's muscular dystrophy; also DUD
DMDS dimethyl disulfide
DMDT dimethoxydiphenyltrichloroethane
DMDZ desmethyldiazepam; also DMD
DME degenerative myoclonus epilepsy
  dimethyl diester
  dimethyl ether (of *d*-tubocurarine)
  diphasic meningoencephalitis
  Director of Medical Education
  dropping mercury electrode
  drug-metabolizing enzyme
  Dulbecco modified Eagle (medium)
  durable medical equipment
DMEM Dulbecco modified Eagle medium
DMF decayed, missing or filled (teeth)
  N,N-dimethylformamide; also DMFA
  diphasic milk fever
DMFA dimethylformamide; also DMF

DMFS decayed, missing, or filled surfaces (permanent teeth)
dmfs decayed, missing, or filled surfaces (deciduous teeth)
DMFT DMF (decayed, missing or filled), used with the tooth as the unit of measurement
DMG dimethylglycine
DMGBL dimethyl-gamma-butyrolactone
DMGG dimethylguanylguanidine
DMH Department of Mental Health
  Department of Mental Hygiene
  diffuse mesangial hypercellularity
  dimethylhydrazine
DMI defense mechanism inventory
  desmethylimipramine (desipramine)
  Diagnostic Mathematics Inventory (psychologic testing)
  diaphragmatic myocardial infarction
  direct migration inhibition
DMKA diabetes mellitus ketoacidosis
DML diffuse mixed (histiocytic-lymphocytic) lymphoma
  distal motor latency
DMM dimethylmyleran
  disproportionate micromelia
DMN dimethylnitrosamine; also DMNA
  dorsal motor nucleus (of vagus nerve)
DMNA dimethylnitrosamine; also DMN
DMO 5,5-dimethyl-2,4-oxazolidinedione (dimethadione)
DMOOC diabetes mellitus out of control
DMP diffuse mesangial proliferation
  dimethyl phosphate
  dimethyl phthalate
  dura mater prosthesis
DMPA depomedroxyprogesterone acetate
DMPE dimethoxyphenylethylamine; also DMPEA
DMPEA dimethoxyphenylethylamine; also DMPE
DMPP dimethylphenylpiperazinium
DMPS dysmyelopoietic syndrome; also DMS
DMR Diploma in Medical Radiology
DMRD Diploma in Medical Radio-Diagnosis (British)
DMRF dorsal medullary reticular formation
DMRT Diploma in Medical Radio-Therapy (British)
DMS delayed microembolism syndrome
  delayed muscle soreness

demarcation membrane system
dense microsphere
Department of Medicine and Surgery
dermatomyositis; also DM
diagnostic medical sonography
diffuse mesangial sclerosis
dimercaptosuccinic acid (succimer); also DMSA
dimethyl sulfate
dimethylsulfoxide; also DMSO
Doctor of Medical Science
dysmyelopoietic syndrome; also DMPS

dms double minute sphere

DMSA dimercaptosuccinic acid (succimer); also DMS

DMSO dimethylsulfoxide; also DMS

DMT dermatophytosis
N,N-dimethyltryptamine
Doctor of Medical Technology

DMTU dimethylthiourea

D,M,V,P disk, macula, vessels, periphery

DMX diathermy, massage, and exercise

DN Deiters' nucleus
dextrose to nitrogen (ratio); also D/N, D:N
diabetic neuropathy
dibucaine number
dicrotic notch
Diploma in Nursing
District Nurse
down
dysplastic nevus

D/N dextrose to nitrogen (ratio); also DN, D:N

D:N dextrose to nitrogen (ratio); also DN, D/N

D&N distance and near (vision)

Dn dekanem [nem: Ger. *Nahrung* (nourishment), *Einheit* (unit), *Milch* (milk)]

dn decinem [nem: Ger. *Nahrung* (nourishment), *Einheit* (unit), *Milch* (milk)]

DNA deoxyribonucleic acid
did not answer
did not appear
did not attend
does not apply

DNAP deoxyribonucleic acid polymerase

DNA-P deoxyribonucleic acid phosphorus

DNAse, DNase deoxyribonuclease

DNB Dictionary of National Biography
dinitrobenzene
Diplomate of the National Board (of Medical Examiners)
dorsal noradrenergic bundle

DNBP dinitrobutylphenol

DNC did not come
dinitrocarbanilide
DNA, collodion, charcoal

DNCB dinitrochlorobenzene

DND died a natural death

DNE Director of Nursing Education
Doctor of Nursing Education

DNF Durand-Nicolas-Favre (disease)

DNFB dinitrofluorobenzene (Sanger's reagent); also DFB

DNI do not intubate

DNIC diffuse noxious inhibitory control

DNJ deoxynojirimycin

DNKA did not keep appointment

DNL diffuse nodular lymphoma
disseminated necrotizing leukoencephalopathy

DNLL dorsal nucleus of lateral lemniscus

DNMR deuterium nuclear magnetic resonance

DNO District Nursing Officer

DNOC dinitro-*ortho*-cresol

DNOCHP dinitro-*o*-cyclohexylphenol

DNP, Dnp deoxyribonucleoprotein
dinitrophenol

DNPH dinitrophenylhydrazine

DNPM dinitrophenolmorphine

DNPT diethylnitrophenyl thiophosphate (parathion); also DNTP

DNR daunorubicin; also D, DAUNO, Dnr, DRB
did not respond
do not report
do not resuscitate
dorsal nerve root

Dnr daunorubicin; also D, DAUNO, DNR, DRB

DNS dansyl; also Dns
de novo synthesis
deviated nasal septum
diaphragmatic nerve stimulation
did not show
Director of Nursing Services
doctor did not see (patient)
Doctor of Nursing Science; also DNSc
do not show
do not substitute
dysplastic nevus syndrome

D₅NS, d₅NS dextrose 5% in normal saline solution; also D5/NS, D5%/NS, D₅NSS

D5/NS dextrose 5% in normal saline; also D₅NS, d₅NS, D5%/NS, D₅NSS

D5%/NS dextrose 5% in normal saline; also D₅NS, d₅NS, D5/NS, D₅NSS

D5.2NS dextrose 5% in one fourth normal saline

D5.4NS dextrose 5% in one half normal saline

Dns dansyl; also DNS

DNSc Doctor of Nursing Science; also DNS

D₅NSS dextrose 5% in normal saline solution; also D₅NS, d₅NS, D5/NS, D5%/NS

DNT did not test

DNTB dinitroblue

DNTP diethylnitrophenyl thiophosphate (parathion); also DNPT

DNUA distillable nonurea adductable

DNV dorsal nucleus of vagus nerve

DO diamine oxidase (histaminase)
diet order
digoxin; also DIG, Dig
dissolved oxygen
disto-occlusal
Doctor of Osteopathy
doctor's orders
doxycycline
drugs only (visits)

D-O directive-organic

D/O disorder

D₀ oxygen diffusion

do the same, as before [L. *dicto*]

DOA date of admission; also D/A
date of arrival
dead on arrival
driver of automobile
duration of action

DOAC Dubois' oleic-albumin complex

DOA-DRA dead on arrival despite resuscitative attempts

DOAP daunorubicin, Oncovin, Ara-C (cytarabine), and prednisone

DOB date of birth; also DB, D/B
dobutamine; also DBM
doctor's order book

DOC date of conception
deoxycholate; also DC
11-deoxycorticosterone
diabetes out of control; also doc, DOOC
died of other causes
diet of choice
drug of choice

doc diabetes out of control; also DOC, DOOC
doctor; also DR, Dr
document
documentation

DOCA deoxycorticosterone acetate

DOCG deoxycorticosterone glucoside; also DCG

DOCLINE Documents On-Line

DOCS, DOCs deoxycorticoids

DOcSc Doctor of Ocular Science; also DOS

DOC-SR desoxycorticosterone secretion rate

DOD date of death
date of discharge
dead of the disease
Department of Defense
died of the disease; also DD
dissolved oxygen deficit
drug overdose

DOE date of examination
Department of Energy
desoxyephedrine hydrochloride
direct observation evaluation (test)
dyspnea on exercise
dyspnea on exertion

DOES disorders of excessive sleepiness

DOET 2,5-dimethoxy-4-ethylamphetamine

DOFOS disturbance of function occlusion syndrome

DOH Department of Health

DOHb Döhle's bodies

DOI date of injury; also DI
died of injuries

DOL day of life (followed by number)

dol dolorimetric unit (of pain intensity)

DOLV double-outlet left ventricle

DOM deaminated *o*-methyl metabolite
Department of Medicine
2,5-dimethoxy-4-methylamphetamine
dissolved organic matter
dominance; also D, dom
dominant; also D, dom

dom domestic
dominance; also D, DOM
dominant; also D, DOM

DOMA dihydroxymandelic acid

DON Determination of Need
diazo-oxonorleucine
Director of Nursing

don until [L. *donec*]

donec alv sol fuerit until the bowels are opened [L. *donec alvus soluta fuerit*]

DOOC diabetes out of control; also DOC, doc

DOOR deafness, onycho-osteodystrophy, and mental retardation (syndrome)

DOP depth of penetration (test)

DOPA, Dopa, dopa dihydroxyphenylalanine (methyldopa)

DOPAC dihydroxyphenylacetic acid

dopase dihydroxyphenylalanine oxidase

DOPC determined osteogenic precursor cell

DOPE disease-oriented physician education

DOPEG dihydroxyphenylglycol; also DHPG

DOPP dihydroxyphenylpyruvate

DOPS diffuse obstructive pulmonary syndrome
dihydroxyphenylserine

Dors dorsal; also D, d

DORV double-outlet right ventricle

DoRx date of treatment; also D/T

DOS date of surgery
day of surgery
deoxystreptamine
disk operating system (computer)
Division of Operational Safety
Doctor of Ocular Science; also DOcSc
Doctor of Optical Science

dos dosage; also D, d
dose; also D, d

DOSC Dubois' oleic serum complex

DOSS Department of Social Services
dioctyl sodium sulfosuccinate (docusate sodium); also DSS
distal over-shoulder strap

DOT date of transcription
date of transfer
died on (operating) table
Doppler ophthalmic test

DOTC Dameshek's oval target cell

DOU direct observation unit

DOV discharged on visit

DOX, Dox doxorubicin; also DOXO, Doxo, DXR

DOXO, Doxo doxorubicin; also DOX, Dox, DXR

DP data processing
deep pulse
definitive procedure
degradation product
degree of polymerization; also dp
deltopectoral
dementia praecox
dense plate
dental prosthesis

dental prosthodontics
developed pressure
dexamethasone pretreatment
diaphragmatic plaque
diastolic pressure
diffuse precipitation
diffusion pressure
digestible protein
diphosgene
diphosphate
dipropionate
directional preponderance
disability pension
discharge planning
discriminating power
disopyramide phosphate
displaced person
distal phalanx
distal pit
distopulpal
docking protein
Doctor of Pharmacy; also DPharm
Doctor of Podiatry
donor's plasma
dorsalis pedis; also dp
driving pressure
dyspnea; also dysp
D-penicillamine; also DPA, d-pen
with proper direction [L. *directione propria*]; also dir prop, dp

dp degree of polymerization; also DP
dorsalis pedis; also DP
with proper direction [L. *directione propria*]; also dir prop, DP

DPA Department of Public Assistance
Designed Plan Agencies (medical records)
dextroposition of aorta
diphenolic acid
diphenylalanine
diphenylamine
dipicolinic acid
dipropylacetate
dual photon absorptiometer
dynamic physical activity
D-penicillamine; also DP, d-pen

DPAT di-*n*-propylaminotetraline

DPB days postburn

DPC delayed primary closure
desaturated phosphatidylcholine
direct patient care
discharge planning coordinator
distal palmar crease

DPD depression pure disease
desoxypyridoxine hydrochloride

DPD—cont'd
diffuse pulmonary disease
diphenamid

DPDL diffuse poorly differentiated (lymphocytic) lymphoma

DPDT, dpdt double-pole double-throw (switch)

DPE Death Personification Exercise (psychology)
dipiperidinoethane

d-pen D-penicillamine; also DP, DPA

DPF Dental Practitioners' Formulary

DPFR diastolic pressure-flow relationship

DPG 2,3-diphosphoglycerate; also 2,3-DPG
displacement placentogram

2,3-DPG 2,3-diphosphoglycerate; also DPG

2,3-DPGM 2,3-diphosphoglycerate mutase

DPGN diffuse proliferative glomerulonephritis

DPGP diphosphoglycerate phosphatase

DPH Department of Public Health
diaphragm; also DI, diaph
diaphragmatic; also DI, diaph
diphenhydramine
diphenylhexatriene
diphenylhydantoin (phenytoin)
Diploma in Public Health
Doctor of Public Health; also DrPH
Doctor of Public Hygiene; also DrPH

DPh Doctor of Philosophy

DPharm Doctor of Pharmacy; also DP

DPhC Doctor of Pharmaceutical Chemistry

DPhc Doctor of Pharmacology

DPHN Department of Public Health Nursing
Doctor of Public Health Nursing

DPI daily permissible intake
days postinoculation
dietary protein intake
disposable personal income
drug prescribing index

DPIF Drug Product Information File

DPJ dementia paralytica juvenilis

DPL diagnostic peritoneal lavage
dipalmitoyl lecithin
distopulpolingual

DPLa distopulpolabial

DPM Diploma in Psychological Medicine
dipyridamole
disabling pansclerotic morphea
discontinue previous medication

disintegrations per minute; also dpm
Doctor of Physical Medicine
Doctor of Podiatric Medicine
dopamine; also DA, DM
drops per minute

dpm disintegrations per minute; also DPM

DPN dermatosis papulosa nigra
diabetic polyneuropathy
diphosphopyridine nucleotide (NAD)

DPN+ oxidized diphosphopyridine nucleotide (NAD+)

DPNase oxidized diphosphopyridine nucleotide nucleosidase

DPNH reduced diphosphopyridine nucleotide (NADH)

DPP deep pseudopupil
differential pulse polarography
dimethoxyphenylpenicillin
dual purpose packaging

DPPC dipalmitoylphosphatidylcholine

DPR Doctor-to-population ratio

DPS dimethyl polysiloxane (simethicone)

dps disintegrations per second

DPSS Department of Public Social Services

DPST, dpst double-pole single-throw (switch)

DPT Demerol, Phenergan, and Thorazine
department; also Dept, dept
dichotic pitch discrimination test
diphosphothiamine
diphtheria-pertussis-tetanus (vaccine)
diphtheric pseudotabes
dipropyltryptamine

DPTI diastolic pressure-time index

DPTP diphtheria, pertussis, tetanus, poliomyelitis (vaccines)

DPTPM diphtheria, pertussis, tetanus, poliomyelitis, measles (vaccines)

DPU delayed pressure urticaria

DPUD duodenal peptic ulcer disease

DPV different pulse voltammetry

DPW distal phalangeal width

DPX dextropropoxyphene

DQ deterioration quotient
developmental quotient

DQE detective quantum efficiency

DR degeneration reaction
Déjérine-Roussy (syndrome)
delivery room
deoxyribose; also d, dRib

diabetic retinopathy; also dr
diagnostic radiology
distribution ratio
diurnal rhythm
doctor; also doc, Dr
donor-related
dorsal raphe
dorsal root; also dr
dose ratio
drug receptor
reaction of degeneration (muscle fibers)

Dr doctor; also doc, DR
rare detail response

dr diabetic retinopathy; also DR
dorsal root; also DR
drachm
drain
dram
dressing(s); also DRSG, drsg, dsg
unusual rare detail response

DRA despite resuscitation attempts
dextran-reactive antibody
disease-resistant antigen
drug-related admissions

DRAM dynamic random access memory

dr ap dram, apothecaries' (weight)

DRAT differential rheumatoid agglutination
test

dr avdp dram, avoirdupois

DRB daunorubicin; also D, DAUNO, DNR,
Dnr
double-ring break (ampoules)

DRBC denatured red blood cell
dog red blood cell; also DRC
donkey red blood cell

DRC damage risk criteria
dendritic reticulum cell
dog red blood cell; also DRBC
dorsal root, cervical; also DRc

DRc dorsal root, cervical; also DRC

dRCA distal right coronary artery

DRE digital rectal examination

DREF dose reduction effectiveness factor

D reg diseased region

DRESS depth-resolved surface coil
spectroscopy

DREZ dorsal root entry zone

DRF daily replacement factor (of lymphocytes)
Deafness Research Foundation
dose range finding
dose-reduction factor

DRG Diagnosis-Related Groups
dorsal respiratory group
dorsal root ganglion

drg drainage; also DRGE, drng
draining; also drng

DRGE drainage; also drg, drng

DrHyg Doctor of Hygiene; also DHg, DHy,
DHyg

DRI Discharge Readiness Inventory

dRib deoxyribose; also d, DR

DRID double radial immunodiffusion
double radioisotope derivative

DRIFT diffuse reflectance infrared Fourier
transform

DRL differential reinforcement of low
(response rates)
dorsal root, lumbar; also DRl

D5RL dextrose 5% in Ringer's lactate solution

DRl dorsal root, lumbar; also DRL

DRME Division of Research in Medical
Education

DRMS drug reaction-monitoring system

DrMT Doctor of Mechanotherapy

DRN dorsal raphe nucleus

dRNA DNA-like ribonucleic acid

DRNDP diribonucleoside-3′,5′-diphosphate

drng drainage; also drg, DRGE
draining; also drg

DRNR certificate in diagnostic radiology with
special competence in nuclear radiology

DRnt diagnostic roentgenology

DRO differential reinforcement of other
(behavior)

DRP digoxin reduction product
dorsal root potential

DrPH Doctor of Public Health; also DPH
Doctor of Public Hygiene; also DPH

DRQ discomfort relief quotient

DRR dorsal root reflex

DRS descending rectal septum
dorsal root, sacral; also DRs
drowsiness
Duane's retraction syndrome
dynamic reflectance spectroscopy
dynamic renal scintigraphy
Dyskinesia Rating Scale

DRs dorsal root, sacral; also DRS

DRSG, drsg dressing(s); also dr, dsg

DRT, DRt dorsal root, thoracic

DRTA distal renal tubular acidosis

DRTS dose record and treatment emergent symptom (scale)

DRUB drug screen–blood

DS dead air space; also D
Debré-Sémélaigne (syndrome)
deep sedative
deep sleep
defined substrate
dehydroepiandrosterone sulfate; also DHAS, DHEAS
Déjérine-Sottas (syndrome)
delayed sensitivity
dendritic spine
density (optical) standard
dental surgery
deprivation syndrome
dermatan sulfate
dermatology and syphilology; also D&S
desynchronized sleep
dextran sulfate
dextrose-saline
dextrose stick
diaphragm stimulation
diastolic (murmur)
difference spectroscopy
diffuse scleroderma
digit span; also DSp
digit symbol (test)
dihydrostreptomycin; also DHS, DHSM, DSM, DST
dilute strength
dioptric strength
Disaster Services (of Red Cross)
discharge summary
discrimination score
discriminative stimulus
disoriented
disseminated sclerosis
dissolved solids
Doctor of Science; also DSc
donor's serum
Doppler sonography
double strength
double subordinance
Down's syndrome
driving signal
drugstore
dry swallow
duration of systole
scale of depression [Ger. *Depressivitätsskala*]

D-S Doerfler-Stewart (test)

D/S dextrose 5% in saline; also D-5-S

D&S dermatology and syphilology; also DS

dextrose in saline
diagnostic and surgical
dilation and suction

D-5-S dextrose 5% in saline (solution); also D/S

Ds associative detail response to white space

D$_S$ sterically related to D-glyceraldehyde (Used in amino acid nomenclature to avoid confusion with carbohydrate nomenclature. The subscript refers to the standard substance "serine".)

ds double-stranded (DNA, RNA)

DSA digital subtraction angiography
digital subtraction arteriography
disease-susceptible antigen

DSACT, D-SACT direct sinoatrial conduction time

DSAP disseminated superficial actinic porokeratosis

DSAS discrete subaortic stenosis

Dsb single-breath diffusing (capacity)

DSBB double sheath bronchial brushing

DSBL disability; also DB, dis
disabled; also dis

DSBT donor-specific blood transfusion

DSC decussation of superior cerebellar (peduncles)
differential scanning colorimeter (calorimetry)
disodium cromoglycate; also DCG, DSCG
Doctor of Surgical Chiropody
Down's syndrome child

DSc Doctor of Science; also DS

DSCF Doppler-shifted constant frequency

DSCG disodium cromoglycate; also DCG, DSC

DSCT dorsal spinocerebellar tract

DSD depressed spectrum disease
depression sine depression
discharge summary dictated
dry sterile dressing

DSDB direct self-destructive behavior

DSDDT double-sampling dye dilution technique

dsDNA double-stranded deoxyribonucleic acid

DSDS daughter sites of dimer strands

DSE digital subtraction echocardiogram
distal stimulating electrode
Doctor of Sanitary Engineering

d seq on the following day [L. *die sequente*]

DSF disulfiram
dry sterile fluff

DSG dry sterile gauze

dsg dressing(s); also dr, DRSG, drsg

DSH deliberate self-harm
dexamethasone-suppressible hyperaldosteronism

DSHR delayed skin hypersensitivity reaction

DSI deep shock insulin
Depression Status Inventory
drug-seeking index

DSIM Doctor of Science in Industrial
Medicine

DSIP delta sleep-inducing peptide

dslv dissolve; also dil, diss

DSM dextrose solution mixture
*Diagnostic and Statistical Manual of Mental
Disorders*
dihydrostreptomycin; also DHS, DHSM, DS,
DST
dried skim milk
German Collection of Microorganisms [Ger.
Deutsche Sammlung von Mikroorganismen]

DSM-III-R *Diagnostic and Statistical Manual
of Mental Disorders*, 3rd Edition

DSML direct suspension microscopic laryngoscopy

DSO distal subungual onychomycosis

DSP decreased sensory perception
delayed sleep phase
dense star polymer
dibasic sodium phosphate
digital signal processor
digital subtraction phlebography

DSp digit span; also DS

DSPC disaturated phosphatidylcholine

DSR distal splenorenal
double simultaneous recording
dynamic spacial reconstructor

DSRF drainage subretinal fluid

DSRNA, dsRNA double-stranded ribonucleic
acid

DSRS distal splenorenal shunt

DSS dengue shock syndrome
Developmental Sentence Scoring
dioctyl sodium sulfosuccinate (docusate
sodium); also DOSS
disability status scale
docusate sodium

DSSEP dermatomal somatosensory evoked
potential

DST desensitization test
desensitization time
dexamethasone suppression test
dihydrostreptomycin; also DHS, DHSM, DS,
DSM
disproportionate septal thickening
donor-specific transfusion

D-state rapid eye-movement sleep

D-S test Doerfler-Stewart test

D-stix Dextrostix

DSU day surgery unit
double setup

DSUH directed suggestion under hypnosis

DSV digital subtraction ventriculography

DSVP downstream venous pressure

DSWI deep surgical wound infection

DSy digit symbol

DT Déjérine-Thomas (syndrome)
delirium tremens; also DTs, DT's, Dts
dental technician
depression of transmission
Dietetic Technician; also Diet Tech
differently tested
digitoxin; also DIG
diphtheria-tetanus (immunization)
diphtheria toxoid; also diph-tox
discharge tomorrow
dispensing tablet
distance test (hearing)
dorsalis tibialis
double tachycardia
doubling time (of tumor size)
duration of tetany; also Dt
dye test

D/T date of treatment; also DoRx
deaths to total (ratio)

D&T diagnosis and treatment
dictated and typed

Dt duration of tetany; also DT

dT deoxythymidine

DTA differential thermoanalysis

DTAA di-tryptophan animal and acetaldehyde

DTB dedicated time block

DTBC *d*-tubocurine; also DTC, dTc

DTBN di-*tert*-butyl nitroxide

DTBP di-*tert*-butyl peroxide; also DBP

DTC day treatment center
differentiated thyroid carcinoma
direct-to-consumer (advertising)
d-tubocurine; also DTBC, dTc

dTc *d*-tubocurine; also DTBC, DTC

DTD, dtd daily therapeutic dose
let such a dose be given [L. *detur talis dosis*]

dTDP deoxythymidine diphosphate

DTE desiccated thyroid extract

2-D TEE two-dimensional transesophageal echocardiography

DTF Debré-De Toni-Fanconi (syndrome)
detector transfer function

DTG derivative thermogravimetry

D-TGA, d-TGA dextrotransposition of the great arteries

DTH delayed-type hypersensitivity (reaction)

dThd thymidine

DTIC dimethyltriazenylimidazole carboxamide (dacarbazine); also DIC

DTIC-ACTD DTIC (dacarbazine) and actinomycin D

DTICH delayed traumatic intracerebral hemorrhage

D time dream time

DTLA Detroit Tests of Learning Aptitude

DTM dermatophyte test medium

DTMA deoxycorticosterone trimethylacetate

DTMC ditrichloromethylcarbinol

DTMP, dTMP deoxythymidine monophosphate

DTMV$_{max}$ diastolic transmembrane voltage, maximum

DTN diphtheria toxin, normal

DTNB dithiodinitrobenzoic acid

DTO deodorized tincture of opium

DTP diphtheria-tetanus-pertussis (vaccine)
distal tingling on percussion (Tinel's sign)

DTPA diethylenetriamine pentaacetic acid; (pentetic acid)

DTPA In 111 the diethylenetriamine pentaacetic acid chelate of indium 111

DTPA In 113m the diethylenetriamine pentaacetic acid chelate of indium 113m

DTPA Tc 99m the diethylenetriamine pentaacetic acid chelate of technetium 99m

DTPT dithiopropylthiamine

DTR deep tendon reflex
direct transverse reaction
registered dietetic technician

DTRTT digital temperature recovery time test

DTS dense tubular system
diphtheria toxin sensitivity
discrete time sample
donor transfusion, specific

DTs, DT's, Dts delirium tremens; also DT

DTT device for transverse traction
diagnostic and therapeutic team
diphtheria-tetanus toxoid
dithiothreitol

dTTP deoxythymidine triphosphate

DTUS diathermy, traction, and ultrasound

DTV due to void

DT-VAC diphtheria-tetanus vaccine

DTVM Diploma in Tropical Veterinary Medicine

DTVMI Developmental Test of Visual Motor Integration

DTVP Developmental Test of Visual Perception

DTX detoxification; also detox
(dimethyltriazeno)imidazole carboxamide

DTZ diatrizoate

DU decubitus ulcer
deoxyuridine; also dU
dermal ulcer
diabetic urine
diagnosis undetermined
diazouracil
diffuse and undifferentiated (lymphoma)
dog unit
dose unit
duodenal ulcer
duroxide uptake
Dutch (rabbit)
optical density unknown

D$_U$ urea dialysance

dU deoxyuridine; also DU

du dial unit

DUA dorsal uterine artery

DUB Dubowitz (score)
dysfunctional uterine bleeding; also DFB

DUD Duchenne's muscular dystrophy; also DMD

dUDP deoxyuridine diphosphate

D$_1$UE diagonal 1 upper extremity

D$_2$UE diagonal 2 upper extremity

DUET drug use education tips

DUF Doppler ultrasonic flowmeter

DUI driving under the influence

DUID driving under the influence of drugs

DUL diffuse undifferentiated lymphoma

dulc sweet [L. *dulcis*]

DUM dorsal unpaired median (axon, neuron)

DUMETi dorsal unpaired median extensor tibiae

dUMP deoxyuridine-5′-monophosphate

DUNHL diffuse undifferentiated non-Hodgkin's lymphoma

duod duodenal; also D
duodenum; also D

dup duplicate
duplication

DUR Drug Utilization Review
duration; also D, d, dur

dur duration; also D, d, DUR
hard [L. *durus*]

dur dol while pain lasts [L. *durante dolore*]; also dur dolor

dur dolor while pain lasts [L. *durante dolore*]; also dur dol

DUS Doppler ultrasound stethoscope

DUSN diffuse unilateral subacute neuroretinitis ("wipe-out" syndrome)

dUTP deoxyuridine triphosphate

DUV damaging ultraviolet
dangerous ultraviolet

DV dependent variable
dilute volume (of solution)
distance vision
distemper virus
domiciliary visit
dorsoventral
double vibrations (unit of frequency of sound waves); also dv
double vision; also dv

D&V diarrhea and vomiting
disks and vessels (ophthalmology)

dv double vibrations (unit of frequency of sound waves); also DV
double vision; also DV

DVA desacetylvinblastine amide (vindesine)
distance visual acuity
duration of voluntary apnea (test)

D/V_A diffusion per unit of alveolar volume

D value decimal reduction time; also D

DVB *cis*-diamminedichloroplatinum, vindesine, and bleomycin
divinylbenzene

DVC direct visualization of vocal cords
divanillalcyclohexanone

DVCC Disease Vector Control Center

DVD dissociated vertical deviation
dissociated vertical divergence
double-vessel disease

DVDALV double-vessel disease with abnormal left ventricle

DVE duck virus enteritis

DVH Division for the Visually Handicapped

DVI atrioventricular sequential (pacemaker code); also DDI
digital vascular imaging (system); also DVIS
Doppler (systolic) velocity index
Doppler (systolic) velocity integral

DVIS digital vascular imaging system; also DVI

DVIU direct vision internal urethrotomy

DVL deep vastus lateralis

DVLP daunomycin, vincristine, L-asparaginase, and prednisone

DVM digital voltmeter
Doctor of Veterinary Medicine

DVMS Doctor of Veterinary Medicine and Surgery

DVN dorsal vagal nucleus

DVP daunorubicin, vincristine and prednisone

DVPA daunorubicin, vincristine, prednisone, and L-asparaginase; also DVPL-ASP, DVPL-Asp

DVPL-ASP, DVPL-Asp daunorubicin, vincristine, prednisone, and L-asparaginase; also DVPA

DVR derotational varus osteotomy
digital vascular reactivity
Doctor of Veterinary Radiology
double valve replacement

DVS Division of Vital Statistics
Doctor of Veterinary Science; also DVSc
Doctor of Veterinary Surgery

DVSA digital venous subtraction angiography

DVSc Doctor of Veterinary Science; also DVS

DVT deep venous thrombosis

DVTS deep venous thromboscintigram

DVXI direct vision times one

DW daily weight
deionized water
dextrose in water; also D/W
distilled water
doing well; also D/W
dry weight
whole response to detail

D/W dextrose in water; also DW
doing well; also DW
dry to wet

D5W, D₅W dextrose 5% in water; also D₅, D5/W, D5&W

D5/W dextrose 5% in water; also D_5, D5W, D_5W, D5&W

D5&W dextrose 5% in water; also D_5, D5W, D_5W, D5/W

dw dwarf (mouse)

DWA died from wounds

DWD died with disease

DWDL diffuse well-differentiated lymphocytic leukemia
diffuse well-differentiated lymphocytic lymphoma

DWI driving while impaired
driving while intoxicated

DWMI deep white-matter infarct

DWRT delayed work recall test

DWS Disaster Warning System

DWT Dichotic Word Test

dwt pennyweight

DX Dextran
diagnosis; also Δ, D, DG, Dg, Diag, diag, Dx, dx
dicloxacillin; also DCL, diclox

Dx, dx diagnosis; also Δ, D, DG, Dg, Diag, diag, DX

DXD, Dxd discontinued; also D/C, D/c'd

DXM dexamethasone (suppression test)

DXR deep x-ray
doxorubicin; also DOX, Dox, DOXO, Doxo

DXRT deep x-ray therapy; also DXT

DXT deep x-ray therapy; also DXRT
dextrose

dXTP deoxyxanthine triphosphate

D-XYL D-xylose (in urine)

DY dense parenchyma
Dyke-Young (syndrome)

Dy dysprosium

dy dystrophia muscularis

DYF drag your feet

dyn dynamics
dynamometer
dyne; also d

dysp dyspnea; also DP

DZ diazepam; also DIAZ, DZP
disease; also D, dis, Dz, dz
dizygotic
dizygous
dizziness
dizzy
Durand-Zunin (syndrome)

Dz, dz disease; also D, dis, DZ

DZAPO daunorubicin, azacytidine, Ara-C (cytarabine), prednisone, and Oncovin

DZP diazepam; also DIAZ, DZ

DZT dizygotic twins

E

E EPSILON, UPPER CASE, fifth letter of the Greek alphabet

ε epsilon, lower case, fifth letter of the Greek alphabet
chain of hemoglobin
dielectric constant
fifth in a series or group
heavy chain of immunoglobulin E
molar absorption coefficient
molar absorptivity
molar extinction coefficient; also E_M
permittivity
specific absorptivity

ε-Acp ε-aminocaproic acid

ε epsilon, lower case, fifth letter of the Greek alphabet, variant

H ETA, UPPER CASE, seventh letter of the Greek alphabet

η eta, seventh letter of the Greek alphabet

η absolute viscosity
apparent (or dynamic) velocity

E air dose
cortisone (compound E)
edema; also ed
einstein (unit of energy)
elastance; also E
electric affinity; also E_0, EA
electric charge; also e
electric field vector
electrode potential
electromagnetic force
electromotive force; also E, $\mathscr{E}$, EMF, emf
electron; also e
embryo; also Emb, emb
emmetropia; also EM, Em
emmetropic
encephalitis
endangered (animal)
endogenous
endoplasm
enema; also En, en, enem
energy; also E
engorged; also ENG
Entamoeba species; also E
enterococcus
enzyme; also enz
eosinophil; also EO, EOS, Eos, eos, eosin
epicondyle
epinephrine; also EPI, epineph
error; also e, e
erythrocyte; also e, Er, er, Erc, ERY, Ery, eryth

erythroid
erythromycin; also EM, ETM
Escherichia species; also E, Esch, Esch
esophagus; also ES, ESO, eso, esoph
esophoria (for distance)
ester; also est
estradiol; also E_2, E-diol
ethanol; also ET, ETH, ETOH, EtOH
ethmoid (sinus)
ethyl; also ET, Et
etiocholanolone; also ETIO
etiology; also ET, et, etio, etiol
exa- (10^{18})
examiner; also exam
exercise; also Ex, ex, exer
expectancy (wave); also E
expected frequency in a cell of a contingency table; also E
experiment; also exp, exper, expt
experimental; also exp, exper, exptl
experimenter
expired (died); also exp
expired (gas); also exp
expired (air)
extension; also EXT, ext
extinction (coefficient)
extraction fraction
extraction ratio; also ER
extralymphatic
eye
glutamic acid (one-letter notation); also GLU, Glu, glu
internal energy
kinetic energy of a particle
mathematical expectation
opposite (stereodescriptor to indicate configuration at a double bond) [Ger. entgegen (opposite)]
redox potential
vectorcardiography electrode (midsternal)
vitamin E

E elastance; also E
electric intensity
electromotive force; also E, $\mathscr{E}$, EMF, emf
energy; also E
Entamoeba species; also E
Escherichia species; also E, Esch, Esch
expectancy (wave); also E
expected frequency in a cell of a contingency table; also E
illumination
oxidation-reduction potential; also $E_o{}^+$, E^o, Eh, E_h, E_h, eH

141

$\mathscr{E}$ electromotive force; also E, *E*, EMF, emf

E* lesion on erythrocyte cell membrane at site of complement fixation

E′ esophoria (for near)

E°, *E*° standard electrode potential
standard reduction potential

E⁻, e⁻ negative electron

E⁺, e⁺ positron (positive electron)

E₁ estrone

E1A early region 1A

E₂ 17-beta-estradiol; also E, E-diol

E₃ estriol; also Es

E₄ esterol

4E four plus edema

e base of natural logarithms (approx. 2.7182818285)
early
egg transfer
electric charge; also E
electron; also E
elementary charge
erg (energy unit)
error; also E, *e*
erythrocyte; also E, Er, er, Erc, ERY, Ery, eryth
from [L. *ex*]; also Ex, ex

e elementary unit of electric charge
error; also E, e

EA early antigen
educational age
egg albumin
elbow aspiration
electric affinity; also E, E₀
electroacupuncture; also EAC, EAP
electroanesthesia
electrophysiologic abnormality
embryonic antibody
embryonic antigen
emergency area
endocardiographic amplifier
enteral alimentation
enteroanastomosis
enzymatic active
epiandrosterone
erythrocyte antibody
erythrocyte antisera
esophageal atresia
esterase activity
estivo-autumnal (malaria)
ethacrynic acid

E → A "E to A" (in pulmonary consolidation, all vowels including "e" heard as "a" through stethoscope)

E&A evaluate and advise

ea each

EAA electroacupuncture analgesia
electrothermal atomic absorption
essential amino acid
excitatory amino acid
extrinsic allergic alveolitis

EAB elective abortion
Ethics Advisory Board
extra-anatomic bypass

EABM electroactive biologic material

EABV effective arterial blood volume

EAC Ehrlich's ascites carcinoma
electroacupuncture; also EA, EAP
erythema action (spectrum)
erythema annulare centrifugum
erythrocyte coated with antibody and complement
eudismic affinity correlation
external auditory canal

EACA epsilon-aminocaproic acid

EACD eczematous allergic contact dermatitis

EACH Essential Access Community Hospital

EAD early afterdepolarization
extracranial arterial disease

ead the same [L. *eadem*]

E-ADD epileptic attentional deficit disorder

EAE experimental allergic encephalitis
experimental allergic encephalomyelitis
experimental autoimmune encephalitis
experimental autoimmune encephalomyelitis

EAEC enteroadherent *Escherichia coli*

EAF emergency assistance to families

EAG electroantennogram
electroatriogram

EAHF eczema, asthma, and hay fever (complex)

EAHLG equine antihuman lymphoblast globulin

EAHLS equine antihuman lymphoblast serum

EAI Employment and Adaption Index
erythrocyte antibody inhibition

EAL electronic artificial larynx

EAM endo-*N*-acetylmuramidase
external acoustic meatus
external auditory meatus

EAMG experimental autoimmune myasthenia gravis

EAN experimental allergic neuritis

EANG epidemic acute non-bacterial gastroenteritis

EAO experimental allergic orchitis

EAP electroacupuncture; also EA, EAC
epiallopregnanolone
erythrocyte acid phosphate
etoposide, Adriamycin, Platinol
evoked action potential

EAPFS electron appearance potential fine
structure

EAQ eudismic affinity quotient

e-aq aqueous electron

EAR electroencephalographic audiometry; also
EEGA
expired air resuscitation

Ea R reaction of degeneration [Ger.
Entartungs-Reaktion]

ear ox ear oximetry

EAST external rotation, abduction, stress test

EAT ectopic atrial tachycardia
Edinburgh Articulation Test
Education Apperception Test
Ehrlich's ascites tumor
electroaerosol therapy
experimental autoimmune thymitis
experimental autoimmune thyroiditis

EATC Ehrlich's ascites tumor cell

EAU experimental autoimmune uveitis

EAV equine abortion virus
extra-alveolar vessel

EAVC enhanced atrioventricular conduction

EAVM extramedullary arteriovenous malformation

EB elbow bearing
elementary body
endometrial biopsy; also EMB
epidermolysis bullosa
Epstein-Barr (virus); also E-B
esophageal body
estradiol benzoate; also E$_2$B
ethidium bromide
Evans blue (dye)

E-B Epstein-Barr (virus); also EB

E$_2$B estradiol benzoate; also EB

EBA epidermolysis bullosa acquisita
epidermolysis bullosa atrophicans
epizootic bovine abortion
erythrocyte-binding antigen
extrahepatic biliary atresia; also EHBA

EBAA Eye Bank Association of America

EBC esophageal balloon catheter

EBCDIC extended binary-coded decimal interchange code

EBD epidermolysis bullosa dystrophica

EBDD epidermolysis bullosa dystrophica
dominant

EBDR epidermolysis bullosa dystrophica
recessive

EBEA Epstein-Barr virus early antigen; also
EBVEA

EBF erythroblastosis fetalis; also EF

EBG electroblepharogram
electroblepharography

EBGS extracorporeal blood gas system

EBI emetine and bismuth iodide
erythroblastic islands
estradiol-binding index

EBK embryonic bovine kidney

EBL enzootic bovine leukosis
erythroblastic leukemia
estimated blood loss

EBL/S estimated blood loss/surgery

EBM electrophysiologic behavior modification
expressed breast milk

EBNA Epstein-Barr virus nuclear antigen; also
EBVNA

E/BOD electrolyte biochemical oxygen
demand

EBP epidural blood patch
estradiol-binding protein

EBPG electron beam pattern generator

EBS elastic back strap
electrical brain stimulation
electrical brain stimulator
epidermolysis bullosa simplex

EBSB equal breath sounds bilaterally

EBSS Earle's balanced salt solution

EBT early bedtime
ethylsulfonylbenzaldehyde thiosemicarbazone
(subathizone)
external beam photon therapy

EBV effective blood volume
Epstein-Barr virus

EB-VCA Epstein-Barr viral capsid antigen

EBV-VCA Epstein-Barr virus, viral capsid
antigen

EBV-VCA Ig Epstein-Barr virus, viral capsid
antigen Ig antibody

EBVDNA Epstein-Barr virus-determinated nuclear antigen

EBVEA Epstein-Barr virus early antigen; also EBEA

EBVNA Epstein-Barr virus nuclear antigen; also EBNA

EBZ epidermal basement zone

EC econazole
effective concentration
effect of closing (of eyes in electroen-cephalography)
ejection click
electrical conductivity
electrochemical
electrochemical detection; also ECD
electron capture
Ellis-van Creveld (syndrome)
embryonal carcinoma
emetic center
endothelial cell
enteric-coated (tablet)
entering complaint
enterochromaffin
entorhinal cortex
entrance compliant
environmental complexity
enzyme code
Enzyme Commission (of the International Union of Biochemistry)
enzyme-treated cell
epidermal cell
epithelial cell
equalization-cancellation
Erb-Charcot (disease, syndrome)
Escherichia coli; Eco
esophageal carcinoma
ether-chloroform (mixture); also E-C
excitation-contraction; also E-C
excitatory center
experimental control
external carotid
external conjugate
extracellular
extracellular compartment
extracellular concentration
extracranial
extruded cell
eye care
eyes closed

E-C ether-chloroform (mixture); also EC
excitation-contraction; also EC

E/C endoscopy/cystoscopy
estriol to creatinine (ratio)
estrogen to creatinine (ratio)

EC$_{50}$ median effective concentration

ECA electric control activity
electrocardioanalyzer
enterobacterial common antigen
epidemiologic catchment area
ethacrynic acid (diuretic)
ethylcarboxylate adenosine
external carotid artery

E-CABG endarterectomy and coronary artery bypass grafting

ECACC European Collection of Animal Cell Cultures

ECAO enteric cytopathogenic avian orphan (virus)

ECAT emission computed axial tomography

ECB electric cabinet bath

ECBD exploration of common bile duct

ECBO enteric cytopathogenic bovine orphan (virus)

ECBV effective circulating blood volume

ECC edema, clubbing, and cyanosis
electrocorticogram; also ECoG
embryonal cell carcinoma
emergency cardiac care
endocervical cone
endocervical curettage
estimated creatinine clearance
external cardiac compression
extracorporeal circulation
extrusion of cell cytoplasm

ECCE extracapsular cataract extraction

ECCLS European Committee for Clinical Laboratory Standards (Kent, England)

ECCO enteric cytopathogenic cat orphan (virus)

ECCO$_2$R extracorporeal carbon dioxide removal

ECD electrochemical detection; also EC
electrochemical detector
electron capture detector
endocardial cushion defect
enzymatic cell dispersion
ethoxycoumarin deethylase

ECDB encourage to cough and deep breathe

ECDEU Early Clinical Drug Evaluation Unit (system)

ECDO enteric cytopathogenic dog orphan (virus)

ECE early childhood education

endocervical ecchymosis
equine conjugated estrogen

ECEMG evoked compound electromyography

ECEO enteric cytopathogenic equine orphan (virus)

ECF East Coast fever
effective capillary flow
eosinophil chemotactic factor
erythroid colony formation
Escherichia coli filtrate
extended care facility
extracellular fluid

ECFA, ECF-A eosinophil chemotactic factor of anaphylaxis

ECF-C eosinophilic chemotactic factor–complement

ECFMG Educational Commission for Foreign Medical Graduates
Educational Council for Foreign Medical Graduates (now: Educational Commission for Foreign Medical Graduates)

ECFMS Educational Council for Foreign Medical Students

ECFV extracellular fluid volume; also EFV

ECG electrocardiogram; also EKG
electrocardiography; also EKG
equine chorionic gonadotropin

ECGF endothelial cell growth factor

ECGS endothelial cell growth supplement

ECH epichlorohydrin
ethylene chlorohydrin
extended care hospital

ECHINO echinocyte

ECHO echocardiogram; also Echo
echocardiography; also Echo
enteric cytopathogenic human orphan (virus); also EcHO
etoposide, cyclophosphamide, hydroxydaunomycin, and Oncovin
ultrasound

EcHO enteric cytopathogenic human orphan (virus); also ECHO

Echo echocardiogram; also ECHO
echocardiography; also ECHO
echoencephalogram; also Echo EG
echoencephalography; also Echo EG

Echo EG echoencephalogram; also Echo
echoencephalography; also Echo

ECI electrocerebral inactivity
eosinophilic cytoplasmic inclusion
extracorporeal irradiation (of blood)

ECIB extracorporeal irradiation of blood

EC-IC extracranial-intracranial

ECIL extracorporeal irradiation of lymph

ECK extracellular potassium [L. *kalium* (potassium)]

ECL electrogenerated chemiluminescence
emitter-coupled logic
enterochromaffin-like (type)
euglobulin clot lysis
extent of cerebral lesion
extracapillary lesions

eclec eclectic

ECLT euglobulin clot lysis time

ECM embryonic chick muscle
erythema chronicum migrans
external cardiac massage
external chemical messenger
extracellular material
extracellular matrix

ECMO enteric cytopathogenic monkey orphan (virus)
extracorporeal membrane oxygenation
extracorporeal membrane oxygenator

ECMP enterocoated microspheres of pancrelipase

ECN extended care nursery

EC No Enzyme Commission Number

Eco *Escherichia coli*; also EC

ECochG electrocochleography

ECOG Eastern Cooperative Oncology Group

ECoG electrocorticogram; also ECC
electrocorticography

econ economic
economics

ECP effector cell precursor
electronic claims processing
endocardial potential
enteric cytopathogenic
eosinophil cationic protein
erythrocyte coproporphyrin
erythroid committed precursor
Escherichia coli polypeptide
estradiol cyclopentanepropionate
external cardiac pressure
external counterpulsation
free cytoporphyrin in erythrocytes

ECPD external counterpressure device

ECPO enteric cytopathogenic porcine orphan (virus)

ECPOG electrochemical potential gradient

ECPR external cardiopulmonary resuscitation

ECR electrocardiographic response
emergency chemical restraint

ECRB extensor carpi radialis brevis

ECRL extensor carpi radialis longus

ECRO enteric cytopathogenic rodent orphan (virus)

ECS elective cosmetic surgery
electrocerebral silence
electroconvulsive shock
electronic claims submission
electroshock; also ES
extracellular space

ECSO enteric cytopathogenic swine orphan (virus)

ECSP epidermal cell surface protein

ECT electroconvulsive therapy
emission computerized tomography
enhanced computerized tomography
enteric-coated tablet
euglobulin clot test
European compression technique (bone screw and internal fixation)
extracellular tissue

ECTA Everyman's Contingency Table Analysis

ECTEOLA epichlorohydrin and tri-ethanolamine

ECU environmental control unit
extended care unit
extensor carpi ulnaris

ECV extracellular volume
extracorporeal volume

ECVD extracellular volume of distribution

ECVE extracellular volume expansion

ECW extracellular water

ED early differentiation; also EDD
ectodermal dysplasia
ectopic depolarization
effective dose
Ehlers-Danlos (disease, syndrome)
elbow disarticulation
electrodiagnosis; also EDX, EDx, El Dx
electrodialysis
electron diffraction
elemental diet
embryonic death
emergency department
emotional disorder
emotional disturbance
emotionally disturbed
end diastole

entering diagnosis
Entner-Doudoroff (metabolic pathway)
enzyme deficiency
epidural
epileptiform discharge
equilibrium dialysis
equine dermis (cells)
erythema dose
erythrocyte density
ethylenediamine; also EDA
ethynodiol
evidence of disease
exertional dyspnea
extensive disease
extensor digitorum
external diameter
external dyspnea
extra-low dispersion

E-D ego-defense

ED$_{50}$ median effective dose

E$_d$ depth dose

ed edema; also E
edition

EDA electrodermal activity
electrodermal audiometry
electrolyte-deficient agar
electron donor-acceptor (interaction)
end-diastolic area
ethylenediamine; also ED

EDAM electron-dense amorphous material

EDAP Emergency Department Approved for Pediatrics

EDB early dry breakfast
ethylene dibromide
extensor digitorum brevis

EDBP erect diastolic blood pressure

EDC effective dynamic compliance
electrodesiccation and curettage; also ED&C
emergency decontamination center
end-diastolic count
estimated date of conception
estimated date of confinement; also EDOC
expected date of confinement
expected delivery, cesarean
extensor digitorum communis

ED&C electrodesiccation and curettage; also EDC

EDCF endothelial-derived contraction factor

EDCI energetic dynamic cardiac insufficiency

EDCS end-diastolic chamber stiffness
end-diastolic circumferential stress

EDD early differentiation; also ED
  effective drug duration
  electrodermal diagnosis
  end-diastolic dimension
  enzyme-digested delta (endotoxin)
  estimated date of delivery
  estimated discharge date
  estimated due date
  expected date of delivery

EDDA expanded duty dental auxiliary

edent edentulous

EDF end-diastolic flow
  eosinophil differentiation factor
  extradural fluid

EDG electrodermography

EDH epidural hematoma
  extradural hematoma

EDICP electron-dense iron-containing particle

EDIM epidemic disease of infant mice
  epizootic diarrhea of infant mice

E-diol estradiol; also E, E_2

EDL end-diastolic load
  end-diastolic segment length
  essential drug list
  estimated date of labor
  extensor digitorum longus

ED/LD emotionally disturbed and learning disabled

EDM early diastolic murmur
  Edmonston (strain)
  extramucosal duodenal myotomy

EDMA ethylene glycol dimethacrylate

EDN electrodesiccation
  eosinophil-derived neurotoxin

EDOC estimated date of confinement; also EDC

EDP electron-dense particle
  electronic data processing
  emergency department physician
  end-diastolic pressure

EDPA ethyldiphenylpropenylamine

EDPT early distal proximal tubule

EDQ extensor digiti quinti

EDR early diastolic relaxation
  edrophonium
  effective direct radiation
  electrodermal response
  electrodialysis with reversed (polarity)

EDRF endothelium-derived relaxing factor

EDS edema disease of swine

  egg drop syndrome
  Ego Development Scale
  Ehlers-Danlos syndrome
  energy-dispersive spectrometer
  excessive daytime sleepiness
  extended data stream
  extradimensional shift

Ed(s) editors

EDT end-diastolic cardiac wall thickness

EDTA ethylenediaminetetraacetic acid (edathamil, edetic acid)

EdU eating disorder unit

educ education

EDV end-diastolic volume

EDVI end-diastolic volume index

EDW estimated dry weight

EDWGT emergency drinking water germicidal tablet

EDWTH end-diastolic wall thickness

EDX electrodiagnosis; also ED, EDx, El Dx
  energy-dispersive x-ray

EDx electrodiagnosis; also ED, EDX, El Dx

EDXA energy-dispersive x-ray analysis

EE embryo extract
  end expiration
  end-to-end (anastomosis); also E-E, ETE
  end-to-end (bite, occlusion)
  energy expenditure
  Enterobacteriaceae enrichment (broth)
  equine encephalitis
  erythematous-edematous
  ethynyl estradiol
  expressed emotion
  external ear
  eyes and ears; also E&E

E-E end-to-end (anastomosis); also EE, ETE
  erythema-edema (reaction)

E&E eyes and ears; also EE

EEA electroencephalic audiometry
  elemental enteral alimentation
  end-to-end anastomosis

EEC ectrodactyly-ectodermal dysplasia-clefting (syndrome)
  enteropathogenic *Escherichia coli*; also EPEC

EECD endothelial-epithelial corneal dystrophy

EECG electroencephalogram; also EEG
  electroencephalography; also EEG

EEDQ ethoxycarbonylethoxydihydroquinoline

EEE Eastern equine encephalomyelitis
  edema, erythema, and exudate

EEE—cont'd
experimental enterococcal endocarditis
external eye examination

EEEP end-expiratory esophageal pressure

EEEV Eastern equine encephalomyelitis virus

EEG electroencephalogram; also EECG
electroencephalography; also EECG

EEGA electroencephalographic audiometry;
also EAR

EEG T Electroencephalographic Technologist

EELS electron energy loss spectroscopy

EEM ectodermal dysplasia, ectrodactyly, macular dystrophy (syndrome)
erythema exudativum multiforme

EEME ethynylestradiol methyl ether

EEMG evoked electromyogram

EENT eye, ear, nose, and throat

EEP end-expiratory pressure
equivalent effective photon

EEPI extraretinal eye position information

EER electroencephalic response
electroencephalographic response

EERP extended endocardial resection procedure

EES erythromycin ethyl succinate
ethyl ethanesulfonate

EESG evoked electrospinogram

EESHRTS Entrance Examination for Schools
of Health-Related Technologies

EEV encircling endocardial ventriculotomy

EF ectopic focus
edema factor
ejection factor
ejection fraction
elastic fiber
elastic fibril
electric field
elongation factor
embedded figures (test)
embryo-fetal
embryo fibroblast
emergency facility
emotional factor
encephalitogenic factor
endothoracic fascia
endurance factor
eosinophilic fasciitis
epithelial focus
equivalent focus
erythroblastosis fetalis; also EBF

erythrocytic fragmentation
essential findings
exophthalmic factor
exposure factor
extended field (radiation therapy)
extrafine
extra food
extrinsic factor

EFA essential fatty acid
extrafamily adoptee

EFAD essential fatty acid deficiency

EFBW estimated fetal body weight

EFC elastin fragment concentration
endogenous fecal calcium
ephemeral fever of cattle

EFDA expanded function dental assistant

EFE endocardial fibroelastosis

eff effect
efferent; also effer
efficient
effusion

effect effective

effer efferent; also eff

EFFU epithelial focus-forming unit

EF-G elongation factor G

EFHBM eosinophilic fibrohistiocytic lesion
of bone marrow

EFL effective focal length
external fluid loss

EFM electronic fetal monitoring
external fetal monitoring

EFP effective filtration pressure
endoneural fluid pressure

EFPS epicardial fat pad sign

EFR effective filtration rate

E FRAG erythrocyte fragility (test)

EFS electric field stimulation

EFT Embedded Figures Test

EFV extracellular fluid volume; also ECFV

EFVC expiratory flow-volume curve

EFW estimated fetal weight

EF/WM ejection fraction/wall motion

EG enteroglucagon
Erb-Goldflam (disease, syndrome)
esophagogastrectomy
esophagogastric
external genitalia

Eg exagram

eg for example [L. *exempli gratia*]

EGA estimated gestational age
evolved gas analysis

EGAT Educational Goal Attainment Tests

EGB eosinophilic granuloma of bone

EGBPS equilibrium-gated blood pool study

EGBUS external genitalia, Bartholin gland,
urethral gland, and Skene (glands); also
EXGBUS

EGC early gastric cancer
epithelioid-globoid cell

EGD esophagogastroduodenoscopy
evolved gas detection

EGDF embryonic growth and development factor

EGF epidermal growth factor

EGFR, EGF-R epidermal growth factor
receptor

EGFRK epidermal growth factor receptor
kinase

EGG electrogastrogram
electrogastrography

EGH equine growth hormone

EGJ esophagogastric junction

EGL eosinophilic granuloma of the lung

EGLT euglobulin lysis time; also ELT

EGM electrogram
extracellular granular material

EGN experimental glomerulonephritis

EGOT erythrocyte glutamic oxaloacetic
transaminase

EGR erythrocyte glutathione reductase

EGRA equilibrium-gated radionuclide
angiography

EGS electric galvanic stimulation
ethylene glycol succinate

EGT ethanol gelation test

EGTA esophageal gastric tube airway
ethyleneglycoltetraacetic acid

EH early healed
educationally handicapped
emotionally handicapped
enlarged heart
enteral hyperalimentation
environment and heredity; also E&H
epidermolytic hyperkeratosis
epoxide hydratase
essential hypertension
extended Hückel (theory)

extramedullary hematopoiesis

E&H environment and heredity; also EH

Eh, E_h, E_h, eH oxidation-reduction potential
(older designation); also E, E_o+ and E°

EHA Environmental Health Agency

EHAA epidemic hepatitis-associated antigen

EHB elevate head of bed

EHBA extrahepatic biliary atresia; also EBA

EHBD extrahepatic bile duct

EHBF estimated hepatic blood flow
exercise hyperemia blood flow; also EXBF
extrahepatic blood flow (clearance)

EHC enterohepatic circulation
enterohepatic clearance
essential hypercholesterolemia
ethylhydrocupreine (optoquine)
extended health care
extrahepatic cholestasis

EH-CF *Entamoeba histolytica*–complement
fixation

EHD electrohemodynamics
epizootic hemorrhagic disease

EHDA ethanehydroxydiphosphonic acid
(etidronate sodium); also EHDP

EHDP ethane hydroxydiphosphate
ethanehydroxydiphosphonic acid (etidronate
sodium); also EHDA

EHDV epizootic hemorrhagic disease virus

EHE epithelioid hemangioendothelioma

EHEC enterohemorrhagic *Escherichia coli*

EHF electrohydraulic fragmentation
epidemic hemorrhagic fever
exophthalmos-hyperthyroid factor
extremely high factor
extremely high frequency

EHH esophageal hiatal hernia

EHL effective halflife (of radioactive substance)
electrohydraulic lithotripsy
endogenous hyperlipidemia
Environmental Health Laboratory
essential hyperlipidemia
extensor hallucis longus

EHME Employee Health Maintenance
Examination

EHMO extended Hückel molecular orbital

EHMS electrohydrodynamic ionization mass
spectrometry

EHNA 9-erythro-2-(hydroxy-3-nonyl)-adenine

EHO extrahepatic obstruction

EHP di (2-ethylhexyl) hydrogen phosphate
Environmental Health Perspectives
excessive heat production
extra high potency

EHPAC Emergency Health Preparedness
Advisory Committee

EHPH extrahepatic portal hypertension

EHPT Eddy hot plate test

EHSDS Experimental Health Services Delivery
System

EHT essential hypertension
extended Hückel theory

EHV electric heart vector
equine herpesvirus

EI electrolyte imbalance
electron impact
electron ionization
emotionally impaired
enzyme inhibitor
eosinophilic index
excretory index
external intervention

E/I expiration to inspiration (ratio)

E&I endocrine and infertility

EIA electroimmunoassay
Electronics Industries Association
enzyme immunoassay
equine infectious anemia
exercise-induced asthma

EIAB extracranial-intracranial arterial bypass

EIAV equine infectious anemia virus

EIB exercise-induced bronchoconstriction
exercise-induced bronchospasm

EIC elastase inhibition capacity
enzyme inhibition complex

EICDT Ego-Ideal and Conscience
Development Test

EICT external isovolumic contraction time

EID egg-infective dose
electroimmunodiffusion
electronic induction desorption
electronic infusion device
emergency infusion device

EIEC enteroinvasive *Escherichia coli*

EIEE early infantile epileptic encephalopathy

EIF, eIF erythrocyte initiation factor
eukaryotic initiation factor

EIM excitability-inducing material

EIMS electron ionization mass spectrometry

EIP elective interruption of pregnancy

end-inspiratory pause
end-inspiratory pressure
extensor indicis proprius

EIPS endogenous inhibitor of prostaglandin
synthase

eIPV enhanced potency inactivated poliovirus

EIRnv extra-incidence rate in non-vaccinated
(groups)

EIRP effective isotropic radiated power

EIRv extra-incidence rate in vaccinated
(groups)

EIS endoscopic injection scleropathy
Environmental Impact Statement
Epidemic Intelligence Service

EISA electroencephalogram interval spectrum
analysis

EIT erythrocyte iron turnover

EIV external iliac vein

EJ ejection (fraction)
elbow jerk; also Ej
external jugular

Ej elbow jerk; also EJ

EJB ectopic junctional beat

EJN external jugular vein

EJP excitation junction potential
excitatory junction potential

ejusd of the same [L. *ejusdem*]

EK enterokinase
erythrokinase

EKC epidemic keratoconjunctivitis

EKG electrocardiogram; also ECG
electrocardiography; also ECG

EKV erythrokeratodermia variabilis

EKY electrokymogram
electrokymography

EL early latent
Eaton-Lambert (syndrome); also E-L
egg lecithin
electroluminescence
elixir; also el, Elix, elix, Elx
erythroleukemia
exercise limit
external lamina

E-L Eaton-Lambert (syndrome); also EL
external lids

El elastase
exaliter

el elbow; also ELB, elb
elixir; also EL, Elix, elix, Elx

ELA endotoxin-like activity

ELAM endothelial cell leukocyte adhesion molecule

ELAS extended lymphadenopathy syndrome

ELAT enzyme-linked antiglobulin test

ELB early light breakfast
elbow; also el, elb

elb elbow; also el, ELB

ELBW extremely low birth weight

ELC expression-linked copy

ELD egg lethal dose

El Dx electrodiagnosis; also ED, EDX, EDx

elec electric; also elect
electricity; also elect
electuary (confection); also elect

Elecs electrolytes; also elytes, LYTES, lytes

elect electric; also elec
electricity; also elec
electuary (confection); also elec

elem elementary

elev elevated
elevation
elevator

ELF elective low forceps (delivery)

ELFA enzyme-linked fluorescence immuno-assay

ELG eligible

ELH egg-laying hormone
endolymphatic hydrops

ELI endomyocardial lymphocytic infiltrates
Environmental Language Inventory
exercise lability index

ELIA enzyme-labeled immunoassay

ELICT enzyme-linked immunocytochemical technique

ELIEDA enzyme-linked immunoelectrodiffusion assay

ELISA enzyme-linked immunosorbent assay

Elix, elix elixir; also EL, el, Elx

ELLIP elliptocyte; also ELLP

ELLP elliptocyte; also ELLIP

ELM Early Language Milestone (scale)
external limiting membrane
extravascular lung mass

ELMT elements (on urinalysis)

ELOP estimated length of program

ELOS estimated length of stay
extralymphatic organ site

ELP early labeled peak
elastase-like protein
electrophoresis; also EP
endogenous limbic potential
Estimated Learning Potential

ELPS excessive lateral pressure syndrome

ELR Equal Listener Response (scale)

ELS Eaton-Lambert syndrome
electron loss spectroscopy
extralobar sequestration

ELSS emergency life support system

ELT euglobulin lysis test
euglobulin lysis time; also EGLT

ELU extended length of utterance

ELV erythroid leukemia virus

Elx elixir; also EL, el, Elix, elix

elytes electrolytes; also Elecs, LYTES, lytes

EM early memory
effective masking
ejection murmur
electromagnetic; also em
electromechanical
electron micrograph
electron microscope; also E/M, EMC, E-MICR
electron microscopic
electron microscopy; also E/M, EMC, E-MICR
electrophoretic mobility; also EPM
Embden-Meyerhof (glycolytic pathway); also E-M
emergency medicine
emmetropia; also E, Em
emotional (disorder)
emotionally (disturbed)
emphysema; also emph
ergonovine maleate
erythema migrans
erythema multiforme
erythrocyte mass
erythromycin; also E, ETM
esophageal manometry
esophageal motility
estramustine
excreted mass
extensive metabolizer(s)
external monitor

E_M molar extinction coefficient; also ϵ

E-M Embden-Meyerhof (glycolytic pathway); also EM

E/M electron microscope; also EM, EMC, E-MICR
electron microscopy; also EM, EMC, E-MICR

E&M endocrine and metabolic

Em emmetropia; also E, EM
exameter

Em² square exameter

Em³ cubic exameter

em electromagnetic; also EM

e/m ratio of electron charge to mass

EMA electronic microanalyzer
emergency assistance
emergency assistant
emergency medical attendant
endomysial antibody
epithelial membrane antigen

EMA-CO etoposide, methotrexate, actinomycin D (dactinomycin), cyclophosphamide, Oncovin

EMAD equivalent mean age at death

EMAP evoked muscle action potential

EMB embryology; also Emb, emb, embryol
endometrial biopsy; also EB
endomyocardial biopsy
engineering in medicine and biology
eosin-methylene blue (agar)
ethambutol (Myambutol)
explosive mental behavior
explosive motor behavior

Emb, emb embolus
embryo; also E
embryology; also EMB, embryol

EMBASE *Excerpta Medica Database*

EMBL European Molecular Biology Laboratory

embryol embryology; also EMB, Emb, emb

EMC electron microscope; also EM, E/M, E-MICR
electron microscopy; also EM, E/M, E-MICR
emergency medical care
encephalomyocarditis
endometrial curettage
essential mixed cryoglobulinemia

EMC&R emergency medical care and rescue

EMCRO Experimental Medical Care Review Organization

EMCV encephalomyocarditis virus

EMD electromechanical dissociation
esophageal mobility disorder

EMEM Eagle's minimal essential medium

EMER electromagnetic molecular electronic resonance

emer emergency; also emerg, EMG

emerg emergency; also emer, EMG

EMF electromagnetic flowmeter
electromotive force; also E, E, $\mathscr{E}$, emf
endomyocardial fibrosis
erythrocyte maturation factor
evaporated milk formula

emf electromotive force; also E, E, $\mathscr{E}$, EMF

EMG electromyelogram
electromyelography
electromyogram
electromyography
emergency; also emer, emerg
essential monoclonal gammopathy
exophthalmos, macroglossia, and gigantism (syndrome)
eye movement gauge

EMGN extramembranous glomerulonephritis

EMGORS electromyogram sensors

EMI Electric and Musical Industries
electromagnetic interference
emergency medical information
enzyme and microbe immobilization

EMIA enzyme membrane immunoassay

EMIC emergency maternal and infant care

E-MICR electron microscope; also EM, E/M, EMC
electron microscopy; also EM, E/M, EMC

EMIT enzyme-multiplied immunoassay test

EMJH Ellinghausen-McCullough-Johnson-Harris (medium)

EML effective mandibular length

EMLB erythromycin lactobionate

EMLD external muscle layer damage

EMM erythema multiforme major

EMMA eye movement measuring apparatus

EMMV extended mandatory minute ventilation

EMO Epstein-MacIntosh-Oxford (inhaler)
exophthalmos, myxedema circumscriptum praetibiale, and osteoarthropathia hypertrophicans (syndrome)

emot emotion
emotional

EMP electrical membrane property
electromagnetic pulse
Embden-Meyerhof-Parnas (pathway)
epimacular proliferation

erythrocyte membrane protein
external membrane protein
extramedullary plasmacytoma

emp a plaster [L. *emplastrum*]
as directed [L. *ex modo prescripto*]

EMPEP erythrocyte membrane protein electrophoretic pattern

emph emphysema; also EM

EMPP ethylmethylpiperidinopropiophenone

emp vesic blistering plaster [L. *emplastrum vesicatorium*]

EMR educable mentally retarded
electromagnetic radiation
emergency mechanical restraint
empty, measure, and record
essential metabolism ratio
ethanol metabolic rate
eye movement recording

EMS early morning specimen
early morning stiffness
electrical muscle stimulation
electromechanical systole
Emergency Medical Services
emergency medical system
endometriosis
eosinophilia myalgia syndrome
ethyl methanesulfonate
extramedullary site

EMSU early morning specimen of urine

EMT emergency medical tag
emergency medical team
Emergency Medical Technician
emergency medical treatment

EMT-A Emergency Medical Technician–Ambulance

EMT-I Emergency Medical Technician–Intermediate

EMT-P Emergency Medical Technician–Paramedic

EMU early morning urine
electromagnetic unit; also emu

emu electromagnetic unit; also EMU

emul emulsion

EMV eye, motor, voice (Glasgow coma scale)

EMVC early mitral valve closure

EMW electromagnetic waves

EN electronarcosis
endocardial; also ENDO
enrolled nurse
enteral nutrition
erythema nodosum

En enema; also E, en, enem

en enema; also E, En, enem
ethylenediamine (in formulas)

E 50% N extension 50% of normal

ENA Emergency Nurses Association
extractable nuclear antibodies
extractable nuclear antigen

END early neonatal death
elective node dissection
- endocrinology; also endocr
endorphin; also EP
enhancement Newcastle's disease

end endoreduplication

ENDO endocardial; also EN
endodontics; also Endo
endoscopy
endotracheal; also Endo, ET

Endo endodontics; also ENDO
endotracheal; also ENDO, ET

endocr endocrine
endocrinology; also END

ENDOR electron nuclear double resonance

endos endosteal

ENE ethylnorepinephrine

ENeG electroneurography; also ENG

enem enema; also E, En, en

ENF Enfamil

ENG electroneurography; also ENeG
electronystagmogram
electronystagmograph
electronystagmography
engorged; also E

ENI elective neck irradiation

ENK enkephalin

ENL erythema nodosum leprosum
erythema nodosum leproticum

enl enlarged
enlargement

ENNS Early Neonatal Neurobehavior Scale

Eno enolase

ENP ethyl-*p*-nitrophenylthiobenzene phosphate
extractable nucleoprotein

ENR eosinophilic non-allergic rhinitis
extrathyroidal neck radioactivity

ENS enteral nutritional support
enteric nervous system
ethylnorsuprarenin

ENT ear, nose, and throat
extranodular tissue

ENTOM entomology
ENV ethylnitrosourea
env envelope (of cell)
environ environment
environmental
enz enzymatic
enzyme; also E
EO effect of opening (eyes)
elbow orthosis
eosinophil; also E, EOS, Eos, eos, eosin
eosinophilia
ethylene oxide; also ETO, EtO, ETOX
eyes open
E_0 electric affinity; also E, EA
epidermis (skin) dose (radiation)
E_0^+, E^o oxidation-reduction potential; also E,
Eh, E_h, E_h, eH
EOA effective orifice area
erosive osteoarthritis
esophageal obturator airway
examination, opinion, and advice
EOB emergency observation bed
EOC enema of choice
EO CT eosinophil count
EOD electrical organ discharge
entry on duty
every other day; also eod
eod every other day; also EOD
EOE ethiodized oil emulsion
EOF end of field
end of file
E of M error of measurement; also EOM
EOG electro-oculogram
electro-oculography
electro-olfactogram
electro-olfactography
EOJ extrahepatic obstructive jaundice
EOL end of life
EOM equal ocular movement
error of measurement; also E of M
external otitis media
extraocular movement
extraocular muscle
EOMA emergency oxygen mask assembly
EOM F & Conj extraocular movements full
and conjugate
EOMI extraocular muscles intact
EOMS extraocular movements
extraocular muscles

EOP efficiency of plating
emergency outpatient
endogenous opioid peptides
EOR emergency operating room
exclusive OR (binary logic)
EORA elderly onset rheumatoid arthritis
EORCT European Organization for Research
in Cancer Therapy
EOS eligibility on-site
eosinophil; also E, EO, Eos, eos, eosin
Eos, eos eosinophil; also E, EO, EOS, eosin
eosin eosinophil; also E, EO, EOS, Eos, eos
EOT effective oxygen transport
EOU epidemic observation unit
EOWPVT Expression One-Word Picture
Vocabulary Test
EP ectopic pregnancy
edible portion
electrophoresis; also ELP
electrophoretic pattern
electrophysiologic
electrophysiology
electroprecipitin
elopement precaution
emergency physician
emergency procedure
endogenous pyrogen
endoperoxide
endorphin; also END
end point
enteropeptidase
environmental protection
enzyme product
eosinophilic pneumonia
eosinophilic pneumonitis
ependymal (cell)
epicardial
epithelial; also Ep, EPI, EPITH, epith
epithelium; also EPI, EPITH, epith
erythrocyte protoporphyrin
erythrophagocytosis
erythropoietic porphyria
erythropoietin; also Ep, EPO
esophageal pressure
esophoria; also ES
evoked potential
extreme pressure
Ep epilepsy; also EPI, epil
epithelial; also EP, EPI, EPITH, epith
erythropoietin; also EP, EPO
E&P estrogen and progesterone
EPA eicosapentaenoic acid

Environmental Protection Agency
erect posterior-anterior (projection)
erythroid-potentiating activity
ethylphenacemide
exophthalmos-producing activity
extrinsic plasminogen activator

EPAP expiratory positive airway pressure

EPAQ Extended Personal Attributes Questionnaire

EPA/RCRA Environmental Protection Agency Resource Conservation and Recovery Act

EPB Environmental Pre-Language Battery
extensor pollicis brevis

EPC electronic pain control
end-plate current
epilepsia partialis continua
external pneumatic compression

EPCA external pressure circulatory assistance

EPCG endoscopic pancreatocholangiography

EPD effective pressor dose

EPDML epidemiologic
epidemiology

EpDRF epithelial-derived relaxant factor

EPE erythropoietin-producing enzyme

EPEA expense per equivalent admission

EPEC enteropathogenic *Escherichia coli*; also EEC

EPEG etoposide; also ETOP, Etop

EPF early pregnancy factor
endocarditis parietalis fibroplastica
endothelial proliferating factor
Enfamil Premature Formula
eosinophil-producing factor
exophthalmos-producing factor

EPG eggs per gram
electropneumogram
electropneumography
ethanolamine phosphoglyceride

EPH edema-proteinuria-hypertension
extensor proprius hallucis

EPI Emotions Profile Index
epilepsy; also Ep, epil
epileptic; also epil
epinephrine; also E, epineph
epithelial; also EP, Ep, EPITH, epith
epithelioid cells
epithelium; also EP, EPITH, epith
epitympanic
evoked potential index
exocrine pancreatic insufficiency
Expanded Program of Immunization

extrapyramidal involvement
Eysenck Personality Inventory

Epi epicardium
epiglottis

epid epidemic

epig epigastric

epil epilepsy; also Ep, EPI
epileptic; also EPI

epineph epinephrine; also E, EPI

EPIS, epis episiotomy
episode
epistaxis

epistom a stopper (on mouth of bottle) [L. *epistomium*]

EPITH, epith epithelial; also EP, Ep, EPI
epithelium; also EP, EPI

EPK early prenatal karyotype

EPL effective patient life
essential phospholipids
extensor pollicis longus
external plexiform layer

EPM Elderfield pyrimidine mustard
electronic pacemaker
electron probe microanalysis
electrophoretic mobility; also EM
energy-protein malnutrition

EPMA electron-probe microanalysis (x-ray)

EPO erythropoietin; also EP, Ep
European Patent Office
exclusive provider organization
expiratory port occlusion

EPP end-plate potential
equal pressure point
erythropoietic protoporphyria

EPPS Edwards Personal Preference Scale

EPQ Eysenck Personality Questionnaire

EPR electron paramagnetic resonance
electrophrenic respiration
emergency physical restraint
estradiol production rate
extraparenchymal resistance

EPROM erasable programmable read-only memory (computer)

EPS elastosis perforans serpiginosa
electrophysiologic study
enzymatic pancreatic secretion
exophthalmos-producing substance
expressed prostatic secretion
extrapyramidal side effect (syndrome)
extrapyramidal signs

EPS—cont'd
extrapyramidal symptoms
extrapyramidal syndrome

ep's epithelial cells

EPSC excitatory postsynaptic current

EPSD E-point to septal distance

EPSDT Early and Periodic Screening,
Diagnosis, and Treatment

EPSE extrapyramidal side effects

EPSEM equal probability of selection method

EPSP 5-enolpyruvylshikimate 3-phosphate
excitatory postsynaptic potential

EPSS E-point septal separation

EPT early pregnancy test
Eidetic Parents Test
endoscopic papillotomy

EPTE existed prior to enlistment

EPTFE expanded polytetrafluoroethylene

EPTS existed prior to service

EPXMA electron probe x-ray microanalyzer

EQ educational quotient
encephalization quotient
energy quotient
equal to
equilibrium; also eq, equil, equilib

Eq equation; also eq, eqn
equivalent; also eq, equiv

eq equal
equation; also Eq, eqn
equilibrium; also EQ, equil, equilib
equivalent; also Eq, equiv

EQA external quality assessment

eqn equation; also Eq, eq

equil equilibrium; also EQ, eq, equilib

equilib equilibrium; also EQ, eq, equil

equip equipment

equiv equivalency
equivalent; also Eq, eq
equivocal

ER early reticulocyte
efficacy ratio
ejection rate
electroresection
emergency room; also er
endoplasmic reticulum; also er
enhanced reactivation
enhancement ratio
environmental resistance
epigastric region
equine rhinopneumonia

equivalent roentgen (unit)
erythrocyte receptor
esophageal rupture
estradiol receptor
estrogen receptor
evoked response
expiratory reserve
extended release (tablet)
extended resistance
external reduction
external resistance
external rotation, also ext rot
extraction ratio; also E
eye research

ER⁻ decreased estrogen receptor

ER⁺ increased estrogen receptor

ER+ estrogen receptor-positive

E&R equal and reactive
examination and report

Er erbium
erythrocyte; also E, e, er, Erc, ERY, Ery, eryth

er emergency room; also ER
endoplasmic reticulum; also ER
erythrocyte; also E, e, Er, Erc, ERY, Ery, eryth
estrogen receptors

ERA electrical response activity
electrical response audiometry
electroencephalic response audiometry
Electroshock Research Association
estradiol receptor assay
estrogen receptor assay
evoked response audiometry

ERB ethnic relational behavior

ERBF effective renal blood flow

ERC endoscopic retrograde cholangiography
enteric cytopathogenic human orphan-rhino-coryza (virus)
equal, reactive, and contracting (pupils)
erythropoietin-responsive cell

Erc erythrocyte; also E, e, Er, er, ERY, Ery, eryth

ERCP endoscopic retrograde cannulation of
pancreatic (duct)
endoscopic retrograde cholangiopancreato-graphy
endoscopic retrograde choledochopancrea-tography

Ercs erythrocytes

ERD early retirement with disability
evoked response detector

ERDA Energy Research and Development Administration

ERE external rotation in extension

ERF Education and Research Foundation
external rotation in flexion

erf error function

ERFC, E-RFC erythrocyte rosette-forming cell

ERG electrolyte replacement with glucose
electron radiography
electroretinogram
electroretinography

erg energy unit; also e

ERH egg-laying release hormone

ERHD exposure-related hypothermia death

ERI Environmental Response Inventory
erythrocyte rosette inhibitor

ERIA electroradioimmunoassay

ER-ICA estrogen receptor–immunocyto-chemical assay

ERL effective refractory length

ERM electrochemical relaxation method
extended radical mastectomy

ERP early receptor potential
effective refractory period (atrial)
emergency room physician
endocardial resection procedure
endoscopic retrograde pancreatography
equine rhinopneumonitis
estrogen receptor protein
event-related brain potential

ERPF effective renal plasma flow

ERPLV effective refractory period of the left ventricle

ERR, err error

ERS endoscopic retrograde sphincterotomy
expression-regulating sequence

ERSP event-related slow-brain potential

ERT esophageal radionuclide transit
estrogen replacement therapy
external radiation therapy

ERV equine rhinopneumonitis virus
expiratory reserve volume

ERY erysipelas
erythrocyte; also E, e, Er, er, Erc, Ery, eryth

Ery erysipelothrix
erythrocyte; also E, e, Er, er, Erc, ERY, eryth

eryth erythema
erythrocyte; also E, e, Er, er, Erc, ERY, Ery

ES Ego Strength (test)
ejection sound
elastic suspensor
electrical stimulation; also Es
electrical stimulus; also Es
electroshock; also ECS
elopement status (psychology)
emergency service
emission spectrometry
emission spectroscopy
endometritis-salpingitis
endoscopic sclerosis
endoscopic sphincterotomy
end stage
end systole
end-to-side (anastomosis); also E-S, ETS
environmental stimulation
enzyme substrate
epileptic syndrome
esophageal scintigraphy
esophagus; also E, ESO, eso, esoph
esophoria; also EP
esterase; also EST
exfoliation syndrome
Expectation Score
experimental study
ex-smoker
exterior surface
extrasystole
soap enema [L. *enema saponis*]; also es

E-S end-to-side (anastomosis); also ES, ETS

Es einsteinium
electrical stimulation; also ES
electrical stimulus; also ES
estriol; also E$_3$

es soap enema [L. *enema saponis*]; also ES

ESA electrosurgical arthroscopy
end-to-side anastomosis

ESAF endothelial cell stimulating angiogenesis factor

ESAP evoked sensory nerve action potention

ESB electrical stimulation of brain

ESC electromechanical slope computer
end-systolic count
erythropoietin-sensitive stem cell

ESCA electron spectroscopy for chemical analysis

ESCC electrolyte steroid cardiopathy by calci-fication
epidural spinal cord compression

ESCH electrolyte steroid-produced cardiopathy characterized by hyalinization

Esch, *Esch* *Escherichia*; also E, *E*

ESCN electrolyte and steroid cardiopathy with necrosis

ESCS Early Social Communication Scale

ESD electronic summation device
electron-stimulated desorption
emission spectrometric detector
end-systolic dimension
environmental sex determination
esophagus, stomach, and duodenum
esterase D
exoskeletal device

ESDIAD electron-stimulated desorption ion angular distribution

ESE electrostatic unit [Ger. *electrostatische Einheit*]

ESEP elbow sensory potential
extreme somatosensory evoked potential

ESF electrosurgical filter
erythropoiesis-stimulating factor
erythropoietic-stimulating factor
external skeletal fixation

ESFL end-systolic force-length (relationship)

ESG electrospinogram
estrogen

ESHAP etoposide, cisplatin, ARA-C, and methylprednisolone

ESI Ego State Inventory
enzyme substrate inhibitor
epidural steroid injection
extent of skin involvement

ES-IMV expiration-synchronized intermittent mandatory ventilation

ESIN elastic stable intramedullary nailing

ESL end-systolic segment length
English as a second language

ESLD end-stage liver disease

ESM ejection systolic murmur
endothelial specular microscope
ethosuximide; also ETX

ESMIS Emergency Medical Services Management Information System

ESN educationally subnormal
estrogen-stimulated neurophysine

ESN(M) educationally subnormal–moderate

ESN(S) educationally subnormal–severe

ESO electrospinal orthosis
esophagoscopy; also eso, esoph
esophagus; also E, ES, eso, esoph

eso esophagoscopy; also ESO, esoph
esophagus; also E, ES, ESO, esoph

esoph esophagoscopy; also ESO, eso
esophagus; also E, ES, ESO, eso

esoph steth esophageal stethoscope

ESP early systolic paradox
effective sensory projection
effective systolic pressure
electrosensitive point
endometritis-salpingitis-peritonitis
end-systolic pressure
eosinophil stimulation promoter
epidermal soluble protein
especially; also esp
evoked synaptic potential
extrasensory perception

esp especially; also ESP

ESPA electrical stimulation-produced analgesia

ESPQ Early School Personality Questionnaire

ESR electric skin resistance
electron spin resonance; also esr
erythrocyte sedimentation rate

esr electron spin resonance; also ESR

ESRD end-stage renal disease

ESRF end-stage renal failure

ESRS extrapyramidal symptom rating scale

ESS empty sella turcica syndrome
endostreptosin
erythrocyte-sensitizing substance
euthyroid sick syndrome
evolutionary stable strategy
excited skin syndrome

ess essence
essential

ess neg essentially negative

EST electroshock therapy
electroshock threshold
endodermal sinus tumor
esterase; also ES
exercise stress test

est ester; also E
estimated
estimation

esth esthetic
esthetics

ESU, esu electrostatic unit (of electrical charge)
electrosurgical unit

E-sub excitor substance

ESV end-systolic ventricular volume
esophageal valve

ESVI end-systolic volume index

ESVS epiurethral suprapubic vaginal suspension

ESWL extracorporeal shock-wave lithotripsy

ESWS end-systolic wall stress

ET Ebbinghaus' Test
edge thickness
educational therapy
effective temperature
ejection time
electroneurodiagnostic technologist
embryo transfer
endotoxin
endotracheal; also ENDO, Endo
endotracheal tube; also ETT
endurance time
enterostomal therapist
enterostomal therapy
epithelial tumor
esotropia
esotropic
essential thrombocythemia
essential tremor
ethanol; also E, ETH, ETOH, EtOH
ethyl; also E, Et
etiocholanolone test
etiology; also E, et, etio, etiol
eustachian tube
exchange transfusion
exercise test
exercise training
exercise treadmill
expiration time
extracellular tachyzoite

ET′ esotropia for near

E(T) intermittent esotropia

E/T effector to target ratio

ET₁ esotropia at near ET_1

ET₃ erythrocyte triiodothyronine ET_3

ET₄ effective thyroxine (test) ET_4

Et ethyl; also E, ET

et and [L. *et*]
etiology; also E, ET, etio, etiol

ETA eicosatetraenoic acid; also ETTA
electron-transfer agent
endotracheal airway
endotracheal aspirates
estimated time of arrival
ethionamide; also ETH
examination thermal analysis

ETAB extrathoracic-assisted breathing

et al and elsewhere [L. *et alibi*]
and others [L. *et alii*]

E₂TBG estradiol-testosterone-binding globulin

ETC estimated time of conception

ET$_C$ corrected ejection time

etc and so forth [L. *et cetera*]

E$_T$CO$_2$ end-tidal carbon dioxide concentration

ETD eustachian tube dysfunction

ETE end-to-end (anastomosis); also EE, E-E

ETEC enterotoxic *Escherichia coli*
enterotoxigenic *Escherichia coli*
enterotoxin of *Escherichia coli*

ETF electron-transferring flavoprotein
eustachian tube function

ETH elixir terpin hydrate
ethanol; also E, ET, ETOH, EtOH
ethionamide; also ETA
ethmoid
Ethrane (enflurane)

eth ether; also Et$_2$O

ETHC, ETH/C elixir terpin hydrate with codeine; also ETHcC

ETHcC elixir terpin hydrate with codeine; also ETHC, ETH/C

ETI ejective time index

ETIO etiocholanolone; also E

etio etiology; also E, ET, et, etiol

etiol etiology; also E, ET, et, etio

ETK erythrocyte transketolase

ETKM every test known to man; also ETKTM

ETKTM every test known to man; also ETKM

ETL expiratory threshold load

ETLC extraction thin-layer chromatography

ETM erythromycin; also E, EM

ETN ethanolamine

Et$_3$N triethylamine

ET-NANB enterically transmitted non-A, non-B hepatitis

ETO estimated time of ovulation
ethylene oxide; also EO, EtO, ETOX
eustachian tube obstruction

EtO ethylene oxide; also EO, ETO, ETOX

Et$_2$O ether; also eth

ETOH, EtOH ethanol; also E, ET, ETH
ethyl alcohol

ETOP elective termination of pregnancy; also ETP

ETOP—cont'd
etoposide; also EPEG, Etop

Etop etoposide; also EPEG, ETOP

ETOX ethylene oxide; also EO, ETO, EtO

ETP elective termination of pregnancy; also ETOP
electron transfer particle
electron transport particle
entire treatment period
ephedrine, theophylline, and phenobarbital
eustachian tube pressure

ETR effective thyroxine ratio
epitympanic recess
estimated thyroid ratio

ETS Educational Testing Service
electrical transcranial stimulation
end-to-side (anastomosis); also ES, E-S

ETT endotracheal tube; also ET
epinephrine tolerance test
esophageal transit time
exercise tolerance test
exercise treadmill test
extrapyramidal thyroxine
extrathyroidal thyroxine

ETTA eicosatetraenoic acid; also ETA

ETTN ethyltrimethylolmethane trinitrate

ETU emergency and trauma unit
emergency treatment unit

ETV educational television
extravascular thermal volume; also EVTV

ETX ethosuximide; also ESM

EU Ehrlich unit
emergency unit
endotoxin unit
entropy unit
enzyme unit
esophageal ulcer
esterase unit
etiology unknown
excretory urography
expected utility

Eu europium
euryon

EUA examination under anesthesia

EUCD emotionally unstable character disorder

EUG extrauterine gestation

EUL expected upper limit

EUM external urethral meatus

EUP extrauterine pregnancy

EURONET European On-Line Network

EUROTOX European Committee on Chronic Toxicity Hazards

EUS external urethral sphincter

eust eustachian

EUV extreme ultraviolet (laser)

EV emergency vehicle
enterovirus
epidermodysplasia verruciformis
esophageal varices
estradiol valerate
eversion; also ev, ever
everted; also ev, ever
evoked (response)
excessive ventilation
expected value
extravascular

eV electron volt; also ev

ev electron volt; also eV
eversion; also EV, ever
everted; also EV, ever

EVA ethylene vinyl acetate
ethyl violet azide (broth)
etoposide, vinblastine, and Adriamycin
equine viral arteritis

EVAC, evac evacuate
evacuated
evacuation

eval evaluate
evaluated
evaluation

EVAP etoposide, vinblastine, Ara-C, Platinol

evap evaporated
evaporation; also evapn

evapn evaporation; also evap

EVCI expected value of clinical information

EVD external ventricular drainage

eve evening

ever eversion; also EV, ev
everted; also EV, ev

EVF ethanol volume fraction

EVG electroventriculogram

EVI endocardial, vascular, interstitial

evisc evisceration

EVLW extravascular lung water

EVM electronic voltmeter
extravascular mass

evol evolution

EVP evoked visual potential

EVR endocardial viability ratio
evoked visual response

EVS endoscopic variceal sclerosis

EVSD Eisenmenger's ventricular septal defect

EVTV extravascular thermal volume; also ETV

EW emergency ward

ew elsewhere

EWB estrogen withdrawal bleeding

EWHO elbow-wrist-hand orthosis

EWI Experimental World Inventory

EWL egg-white lysozyme
evaporation water loss
evaporative water loss
list of adjectives [Ger. *Eigenschaftswörter* (adjectives), *Liste* (list)]

EWSCLs extended-wear soft contact lenses

EWT erupted wisdom teeth

E(X) expected value of the random variable X

Ex, ex exacerbation
exaggerated; also exag
examination; also exam
examine; also exam
examined; also exam
example
excision; also exc
exercise; also E, exer
exophthalmos
exposure; also exp
extract; also EXT, ext
extraction; also EXT
from [L. *ex*]; also e

ex aff of affinity [L. *ex affinis*]

EXAFS extended x-ray absorption fine structure (spectroscopy)

exag exaggerated; also Ex, ex

exam examination; also Ex, ex
examine; also Ex, ex
examined; also Ex, ex
examiner; also E

ex aq in water [L. *ex aqua* (from water)]

EXBF exercise hyperemia blood flow; also EHBF

exc except
excision; also Ex, ex

EXD ethylxanthic disulfide

exec executive

ExEF ejection fraction during exercise

EXELFS extended electron-loss fine structure

exer exercise; also E, Ex, ex

EXGBUS external genitalia, Bartholin gland, urethral gland, and Skene gland; also EGBUS

ex gr of the group of [L. *ex grupa*]

exhib let it be given [L. *exhibeatur*]

exist existing

EXO exonuclease
exophoria

EXP experienced
exploration; also exp
expose; also exp

Exp expectorant; also exp, expec, expect
expiration; also expir
expiratory; also expir
expire; also expir

exp expected
expectorant; also Exp, expec, expect
experiment; also E, exper, expt
experimental; also E, exper, exptl
expired (died); also E
expired (gas); also E
exploration; also EXP
exploratory
exponent
exponential function
expose; also EXP
exposed
exposure; also Ex, ex

expec expectorant; also Exp, exp, expect

expect expectorant; also Exp, exp, expec

exper experiment; also E, exp, expt
experimental; also E, exp, exptl

ExPGN extracapillary proliferative glomerulonephritis

expir expiration; also Exp
expiratory; also Exp
expired; also Exp

exp lap exploratory laparotomy

expn expression

expt experiment; also E, exp, exper

exptl experimental; also E, exp, exper

exptlly experimentally

EXREM external radiation-emission-man (radiation dose)

EXS externally supported
extrinsically supported

exsicc dried out [L. *exsiccatus*]

EXT extension; also E, ext

external; also ext
extract; also Ex, ex, ext
extraction; also Ex, ex
extremity; also ext, extr

ext extension; also E, EXT
extensor
exterior
external; also EXT
extract; also Ex, ex, EXT
extremity; also EXT, extr
spread [L. *extende*]

ext aud external auditory

extd extended
extracted

extern externally

Ext FHR external fetal heart rate

ext fd fluid extract

extr extremity; also EXT, ext

extrap extrapolate
extrapolation

extrav extravasation

ext rot external rotation; also ER

EXTUB extubation

EXU excretory urogram

EY egg yolk
epidemiology year

EYA egg yolk agar

Ez eczema

F

F bioavailability
brother [L. *frater*]
conjugative plasmid in F+ bacterial cells
degree of fineness of abrasive particles (less fine than "FF")
facial
facies
factor; also Fac
Fahrenheit; also Fahr
failure
fair
false
familial; also Fam, fam
family; also Fam, fam
farad; also f, far
Faraday's constant; also *F*
faradic; also f, far
fascia
fasting
fat (dietary)
father; also fa, FR
fecal
feces
feet; also f, ft
Fellow
female; also Fe, fe, FEM, fem
fermentative
fermi
fertility; also fert
fetal
fibroblast
fibrous (insulin, protein)
Ficoll
field of vision
filament; also fil
Filaria species; also *F*
fine
finger
firm
flexed
flexion; also f, fl, flex
flow (of blood)
fluid; also f, Fl, fl, FLD, fld
fluoride; also F −
fluorine
flutter wave
focal length; also f, FL
focus
foil
fontanel
foot; also f, ft

foramen; also FA
force; also *F*
form; also f
formula; also for, form
formulary
fossa
Fourier
fractional; also fract, FX, fx
fracture; also Fr, frac, fract, Frx, Fx, fx, FXR
fragment of antibody
free
free energy; also *F*
French (gauge, scale); also FR, Fr
frequency; also f, *f*, freq
frequent; also f, freq
frontal
frontal electrode placement (in electroencephalography)
full (diet)
function; also fn, func, funct, FXN
fundus; also Fd
Fusiformis species; also *F*
fusion beat
Fusobacterium species; also *F*
gilbert (unit of magnetomotive force); also *F*
hydrocortisone (compound F)
inbreeding coefficient
let there be made [L. *fiat, fiant*]; also f, ft
luminous flux; also *F*
make [L. *fac*]; also f
phenylalanine (one-letter notation); also P, PA, PHA, PHE, Phe
son [L. *filius*]
variance ratio
vectorcardiography electrode (left foot)
visual field

F Faraday's constant; also F
Filaria species; also F
force; also F
free energy; also F
F statistic (variance ratio)
Fusiformis species; also F
Fusobacterium species; also F
gilbert (unit of magnetomotive force); also F
luminous flux; also F

𝔉 Fourier transform; also FT

F′ hybrid F plasmid
secondary focal point (of lens)

°F degree Fahrenheit

F+ bacterial cell with an F plasmid

F⁺ —cont'd
  good form response

F⁻ bacterial cell lacking an F plasmid
  fluoride; also F
  poor form response

F/ full upper denture

/F full lower denture

(F) final

F₁, F₂, etc. first, second, etc. filial generation

F₃ trifluorothymidine

FI thru FXIII factor I through factor XIII
  (blood coagulation)

F344 Fischer 344 (rat)

f atomic orbital with angular momentum quan-
    tum number 3
  breathing frequency
  farad; also F, far
  faradic; also F, far
  fasting
  feet; also F, ft
  femto- (10⁻¹⁵)
  fingerbreadth; also FB, fb
  fission
  flexion; also F, fl, flex
  fluid; also F, Fl, fl, FLD, fld
  focal length; also F, FL
  following; also ff, fol
  foot; also F, ft
  form; also F
  fostered (experimental animal)
  frequency; also F, *f*, freq
  frequent; also F, freq
  frequently
  let there be made [L. *fiat, fiant*]; also F, ft
  make [L. *fac*]; also F
  respiratory frequency

f frequency; also F, f, freq
  furanose

F-12, f-12 freon

FA false aneurysm
  Families Anonymous
  Fanconi's anemia
  far advanced
  fatty acid
  febrile antigen
  femoral artery
  fertilization antigen
  fetal age
  fibrinolytic activity
  fibroadenoma
  fibrosing alveolitis

  field ambulance
  filterable agent
  filterable air
  filtered air
  first aid
  fluorescein angiography, also FL Ang
  fluorescent antibody (technique)
  fluorescent assay
  fluoroalanine
  folic acid
  follicular area
  foramen, also F
  Forbes-Albright (syndrome)
  forearm; also Fo
  fortified aqueous (solution)
  free acid
  Freund's adjuvant
  Friedreich's ataxia
  functional activities
  fusaric acid
  fusidic acid

F/A fetus active

fa father; also F, FR
  fatty (rat)

FAA folic acid antagonist
  formalin, acetic acid, and alcohol (solution)

FAAD fetal activity acceleration determination;
  also FAD

FAAN Fellow of the American Academy of
  Nursing

FAAP family assessment adjustment pass

FAB fast atom bombardment
  formalin ammonium bromide
  fragment of immunoglobulin G involved in
    antigen binding; also Fab
  French-American-British (classification sys-
    tem for certain leukemias)
  functional arm brace

Fab fragment of immunoglobulin G involved in
  antigen binding; also FAB

F(ab)₂ fragment of an immunoglobulin G molecule

F(ab′)₂ fragment of immunoglobulin G after
  digestion with the enzyme pepsin

FABER flexion in abduction and external rotation

Fabere flexion, abduction, external rotation,
  and extension

FABF femoral artery blood flow

FAB-MS, FAB/MS fast atom bombardment
  mass spectrometry

FABP fatty acid-binding protein
folic acid-binding protein

FAC femoral arterial cannulation
ferric ammonium citrate
fetal abdominal circumference
fluorouracil, Adriamycin, and cyclophosphamide
fractional area concentration
free available chlorine

Fac factor; also F

FACA Fellow of the American College of Anesthesiologists

Facb fragment, antigen, and complement binding

FACC Fellow of the American College of Cardiology

FACCP Fellow of the American College of Chest Physicians

FACES unique facies, anorexia, cachexia, and eye and skin (syndrome)

FACD Fellow of the American College of Dentists

FACFS Fellow of the American College of Foot Surgeons

FACH forceps to after-coming head

FACHA Fellow of the American College of Hospital Administrators

FACHCA Foundation of American College of Health Care Administrators

FAC-LEV fluorouracil, Adriamycin, cyclophosphamide, and levamisole

FACMTA Federal Advisory Council on Medical Training Aids

FACNHA Foundation of American College of Nursing Home Administrators (now: FACHCA, Foundation of American College of Health Care Administrators)

FACOG Fellow of the American College of Obstetricians and Gynecologists

FACOSH Federal Advisory Committee on Occupational Safety and Health

FACP Fellow of the American College of Physicians
Ftorafur, Adriamycin, cyclophosphamide, and platinol

FACR Fellow of the American College of Radiologists

FACS Fellow of the American College of Surgeons
fluorescence-activated cell sorter

fluorouracil, Adriamycin, cyclophosphamide, and streptozocin

FACSM Fellow of the American College of Sports Medicine

FACT Flanagan Aptitude Classification Test

FAD familial Alzheimer dementia
familial autonomic dysfunction
Family Assessment Device
fetal abdominal diameter
fetal activity acceleration determination; also FAAD
flavin adenine dinucleotide; also FADN

FADF fluorescent antibody dark-field

FADH flavin adenine dinucleotide (reduced form); also $FADH_2$

FADH$_2$ flavin adenine dinucleotide (reduced form); also FADH

FADIR flexion in adduction and internal rotation

Fadire flexion, adduction, internal rotation, and extension

FADN flavin adenine dinucleotide; also FAD

FADU fluorometric analysis of DNA unwinding

FAE fetal alcohol effect
fetal alcohol-exposed

FAF fatty acid free
fibroblast-activating factor

FAGA full-term appropriate for gestational age

FAH Federation of American Hospitals (now: FAHS, Federation of American Health Systems)

Fahr Fahrenheit; also F

FAHS Federation of American Health Systems

FAI first aid instruction
functional aerobic impairment
functional assessment inventory

FAJ fused apophyseal joints

FALG fowl anti-mouse lymphocyte globulin

FALL fallopian

FALP fluoro-assisted lumbar puncture

FAM fluorouracil, Adriamycin, and mitomycin C

Fam, fam familial; also F
family; also F

FAMA Fellow of the American Medical Association
fluorescent antibody to membrane antigen (test)

fam doc family doctor; also FD

FAME fatty acid methyl ester
fluorouracil, Adriamycin, and methyl CCNU (semustine); also FAMe

FAMe fluorouracil, Adriamycin, and methyl CCNU (semustine); also FAME

fam hist family history; also FH, FH$_x$

FAMMM familial atypical mole malignant melanoma
familial atypical multiple mole melanoma (syndrome)

fam per par familial periodic paralysis

fam phys family physician; also FP

FAM-S fluorouracil, Adriamycin, mitomycin C, and streptozotocin

FAN fuchsin, amido black, and naphthol yellow

FANA fluorescent antinuclear antibody

FANCAP fluids, aeration, nutrition, communication, activity, and pain

FANCAS fluids, aeration, nutrition, communication, activity, and stimulation

F and R force and rhythm (of pulse); also F&R

FANPT Freeman Anxiety Neurosis and Psychosomatic Test

FANS Fellow of the American Neurological Society

FANSS & M fundus anterior, normal size and shape, and mobile

FAO Food and Agriculture Organization

FAOTA Fellow of the American Occupational Therapy Association

FAP familial adenomatous polyposis
familial amyloid polyneuropathy
fatty acid poor
fatty acids polyunsaturated
femoral artery pressure
fibrillating action potential
fixed action pattern
fluorouracil, Adriamycin, Platinol
frozen animal procedure

FAPA Fellow of the American Psychiatric Association
Fellow of the American Psychoanalytical Association

FAPHA Fellow of the American Public Health Association

FAQ Family Attitudes Questionnaire

FAR flight aptitude rating
fractional albuminuria rate

F^{AR} immediate good function followed by accelerated rejection

far farad; also F, f
faradic; also F, f

FARS Fatal Accident Reporting System

FAS fatty acid synthetase
Federation of American Scientists
fetal alcohol syndrome

FASC free-standing ambulatory surgical center

fasc bundle [L. *fascis*]
fascicle
fasciculation
fasciculus

FASEB Federation of American Societies for Experimental Biology

FASF Factor Analyzed Short Form

FAST Filtered Audiometer Speech Test
flow-assisted short term (balloon catheter)
fluorescent allergosorbent test
fluorescent antibody staining technique

FAT family attitudes test
fast axoplasmic transport
fluorescent antibody technique
fluorescent antibody test
fluorouracil, Adriamycin, and trazinate
food awareness training

FATG fat globules

F$_1$ATPase F$_1$ adenosine triphosphatase

FATSA Flowers Auditory Test of Selective Attention

FAV feline ataxia virus
floppy aortic valve
fowl adenovirus

FAZ Fanconi-Albertini-Zellweger (syndrome)
foveal avascular zone

FB factor B
fasting blood
feedback
fiberoptic bronchoscope; also Fib bronc, FOB
fiberoptic bronchoscopy; also Fib bronc, FOB
fingerbreadth; also f, fb
foreign body; also fb

F/B forward bending

fb fingerbreadth; also f, FB
foreign body; also FB

f-b face-bow

FBA fecal bile acid

FBC full blood count
functional bactericidal concentration

FBCOD foreign body of the cornea, right eye [L. *oculus dexter* (right eye)]

FBCOS foreign body of the cornea, left eye [L. *oculus sinister* (left eye)]

FBCP familial benign chronic pemphigus

FBD fibrocystic breast disease
functional bowel disease
functional bowel disorder

FBE full blood examination

FBEC fetal bovine endothelial cell

FBF forearm blood flow

FBG fasting blood glucose
fibrinogen; also fbg, FG, FGN, FI, FIB, fib
foreign-body-type granuloma

fbg fibrinogen; also FBG, FG, FGN, FI, FIB, fib

FBH familial benign hypercalcemia

FBHH familial benign hypocalciuric hypercalcemia

FBI flossing, brushing, and irrigation

FBL fecal blood loss
follicular basal lamina

FBL-G Freiburg Complaint List, General Form [Ger. *Freiburger Beschwerdenliste Gesamtform*]

FBL-W Freiburg Complaint List, Repeat Form [Ger. *Freiburger Beschwerdenliste Wiederholungsform*]

FBM fetal breathing movement

FBN Federal Bureau of Narcotics

FBP femoral blood pressure
fibrin breakdown product(s)
fibrinogen breakdown product(s)

FBR fresh-blood reaction [Ger. *Frischblut* (fresh blood)]

FBRCM fingerbreadth below right costal margin

FBS fasting blood sugar
feedback signal
feedback system
fetal bovine serum

FBSS failed back surgery syndrome

FBU fingers below umbilicus (measurement); also F↓U

FBW fasting blood work

FC family conference
fasciculus cuneatus
fast component (of neuron)
febrile convulsion
fecal coliform (agar, broth)
feline conjuctivitis
ferric citrate
fever and chills; also F/C
fibrocystic

fibrocyte
financial class
finger clubbing
finger counting
flexion contracture
flow cytometry; also FCM
flucytosine
Foley catheter; also F cath
form response determined by color
foster care
free cholesterol
frontal cortex; also FCx
functional capacity
functional class

F/C fever and chills; also FC
flare and cell; also F + C

F&C foam and condom

F+C flare and cell; also F/C

5-FC 5-fluorocytosine

Fc centroid frequency
foot-candle; also fc, ftc
fragment, crystallizable (of immunoglobulin G molecules)
shade response to black areas

Fc′ fragment crystallized in minute quantities (by papain digestion of immunoglobulin G molecules)
shade response to light gray area

fc foot-candle; also Fc, ftc

FCA ferritin-conjugated antibodies .
fracture, complete, angulated
Freund's complete adjuvant; also CFA

FCAP Fellow of the College of American Pathologists

F cath Foley catheter; also FC

FCC familial colonic cancer
Federal Communications Commission
femoral cerebral catheter
follicular center cells
Food Chemical Codex
fracture complete and compound
fracture compound and comminuted

fcc face-centered-cubic

FCCC fracture complete, compound, and comminuted

FCCL follicular center cell lymphoma

FCCP trifluoromethoxycarbonylcyanide phenylhydrazone

FCD feces collection device
fibrocystic disease
fibrocystic dysplasia

FCD—cont'd
  focal cytoplasmic degradation
  fracture complete and deviated
FCDB fibrocystic disease of breast
FCE fluorouracil, cisplatin, and etoposide
FCF fetal cardiac frequency
  fibroblast chemotactic factor
FCFC fibroblast colony-forming cells
FCG French catheter gauge
FCGP Fellow of the College of General
  Practitioners
FCH familial combined hyperlipidemia; also
  FCHL
FCHL familial combined hyperlipidemia; also
  FCH
FCI fixed cell immunofluorescence
  food-chemical intolerance
fCi femtocurie
F-CL fluorouracil and calcium leucovorin
fcly face lying (position)
FCM fetal cardiac motion
  flow cytometric
  flow cytometry; also FC
FCMC family-centered maternity care
FCMD Fukuyama-type congenital muscular
  dystrophy
FCMN family-centered maternity nursing
FCMW Foundation for Child Mental Welfare
  (inactive)
FCP fasting chemistry profile
  final common/pathway
  fluorouracil, cyclophosphamide, and pred-
  nisone
  Functional Communication Profile (of
  aphasic adults)
FCPS Fellow of the College of Physicians and
  Surgeons
FCP(SA) Fellow of the College of Physicians
  of South Africa
FCR flexor carpi radialis
  fractional catabolic rate
FcR Fc receptor
FCRA fecal collection receptacle assembly
FCRB flexor carpi radialis brevis
FCRC Frederick Cancer Research Center
FCS fecal containment system
  feedback control system
  fetal calf serum
FCSNVD fever, chills, sweating, nausea, vom-
  iting, and diarrhea

FCT film-coated tablet
  food composition table
FCU flexor carpi ulnaris
FCV feline calicivirus
FCVD fracture complete and varus deformity
FCVDS Framingham Cardiovascular Disease
  Survey
FCx frontal cortex; also FC
FD failure to descend; also FTD
  familial dysautonomia
  family doctor; also fam doc
  fan douche
  fatal dose
  fetal danger
  fetal demise
  fetal distress
  fibrinogen derivation
  field desorption
  Filatov-Dukes (disease)
  fixed and dilated; also F&D
  fluorescence depolarization
  fluoroDOPA
  fluphenazine decanoate; also FPZ-D
  focal disease
  focal distance
  Folin-Denis (assay)
  follicular diameter
  foot drape
  forceps delivery
  freedom from distractibility
  freeze-dried
  frequency deviation
  full denture
F/D fracture/dislocation; also Fx-dis
F&D fixed and dilated; also FD
FD$_{50}$ median fatal dose
Fd amino-terminal portion of heavy chain of
  immunoglobulin
  ferredoxin
  fundus; also F
FDA fluorescein diacetate
  Food and Drug Administration
  right fronto-anterior (position of fetus) [L.
  frontodextra anterior]
FDB flexor digitorum brevis
FDBL fecal daily blood loss
FDC frequency dependence of compliance
  perfluorodecalin (blood substitute)
FD&C Food, Drug, and Cosmetic (Act)
FDCA Federal Food, Drug, and Cosmetic Act;
  also FFDCA

FDCPA Food, Drug, and Consumer Product Agency

FDCT Franck Drawing Completion Test

FDD Food and Drugs Directorate

FD&D food, drug, and cosmetic dyes

FDDC ferric dimethyldithiocarbonate

FDDQ Freedom from Distractibility Deviation Quotient

FDDS Family Drawing Depression Scale

FDE female day-equivalent
final drug evaluation

FDF fast death factor
further differentiated fibroblast

FDG Fibiger-Debré-Gierki (syndrome)
fluorodeoxyglucose

FDG, fdg feeding

FDGF fibroblast-derived growth factor

FDH familial dysalbuminemic hyper-thyroxinemia
formate dehydrogenase

FDI first dorsal interosseus
International Dental Federation (London, England) [Fr. *Fédération Dentaire Internationale*]

FDIM fluorescence digital imaging microscopy

FDIU fetal death in utero

FDL flexor digitorum longus

FDLMP first day of last menstrual period

FDLV fer de lance virus

FDM fetus of diabetic mother

FDNB 1-fluoro-2,4-dinitrobenzene (Sanger's reagent)

FDP fibrin degradation product(s); also fdp
fibrinogen degradation product(s); also fdp
flexor digitorum profundus
fructose 1,6-diphosphate
right frontoposterior (position of fetus) [L. *frontodextra posterior*]

fdp fibrin degradation product(s); also FDP
fibrinogen degradation product(s); also FDP

FDPALD fructose diphosphate aldolase

FDPase fructose diphosphatase

FDQB flexor digiti quinti brevis

FDR fractional disappearance rate
frequency dependence of resistance

FDS Fellow in Dental Surgery
flexor digitorum sublimis
flexor digitorum superficialis
for duration of stay

FDT right frontotransverse (position of fetus) [L. *frontodextra transversa*]

F₃dTMP trifluorothymidylate

FdUMP fluorodeoxyuridine monophosphate

FDV Friend's disease virus

FDZ fetal danger zone

FE fatty ester
fecal emesis
fetal erythrocyte
fetal erythroblastosis
fluid extract; also fld ext, fldxt, fl ext
fluorescing erythrocyte
forced expiratory
formalin and ethanol
freely eating

Fe female; also F, fe, FEM, fem
iron [L. *ferrum*]; also Fer

Fe⁵⁹ radioactive iron; halflife, 45.1 ± .05 days

fe female; also F, Fe, FEM, fem

feb febrile
fever [L. *febris*]; also fev, fv

FEBA factor eight bypassing activity

feb dur while the fever lasts [L. *febre durante*]

FEBP fetal estrogen-binding protein

FEBS Federation of European Biochemical Societies (Strasbourg, France)

FEC fluorouracil, epirubicin, and cyclophos-phamide
fluorouracil, etoposide, and cisplatin
forced expiratory capacity
free erythrocyte coproporphyrin; also FECP
freestanding emergency center
Friend's erythroleukemia cell; also FELC

FECG fetal electrocardiogram; also FEKG

F_{ECO2} fractional concentration of carbon dioxide in expired gas

FECP free erythrocyte coproporphyrin; also FEC

FECT factor VIII correctional time
fibroelastic connective tissue

FECV feline enteric coronavirus
functional extracellular fluid volume

FED final evaluation day

FeD iron deficiency [L. *ferrum* (iron)]; also Fe def

Fe def iron deficiency [L. *ferrum* (iron)]; also FeD

FEE forced equilibrating expiration

FEEG fetal electroencephalogram

FEF Family Evaluation Form
  forced expiratory flow (rate)

FEF$_{50}$ forced expiratory flow after 50% of vital
  capacity has been expelled

FEF$_{50}$/FIF$_{50}$ ratio of expiratory flow to inspiratory flow at 50% of forced vital capacity

FEFV forced expiratory flow volume

FEHBP Federal Employee Health Benefits
  Program

FEI factor eight inhibitor

FEIBA factor VIII inhibitor bypassing activity

FEKG fetal electrocardiogram; also FECG

FEL familial erythrophagocytic lymphohistio-
  cytosis

FELC Friend's erythroleukemia cell; also FEC

FeLV feline leukemia virus; also FLV

FEM female; also F, Fe, fe, fem
  femoral; also fem
  femur; also fem
  finite element method
  fluid-electrolyte malnutrition

fem female; also F, Fe, fe, FEM
  feminine
  femoral; also FEM
  femur; also FEM
  thigh [L. *femoris*]

fem intern at inner side of thighs [L. *femoribus
  internis*]

Fem-pop, fem-pop femoral-popliteal; also F-P

FEN fluid, electrolytes, and nutrition

FENa, FE$_{Na}$ excreted fraction of filtered
  sodium [L. *natrium* (sodium)]

FENF fenfluramine

F$_{EO2}$ fractional concentration of oxygen in
  expired gas

FEP fluorinated ethylene-propylene (polymer)
  free erythrocyte porphyrin
  free erythrocyte protoporphyrin; also FEPP

FEPB functional electronic peroneal brace

FEPP free erythrocyte protoporphyrin; also
  FEP

FER flexion, extension, and rotation
  fractional esterification rate

Fer iron [L. *ferrum*]; also Fe

fert fertility; also F
  fertilized

ferv boiling, hot [L. *fervens*]

FES Family Environment Scale
  fat embolism syndrome

flame emission spectrophotometry
flame emission spectroscopy
forced expiratory spirogram
functional electrical stimulation

FESA finite element stress analysis

FeSV feline sarcoma virus

FET field-effect transistor
  Fisher exact test
  fixed erythrocyte turnover
  forced expiratory time

fet fetus

FETE Far Eastern tick-borne encephalitis

FETI fluorescence energy transfer immunoassay

Fe/TIBC iron saturation of serum transferrin
  (TIBC: total iron binding capacity)

FETS, FETs forced expiratory time, in seconds

FEUO for external use only

FEV familial exudative vitreoretinopathy
  forced expiratory volume

fev fever; also feb, fv

FEV$_1$ forced expiratory volume in one second

FEVB frequency ectopic ventricular beat

FEV$_t$ forced expiratory volume timed

FEV$_1$/VC ratio of one-second forced expiratory
  volume to vital capacity

FEXE formalin, ethanol, xylol, and ethanol

FeZ iron zone [L. *ferrum* (iron)]

FF degree of fineness of abrasive particles
  (more fine than "F")
  fat fraction
  fat-free
  father factor
  fear of failure
  fecal frequency
  fertility factor
  fields of Forel
  filtration factor
  filtration fraction
  fine fiber
  fine fraction
  finger flexion
  finger-to-finger; also f → f
  fixation fluid
  fixing fluid
  flat feet
  flip-flop (electronic logic circuitry)
  fluorescent focus
  force fluids; also ff
  forearm flow
  forward flexion

forward flexion
foster father
Fox-Fordyce (disease)
free fraction
fresh frozen
fundus firm; also ff
further flexion

F&F filiform bougie and follower
fixes and follows

fF ultrafine fiber
ultrafine fraction

ff following; also f, fol
force fluids; also FF
fundus firm; also FF

f-f finger-to-finger; also FF

FFA female-female adaptor
free fatty acid

FFAP free fatty acid phase

FFB fast feedback
flexible fiberoptic bronchoscopy

FFC fixed flexion contracture
free from chlorine

FFCS forearm flexion control strap

FFD fat-free diet
focus-film distance

FFDCA Federal Food, Drug, and Cosmetic
Act; also FDCA

FFDW fat-free dry weight

FFE fecal fat excretion

FFEM freeze fracture electron microscopy

FFF degree of fineness of abrasive particles
(more fine than "FF")
field-flow fractionation
flicker fusion frequency (test)

FFG free fat graft

FFI fast food intake
free from infection
fundamental frequency indicator

FFIT fluorescent focus inhibition test

FFM fat-free mass
five-finger movement

FFP fresh frozen plasma

FFPS Fellow of the Faculty of Physicians and
Surgeons

FFR freedom from relapse
frequency-following response

FFROM full, free range of motion

FFS failure of fixation suppression
fat-free solid
fat-free supper

fee for service
flexible fiberoptic sigmoidoscopy

FFT fast Fourier transform
flicker fusion test
flicker fusion threshold

FFTP first full-term pregnancy

FFU focus-forming unit

FFW fat-free weight

FFWC fractional free-water clearance

FFWW fat-free wet weight

FG fasciculus gracilis
fast-glycolytic (muscle fiber)
fast green
Feeley-Gorman (agar); also F-G
fibrin glue
fibrinogen; also FBG, fbg, FGN, FI, FIB, fib
field gain
Flemish giant (rabbit)
French gauge

F-G Feeley-Gorman (agar); also FG

fg femtogram

FGAR formylglycinamide ribonucleotide

FGB fully granulated basophil

FGC fibrinogen gel chromatography

FGD fatal granulomatous disease

FGDS fibrogastroduodenoscopy

FGF father's grandfather
fibroblast growth factor
fresh gas flow

FGG focal global glomerulosclerosis
fowl gamma-globulin

FGL fasting gastrin level

FGLU fasting glucose

FGM father's grandmother

FGN fibrinogen; also FBG, fbg, FG, FI, FIB,
fib
focal glomerulonephritis

FGP fundic gland polyps

FGRN finely granular

FGS fibrogastroscopy
focal glomerular sclerosis

FGT female genital tract
fluorescent gonorrhea test

FGT-H fluorescence gonorrhea test–heated

FGU French gauge, urodynamic

FH familial hypercholesterolemia; also FHC
family history; also fam hist, FH_X
Fanconi-Hegglin (syndrome)
fasting hyperbilirubinemia

FH—cont'd
favorable histology
femoral hypoplasia
fetal head
fetal heart; also FHT
fibromuscular hyperplasia; also FMH
Ficoll-Hypaque (technique)
floating hospital
follicular hyperplasia
Frankfort's horizontal (plane of skull)
fundal height

fh fostered by hand (experimental animal)
let a draught be made [L. *fiat haustus*]

FH₄ folacin
tetrahydrofolic acid

FHA familial hypoplastic anemia
filamentous hemagglutinin
filterable hemolytic anemia
fimbrial hemagglutinin

FHC familial hypercholesterolemia; also FH
familial hypocalcemia
familial hypocalciuria
family health center
Ficoll-Hypaque centrifugation
Fuchs' heterochromic cyclitis

FHCH fortified hexachlorocyclohexane

FHD family history of diabetes

FHF fetal heart frequency
fulminant hepatic failure

FHH familial hypocalciuric hypercalcemia
family history of hirsutism
fetal heart heard

FHI Family Health International
Fuchs' heterochromic iridocyclitis

FHIF fibroblast human interferon

FHIP family health insurance plan

FHL flexor hallucis longus
functional hearing loss

FHLDL familial hypercholesterolemia, low
density lipoprotein

FHM fathead minnow (cells)
fetal heart motion

FH-M fumarate hydratase, mitochondrial

FHMI family history of mental illness

FHN family history negative

FHNH fetal heart not heard

FHP family history positive

FHR familial hypophosphatemic rickets
fetal heart rate
fetal heart rhythm

FHRDC family history, research diagnostic
criteria

FHR-NST fetal heart rate non-stress test

FHS fetal heart sound
fetal hydantoin syndrome

FH-S fumarate hydratase, soluble

FHT fetal heart; also FH
fetal heart tone

FHTG familial hypertriglyceridemia

FH-UFS femoral hypoplasia–unusual facies
syndrome

FHVP free hepatic vein pressure
free hepatic venous pressure

FHₓ family history; also fam hist, FH

FI fasciculus interfascicularis
fever caused by infection
fibrinogen; also FBG, fbg, FG, FGN, FIB, fib
fibula, complete (congenital absence of limb)
fiscal intermediary
fixed internal
fixed interval (schedule)
flame ionization
forced inspiration
fronto-iliacus
functional inquiry

fi fibula, incomplete (congenital absence of
limb)

FIA flow injection analysis
fluorescent immunoassay
Freund's incomplete adjuvant; also ICFA

FIAC
2′-fluoro-2′-deoxy-5-iodoarabinoside C
2-fluoro-5-iodoaracytosin

FIAT Field Information Agency, Technical

FIAU 2′-fluoro-2′-deoxy-5-iodoarabinoside U

FIB fibrin
fibrinogen; also FBG, fbg, FG, FGN, FI, fib
fibrositis
fibula

fib fiber
fibrillation; also fibrill
fibrinogen; also FBG, fbg, FG, FGN, FI, FIB

fibrill fibrillation; also fib

Fib bronc fiberoptic bronchoscope; also FB,
FOB
fiberoptic bronchoscopy; also FB, FOB

FIC Fellow of the Institute of Chemistry
functional inhibitory concentration

FICA Federal Insurance Contributions Act

FICO₂, FI_CO2 fractional concentration of carbon dioxide in inspired gas

FICD Fellow of the International College of Dentists

FICS Fellow of the International College of Surgeons

FID father in delivery
flame ionization detector
free induction decay
fungal immunodiffusion

FIF feedback inhibition factor
forced inspiratory flow
formaldehyde-induced fluorescence
human fibroblast interferon; also FIFN

FIFN human fibroblast interferon; also FIF

FIFR fasting intestinal flow rate

Fig figure

FIGE field inversion gel electrophoresis

FIGD familial idiopathic gonadotropin deficiency

FIGLU formiminoglutamic acid

FIGO International Federation of Gynecology and Obstetrics (London, England)

FIH fat-induced hyperglycemia

FIL father-in-law

fil filament; also F

FILAR filariasis

filt filter
filtration

FIM field ion microscopy
functional independence measure

FIME fluorouracil, ICRF-159 (razoxane), and methyl-CCNU (semustine)

FIMLT Fellow of the Institution of Medical Laboratory Technology

FIN fine intestinal needle

FIO2, FIO₂, FI_O2 forced inspiratory oxygen fraction of inspired oxygen

FIP feline infectious peritonitis

FIPT feline infectious periarteriolar transudate

FIPV feline infectious peritonitis virus

FIQ full scale intelligence quotient

FIR far infrared
fold increase in resistance

FIRA falciparum interspersed repeat antigen

FIRDA frontal irregular rhythmic delta activity (electroencephalography)

FIRO-B Fundamental Interpersonal Relations Orientation–Behavior

FIRO-F Fundamental Interpersonal Relations Orientation–Feelings

FIS forced inspiratory spirogram

FISP fast imaging with steady-state precision

FISS Flint Infant Security Scale

Fiss, fiss fissure

fist fistula

FIT Flanagan Industrial Tests
fluorescein isothiocyanate; also FITC
fusion-inferred threshold (test)

FITC fluorescein isothiocyanate; also FIT
fluorescein isothiocyanate, conjugated

FITT frequency, intensity, time, and type (exercise)

FIUO for internal use only

FIV₁ forced inspiratory volume in one second

FIVC forced inspiratory vital capacity

F-J Fisher-John (melting point method)

FJN familial juvenile nephrophthisis

FJP familial juvenile polyposis

FJRM full joint range of motion; also FJROM

FJROM full joint range of motion; also FJRM

FJS finger joint size

FK Feil-Klippel (syndrome)
feline kidney
Foster-Kennedy (syndrome)
functioning kasai (Belgian Congo anemia)

FKQCP Fellow of the King and Queen's College of Physicians (of Ireland)

FL factor level
fatty liver
feline leukemia
femur length
fetal length
fibers of Luschka
fibroblast-like
Fiessinger-Leroy (syndrome)
filtered load; also Fl, fl
filtration leukapheresis
flavomycin
fluorescein
flutamide and leuprolide acetate
focal length; also F, f
follicular lymphoma
Friend's leukemia
frontal lobe
full liquids (diet)
functional length

Fl filtered load; also FL, fl
florentium
fluid; also F, f, fl, FLD, fld
fluorescence; also fl, fluores
fluorescent; also fl, fluores

fl femtoliter; also fL
filtered load; also FL, Fl
flank
flexible
flexion; also F, f, flex
flourished (in historical dates)
fluid; also F, f, Fl, FLD, fld
fluorescence; also Fl, fluores
fluorescent; also Fl, fluores
flutter

fL femtoliter; also fl

FL-2 feline lung (cell)

FLA fluorescent-labeled antibody
left fronto-anterior (position of fetus) [L.
frontolaeva anterior]

Fla, fla let it be done according to rule of the
art [L. *fiat lege artis*]

flac flaccid
flaccidity

Fl Ang fluorescein angiography; also FA

FLASH fast low-angle shot

flav yellow [L. *flavus*]

FLC fatty liver cell
fetal liver cell
Friend's leukemia cell; also FL

FLD fatty liver disease
fibrotic lung disease
fluid; also F, f, Fl, fl, fld
flutamide and leuprolide acetate depot

fld field
fluid; also F, f, Fl, fl, FLD

fld ext fluid extract; also FE, fldxt, fl ext

fl dr fluid dram

fld rest fluid restriction; also FR

fl drs fluff dressing

fldxt fluid extract; also FE, fld ext, fl ext

FLe fluourouracil and levamisole

FLES Fairview Language Evaluation Scale

FLEX Federation licensing examination

flex flexion; also F, f, fl
flexor

flex sig flexible sigmoidoscopy; also FS

fl ext fluid extract; also FE, fld ext, fldxt

FLGA full-term, large for gestational age

FLK fetal lamb kidney
funny-looking kid (syndrome)

FLKS fatty liver and kidney syndrome

FLM fasciculus longitudinalis medialis

floc flocculation; also flocc

flocc flocculation; also floc

flor flowers [L. *flores*] (mineral substance in
powdery state after sublimation)

fl oz fluid ounce

FLP left frontoposterior (position of fetus) [L.
frontolaeva posterior]

FLPR flurbiprofen

FLR Fiessinger-Leroy-Reiter (syndrome)

FLS fatty liver syndrome
Fellow of the Linnean Society
fibrous long-spacing (collagen)
flashing lights and/or scotoma
flow-limiting segment
Functional Life Scale

FLSA follicular lymphosarcoma

FLSP fluorescein-labeled serum protein

FLT left frontotransverse (position of fetus) [L.
frontolaeva transversa]

FLTA Fullerton Language Test for Adolescents

FLTAC Fisher-Longemann Test of Articulation
Competence

FLU fluphenazine; also FPZ

flu influenza

FLU A influenza A

fluor fluorometry

fluores fluorescence; also Fl, fl
fluorescent; also Fl, fl

fluoro fluoroscopy; also FX

fl up flare-up
follow-up; also FU, F/U

FLV feline leukemia virus; also FeLV
Friend's leukemia virus

FLW fasting laboratory work

FLZ flurazepam

FM face mask
facilities management
fathom
feedback mechanism
fetal movement
fibromuscular
filtered mass
fine motor
flavin mononucleotide; also FMN
flowmeter

fluid movement
fluorescent microscopy
foramen magnum
forensic medicine
formerly married
foster mother
frequency modulation
Friend-Moloney (antigen)
functional movement
Fusobacterium micro-organisms
make a mixture [L. *fiat mixtura*]; also fm

F&M firm and midline (uterus)

Fm fermium

fm femtometer
from; also fr
make a mixture [L. *fiat mixtura*]; also FM

fm² square femtometer

fm³ cubic femtometer

FMA Frankfort-mandibular plane angle

FMAC fetal movement acceleration (test)

FMAU 2′-fluoro-2′-deoxy-5-methylarabino-
side U

FMB full maternal behavior

FMC family medicine center
fetal movement count
flight medicine clinic
focal macular choroidopathy
Foundation for Medical Care

FMD family medical doctor
fibromuscular dysplasia
foot-and-mouth disease

FMDV foot-and-mouth disease virus

FME full-mouth extraction

FMEL Friend's murine erythroleukemia

FMEN familial multiple endocrine neoplasia

FMET, F-met, fMet formylmethionine

FMF familial Mediterranean fever
fetal movement felt
flow microfluorometry
forced midexpiratory flow

FMFD1 familial multiple factor deficiency 1

FMG fine mesh gauze
foreign medical graduate

FMGEMS Foreign Medical Graduate
Examination in Medical Sciences

FMH family medical history
fat-mobilizing hormone
fetomaternal hemorrhage
fibromuscular hyperplasia; also FH

FMIR frustrated multiple internal reflexion

FML flail mitral leaflet
fluorometholone

FMLP, f-MLP formyl-methionyleucyl-
phenylalanine

FMN first malignant neoplasm
flavin mononucleotide; also FM
frontomaxillo-nasal (suture)

FMNH flavin mononucleotide (reduced form);
also FMNH₂

FMNH₂ flavin mononucleotide (reduced form);
also FMNH

FMO frontier molecule orbital (theory)

Fmoc 9-fluoromethoxycarbonyl

fmol femtomole

FMP fasting metabolic panel
first menstrual period

FMR fetal movement record
Friend-Moloney-Rauscher (antigen)

FMRF Phe-Met-Arg-Phe (phenylalanine-
methionine-arginine-phenylalanine)

FMS fat-mobilizing substance
financial management system
fluorouracil, mitomycin, and streptozocin
Frankfurt-Marburg syndrome
full-mouth series (dental x-ray films)

FMSTB Frostig Movement Skills Test Battery

FMU first morning urine

FMULC free monoclonal urinary light chain

FMV fluorouracil, methyl-CCNU (semustine),
and vincristine

FMX full-mouth x-ray

FN facial nerve
false negative; also Fneg
fastigial nucleus
fibronectin
final nitrogen
finger-to-nose (coordination test); also F-N,
F → N, FTN
first nucleotide
flip number (number of times an animal can
right itself when placed on its back)
fluoride number

F-N finger-to-nose (coordination test); also FN,
F → N, FTN

F → N finger-to-nose (coordination test); also
FN, F-N, FTN

fn function; also F, func, funct, FXN

FNA fine-needle aspiration

FNa filtered sodium [L. *natrium* (sodium)]

FNAB fine-needle aspiration biopsy

FNAC fine-needle aspiration cytology

FNC fatty nutritional cirrhosis

FNCJ fine-needle catheter jejunostomy

FND febrile neutrophilic dermatosis
frontonasal dysplasia

Fneg false negative; also FN

FNF false-negative fraction
femoral neck fracture
finger-to-nose-to-finger (coordination test)

FNH focal nodular hyperplasia

FNP Family Nurse Practitioner

fn p fusion point; also FP, fu p

FNR false-negative rate

FNS food and nutrition services
functional neuromuscular stimulation

FNT false neurochemical transmitter
finger-to-nose test

FNTC fine needle transhepatic cholangiography

FO fast oxidative
fiberoptic
focus out
foot orthosis
foramen ovale
forced oscillation
foreign object
fronto-occipital (fetal position)

Fo fomentation
fomenting
forearm; also FA
forearm amputation

FOAVF failure of all vital forces

FOB father of baby
fecal occult blood
feet out of bed
fiberoptic bronchoscope; also FB, Fib bronc
fiberoptic bronchoscopy; also FB, Fib bronc
foot of bed
foreign object/body

FOBT fecal occult blood test

FOC father of child
fluid of choice
frequency of contact (scale)
fronto-occipital circumference

FOCAL formula calculation (computer language)

FOCMA feline oncornavirus-associated cell membrane antigen

FOD free of disease

FOEB feet over edge of bed

FOG fast-oxidative-glycolytic (muscle fiber)
Fluothane, oxygen, and gas (nitrous oxide)
full-on gain

FOI flight of ideas

fol following; also f, ff
leaves [L. *folia*]

FOM figure of merit (measure of diagnostic value per radionuclide radiation dose)
floor of mouth

FOMI fluorouracil, Oncovin, and mitomycin C

FONAR Focusing Magnetic Nuclear Magnetic Resonance

FOOB fell out of bed

FOOSH fell on outstretched hand

FOP fibrodysplasia ossificans progressiva
forensic pathology

FOPR full outpatient rate

FOR, For forensic

for foreign
formula; also F, form

form formula; also F, for

fort strong [L. *fortis*]

FORTRAN formula translation (computer language)

Forum The Forum for Health Care Planning

FOS fiberoptic sigmoidoscope
fiberoptic sigmoidoscopy
fissura orbitalis superior
fractional osteoid surface
full of stool

found foundation

FOV field of view

FOVI field of vision intact

FOW fenestrated oval window
fenestration open window

FP false positive
family physician; also fam phys
family planning
family practice
family practitioner
Fanconi-Petrassi (syndrome)
fibrinolytic potential
fibrinopeptide
filling pressure
filter paper
final pressure
first pass
fixation protein
flat plate
flavin phosphate

flavoprotein
flexor profundus
fluid pressure
fluorescence polarization
food poisoning
forearm pronated; also fp
freezing point; also Fp, fp
frontoparietal
frozen plasma
full period
fundal pressure
fusion point; also fn p, fu p

F-P femoral-popliteal; also Fem-pop, fem-pop

F/P fluid to plasma (ratio)
fluorescein to protein (ratio)

F-1-P fructose-1-phosphate

F-6-P fructose-6-phosphate

Fp filtered phosphate
freezing point; also FP, fp
frontal polar (electrode placement in electroencephalography)

fp flexor pollicis
foot-pound; also ft lb, ft-lb
forearm pronated; also FP
freezing point; also FP, Fp
let a potion be made [L. *fiat potio*]
let a powder be made [L. *fiat pulvis*]; also ft
pulv

FPA Family Planning Association
fibrinopeptide A; also fpA
filter paper activity
fluorophenylalanine

fpA fibrinopeptide A; also FPA

FPAL full-term deliveries, premature deliveries, abortion(s), living children

FPB femoral popliteal bypass
fibrinopeptide B
flexor pollicis brevis

FPC familial polyposis coli
family planning clinic
family practice center
fish protein concentrate
forced pair copulation
frozen packed cells

FPCL fibroblast-populated collagen lattice

FPD fetopelvic disproportion
fixed partial denture
flame photometric detector

FPDD familial pure depressive disease

FPE first-pass effect

FPF false-positive fraction

fibroblast pneumocyte factor

FPG fasting plasma glucose
fluorescence plus Giemsa (stain)
focal proliferative glomerulonephritis; also
FPGN

FPGN focal proliferative glomerulonephritis;
also FPG

FPH$_2$ flavin phosphate (reduced form)

FPHA family planning health assistant

FPHE formalin-treated pyruvaldehyde-stabi-
lized human erythrocytes

FPHx family psychiatric history

FPI femoral pulsatility index
formula protein intolerance
Freiburger Personality Inventory

FPIA fluorescence-polarization immunoassay

f pil let pills be made [L. *fiant pilulae*]; also
ft pil

f pil xi make 11 pills [L. *fac pilulas xi*]

FPK fructose-6-phosphokinase

FPL fasting plasma lipid
flexor pollicis longus

FPLA fibrin plate lysis area

FPLC fast protein liquid chromatography

FPM filter paper microscopic (test)
full passive movements

fpm feet per minute

FPN ferric chloride, perchloric acid, and nitric
acid (solution)

FPNA first-pass nuclear angiocardiography

FPO freezing point osmometer

FPP free portal pressure

FPPH familial primary pulmonary hypertension

FPR fluorescence photobleaching recovery
fractional proximal resorption

FPRA first-pass radionuclide angiogram

FPS fetal polychlorinated biphenyl syndrome
footpad swelling
foot-pound-second (system); also fps

fps feet per second
foot-pound-second (system); also FPS
frames per second

FPT fixed parenchymal turnover

FPU Family Participation Unit

FPV fowl pest virus
fowl plague virus

FPVB femoral-popliteal vein bypass

FPZ fluphenazine; also FLU
FPZ-D fluphenazine decanoate; also FD
FR failure rate (contraception)
family report
father; also F, fa
Favre-Racouchot (syndrome)
feedback regulation
feedback regulator
fibrinogen related
Fisher-Race (notation)
fixed ratio
flocculation reaction
flow rate
fluid restriction; also fld rest
fluid retention
framework region
free radical
French (gauge, scale); also F, Fr
frequency of respiration
frequent relapses
Friend (virus)
full range
functional residual (capacity)
reticular formation [L. *formatio reticularis*]
F&R force and rhythm (of pulse); also F and R
Fr fracture; also F, frac, fract, Frx, Fx, fx, FXR
francium
franklin (unit charge)
French (gauge, scale); also F, FR
fr fried
from; also fm
FRA fibrinogen-related antigen
fluorescent rabies antibody
fra fragile site (chromosome in cytogenetics)
frac fracture; also F, Fr, fract, Frx, Fx, fx, FXR
FRACON framycetin, colistin, and nystatin
fract fractional; also F, FX, fx
fracture; also F, Fr, frac, Frx, Fx, fx, FXR
fract dos in divided doses [L. *fracta dosi*]
FRACTS fractional urines
frag fragile
fragility
fragment
FRAP fluorescence recovery after photobleaching
fluorescence redistribution after photobleaching
fluoride-resistant acid phosphatase
FRAT free radical assay technique
fra(X) fragile X (chromosome, syndrome)
FRBB, Fr BB fracture of both bones; also Fx BB

FRBS fast red B salt
FRC frozen red cells
functional reserve capacity (of lungs)
functional residual capacity (of lungs)
FRCD fixed ratio combination drugs
FRCP Fellow of the Royal College of Physicians (London)
FRCP(C) Fellow of the Royal College of Physicians of Canada
FRCP(E) Fellow of the Royal College of Physicians of Edinburgh
FRCP(Glasg) Fellow of the Royal College of Physicians and Surgeons of Glasgow qua Physician
FRCPI Fellow of the Royal College of Physicians in Ireland
FRCS Fellow of the Royal College of Surgeons
FRCS(C) Fellow of the Royal College of Surgeons of Canada
FRCS(E) Fellow of the Royal College of Surgeons of Edinburgh
FRCS(Glasg) Fellow of the Royal College of Physicians and Surgeons of Glasgow qua Surgeon
FRCSI Fellow of the Royal College of Surgeons in Ireland
FRCVS Fellow of the Royal College of Veterinary Surgeons
FRD flexion-rotation-drawer
FRE Fischer rat embryo
flow-related enhancement
FREIR Federal Research on Biological and Health Effects of Ionizing Radiation
frem vocal fremitus [L. *fremitus vocalis*]
freq frequency; also F, f, *f*
frequent; also F, f
FRF fasciculus retroflexus
filtration replacement fluid
follicle-releasing factor
follicle-stimulating hormone-releasing factor; also FSH-RF
FRFPS Fellow of the Royal Faculty of Physicians and Surgeons
FRFPSG Fellow of the Royal Faculty of Physicians and Surgeons of Glasgow
FRH follicle-stimulating hormone-releasing hormone; also FSH-RH
FRh fetal Rhesus kidney (cell line)
FRhL fetal Rhesus lung

FRHS fast-repeating high sequence

FRI Fermentation Research Institute (Japan)

frict friction; also Fx

Fried Friedman (test for pregnancy)

frig cold [L. *frigidus*]

FRJM full range of joint movement

FRM full range of motion; also FROM

FRN fully resonant nucleus

FRNS frequently relapsing nephrotic syndrome

FROM full range of motion; also FRM

FROS front routing of signal

FRP follicular regulatory protein
functional refractory period

Fr pat French patent

FRPS functional resting position splint

FR r, fr r friction rub

FRS Fellow of the Royal Society
ferredoxin-reducing substance
first rank symptom
furosemide; also FSM, FUR

FRSC Fellow of the Royal Society (Canada)

FRSE Fellow of the Royal Society of
Edinburgh

FRT Family Relations Test
full recovery time

Fru, fru fructose

frust in small pieces [L. *frustillatim*]

FRV functional residual volume

Frx fracture; also F, Fr, frac, fract, Fx, fx, FXR

FS factor of safety
Fanconi's syndrome
Felty's syndrome
fetoscope
fibrosarcoma
field stimulation
fine structure
fingerstick
fire setter (psychology)
Fisher's syndrome
flexible sigmoidoscopy; also flex sig
food service
forearm supination
foreskin
Fourier series
fracture, simple
fracture site
fragile site
Freeman-Sheldon (syndrome)
Friesinger's score
frozen section; also FX, fx, FZ

full and soft (diet); also F&S
full-scale (IQ)
full strength
functional shortening
functional study
human foreskin (cells)

F/S female, spayed (animal)

F&S full and soft (diet); also FS

FSA fetal sulfoglycoprotein antigen

fsa let it be made skillfully [L. *fiat secundum
artem*]; also fsar

fsar let it be made according to the rules of
the art [L. *fiat secundum artis regulas*];
also fsa

FSB fetal scalp blood
Fokes' sentence builder
full spine board

FSBG fingerstick blood gas

FSBM full-strength breast milk

FSBT Fowler's single breath test

FSC Forer Sentence Completion (Test)
fracture simple and comminuted
fracture simple and complete
free secretory component
free-standing clinic

FSCC fracture simple, complete, and
comminuted

FSD focal-skin distance
fracture simple and depressed
full-scale deflection

FSDQ Frost Self-Description Questionnaire

FSE fetal scalp electrode
filtered smoke exposure

FSF fibrin stabilizing factor (factor XIII)

FSG fasting serum glucose
focal sclerosing glomerulonephritis; also
FSGN
focal segmental glomerulosclerosis; also
FSGS

FSGA full-term, small for gestational age

FSGHS focal segmental glomerular hyalinosis
and sclerosis

FSGN focal sclerosing glomerulonephritis;
also FSG

FSGO floating spherical Gaussian orbital
(method)

FSGS focal segmental glomerulosclerosis;
also FSG

FSH fascioscapulohumeral
focal and segmental hyalinosis

FSH—cont'd
follicle-stimulating hormone

FSH/LH-RH follicle-stimulating hormone and luteinizing hormone-releasing hormone

FSHMD facioscapulohumeral muscular dystrophy

FSH-RF follicle-stimulating hormone-releasing factor; also FRF

FSH-RH follicle-stimulating hormone-releasing hormone; also FRH

FSI foam stability index
Food Sanitation Institute
Function Status Index

FSIA foot shock-induced analgesia

FSIQ Full-Scale Intelligence Quotient

FSL fasting serum level
fixed slit light

FSLA fibroblast somatomedin-like activity

FSM furosemide; also FRS, FUR

FSMB Federation of State Medical Boards (of the United States)

F-SM/C fungus, smear and culture

FSP familial spastic paraplegia
fibrinogen split product(s)
fibrinolytic split product(s)
fibrin split product(s)
fine suspended particulate
free secretory piece

F-SP special form (taxonomy) [L. *forma specialis*]

FSR film screen radiography
fragmented sarcoplasmic reticulum
fusiform skin revision

FSR-3 isoniazid

FSS Familiar Sensory Stimulation
Fear Survey Schedule
focal segmental sclerosis
Freeman-Sheldon syndrome
French steel sound
front support strap
full-scale score
functional systems scale

FSST Full-Scale Score Total

FST foam stability test

FSU family service unit

FSV feline fibrosarcoma virus
Fujinami sarcoma virus

FSW field service worker

FT false transmitter
family therapy

Fanconi-De Tari (syndrome)
fast twitch
feeding tube
ferritin; also F_t
ferromagnetic tamponade
fetal tonsil
fibrous tissue
filling time
finger tapping
fingertip
follow through (after barium meal)
formol toxoid
Fourier transform; also $\mathcal{T}$
free thyroxine
full term
function test

FT-3, FT₃ free triiodothyronine

FT-4, FT₄ free (unbound) thyroxine

F_t ferritin; also FT

ft feet; also F, f
foot; also F, f
let there be made [L. *fiat, fiant*]; also F, f

ft² square feet

ft³ cubic feet

FTA fluorescein treponema antibody (test)
fluorescent titer antibody
fluorescent treponemal antibody

FTA-AB fluorescent treponemal antibody absorption (test); also FTA-ABS, FTA-Abs

FTA-ABS, FTA-Abs fluorescent treponemal antibody absorption (test); also FTA-AB

F-TAG fast-binding target-attaching globulin

FTAT fluorescent treponemal antibody test

FTB fingertip blood

FTBD fit to be detained
full-term, born dead

FTBE focal tick-borne encephalitis

FTBS Family Therapist Behavioral Scale

FTC frames to come (optometry)
frequency threshold curve

ftc foot-candle; also Fc, fc

ft catpl let a poultice be made [L. *fiat cataplasma*]; also ft cerat

ft cerat let a poultice be made [L. *fiat ceratum*]; also ft catpl

ft collyr let an eyewash be made [L. *fiat collyrium*]

FTD failure to descend; also FD
femoral total density
folic acid and thymidine (medium)

FTE full-time equivalent

ft emuls let an emulsion be made [L. *fiat emulsio*]

ft enem let an enema be made [L. *fiat enema*]

FTF finger-to-finger (test)

FTFTN finger-to-finger-to-nose (test)

FTG full-thickness graft
gigantocellular tegmental field (unit)

ft garg let a gargle be made [L. *fiat gargarisma*]

FTI free thyroxine index; also FT_4I

FT_3I free triiodothyronine index

FT_4I free thyroxine index; also FTI

FT-ICR Fourier transform–ion cyclotron resonance

ft infus let an infusion be made [L. *fiat infusum*]

ft injec let an injection be made [L. *fiat injectio*]

FTIR Fourier transform infrared
functional terminal innervation ratio

FTKA failed to keep appointment

FTLB full-term, live birth

ft lb, ft-lb foot-pound; also fp

FTLE full-thickness local excision

FTLFC full-term, living female child

ft linim let a liniment be made [L. *fiat linimentum*]

FTLMC full-term, living male child

FTLV feline T-lymphotropic virus

FTM fluid thioglycollate medium
fractional test meal

ft mas let a mass be made [L. *fiat massa*]

ft mas div in pil let a mass be made and divided into pills [L. *fiat massa dividenda in pilulae*]

ft mixt let a mixture be made [L. *fiat mixtura*]

FTMS Fourier transform mass spectrometry

FTN finger-to-nose (coordination test); also FN, F-N, F ➡ N
full term nursery

FTNB full-term newborn

FTND full-term, normal delivery

FT-NMR Fourier transform–nuclear magnetic resonance

FTNS functional transcutaneous nerve stimulation

FTNSD full-term, normal, spontaneous delivery

FTO fructose-terminated oligosaccharide

FTP failure to progress (in labor)

FTPA perfluorotripropylamine (blood substitute)

ft pil let pills be made [L. *fiat pilulae*]; also f pil

ft pulv let a powder be made [L. *fiat pulvis*]; also fp

FTR for the record
fractional turnover rate

FTS Family Tracking System
feminizing testis syndrome
fingertips
serum thymic factor [Fr. *facteur thymique sérique*]

FTSG full-thickness skin graft

ft solut let a solution be made [L. *fiat solutio*]

ft suppos let a suppository be made [L. *fiat suppositorium*]

FTT failure to thrive
fat tolerance test
fraternal twins raised together
fructose tolerance test

ft troch let lozenges be made [L. *fiat trochisci*]

FTU fluorescence thiourea

ft ung let an ointment be made [L. *fiat unguentum*]

FTX field training exercise

FU Farmacopea Ufficiale (della Repubblica Italiana)
fecal urobilinogen
Finsen unit; also Fu
fluorouracil
follow-up; also fl up, F/U
fractional urinalysis
fundus at umbilicus; also F/U

F/U follow-up; also fl up, FU
fundus at umbilicus; also FU

F&U flanks and upper quadrants

F ↑ U fingers above umbilicus (measurement)

F ↓ U fingers below umbilicus (measurement); also FBU

5-FU 5-fluorouracil

FU-I, FU-II, etc first, second, etc, set of follow-up data

Fu Finsen unit; also FU

FUB found under bridge
functional uterine bleeding

FUBT fulguration of urinary bladder tumor

FUC fucosidase

Fuc fucose

FU_{CO} functional uptake of carbon monoxide

FUDR floxuridine
fluorodeoxyuridine; also FUdR
5-fluorouracil deoxyribonucleoside; also
FUdR

FUdR fluorodeoxyuridine; also FUDR
5-fluorouracil deoxyribonucleoside; also
FUDR

FUE fever of unknown etiology

FUFA free volatile fatty acid

fulg fulguration

FUM 5-fluorouracil and methotrexate
fouled-up mess
fucked-up mess
fumarase
fumarate
fumigation

FUMP fluorouridine monophosphate

FUN follow-up note

func function; also F, fn, funct, FXN
functional; also funct

funct function; also F, fn, func, FXN
functional; also func

FUNG-C fungus culture

FUNG-S fungus smear

FUO fever of undetermined origin
fever of unknown origin

FUOV follow-up office visit

fu p fusion point; also fn p, FP

FUR fluorouracil riboside
fluorouridine
furosemide; also FRS, FSM

FURAM Ftorafur, Adriamycin, and mitomycin C

FUS feline urologic syndrome
fusion

FUT fibrinogen uptake test

FUTP fluorouridine triphosphate

FUVAC fluorouracil, vinblastine, Adriamycin,
and cyclophosphamide

FV facial vein
Fahr-Volhard (disease)
femoral vein
flow volume
fluid volume

formaldehyde vapors
Friend's virus

fv fever; also feb, fev

FVA, FV-A Friend's virus anemia

FVC false vocal cord
forced expiratory vital capacity
forced vital capacity

FVC₁ forced vital capacity in one second

FVD fibrovascular tissue on disk

FVE fibrovascular tissue elsewhere
forced volume, expiratory

FVFR filled voiding flow rate

FVH focal vascular headache

FVL femoral vein ligation
flow volume loop
force, velocity, length

FVM familial visceral myopathy

FVP, FV-P Friend's virus polycythemia

FVR feline viral rhinotracheitis
forearm vascular resistance

fvs let the patient be bled [L. *fiat venae sectio*]
let there be a cutting of a vein [L. *fiat venae
sectio*]

FW Falconer-Weddell (syndrome)
Felix-Weil (reaction)
Folin-Wu (method)
forced whisper
fracturing wall
fragment wound
Friderichsen-Waterhouse (syndrome)

Fw F wave (fibrillatory wave, flutter wave)

fw fresh water

FWB full weight bearing

FWHH full width at half height (spectrometry)

FWHM full width of line-spread function half-
maximum height (of a curve)
full width of photopeak measured at half
maximum count (tomography)

FWLS fever without localizing signs

FWPCA Federal Water Pollution Control
Administration

FWR Felix-Weil reaction
Folin-Wu reaction

FWW front wheel walker

FX factor X
fluoroscopy; also fluoro
fornix
fractional; also F, fract, fx
frozen section; also FS, fx, FZ

Fx fractional urine
  fracture; also F, Fr, frac, fract, Frx, fx, FXR
  friction; also frict
fx fractional; also F, fract, FX
  fracture; also F, Fr, frac, fract, Frx, Fx, FXR
  frozen section; also FS, FX, FZ
Fx BB fracture of both bones; also FRBB,
  Fr BB
Fx-dis fracture-dislocation; also F/D
FXN function; also F, fn, func, funct
FXR fracture; also F, Fr, frac, fract, Frx, Fx, fx
FY fiber year
  fiscal year
  framycetin
  full year

Fy antigen in the Duffy blood group system
Fy^a antigen in the Duffy blood group system
Fy^b antigen in the Duffy blood group system
FYI for your information
F-Y test fibrinogen qualitative test
FZ focal zone
  frozen section; also FS, FX, fx
  furazolidone
FZRC frozen section red blood cell
Fz frontal midline (placement of electrodes in
  electroencephalography)

G

Γ GAMMA, UPPER CASE, third letter of the Greek alphabet

γ gamma, lower case, third letter of the Greek alphabet

10^{-4} gauss

carbon separated from the carboxyl group by two other carbon atoms

constituent of gamma protein plasma fraction

done

gamma chain of fetal hemoglobin

heavy chain of immunoglobulin G

microgram (former symbol, now μg)

photon (gamma ray)

plasma protein (globulin)

third in a series or group

γ-**Abu** gamma-aminobutyric acid; also GABA

γ-**BHC** gamma-benzene hexachloride (lindane); also GBH

γ**G** immunoglobulin G; also G

γ**GT** gamma-glutamyltranspeptidase; also GGT, GGTP

γ-**HCD** gamma-heavy chain disease

γ hexachlorocyclohexane (lindane); also HCC, HCH

G conductance; also G
gallop (heart sound)
ganglion; also gang, gangl
gap (in cell cycle)
gas; also g
gastrin
gauge; also g, ga
gauss; also Gs
gender; also g, GEN
geometric efficiency
Gibbs free energy; also G
Giemsa (banding stain)
giga- (10^9)
gingiva; also GIN, GING, ging
gingival; also GIN, GING, ging
glabella; also Gl
globular (protein)
globulin; also GLB, Glob, glob
glucose; also Glc, GLU, Glu, glu, Gluc, gluc
glycine (one-letter notation); also GLY, Gly, gly
glycogen
gold inlay
gonidial (bacterial colony)
good; also gd
goose

grade; also gr
Gräfenberg's spot
gram; also g, gm
gram (stain)
gravida (pregnant)
gravitational constant; also G
gravity unit (multiples of gravitational pull); also g
Greek; also Gr
green; also GRN, Grn
Gross' (leukemia antigen)
guanidine; also Gdn
guanine; also Gua
guanosine; also Guo
gynecology; also GYN, gyn
immunoglobulin G; also γG
in electrocardiography, a symbol for ventricular gradient, usually as projected on the frontal plane of the body; also g

G conductance; also G
G force (multiples of gravitational pull)
Gibbs free energy; also G
gravitational constant; also G

G- gram-negative; also GM-, GN, gr-, GrN

G+ gram-positive; also GM+, GP, gr+, GrP

G° standard free energy

G₀ quiescent phase of cells leaving the mitotic cycle

G1 grid 1 (in electroencephalography)

G₁ presynthetic gap (the period that follows cell division and precedes DNA replication)

G1 thru G4 grade 1 through grade 4 (heart murmur)

G2 grid 2 (in electroencephalography)

G₂ postsynthetic gap (the period between DNA replication and the onset of mitosis)

G-4, G₄ dichlorophen (dihydroxydichlorodiphenylmethane)

G-11, G₁₁ hexachlorophene

GI, GII, GIII, etc primigravida, secundigravida, tertigravida, etc; also grav 1, grav 2, grav 3, etc

g acceleration due to gravity (9.80665 m/s^2)
gas; also G
gauge; also G, ga
gender; also G, GEN
grain; also GR, gr
gram; also G, gm

gravity; also gr, grav
gravity unit (multiples of gravitational pull); also G
great; also gr, gt
group; also GP, gp, grp
in electrocardiography, a symbol for ventricular gradient, usually as projected on the frontal plane of the body; also G
ratio of magnetic moment of a particle to Bohr magneton

g relative centrifugal force

g% grams percent (grams per deciliter); also g/dL, g/dl, gm%

GA airway conductance; also GAW, Gaw
Gamblers Anonymous
gastric analysis
gastric antrum
general anesthesia; also gen-an
general appearance
gentisic acid
gestational age
Getting Along (psychologic test)
ginger ale; also G'ale
gingivo-axial
glucoamylase
glucose/acetone
glucuronic acid; also GlcUA, GluA
Golgi's apparatus
gramicidin A
granulocyte adherence
granuloma annulare
guessed average
gut associated

Ga gallium
granulocyte agglutination

ga gauge; also G, g

GAA gossypol acetic acid

GABA gamma-aminobutyric acid; also γ-Abu

GABA-Ch gamma-aminobutyrylcholine

GABA-T gamma-aminobutyric acid transaminase

GABHS group A beta-hemolytic streptococcus; also GABS

GABOA gamma-amino-beta-hydroxybutyric acid

GABOB gamma-amino-beta-hydroxybutyric

GABS group A beta-hemolytic streptococcus; also GABHS

G Acid 2-naphthol-6,8-disulfonic acid

GAD generalized anxiety disorder
glutamic acid decarboxylase

GADH gastric alcohol dehydrogenase

GADS gonococcal arthritis/dermatitis syndrome

GAF giant axon formation
Global Assessment of Functioning

GAG glycosaminoglycan

GAHS galactorrhea-amenorrhea hyperprolactinemia syndrome

GAI guided affective imagery

GAIPAS General Audit Inpatient Psychiatric Assessment Scale

GAL galactosemia
galactosyl
gallus adeno-like (virus)
glucuronic acid lactone

Gal, gal galactose
gallon

G-ALB globulin-albumin

G'ale ginger ale; also GA

GALK galactokinase; also GK

gal/min gallons per minute; also g/m

GalN galactosamine

GalNAc N-acetyl-D-galactosamine

gal-1-P galactose-1-phosphate

GALT galactose-1-phosphate uridyltransferase
gut-associated lymphoid tissue

GAL TT galactose tolerance test

GALV gibbon ape leukemia virus

GaLV gibbon ape lymphosarcoma virus

Galv, galv galvanic
galvanism
galvanized

GAMG goat anti-mouse immunoglobulin G

GAN giant axonal neuropathy

G and D growth and development; also GD, G&D

gang ganglion; also G, gangl
ganglionic; also gangl

gangl ganglion; also G, gang
ganglionic; also gang

GAP Gardner Analysis of Personality (Survey)
glyceraldehyde phosphate
gonadotropin-releasing hormone associated peptide

GAPD glyceraldehyde-3-phosphate dehydrogenase; also GAPDH

GAPDH glyceraldehyde-3-phosphate dehydrogenase; also GAPD

GAPO growth retardation, alopecia, pseudoanodontia, and optic atrophy (syndrome)

GAR genitoanorectal (syndrome)
goat anti-rabbit (gamma globulin)

Garg, garg gargle

GARGG goat anti-rabbit gamma globulin

GAS gastric acid secretion
gastroenterology; also Gastro, gastro, GE
general adaptation syndrome
generalized arteriosclerosis
Glasgow Assessment Schedule
Global Assessment Scale
group A streptococcus

GASA growth-adjusted sonographic age

Gas Anal F&T gastric analysis, free and
total

GAST gastrocnemius (muscle); also gastroc

Gastro, gastro gastroenterology; also GAS,
GE
gastrointestinal; also GI

gastroc gastrocnemius (muscle); also GAST

GAT gas antitoxin
gelatin agglutination test
Gerontological Apperception Test
gonorrhea antibody test
group adjustment therapy

GATase 6-alkyl guanine alkyl transferase

GATB General Aptitude Test Battery

GAU geriatric assessment unit

gav gavage

GAW, Gaw airway conductance; also GA

GAZT glucuronide derivative of azidothymidine

GB gallbladder
Gilbert-Behçet (syndrome)
glass bead
glial bundle
goofball (barbiturate pill)
Gougerot-Blum (syndrome)
Guillain-Barré (syndrome)

G&B good and bad (days)

GBA ganglionic blocking agent
gingivobuccoaxial

GBBS group B beta-hemolytic streptococcus;
also GBS

GBCE Grassi Basic Cognitive Evaluation

GBD gallbladder disease
gender behavior disorder
glassblower's disease
granulomatous bowel disease

GBE *Ginkgo biloba* extract

GBG glycine-rich beta-glycoprotein

gonadal steroid-binding globulin; also GSBG

GBGase glycine-rich beta glycoproteinase

GBH gamma-benzene hexachloride (lindane);
also γ-BHC
graphite, benzalkonium, heparin

GBI globulin-bound insulin

GBIA Guthrie's bacterial inhibition assay

GBL gamma-butyrolactone
glomerular basal lamina

GBM glioblastoma multiforme
glomerular basement membrane

GBMI guilty but mentally ill

GBP galactose-binding protein
gastric bypass
gated blood pool
glycophorin-binding protein

GBPS gallbladder pigment stones

GBq gigabequerel

GBS gallbladder series
gastric bypass surgery
glycerine-buffered saline
group B beta-hemolytic streptococcus; also
GBBS
Guillain-Barré syndrome

GBSS Grey's balanced saline solution
Guillain-Barré-Strohl syndrome

GC ganglion cell
gas chromatography
gel chromatography
general circulation
general condition
geriatric care
geriatric chair (Gerichair)
glucocorticoid
glycocholate
goblet cell
Golgi's complex
gonococcal
gonococcus; also GN
gonorrhea (gonococcus infection)
gonorrhea culture
good condition
Gougerot-Carteaud (syndrome)
graham crackers
granular casts
granular cysts
granule cell
granulocyte cytotoxic
granulomatous colitis
granulosa cell
guanine cytosine
guanylate cyclase

G-C gram-negative cocci; also GNC

G+C gram-positive cocci; also GPC

Gc gigacycle
group-specific component

GCA gastric cancerous area
giant cell arteritis

g-cal gram calorie (small calorie); also gm cal

GCB gonococcal base

GCDFP gross cystic disease fluid protein

GCDP gross cystic disease protein

GCF greatest common factor

GCFT gonococcal complement-fixation test
gonorrhea complement-fixation test

GCI General Cognitive Index

GCII glucose-controlled insulin infusion

GCIIS glucose-controlled insulin infusion
system

GCM good control maintained

g-cm gram-centimeter

GC-MS, GC/MS gas chromatography–mass
spectrometry

GCN giant cerebral neuron

GCP good clinical practice

GCR glucocorticoid receptor; also GR
Group Conformity Rating

GCRC General Clinical Research Centers

GCS general clinical service
Generalized Contentment Scale
Glasgow Coma Scale
glucocorticosteroid
glutamylcysteine synthetase

Gc/s gigacycles per second

GCSA Gross cell surface antigen

GCSF granulocyte cell-stimulating factor

G-CSF granulocyte colony-stimulating factor

GCT general care and treatment
giant cell thyroiditis
giant cell tumor

GCU gonococcal urethritis; also GU

GCV great cardiac vein

GCVF great cardiac vein flow

GCW glomerular capillary wall

GCWM General Conference on Weights and
Measures

GD gastroduodenal
general diagnostics
general dispensary
general duties
gestational day

Gianotti's disease
gonadal dysgenesis
Graves' disease
growth and development; also G and D, G&D

G&D growth and development; also GD,
G and D

Gd gadolinium

gd good; also G

GDA gastroduodenal artery
germine diacetate

GDB gas-density balance
Genome Database
guide dogs for the blind

GDC General Dental Council   *+ GDC coils (brain)*
giant dopamine-containing cell

GDE granular diatomaceous earth

GDF gel diffusion precipitin; also GDP

GDH glucose dehydrogenase
glutamate dehydrogenase; also GLD, GLDH,
GMD
glutamic acid dehydrogenase
glycerophosphate dehydrogenase; also GPD
glycol dehydrogenase
gonadotropic hormone; also GTH
growth and differentiation hormone (in
insects)

GDID genetically determined immunodeficiency disease

g/dL, g/dl grams per deciliter; also g%, gm%

GDM gestational diabetes mellitus

GDMO General Duties Medical Officer

Gdn guanidine; also G

gdn guardian

GdNPF glia-derived neurite-promoting factor

GDP gastroduodenal pylorus
gel diffusion precipitin; also GDF
good design practice
guanosine diphosphate

GDS Gesell Developmental Schedules
Global Deterioration Scale
gradual dosage schedule

GDT gel development time

GDW glass-distilled water

GE gainfully employed
gamma-endorphin
Gänsslen-Erb (syndrome)
gastric emptying
gastroemotional
gastroenteritis
gastroenterology; also GAS, Gastro, gastro
gastroenterostomy

GE—cont'd
gastroesophageal
gastrointestinal endoscopy
gel electrophoresis
generalized epilepsy
generator of excitation
gentamicin; also GENT, gent, GM
glandular epithelium
Gsell-Erdheim (syndrome)

G/E granulocyte to erythroid (ratio)

Ge Gerbich red cell antigen
germanium

GEC galactose elimination capacity
glomerular epithelial cell

GEE glycine ethyl ester

GEF glosso-epiglottic fold
gonadotropin-enhancing factor

GEFT Group Embedded Figures Test

GEH glycerol ester hydrolase

GEJ gastroesophageal junction

gel gelatin

gel quav in any kind of jelly [L. *gelatina quavis*]

gem- geminal (indicates that the two substituents in a disubstituted compound are on the same atom)

GEMS good emergency mother substitute

GEN gender; also G, g
generation
genetic(s); also Gen, genet
genital; also gen, genit
genitalia; also gen, genit

Gen genetic(s); also GEN, genet
genus; also gen

gen general; also gen'l
genital; also GEN, genit
genitalia; also GEN, genit
genus; also Gen

gen-an general anesthesia; also GA

GEN/ENDO general anesthesia with endotracheal intubation

genet genetic(s) also GEN, Gen

gen et sp nov new genus and species [L. *genus et species nova*]

genit genital; also GEN, gen
genitalia; also GEN, gen

gen'l general; also gen

gen nov new genus [L. *genus novum*]

gen proc general procedure

GENPS genital neoplasm-papilloma syndrome

GENT, gent gentamicin; also GE, GM

GENTA/P gentamicin peak (level)

GENTA/T gentamicin trough (level)

geol geological

GEP gastroenteropancreatic

GEPG gastroesophageal pressure gradient

GER gastroesophageal reflux; also GOR
geriatric(s); also ger, geriat
granular endoplasmic reticulum

Ger German

ger geriatric(s); also GER, geriat

GERD gastroesophageal reflux disease; also GRD

geriat geriatric(s); also GER, ger

GERL Golgi-associated endoplasmic reticulum lysosome

Geront gerontologic
gerontologist
gerontology

Ger pat German patent

GES glucose-electrolyte solution
Group Encounter Survey
Group Environment Scale

GEST, gest gestation

GET gastric emptying time
graded treadmill exercise test

GET$^{1}/_{2}$ gastric emptying half-time

GETA general endotracheal anesthesia

GEU gestation, extrauterine

Gev, GeV giga electron volts; also GiV

GEX gas exchange

GF gastric fistula
gastric fluid; also Gf
germ-free
glass factor (tissue culture)
globule fibril
glomerular filtrate
glomerular filtration
gluten-free
grandfather; also GR-FR
griseofulvin
growth factor
growth failure
growth fraction

G-F globular-fibrous (protein)

Gf gastric fluid; also GF

gf gram-force

GFA glial fibrillary acidic (protein)
global force applicator

G factor general factor (single variance common to different intelligence tests)

GFAP glial fibrillary acidic protein

GFCL giant follicular cell

GFD gluten-free diet
Goodenough Figure Drawing

GFFS glycogen- and fat-free solid

GFH glucose-free Hanks (solution)

GFI glucagon-free insulin
ground-fault interrupter

GFL giant follicular lymphoma

GFM good fetal movement

GFP gamma-fetoprotein
gel-filtered platelet
glomerular filtered phosphate

GFR glomerular filtration rate
grunting, flaring, and retracting (neonate)

GFS global focal sclerosis

GFTA Goldman-Fristoe Test of Articulation

G-F-W Goldman-Fristoe-Woodcock (Auditory Skills Test Battery)

GG gamma globulin
genioglossus
glyceryl guaiacolate
glycylglycine
guar gum

Gg gigagram

GGA general gonadotropic activity

GGCT ground glass clotting time

GGE generalized glandular enlargement
gradient gel electrophoresis

GGF glial growth factor

GGFC gamma globulin-free calf (serum)

GGG cambogia (gamboge)
gamboge [L. *gummi guttae gambiae*]
glycine-rich gamma-glycoprotein

GG or S glands, goiter, or stiffness (of neck); also GGS

GGM glucose-galactose malabsorption

GGPNA gamma-glutamyl-*para*-nitroaniline

GGS glands, goiter, or stiffness (of neck); also GG or S

GGT gamma-glutamyltransferase; also GT
gamma-glutamyltranspeptidase; also GGTP, γGT

GGTP gamma-glutamyltranspeptidase; also GGT, γGT

GGVB gelatin, glucose, and veronal buffer

GH Gee-Herter (disease)
general health
general hospital
genetically hypertensive (rat)
genetic hypertension
geniohyoid
Gilford-Hutchinson (syndrome)
glenohumeral
good health
Gougerot-Hailey (syndrome)
growth hormone

GHAA Group Health Association of America

GHAG general high altitude questionnaire

GHB gamma-hydroxybutyrate
gamma-hydroxybutyric acid; also GHBA

GHb glycohemoglobin; also GLYCOS Hb, Hb A1c
glycosylated hemoglobin; also GLYCOS Hb, Hb A1c

GHBA gamma-hydroxybutyric acid; also GHB

GHD growth hormone deficiency

GHDT Goodenough-Harris Drawing Test

GH-IH growth hormone-inhibiting hormone

GHK Goldman-Hodgkin-Katz (equation)

GHPP Genetically Handicapped Persons Program

GHQ General Health Questionnaire

GHR granulomatous hypersensitivity reaction

GHRF, GH-RF growth hormone-releasing factor; also GRF

GHRH, GH-RH growth hormone-releasing hormone; also GRH

GHRIF, GH-RIF growth hormone release-inhibiting factor; also GRIF

GHRIH, GH-RIH growth hormone release-inhibiting hormone; also GRIH

GHV goose hepatitis virus

GHz gigahertz

GI gastrointestinal; also Gastro, gastro
gelatin heart infusion (medium)
gingival index
globin insulin
glomerular index
glucose intolerance
granuloma inguinale
growth inhibiting
growth inhibition

Gi good impression (California Psychological Inventory)

gi gill (1/4 pint); also gl

GIA gastrointestinal anastomosis

GIB gastric ileal bypass
gastrointestinal bleeding

GIBB GenInfo Backbone (database)

GIBF gastrointestinal bacterial flora

GIC gastric interdigestive contraction
general immunocompetence

GICA gastrointestinal cancer
gastrointestinal cancer antigen
gastrointestinal carcinoma-associated
(antigen)

GID gender identity disorder

GIDA Gastrointestinal Diagnostic Area

GIF glucosylisoflavonoid
gonadotropin-inhibitory factor (somatostatin)
growth hormone-inhibiting factor

GIFT gamete intrafallopian transfer
granulocyte immunofluorescence test

GIGO garbage in, garbage out (computers)

GIH gastric inhibitory hormone
gastrointestinal hemorrhage
gastrointestinal hormone
growth-inhibiting hormone

GII gastrointestinal infection

GIK glucose-insulin-potassium (solution) [L.
kalium (potassium)]

GILCU gradual increase in length and complexity of utterance

GIM gonadotropin-inhibiting material
Grace's insect medium

GIN gingiva; also G, GING, ging
gingival; also G, GING, ging

GING gingiva; also G, GIN, ging
gingival; also G, GIN, ging

ging gingiva; also G, GIN, GING
gingival; also G, GIN, GING
gum [L. *gingiva*]

g-ion gram-ion

GIP gastric inhibitory peptide
gastric inhibitory polypeptide
giant cell interstitial pneumonia
giant cell interstitial pneumonitis
glucose-dependent insulin-releasing peptide
glucose insulinotropic peptide
gonorrheal invasive peritonitis
good import practice

GIR global improvement rating

GIS gas in stomach
gastrointestinal series
gastrointestinal symptom
gastrointestinal system

Gener Identity Service

GISSI Gruppo Italiano per lo Studio Della
Streptochinase Nell' Infarto Miocardico

GIT gastrointestinal tract
glutathione-insulin transhydrogenase

GITS gastrointestinal therapeutic system

GITSG Gastrointestinal Tumor Study Group

GITT gastrointestinal transit time
glucose-insulin tolerance test

GIV gastrointestinal virus

GiV giga electron volts; also Gev, GeV

giv give
given

GIWU gastrointestinal work-up

GIX, Gix DFDT (difluorodiphenyltrichloroethane, an insecticidal compound)

GJ gap junction
gastric juice
gastrojejunostomy

GK galactokinase; also GALK
Gasser-Karrer (syndrome)
glomerulocystic kidney
glycerol kinase

GKA guinea pig keratocyte

GKN glucose-potassium-sodium [L. *kalium*
(potassium), *natrium* (sodium)]

GL gastric lavage
Gilbert-Lereboullet (syndrome)
gland; also gl
glomerular layer
glycolipid
glycosphingolipid
granular layer; also GRL
greatest length (an axis of measurement used
for small flexed embryos)
gustatory lacrimation

Gl beryllium [L. *glucinium*]
gigaliter
glabella; also G

gl gill (1/4 pint); also gi
gland; also GL

g/L, g/l grams per liter; also gm/L, gm/l

GLA alpha-galactosidase
gamma-carboxyglutamic acid; also Gla
gamma-linolenic acid
giant left atrium
gingivolinguoaxial
D-glucaric acid

Gla gamma-carboxyglutamic acid; also GLA

glac glacial

GLAD gold-labeled antigen detection (technique)

gland glandular

GLAT glutamic acid, lysine, alanine, and tyrosine

glau glaucoma; also glc

GLB globulin; also G, Glob, glob

GLC gas-liquid chromatography

Glc glucose; also G, GLU, Glu, glu, Gluc, gluc

glc glaucoma; also glau

GlcA gluconic acid

GLC/MS gas-liquid chromatography/mass spectrometry

GlcN glucosamine

GlcNAc N-acetyl-D-glucosamine

GlcUA glucuronic acid; also GA, GluA

GLD globoid leukodystrophy
glutamate dehydrogenase; also GDH, GLDH, GMD

GLDH glutamate dehydrogenase; also GDH, GLD, GMD

GLH germinal layer hemorrhage
giant lymph node hyperplasia; also GLNH

GLI glicentin
glucagon-like immunoreactivity

GLIM generalized linear interactive model

glio glioma

GLL glabellolambda line (craniometric point)

GLM general linear model

GLN glutamine; also Gln, GLU, Glu, glu, Q

Gln glucagon; also GN
glutamine; also GLN, GLU, Glu, glu, Q
glutaminyl

GLNH giant lymph node hyperplasia; also GLH

GLO, Glo glyoxalase

GLO1 glyoxalase 1

Glob, glob globular
globulin; also G, GLB

GLP Gambro Liendia Plate
glucose-L-phosphate
glycolipoprotein
good laboratory practice
group-living program

GLPP, GL-PP glucose, postprandial

GLR graphic level recorder

GLS generalized lymphadenopathy syndrome
guinea pig lung strip

GLTN glomerulotubulonephritis

GLTT glucose-lactate tolerance test

GLU, glu glucose; also G, Glc, Glu, Gluc, gluc
glucuronidase
glutamic acid; also E, Glu
glutamine; also GLN, Gln, Glu, Q

Glu glucose; also G, Glc, GLU, glu, Gluc, gluc
glutamic acid; also E, GLU, glu
glutamine; also GLN, Gln, GLU, glu, Q
glutamyl

GLU-5 five-hour glucose tolerance test

GluA glucuronic acid; also GA, GlcUA

GLUC glucosidase

Gluc, gluc glucose; also G, Glc, GLU, Glu, glu

GLUC-S urine glucose spot (test)

glucur glucuronide

glu ox glucose oxidase

GLUT glucose transporter

glut gluteal

GLV Gross' leukemia virus

Glx symbol for glutamine (Gln) or glutamic acid (Glu) (to denote uncertainty between the two); also Z

GLY, gly glycerite; also glyc
glycerol; also glyc, Gro
glycine; also G, Gly
glycocoll
glycyl

Gly glycine; also G, GLY, gly
glycinyl

glyc glyceride
glycerine
glycerite; also GLY, gly
glycerol; also GLY, gly, Gro

GLYCOS Hb glycohemoglobin; also GHb, Hb A1c
glycosylated hemoglobin; also GHb, Hb A1c

GM gastric mucosa
Geiger-Müller (counter); also G-M
general medical
general medicine
genetic manipulation
gentamicin; also GE, GENT, gent
geometric mean
giant melanosome
grand mal
grandmother; also GR-MO
grand multiparity
granulocyte-macrophage
granulocyte-monocyte
gross motor
growth medium
monosialoganglioside (genetic marker)

GM- gram-negative; also G-, GN, gr-, GrN

GM+ gram-positive; also G+, GP, gr+, GrP

G-M Geiger-Müller (counter); also GM

Gm gamma (allotype marker on heavy chain of immunoglobins)
gigameter

Gm^2 square gigameter

Gm^3 cubic gigameter

gm gram; also G, g

g/m gallons per minute; also gal/min

g-m gram-meter; also gm-m

gm% grams percent (grams per deciliter); also g%, g/dL, g/dl

GMA glyceryl methacrylate
glycol methacrylate
gross motor activity

GMB gastric mucosal barrier
granulomembranous body

GMBF gastric mucosal blood flow

GMC ganglion mother cell
general medical clinic
General Medical Council (British)
grivet monkey cell

gm cal gram calorie (small calorie); also g-cal

GMCD grand mal convulsive disorder

GM-CFU granulocyte-macrophage colony-forming unit

GM-CSF granulocyte-macrophage colony-stimulating factor

GMCU gracilis myocutaneous unit

GMD geometric mean diameter
glutamate dehydrogenase; also GDH, GLD, GLDH
glycopeptide moiety modified derivative

GME graduate medical education

GMENAC Graduate Medical Education National Advisory Committee

GMEPP giant miniature end-plate potential

GMH germinal matrix hemorrhage

GMK green monkey kidney (cells, culture medium)

GML glabellomeatal line (craniometric point)
gut mucosal lymphocyte

g/mL, g/ml grams per milliliter

gm/L, gm/l grams per liter; also g/L, g/l

GMM Goldberg-Maxwell-Morris (syndrome)

gm-m gram-meter; also g-m

GMO general medical officer

g-mol gram-molecular mole

GMP good manufacturing practice
guanosine 5′-monophosphate
guanosine 5′-phosphoric acid
guanylic acid

G-MP G-myeloma proteins

3′,5′-GMP cyclic guanosine monophosphate

GMR gallops, murmurs, or rubs

GMS general medical service(s)
glyceryl monostearate
Gomori's methenamine silver (stain)

GM&S general medical and surgical
general medicine and surgery

GMT geometric mean antibody titer
gingival margin trimmer
Greenwich Mean Time

GMTs geometric mean antibody titers

GMV gram-molecular volume

GMW gram molecular weight

GN Gandy-Nanta (disease)
gaze nystagmus
glomerulonephritis
glucagon; also Gln
glucose to nitrogen (ratio in urine); also G/N, G:N
gnotobiote
gonococcus; also GC
graduate nurse
gram-negative; also G-, GM-, gr-, GrN

G/N glucose to nitrogen (ratio in urine); also GN, G:N

G:N glucose to nitrogen (ratio in urine); also GN, G/N

Gn gnathion
gonadotropin

GNA general nursing assistance

GNB gram-negative bacilli

GNBM gram-negative bacillary meningitis

GNC general nursing care
General Nursing Council
glandular neck cell
gram negative cocci; also G-C

GNCA gastric noncancerous area

GND gram-negative diplococcus

gnd ground; also grd

GNID gram-negative intracellular diplococci

GNP Gerontologic Nurse Practitioner

GNR gram-negative rod; also G-R

G/Nr glucose to nitrogen ratio (in urine)

GnRF, Gn-RF gonadotropin-releasing factor; also GRF

GnRH, Gn-RH gonadotropin-releasing hormone; also GRH

GNS gerontologic nurse-specialist

G/NS glucose in normal saline

GNTP Graduate Nurse Transition Program

GO glucose oxidase; also GOD
gonorrhea
Gordon-Overstreet (syndrome)

G&O gas and oxygen

Go Golgi
gonion

GOAT Galveston Orientation and Amnesia Test

GOBAB gamma-hydroxy-beta-aminobutyric acid

GOD generation of diversity
glucose oxidase; also GO

GOD/POD glucose oxidase-peroxidase (method)

GOE gas, oxygen, and ether (anesthesia)

GOG Gynecologic Oncology Group (of National Cancer Institute)

GOH geroderma osteodysplastica hereditaria

GΩ gigohm (one billion ohms)

GOK God only knows

GOL glabello-opisthion line (craniometric point)

GON gonococcal ophthalmia neonatorum

Gonio gonioscopy

GOO gastric outlet obstruction

GOQ glucose oxidation quotient

GOR gastroesophageal reflux; also GER
general operating room

GORT Gilmore Oral Reading Test
Gray Oral Reading Test

GOT glucose oxidase test
glutamic-oxaloacetic transaminase (aspartate aminotransferase)
goals of treatment

GOTM, GOT-M glutamic-oxaloacetic transaminase, mitochondrial

GOT-S glutamic-oxaloacetic transaminase, soluble

govt government

GP gastroplasty
general paralysis
general paresis
general practice
general practitioner
general proprioception
general purpose
genetic prediabetes
geometric progression
globus pallidus
glucose phosphate
glucose production
glutathione peroxidase; also GPx
glycerophosphate
glycopeptide
glycoprotein; also gp
Goodpasture's (syndrome)
gram-positive; also G+, GM+, gr+, GrP
group; also g, gp, grp
guinea pig
gutta-percha (coagulated milky juice of various tropical trees of the family Sapotaceae)

G/P gravida/para

G-1-P glucose-1-phosphate

G3P, G-3-P glyceraldehyde 3-phosphate
glycerol 3-phosphate

G6P, G-6-P glucose-6-phosphate

gp glycoprotein; also GP
group; also g, GP, grp

GPA glutaraldehyde, picric acid, acetic acid
grade point average
guinea pig albumin
pregnant, birth, miscarriage [L. *gravida* (pregnant), *partus* (birth), *abortus* (miscarriage)] (subscript numbers after each category); also GrPAB

GPAIS guinea pig anti-insulin serum

G6PASE, G-6-Pase glucose-6-phosphatase

GPB glossopharyngeal breathing

GPBP guinea pig myelin basic protein

GPC gastric parietal cell
gel permeation chromatography
giant papillary conjunctivitis
glycerophosphorylcholine
gram-positive cocci; also G+C
granular progenitor cell
guinea pig complement

GPCI geographic practice cost index

GPC/TP glycerophosphorylcholine to total phosphate (ratio)

GPD glucose phosphate dehydrogenase; also GPDH
glycerophosphate dehydrogenase; also GDH
guinea pig dander

G6PD, G-6-PD glucose-6-phosphate dehydrogenase; also G-6-PDH

GPDH glucose phosphate dehydrogenase; also GPD

G-6-PDH glucose-6-phosphate dehydrogenase; also G6PD, G-6-PD

G6PDA glucose-6-phosphate dehydrogenase enzyme variant A; also G-6-PDHA

G-6-PDHA glucose-6-phosphate dehydrogenase enzyme variant A; also G6PDA

GPE glycerylphosphorylethanolamine
guinea pig embryo

GPF glomerular plasma flow
granulocytosis-promoting factor
guinea-pig fibrinogen

GPG growth-promoting genes

GPGG guinea pig gamma globulin

GPHN giant pigmented hairy nevus

GPHLV guinea pig herpes-like virus

GPHV guinea pig herpesvirus

GPI general paralysis of the insane
general paresis of the insane
Gingival-Periodontal Index
glucosephosphate isomerase
Gordon Personal Inventory
guinea pig ileum

GPIMH guinea pig intestinal mucosal homogenate

GPIPID guinea pig intraperitoneal infectious dose

GPK guinea pig kidney (antigen)

GPKA guinea pig kidney absorption (test)

G-PLT giant platelet(s)

GPLV guinea pig leukemia virus

Gply gingivoplasty

GPM general preventive medicine
giant pigment melanosome

GPMAL gravida, para, multiple births, abortions, live births

GPMSP good postmarketing surveillance practice

GPN Graduate Practical Nurse

GPO group purchasing organization

GPP Gordon Personal Profile

GPPQ General Purpose Psychiatric Questionnaire

GPR good partial response
gram-positive rod; also G+R

GPRBC guinea-pig red blood cell

GPS Goodpasture's syndrome
gray platelet syndrome
guinea pig serum
guinea pig spleen

GPT glutamic pyruvic transaminase (alanine aminotransferase)
guinea pig trachea

GpTh group therapy; also GT

GPTSM guinea pig tracheal smooth muscle

GPU guinea pig unit

GPUT galactose phosphate uridyl transferase

GPx glutathione peroxidase; also GP

GQAP general question-asking program

GR gamma-ray
gamma roentgen; also gr
gastric resection
generalized rash
general relief
general research
glucocorticoid receptor; also GCR
glucose response
glutathione reductase; also GSR
good recovery
grain; also g, gr
granulocyte
gravid; also gr, Grav, grav

G-R gram-negative rod; also GNR

G+R gram-positive rod; also GPR

Gr Greek; also G

gr gamma roentgen; also GR
grade; also G
graft
grain; also g, GR
gravid; also GR, Grav, grav
gravity; also g, grav
gray
great; also g, gt
gross; also GRS

gr- gram-negative; also G-, GM-, GN, GrN

gr+ gram-positive; also G+, GM+, GP, GrP

GRA gated radionuclide angiography
glycyrrhizic acid
Gombart's reducing agent
gonadotropin-releasing agent

GRA+ Gombart's reducing agent–positive

Gra glyceraldehyde

Grad by degrees [L. *gradatim*]; also grad

grad by degrees [L. *gradatim*]; also Grad
gradient
gradually
graduate

GRAE generally recognized as effective

GRAN Gombart's reducing agent–negative

gran granulated
granule

GRAR generally recognized as reasonable

GRAS generally recognized as safe

GRASE generally recognized as safe and effective

Grav gravid; also GR, gr, grav

grav gravid; also GR, gr, Grav
gravity; also g, gr

grav 1, grav 2, grav 3, etc first, second, third, etc, pregnancy; also GI, II, III, etc
pregnant once, twice, etc
primigravida, secundigravida, tertigravida, etc.; also GI, GII, GIII, etc.

GRD beta-glucuronidase; also GRS, GUSB
gastroesophageal reflux disease; also GERD
gender role definition

grd ground; also gnd

GRE glucocorticoid responsive element
gradient-echo
Graduate Record Examination

GREAT Graduate Record Examination Aptitude Test

GRF gonadotropin-releasing factor; also GnRF, Gn-RF
growth hormone-releasing factor; also GHRF, GH-RF

GR-FeSV Gardner-Rasheed feline sarcoma virus

GR-FR grandfather; also GF

GRG glycine-rich glycoprotein

GRH gonadotropin-releasing hormone; also GnRH, Gn-RH
growth hormone-releasing hormone; also GHRH, GH-RH

Gri glyceric acid

GRID gay-related immune disease

GRIF growth hormone release-inhibiting factor; also GHRIF, GH-RIF

GRIH growth hormone release-inhibiting hormone; also GHRIH, GH-RIH

GRIP graphics interaction with proteins (system)

GRL granular layer; also GL

GR-MO grandmother; also GM

gr m p ground in a coarse way [L. *grosso modo pulverisatum*]

GRN granules
green; also G, Grn

Grn glycerone
green; also G, GRN

GrN gram-negative; also G-, GM-, GN, gr-

Gro glycerol; also GLY, gly, glyc

gros coarse [L. *grossus*]

GRP gastrin-releasing peptide

GrP gram-positive; also G+, GM+, GP, gr+

grp group; also g, GP, gp

GrPAB pregnant, birth, miscarriage [L. *gravida* (pregnant), *partus* (birth), *abortus* (miscarriage)] (subscript numbers after each category); also GPA

GRPS glucose-Ringer-phosphate solution

GRS beta-glucuronidase; also GRD, GUSB
geriatric rating scale
gross; also gr

GRS&MIC gross and microscopic

GRT gastric residence time
Graduate Respiratory Therapist

GrTr graphite treatment

GRW giant ragweed (test)

gr wt gross weight

GS gallstone
Gardner's syndrome
gastric shield
gastrocnemius soleus
generalized seizure
general surgery
Gilbert's syndrome
Glanzmann-Saland (syndrome)
glomerular sclerosis
glucagon secretion
glutamine synthetase
goat serum
Goldenhar syndrome
Gougerot-Sjögren (syndrome)
graft survival
Gram's stain
granulocyte substance
grip strength
Grönblad-Strandberg (syndrome)
group section
group specific; also gs
Guérin-Stern (syndrome)

G/S glucose and saline

Gs gauss; also G

gs group specific; also GS

g/s gallons per second

GSA general somatic afferent (nerve)
Gross sarcoma virus antigen
group-specific antigen
guanidinosuccinic acid

GSB graduated spinal block

GSBG gonadal steroid-binding globulin; also GBS

GSC gas-solid chromatography
gravity-settling culture (plate)

G-SC guanosine-coupled spleen cell

GSCN giant serotonin-containing neuron; also GSN

GSD genetically significant dose (of mutagenic radiation)
glutathione synthetase deficiency
glycogen storage disease

GSE general somatic efferent (nerve)
genital self-examination
gluten-sensitive enteropathy
grip strong and equal

GSF galactosemic fibroblast
genital skin fibroblast

GSH glomerulus-stimulating hormone
golden Syrian hamster
growth-stimulating hormone
reduced glutathione

GSHP reduced glutathione peroxidase; also GSH-Px

GSH-Px reduced glutathione peroxidase; also GSHP

GSHV ground squirrel hepatitis virus

GSI genuine stress incontinence

GSK glycogen synthetase kinase

GSL general sales list

GSN giant serotonin-containing neuron; also GSCN

GSP galvanic skin potential
general survey panel
glycogen synthetase phosphatase
glycosylated serum protein

GSPN greater superficial petrosal neurectomy

GSR galvanic skin resistance
galvanic skin response
generalized Shwartzman reaction
glutathione reductase; also GR

GSS gamete-shedding substance
Gerstmann-Sträussler syndrome

GSSG oxidized glutathione

GSSG-R oxidized glutathione reductase

GSSI Global Sexual Satisfaction Index

GSSR generalized Sanarelli-Shwartzman reaction

GST glutathione-*S*-transferase
gold salt therapy
gold sodium thiomalate; also GSTM

graphic stress telethermometry
graphic stress thermography
group striction

GSTM gold sodium thiomalate; also GST

GSW gunshot wound

GSWA gunshot wound to abdomen; also GWA

GT gait; also gt
gait training
galactosyl transferase
gamma-glutamyltransferase; also GGT
Gamow-Teller
gastrostomy
gastrostomy tube; also G-tube
Gee-Thaysen (disease)
generation time
genetic therapy
gingiva treatment
Glanzmann's thrombasthenia
glucagon test
glucose tolerance
glucose transport
glucuronyl transferase
glutamyl transpeptidase; also GTP
glycityrosine
grand total
granulation tissue; also g/t
greater trochanter
great toe
group tensions
group therapy; also GpTh

G&T gowns and towels

GT1 thru GT10 glycogen storage disease, types 1 through 10

gt drop [L. *gutta*]
gait; also GT
great; also g, gr

g/t granulation time
granulation tissue; also GT

GTB gastrointestinal tract bleeding

GTC generalized tonic-clonic (seizure)

GTCS generalized tonic-clonic seizure

GTD gestational trophoblastic disease

GTF gastrostomy tube feedings
glucose tolerance factor
glucosyltransferase

GTG Giemsa banding technique
gold thioglucose

GTH gonadotropic hormone; also GDH

GTM grade, location, lymph node involvement, and metastases (Surgical Staging System for bone sarcomas)

GTN gestational trophoblastic neoplasia
gestational trophoblastic neoplasm
glomerulo-tubulo-nephritis
glyceryl trinitrate (nitroglycerin)

GTO Gaussian-type orbital
Golgi tendon organ

GTP glutamyl transpeptidase; also GT
guanosine triphosphate

GTR galvanic tetanus ratio
generalized time reflex
granulocyte turnover rate

GTS Gilles de la Tourette's syndrome
glucose transport system

gts drops [L. *guttae*]; also gtt, GTTS, gtts

GTSTD Grid Test of Schizophrenic Thought
Disorder

GTT gelatin-tellurite-taurocholate (agar)
glucose tolerance test

gtt drops [L. *guttae*]; also gts, GTTS, gtts

GTTS, gtts drops [L. *guttae*]; also gts, gtt

GTT3H glucose tolerance test, 3 hours

G-tube gastrostomy tube; also GT

GU gastric ulcer
genitourinary
glucose uptake
glycogenic unit
glycogen unit
gonococcal urethritis; also GCU
gravitational ulcer

[G]u concentration of glucose in urine

GUA group of units of analysis

Gua guanine; also G

guid guidance

GUK guanylate kinase

Gul gulose

GULHEMP general physique, upper extremity,
lower extremity, hearing, eyesight, mental-
ity, and personality

Guo guanosine; also G

GUS genitourinary sphincter
genitourinary system

GUSB beta-glucuronidase; also GRD, GRS

gutt to the throat [L. *gutturi*]

guttat drop by drop [L. *guttatim*]

gutt quibusd with a few drops [L. *guttis
quibusdam* (with certain drops)]

GV gastric volume
gentian violet
germinal vesicle

granulosis virus
griseoviridin
Gross' virus (nodule)

GVA general visceral afferent (nerve)

GVB gelatin-veronal buffer

GVBD germinal vesicle breakdown

GVE general visceral efferent (nerve)

GVF Goldmann's visual fields
good visual fields

GVG gamma-vinyl-gamma-aminobutyric acid

GVH, GvH graft-versus-host (disease, reaction)

GVHD, GvHD graft-versus-host disease

GVHR, GvHR graft-versus-host reaction

GVTY gingivectomy

GW germ warfare
gigawatt
glycerin in water
gradual withdrawal
Gray-Wheelwright
group work

G/W glucose in water

G&W glycerin and water

GWA gunshot wound to abdomen; also GSWA

GWBS global ward behavior scale

GWE glycerin and water enema

GWG generalized Wegener granulomatosis

GWT gunshot wound of the throat

GX glycinexylidide

GX EKG graded exercise electrocardiogram

GXP graded exercise program

GXT graded exercise test

GY gynecologic disease

Gy gray (unit of absorbed dose of ionizing
radiation)

GYN, gyn gynecologic
gynecologist
gynecology; also G

GYS guaranteed yield strength

GZ Guilford-Zimmerman (personality test)

GZAS Guilford-Zimmerman Aptitude Survey

GZTS Guilford-Zimmerman Temperament
Survey

H

a draft, a drink [L. *haustus*]; also h, haust, ht
bacterial flagellar antigen [Ger. *Hauch* (breath)]; also *H*
deflection of His' bundle in electrogram (spike)
electrically induced spinal reflex
enthalpy (physics); also *H*
Fraunhofer's line (at wavelength 3968, due to calcium)
fucosal transferase-producing gene
Hancock
Hartnup's (disease)
head; also HD, hd, he
hearing
heart; also He, HT, Ht, ht
heavy
heavy chain (immunoglobulin); also HC
heelstick; also HS
height; also h, Hgt, HT, Ht, ht
hemagglutination; also HA
hemagglutinin; also HA
hemisphere; also hemi
hemolysis; also HEM, Hem, HL
hemolytic; also HEM, Hem
henry (unit of electric inductance); also h
heparin; also HEP, HP
hernia; also her, hern
herniated; also her, hern
herniation; also her, hern
heroin
hetacillin
high; also h
histidine (one-letter notation); also HI, Hi, HIS, His, Hist, hist
history; also Hist, hist, Hx, hx, Hy
Hoffmann (reflex); also Hoff
Holzknecht (unit)
homosexual; also HOMO, homo, HS
horizontal; also h, hor, horiz
hormone
horse; also Ho
hospital; also Hosp, hosp
hospitalization; also Hosp, hosp, HX
hot; also Ht
Hounsfield (unit); also HU
hour; also h, HR, hr
human; also h, Hu
husband; also husb
hydrogen
hydrolysis
hydroxydaunomycin (doxorubicin)
hygiene; also Hyg, hyg

hygienic; also Hyg, hyg
hygienist; also Hyg, hyg
hyoscine (scopolamine)
hypermetropia; also h, Hy
hyperopia; also h, Hy
hyperopic; also h, Hy
hyperphoria; also HP
hyperplasia
hypochondriac
hypodermic; also (H), h, hyp
hypothalamus; also HT, Ht, Hth, Hyp, hyp
magnetization
motile or flagellate type of microorganism [Ger. *Hauch* (breath)]; also *H*
oersted (unit of magnetic field intensity); also *H*
patient's home
region of sarcomere containing only myosin filaments [Ger. *heller* (lighter)]
vectorcardiography electrode (neck)

H bacterial flagellar antigen [Ger. *Hauch* (breath)]; also H
enthalpy (physics); also H
Hemophilus species
motile or flagellate type of microorganism [Ger. *Hauch* (breath)]; also H
oersted (unit of magnetic field intensity); also H

(H) hip
hypodermic; also H, h, hyp

H+ hydrogen ion

[H+] hydrogen ion concentration

H_0 null hypothesis

H1, ^{1}H, H^1 protium (ordinary or light hydrogen, hydrogen-1)

H-1 parvovirus

H_1 alternative hypothesis
histamine receptor type 1

H^2 hiatal hernia; also HH

H_2 histamine; also HA, Hi, Hist, hist

H2, ^{2}H, H^2 deuterium (heavy hydrogen, hydrogen-2)

H3, ^{3}H, H^3 tritium (hydrogen-3)

H-3 fumagillin

H_3 procaine hydrochloride

h a draft, a drink [L. *haustus*]; also H, haust, ht
at bedtime [L. *hora decumbendi* (hour of lying down), *hora somni* (hour of sleep)]; also hd, hor decub, HS, hs, hor som, h som

coefficient of heat transfer
hand-rearing (of experimental animals)
hecto (10^2)
height; also H, Hgt, HT, Ht, ht
henry; also H
heteromorphic region
high; also H
horizontal; also H, hor, horiz
hour; also H, HR, hr
human; also H, Hu
human response
hundred
hypermetropia; also H, Hy
hyperopia; also H, Hy
hyperopic; also H, Hy
hypodermic; also H, (H), hyp
negatively staining region of chromosome
Planck's constant; also *h*
quantum constant
specific enthalpy

h Planck's constant; also h

HA abbreviation for an acid
hallux abductus
halothane anesthesia
H antigen [Ger. *Hauch* (breath)]
Hartley (guinea pig)
headache; also H/A
hearing aid
heated
heated aerosol; also ht aer
height age
hemadsorbent
hemadsorption (test)
hemagglutinating activity
hemagglutinating antibody
hemagglutinating antigen
hemagglutination; also H
hemagglutinin; also H
hemolytic anemia
hemophiliac with adenopathy
hepatic adenoma
hepatic artery
hepatitis A
hepatitis-associated (virus)
herpangina
heterophil antibody
Heyden antibiotic
high anxiety
hippuric acid
histamine; also H_2, Hi, Hist, hist
histidine ammonia-lyase
histocompatibility antigen
Horton's arteritis
hospital acquired

hospital administration; also HAD, HAd
hospital administrator; also HAD, HAd
hospital admission
hospital apprentice
household activity
hyaluronic acid
hydroxyanisole
hydroxyapatite; also HAP
hyperalimentation; also HAL, hyperal, hyper-al
hyperandrogenism
hypermetropic astigmatism
hyperopia, absolute
hypersensitivity alveolitis
hypothalamic amenorrhea

H/A headache; also HA
head to abdomen (ratio)

HA1 hemadsorption virus, type 1

HA2 hemadsorption virus, type 2

Ha absolute hypermetropia
hahnium
hamster

H/a home with advice

HAA hearing aid amplifier
hemolytic anemia antigen
hepatitis A antibody; also HAAb
hepatitis-associated antigen
hospital activity analysis

HAAb hepatitis A antibody; also HAA

HAAg hepatitis A antigen

HABA hydroxybenzeneazobenzoic acid; also HBABA

HABF hepatic artery blood flow

HAb horizontal abduction

HAd horizontal adduction

habit habitat

habt let the patient have [L. *habeatur*]

HAC hexamethylmelamine, Adriamycin, and cyclophosphamide

HAc acetic acid

HAChT high-affinity choline transport

HACR hereditary adenomatosis of colon and rectum

HACS hyperactive child syndrome

HAD hearing aid dispenser
hemadsorption; also HAd
hexamethylmelamine, Adriamycin, and *cis*-diamminedichloroplatinum (cisplatin)
hospital administration; also HA, HAd
hospital administrator; also HA, HAd

HAD—cont'd
  human adjuvant disease
  hypophysectomized alloxan diabetic

HAd hemadsorption; also HAD
  hospital administration; also HA, HAD
  hospital administrator; also HA, HAD

HADD hydroxyapatite deposition disease

HAd-I hemadsorption inhibition

HAE health appraisal examination
  hearing aid evaluation
  hepatic artery embolization
  hereditary angioedema
  hereditary angioneurotic edema; also HANE

HAF hepatic arterial flow

HaF Hageman factor (coagulation factor XII);
  also HF

HAFOE high air flow oxygen enrichment

HAFP human alpha-fetoprotein

HAG heat-aggregated globulin

HAGG hyperimmune anti-variola gamma
  globulin

HAHTG horse antihuman thymus globulin

HAI hemagglutination inhibition; also HI
  hemagglutinin inhibition
  hepatic arterial infusion

H&A Ins health and accident insurance

HAIR-AN hyperandrogenism, insulin resistance, and acanthosis nigricans (syndrome)

HaK hamster kidney

HAL haloperidol; also HL
  halothane; also hal, HALO
  hepatic artery ligation
  hyperalimentation; also HA, hyperal,
  hyper-al

Hal halogen

hal halothane; also HAL, HALO

halluc hallucination

HALO halothane; also HAL, hal
  hemorrhage, abruption, labor, placenta previa
  with mild bleeding

HALP hyperalphalipoproteinemia

HALT Heroin Antagonist and Learning
  Therapy

HaLV hamster leukemia virus

HAM hearing aid microphone
  helical axis of motion
  hexamethylmelamine, Adriamycin, and melphalan
  human albumin microsphere(s)
  human alveolar macrophage

hypoparathyroidism, Addison's disease, and
  mucocutaneous candidiasis (syndrome)

HAMA Hamilton Anxiety (Scale)
  human anti-mouse antibody
  hydroxy-aluminum magnesium aminoacetate

HAMD Hamilton Depression (Scale)

HAMM human albumin minimicrosphere

Hams hamstrings; also HS

HaMSV Harvey murine sarcoma virus

HAN heroin-associated nephropathy
  hyperplastic alveolar nodule

HANA hemagglutinin neuraminidase; also HN

H and D Hunter and Driffield (curve, radiology); also H&D

H and E hematoxylin and eosin (stain); also
  H&E

H and P history and physical (examination);
  also H&P, H+P, HPE

H and V hemigastrectomy and vagotomy;
  also H&V

Handicp handicapped; also HC, HCAP, HCP

HANE hereditary angioneurotic edema; also
  HAE

HANES Health and Nutrition Examination
  Survey

HANP human atrium natriuretic peptide

H antigens flagella antigens of motile bacteria
  [Ger. *Hauch* (breath)]

HAP Handicapped Aid Program
  haptoglobin; also HAPTO, HP, Hp, Hpb, Hpt
  held after positioning
  heredopathia atactica polyneuritiformis
  high-amplitude peristalsis
  histamine acid phosphate
  hospital-acquired pneumonia
  humoral antibody production
  hydrolyzed animal protein
  hydroxyapatite; also HA

HAPA hemagglutinating anti-penicillin antibody

HAPC hospital-acquired penetration contact

HAPE high-altitude pulmonary edema; also
  HAPO

HAPO high-altitude pulmonary (o)edema; also
  HAPE

HAPS hepatic arterial perfusion scintigraphy

HAPTO haptoglobin; also HAP, HP, Hp, Hpb,
  Hpt

HAQ Headache Assessment Questionnaire

HAR high-altitude retinopathy

Har homoarginine

HAREM heparin assay rapid easy method

HARH high-altitude retinal hemorrhage

HARM heparin assay rapid method

harm harmonic

HARPPS heat, absence of use, redness, pain, pus, swelling (symptoms of infection)

HARS Hamilton Anxiety Rating Scale

HAS Hamilton Anxiety Scale
health advisory service
highest asymptomatic (dose)
hospital adjustment scale
hospital administrative service
hospital advisory service
hyperalimentation solution
hypertensive arteriosclerotic

HASCHD hypertensive arteriosclerotic heart disease; also HASHD

HASCVD hypertensive arteriosclerotic cardiovascular disease

HASHD hypertensive arteriosclerotic heart disease; also HASCHD

HASP Hospital Admissions and Surveillance Program

HAsP health aspects of pesticides

HAT Halstead Aphasia Test
harmonic attenuation table
harmonic attenuation test
head, arms, and trunk
heterophil antibody titer
hospital arrival time
hypoxanthine, aminopterin, and thymidine (medium)
hypoxanthine, azaserine, and thymidine

HATG horse anti-human thymocyte globulin

HATH Heterosexual Attitudes Toward Homosexuality (scale)

HATT hemagglutination treponemal test

HATTS hemagglutination treponemal test for syphilis

HAU hemagglutinating unit; also HU

haust a draft, a drink [L. *haustus*]; also H, h, ht

HAV hallux abducto valgus
hemadsorption virus
hepatitis A virus
high-activity variant (cells)

HAVAB hepatitis A virus antibody

HAWIC Hamburg-Wechsler Intelligence Test for Children

HB head backward
health board
heart block; also hb
heel-to-buttock
held backward
hemoglobin; also Hb, Hbg, hemo, HG, Hg, hg, HGB, Hgb
hemolysis blocking
hepatitis B
highball
His's bundle
hold breakfast
hospital bed
housebound
Hutchinson-Boeck (disease)
hybridoma bank
hyoid body

HB-8 hexagonal bipyramidal

HB-9 heptagonal bipyramidal

HB1° first-degree heart block

HB2° second-degree heart block

HB3° third-degree heart block

Hb hemoglobin; also HB, Hbg, hemo, HG, Hg, hg, HGB, Hgb

H-2*b* mouse cells

hb heart block; also HB

HBA hemoglobin alpha (α) chain

HbA hemoglobin A (normal adult hemoglobin)

Hb A° hemoglobin determination

HbA$_1$ major fraction of adult hemoglobin

HbA$_2$ minor fraction of adult hemoglobin

HBAb, HBAB hepatitis B antibody

HBABA hydroxybenzeneazobenzoic acid; also HABA

HBAC hyperdynamic beta-adrenergic circulatory

Hb A1c glycohemoglobin; also GHb, GLYCOS Hb
glycosylated hemoglobin; also GHb, GLYCOS Hb

HBAg, HbAg, HB-Ag hepatitis β antigen

HbAS heterozygosity for hemoglobin A and hemoglobin S (sickle-cell trait)

HBB hemoglobin beta (·) chain
hospital blood bank
hydroxybenzyl benzimidazole

HbB hemoglobin in the blood

HbBC hemoglobin-binding capacity

HBBW hold breakfast for blood work

HB$_c$ hepatitis B core (antibody, antigen)

HbC hemoglobin C

HB$_c$Ab, HBcAb, HBCAB antibody to the hepatitis · core antigen

HB$_c$Ag, HBcAg, HBCAG hepatitis b core antigen

HBCG heat-aggregated bacille Calmette-Guérin

HbCO carboxyhemoglobin (carbon monoxide hemoglobin)

HB core hepatitis core (antibody, antigen)

Hb CS hemoglobin Constant Spring

HbCV *Haemophilus influenzae b* conjugate vaccine
hepatitis B conjugate vaccine

HBD has been drinking
hemoglobin delta (δchain
hydroxybutyrate dehydrogenase; also HBDH, HOBDH
hydroxybutyric dehydrogenase; also HBDH, HDBD, HDBH
hypophosphatemic bone disease

HbD hemoglobin D

HBDH hydroxybutyrate dehydrogenase; also HBD, HOBDH
hydroxybutyric dehydrogenase; also HBD, HDBD, HDBH

HBDT human basophil degranulation test

HBE hemoglobin epsilon ∈ chain
His' bundle electrogram

HbE hemoglobin E

HBE$_1$ His' bundle electrogram, distal

HBE$_2$ His' bundle electrogram, proximal

HB$_e$ hepatitis B early (antibody, antigen)

HB$_e$Ab, HBeAb, HBEAB antibody to the hepatitis B early antigen

HB$_e$Ag, HBeAg, HBEAG hepatitis B early antigen

HBF fetal hemoglobin; also HbF, Hb F
hand blood flow
hemispheric blood flow
hemoglobinuric bilious fever
hepatic blood flow
hypothalamic blood flow

HbF, Hb F fetal hemoglobin; also HBF
hemoglobin F

HBG1 hemoglobin gamma (γ) chain A

HBG2 hemoglobin gamma (γ) chain G

Hbg hemoglobin; also HB, Hb, hemo, HG, Hg, hg, HGB, Hgb

HBGA had it before, got it again

HBGF heparin-binding growth factor

HBGM home blood glucose monitoring

HBGS human blood group substance

HbH hemoglobin H

HBHC home-based hospital care

Hb-Hp hemoglobin-haptoglobin (complex)

HBI hemibody irradiation
hepatobiliary imaging; also HI
high serum-bound iron

HBID hereditary benign intraepithelial dyskeratosis

HBIG, HBIg hepatitis B immune globulin
hepatitis B immunoglobulin

Hb$_{Kansas}$ mutant hemoglobin with low affinity for oxygen

HBL hepatoblastoma

HBLA human B-lymphocyte antigen

Hb$_{Lepore}$ hemoglobin Lepore

HBLLSB heart best at left lower sternal border

HBLUSB heart best at left upper sternal border

HBLV human B-lymphotropic virus

HBM Health Belief Model
hypertonic buffered medium

HbM hemoglobin M

HbMet methemoglobin; also HiHb, Met-Hb, MHB, MHb

HBO hyperbaric oxygen; also HBO$_2$, HO
hyperbaric oxygenation
oxyhemoglobin (oxygenated hemoglobin); also HbO$_2$

HbO$_2$ oxyhemoglobin (oxygenated hemoglobin); also HBO
hyperbaric oxygen; also HBO, HO

HbOC oligosaccharide-CRM$_{197}$ conjugate *Haemophilus influenzae b* vaccine

HBOT hyperbaric oxygen therapy

HBP hepatic binding protein
high blood pressure

HbP primitive (fetal) hemoglobin

HBPM home blood pressure monitoring

HbPV *Haemophilus influenzae b* polysaccharide vaccine

HBr hydrobromic acid

HbR methemoglobin reductase

HBS Health Behavior Scale
hepatitis B surface (antibody, antigen); also HB$_s$
hyperkinetic behavior syndrome

HbS sickle-cell hemoglobin; also Hb S
sulfhemoglobin

Hb S sickle-cell hemoglobin; also HbS

HB$_s$ hepatitis B surface (antibody, antigen);
also HBS

HB$_s$A hepatitis B surface-associated

HB$_s$Ab, HBsAb, HBSAB antibody to the
hepatitis B surface antigen

HB$_s$Ag, HBsAg, HBSAG hepatitis B surface
antigen

HBsAg/adr hepatitis B surface antigen mani-
festing group-specific determinant *a* and
subtype-specific determinants *d* and *r*

HBSC hemopoietic blood stem cell

HbSC sickle-cell hemoglobin C

HBSS Hank's balanced salt solution

HbSS homozygosity for hemoglobin S

HBSSG Hank's balanced salt solution plus
glucose

HBT human brain thromboplastin
human breast tumor

HBV hepatitis B vaccine
hepatitis B virus
honey-bee venom

HBVP hepatitis B virus polymerase

HBW high birth weight

H/BW heart to body weight (ratio)
height to body weight (ratio)

HBZ hemoglobin zeta (ζ) chain

HbZ hemoglobin Z (Zürich)
hemoglobin

HC hair cell
hairy cell
handicapped; also Handicp, HCAP, HCP
head check
head circumference
head compression
healthy control
heart cycle
heat conservation
heavy chain (immunoglobulin); also H
heel cord
hemoglobin concentration
hemorrhage, cerebral
heparin cofactor
hepatic catalase
hepatocellular cancer
hereditary coproporphyria; also HCP
Hickman catheter
high calorie; also hg-cal

hippocampus; alsp Hip
histamine challenge
histochemistry
home call
home care
homocystinuria; also HCU
Hospital Corps
hospital course
hospitalized controls
house call
Huntington's chorea
hyaline casts
hydranencephaly
hydraulic concussion
hydrocarbon
hydrocodone
hydrocortisone; also HCT, Hyd
hydrophobic cellulose
hydroxycorticoid; also HOC
hyoid cornu
hypercholesterolemia
hypertrophic cardiomyopathy; also HCM

H&C hot and cold

Hc hematocrit; also C, Crit, crit, H'crit, HCT,
Hct, hemat, HMT
hydrocolloid

HCA health care aide
heart cell aggregate
hepatocellular adenoma
home care aide
Hospital Corporation of America
hydrocortisone acetate

HCAP handicapped; also Handicp, HC, HCP

H-CAP hexamethylmelamine, cyclophosphamide, Adriamycin, and Platinol (cisplatin)

HCB hexachlorobenzene

HCC heat conservation center
hepatitis contagiosa canis (virus)
hepatocellular carcinoma
hepatoma carcinoma cell
hexachlorocyclohexane (lindane); also HCH,
γ-HCH
history of chief complaint
hydroxycholecalciferol (vitamin D)

25-HCC 25-hydroxycholecalciferol

HCD health care delivery
heavy-chain disease (protein)
high caloric density
high-carbohydrate diet
homologous canine distemper (antiserum)
hydrocolloid dressing

HCF hereditary capillary fragility
high carbohydrate, high fiber (diet)
highest common factor
hypocaloric carbohydrate feeding

HCFA Health Care Financing Administration

HCFSH human chorionic follicle-stimulating
hormone

HCFU hexylcarbamoylfluorouracil (carmofur-
antineoplastic)

HCG, hCG human chorionic gonadotropin

hCG-α subunit chorionic gonadotropin–alpha
subunit

hCG-β subunit chorionic gonadotropin–beta
subunit

HCGN hypocomplementemic glomerulonephritis

HCGPF hematopoietic cell growth potentiating
factor

HCH hexachlorocyclohexane (lindane); also
HCC, γ-HCH

γ-HCK hexachlorocyclohexane (lindane); also
HCC, HCH

Hch hemochromatosis

HCHO formaldehyde

HCI hemocytology index

Hcimp hydrocolloid impression

HCIS Health Care Information System

HCL hairy-cell leukemia
hard contact lens
human cultured lymphoblasts

HCLF high carbohydrate, low fiber (diet)

HCLs hard contact lenses

HCM health care maintenance
health care management
hypertrophic cardiomyopathy; also HC

HCMM hereditary cutaneous malignant
melanoma

HCMV human cytomegalovirus

HCN hereditary chronic nephritis
hydrocyanic acid
hydrogen cyanide

HCO carbohydrate

HCO₃- bicarbonate radical

HCP handicapped; also Handicp, HC, HCAP
hepatocatalase peroxidase
hereditary coproporphyria; also HC
hexachlorophene
high cell passage

H&CP hospital and community psychiatry

HCP-SAD high cell passage Street-Alabama-
Dufferin (strain)

HCQ hydroxychloroquine

HCR heme-controlled repressor
host-cell reactivation
human-controlled repressor
hydrochloric acid
hysterical conversion reaction

HCRE Homeopathic Council for Research and
Education

H'crit hematocrit; also C, Crit, crit, Hc, HCT,
Hct, hemat, HMT

HCS Hajdu-Cheney syndrome
Harvey Cushing Society
health care support
hourglass contraction of stomach
human chorionic somatomammotropin
(human placental lactogen); also hCS,
HCSM, hCSM
human chorionic somatotropin
human cord serum
hydroxycorticosteroid

17-HCS 17-hydroxycorticosteroids

hCS human chorionic somatomammotropin
(human placental lactogen); also HCS,
HCSM, hCSM

HCSD Health Care Studies Division

HCSM, hCSM human chorionic somatomammotropin (human placental lactogen); also
HCS, hCS

HCT Health Check Test
heart-circulation training
hematocrit; also C, Crit, crit, Hc, H'crit, Hct,
hemat, HMT
histamine challenge test
historic control trial
homocytotropic
human calcitonin; also hCT
human chorionic (placental) thyrotropin; also
hCT
hydrochlorothiazide; also HCTZ
hydrocortisone; also HC, Hyd
hydroxycortisone

Hct hematocrit; also C, Crit, crit, Hc, H'crit,
HCT, hemat, HMT

hCT human calcitonin; also HCT
human chorionic thyrotropin; also HCT

hct hundred count

HCTC Health Care Technology Center

HCTD hepatic computed tomographic density
high cholesterol and tocopherol deficient

HCTS high cholesterol and tocopherol supplemented

HCTU home cervical traction unit

HCTZ hydrochlorothiazide; also HCT

HCU homocystinuria; also HC
hyperplasia cystica uteri

HCV hepatitis C virus
human coronavirus

HCVD hypertensive cardiovascular disease; also HTCVD

HCVR hypercapnic ventilatory response

HCVS human corona virus sensitivity

HCW health care worker

HCWs health care workers

Hcy hemocyanin
homocysteine

HD Haab-Dimmer (syndrome)
Hajna-Damon (broth)
haloperidol decanoate; also HLD, HL-D
Hanganatziu-Deicher (reaction, test)
Hansen's disease
hard corn [L. *heloma durum*]
head; also H, hd, he
hearing distance
heart disease
helium dilution
hemidiaphragm
hemodialysis
hemolytic disease
hemolyzing dose
herniated disc
high density
high dosage
high dose
hip disarticulation
Hirschsprung's disease
histidine decarboxylase; also HDC
Hodgkin's disease
hormone dependent
hospital day; also HOD
house dust
human diploid (cell)
Huntington's disease
hydatid disease
hydroxydopamine; also HDA
hypnotic dosage

HD# hospital day number

H&D Hunter and Driffield (curve, radiology); also H and D

HD$_{50}$ hemolyzing dose of complement that lyses 50% of sensitized red blood cells

hd at bedtime [L. *hora decumbendi* (hour of lying down)]; also h, hor decub
head; also H, HD, he

HDA hydroxydopamine; also HD

HDAC high-dose cytarabine (Ara-C); also HDARAC

HDARAC high-dose cytarabine (Ara-C); also HDAC

HDBD hydroxybutyric dehydrogenase; also HBD, HBDH, HDBH

HDBH hydroxybutyric dehydrogenase; alsoHBD, HBDH, HDBD

HDC histidine decarboxylase; also HD
human diploid cell
hypodermoclysis

HDCS human diploid cell strain
human diploid cell system

HDCSV human diploid cell strain vaccine

HDCV human diploid cell rabies vaccine

HDD half-dose depth
high-dose depth

HDF high dry field (microscope)
host defensive factor
human diploid fibroblast

HDFL human development and family life

HDFP Hypertension Detection and Follow-up Program

HDG high-dose group

HDH heart disease history
Hostility and Direction of Hostility (questionnaire); also HDHQ

HDHQ Hostility and Direction of Hostility Questionnaire; also HDH

HDI hemorrhagic disease of infants

HDL high-density lipoprotein; also HDLP

HDL$_1$ Lp(a) lipoprotein

HDL-C high-density lipoprotein cholesterol

HDL-c high-density lipoprotein–cell surface (receptor)

HDLP high-density lipoprotein; also HDL

HDLS hereditary diffuse leukoencephalopathy with spheroids

HDLW hearing distance, left, watch (distance from which watch ticking is heard by left ear)

HDM hexadimethrine

HDMP high-dose methylprednisolone

HDMTX high-dose methotrexate

HDMTX-CF high-dose methotrexate and cit-rovorum factor

HDMTX/LV high-dose methotrexate and leu-covorin

HDN hemolytic disease of the newborn
 high-density nebulizer

hDNA deoxyribonucleic acid, histone

HDP hexose diphosphate
 high-density polyethylene
 hydroxydimethylpyrimidine

HDPAA heparin-dependent platelet-associated antibody

HDR Harrington distraction rod

HDRF Heart Disease Research Foundation

HDRS Hamilton Depression Rating Scale; also HDS

HDRV human diploid rabies vaccine

HDRW hearing distance, right, watch (distance from which watch ticking is heard by right ear)

HDS Hamilton Depression Rating Scale; also HDRS
 Healthcare Data Systems
 Health Data Services
 health delivery system
 herniated disc syndrome
 Hospital Discharge Survey

HDU head-drop unit (curare standard)
 hemodialysis unit

HDV hepatitis delta virus
 hepatitis virus, type D
 hepatocyte-directed vesicle
 human delta virus

HDW hearing distance with watch

HDZ hydralazine; also HYD

HE hard exudate; also HEx
 hektoen enteric (agar)
 hemagglutinating encephalomyelitis
 hemoglobin electrophoresis
 hepatic encephalopathy
 hepatoma
 hereditary elliptocytosis
 hollow enzyme
 human enteric (virus)
 hyperextension
 hypogonadotropic eunuchoidism
 hypophysectomy; also hyp
 hypoxemic episode

H-E heat exchanger

H&E hematoxylin and eosin (stain); also H and E

 hemorrhage and exudate
 heredity and environment

He heart; also H, HT, Ht, ht
 Hedstrom number
 helium

^{3}He helium-3

^{4}He helium-4

he head; also H, HD, hd

HEA hexone-extracted acetone
 human erythrocyte antigen

HEADSS home life, education level, activities, drug use, sexual activity, suicide ideation/attempts (adolescent medical history)

HEAL Health Education Assistance Loan

HEART Health Evaluation and Risk Tabulation

HEAT human erythrocyte agglutination test

HEB hematoencephalic barrier (blood-brain barrier)

hebdom a week [L. *hebdomata*]
 first week of life [L. *hebdomas* (the seventh day of a disease, supposed to be a critical period)]

HEC hamster embryo cell
 Health Education Council
 health evaluation center
 human endothelial cell
 human enteric coronavirus
 hydroxyergocalciferol

HECT head equivalent computed tomography

HED hydrotropic electron donor
 skin erythema dose [Ger. *Hauterythemdosis*]
 unit skin dose (of x-rays) [Ger. *Hauteinheitisdosis*]

HeD helper determinant

HEDSPA ^{99m}Tc-etidronate (bone-imaging agent)

HEDTA *N*-hydroxyethylenediaminetriacetic acid

HEEDTA *N*-hydroxyethylethylenediaminetri-acetate

HEENT head, ears, eyes, nose, and throat

HEEP health effects of environmental pollutants

HEF hamster embryo fibroblast

HEG hemorrhagic erosive gastritis

HEHR highest equivalent heart rate

HEI high-energy intermediate
 homogeneous enzyme immunoassay

human embryonic intestine (cell)

HE inj hyperextension injury

HEIR health effects of ionizing radiation
high-energy ionizing radiation

HEIS high-energy ion scattering

HEK human embryo kidney (cell culture)
human embryonic kidney

HEL hen egg-white lysozyme; also HEWL
human embryo lung (cell culture)
human embryonic lung (cell)
human erythroleukemia
human erythroleukemia line

HeLa cells of the first continuously cultured
human cervical carcinoma cell line used for
tissue cultures (named for patient, Henrietta
Lacks)

HELF human embryonic lung fibroblast

HELLP hemolysis, elevated liver enzymes, and
low platelet (count)

HELM helmet cell

HELP Hawaii Early Learning Profile
Health Education Library Program
Health Emergency Loan Program
Health Evaluation and Learning Program
heat escape lessening posture
Heroin Emergency Life Project
Hospital Equipment Loan Project

HEM, Hem hematologist; also hemat, hematol
hematology; also hemat, hematol
hemolysis; also H, HL
hemolytic; also H
hemorrhage; hemorr
hemorrhoid

hem hematuria

HEMA hydroxyethylmethacrylate

hemat hematocrit; also C, Crit, crit, Hc, H'crit,
HCT, Hct, HMT
hematologist; also HEM, Hem, hematol
hematology; also HEM, Hem, hematol

hematem hematemesis

hematol hematologist; also HEM, Hem, hemat
hematology; also HEM, Hem, hemat

hemi hemiparalysis
hemiparesis; also HP
hemiplegia; also HP, Hp
hemiplegic
hemisphere; also H

hemo hemoglobin; also HB, Hb, Hbg, HG, Hg,
hg, HGB, Hgb
hemophilia

hemocyt hemocytometer

hemorr hemorrhage; also HEM, Hem

HEMOSID hemosiderin

HEMPAS hereditary erythroblastic multinuclearity associated with positive acidified
serum
hereditary erythrocytic multinuclearity associated with positive acidified serum

HEMRI hereditary multifocal relapsing
inflammation

HEMS helicopter emergency medical services

HEN hemorrhages, exudates, and/or nicking

HEP hemolysis end point
heparin; also H, HP
hepatic
hepatoerythropoietic porphyria
high egg passage (attenuated virus vaccine)
high-energy phosphate
histamine equivalent prick
human epithelial (cell); also HEp

HEp human epithelial (cell); also HEP

HEp-1 human cervical carcinoma cells

HEp-2 human laryngeal tumor cells

hEP human endorphin

hep hepatitis

HEPA hamster egg penetration assay
high-efficiency particulate air (filter)

HEP-AC hepatitis battery-acute

HEPES N-(2-hydroxyethyl)piperazine-N'-2-
ethanesulphonic acid (buffer)

Hep/Clav hepatoclavicular

HEPM human embryonic palatal mesenchymal
(cell)

HEPP human IgE pentapeptide

HEPPS N-(2-hydroxyethyl)piperazine-N'-3-
propanesulphonic acid

HEPT 1-(2-hydroxyethoxymethyl)-6-phenylth-
iothymine

HER hemorrhagic encephalopathy of rats
human estrogen receptor

her hernia; also H, hern
herniated; also H, hern
herniation; also H, hern

herb recent of fresh herbs [L. *herbarium recen-
tium*]

hered hereditary
heredity

hern hernia; also H, her
herniated; also H, her
herniation; also H, her

HERP human exposure dose/rodent potency

HERS Health Evaluation and Referral Service

HES (acute) hypereosinophilic syndrome
health examination survey
hematoxylin-eosin stain
human embryonic skin
human embryonic spleen
hydroxyethyl starch (hetastarch)

HET Health Education Telecommunications
helium equilibration time

Het heterophil (antibody)

het heterozygous

HETE hydroxyeicosatetraenoic (acid)

HETP height equivalent to a theoretical plate
(gas chromatography)
hexaethyltetraphosphate

HEV health and environment
hemagglutination encephalomyelitis virus
hepatoencephalomyelitis virus
high endothelial venule(s)
human enteric virus

HEW Department of Health, Education, and
Welfare (now: HHS, Department of Health
and Human Services)

HEWL hen egg-white lysozyme; also HEL

HEX hexosaminidase

HEx hard exudate; also HE

Hex hexamethylmelamine; also HM, HMM,
Hmm, HXM

HEX A hexosaminidase A (alpha-subunit)

Hexa-CAF Hexalen, cyclophosphamide,
Adrucil, and Folex
hexamethylmelamine, cyclophosphamide,
Amethopterin, and fluorouracil

HEX B hexosaminidase B (beta-subunit)

HF Hageman factor (coagulation factor
XII);also HaF
half; also hf
haplotype frequency
hard feces
hard filled (capsule)
harvest fluid
hay fever
head forward
head of fetus
heart failure
helper factor
hemofiltration
hemorrhagic factor
hemorrhagic fever
hepatocyte function
Hertz frequency

high-fat (diet)
high flow
high frequency; also hf
hollow filter (dialyzer)
hot fomentation
house formula
human fibroblast
human foreskin
hydrogen fluoride (catalyst)
hyperflexion

H/F HeLa/fibroblast (hybrid)

Hf hafnium

hf half; also HF
high frequency; also HF

HFAK hollow-fiber artificial kidney

HFB heptafluorobutyric (acid)

HFC hand-filled capsule
high-frequency current
histamine-forming capacity

HFCS high-fructose corn syrup

HFCWC high-frequency chest wall compression

HFD hemorrhagic fever of deer
high-fiber diet
high forceps delivery
hospital field director
Human Figure Drawing

HFDK human fetal diploid kidney (cell)

HFDL human fetal diploid lung (cell)

HFEC human foreskin epithelial cell

HFF human foreskin fibroblast

HFFTTA hypermobile flat foot with tight
tendo Achillis

HFHL high-frequency hearing loss

HFI hereditary fructose intolerance
human fibroblast interferon; also HFIF

HFIF human fibroblast interferon; also HFI

HFJV high-frequency jet ventilation

HFL human fetal lung

HFM hemifacial microsomia; also HM

HFMB hollow-fiber membrane bioreactor

HFO hard food orientation
high-frequency oscillation

H$_4$folate tetrahydrofolate

HFOV high-frequency oscillatory ventilation

HFP hexafluoropropylene
hypofibrinogenic plasma

HFPPV high-frequency positive pressure ventilation

HFR heart frequency
high-frequency recombination; also Hfr

Hfr high-frequency recombination; also HFR

HFRS hemorrhagic fever with renal syndrome

HFS hemifacial spasm
high-frequency stimulus
Hospital Financial Support

hfs hyperfine structure

hFSH, HFSH human follicle-stimulating hormone

HFST hearing-for-speech test

HFT high-frequency transduction (lysate)
high-frequency transfer (sex factor)

HFUPR hourly fetal urine production rate

HFV high-frequency ventilation

HG hand grip (exercise)
hemoglobin; also HB, Hb, Hbg, hemo, Hg,
hg, HGB, Hgb
herpes genitalis
herpes gestationis
Herter-Gee (syndrome)
Heschl's gyrus
high glucose
human gonadotropin
human growth (factor)
Hutchinson-Gilford (disease/syndrome)
hypoglycemia

Hg hectogram; also hg
hemoglobin; also HB, Hb, Hbg, hemo, HG,
hg, HGB, Hgb
mercury [L. *hydrargyrum* (silver water)]; also
hydrarg

hg hectogram; also Hg
hemoglobin; also HB, Hb, Hbg, hemo, HG,
Hg, HGB, Hgb
hyperglycemic (factor)

HGA homogentisic acid
homogentisic acid oxidase (homogentisate
oxygenase)

HGB, Hgb hemoglobin; also HB, Hb, Hbg,
hemo, HG, Hg, hg

hg-cal high calorie; also HC

HGF human growth factor
hyperglycemic-glycogenolytic factor
(glucagon)

Hg-F hemoglobin, fetal

HGG herpetic geniculate ganglionitis
human gamma globulin; also hGG

hGG human gamma globulin; also HGG

HGH, hGH high growth hormone
human growth hormone

hGHr human growth hormone recombinant

HGI hostility-guilt inventory

HGM hog gastric mucin
human glucose monitoring

HGMCR human genetic mutant cell repository

HGO hepatic glucose output
hip guidance orthosis

HGP hepatic glucose production
Human Genome Project
hyperglobulinemia purpura

HGPRT hypoxanthine-guanine phosphoribosyltransferase; also HG-PRTase

HG-PRTase hypoxanthine-guanine phosphoribosyltransferase; also HGPRT

HGSHS Harvard Group Scale of Hypnotic
Susceptibility

Hgt height; also H, h, HT, Ht, ht

HH halothane hepatitis
hard of hearing; also HOH
Head-Holmes (syndrome)
healthy hemophiliac
Henderson and Haggard (inhaler)
hiatal hernia; also H^2
holistic health
home health
home help
Hunter-Hurler (syndrome)
hydroxyhexanamide
hypergastronemic hyperchlorhydria
hyperhidrosis
hypogonadotropic hypogonadism
hyporeninemic hypoaldosteronism

H/H hemoglobin and hematocrit; also H&H

H-H Henderson-Hasselbalch (equation)

H&H hemoglobin and hematocrit; also H/H

Hh hemopoietic histocompatibility

HHA Health Hazard Appraisal
hereditary hemolytic anemia
Home Health Agency
hypothalamic hypophyseal adrenal (system)

HHAA hypothalamo-hypophyseal-adrenal
axis

HHB, HHb deoxyhemoglobin
hypohemoglobinemia
reduced hemoglobin
un-ionized hemoglobin

HHC hemoglobin-haptoglobin complex
home health care

HHCS high-altitude hypertrophic cardiomyopathy syndrome

HHD high heparin dose

HHD—cont'd
home hemodialysis
hypertensive heart disease; also HTHD

HHE health hazard evaluation
hemiconvulsion-hemiplegia-epilepsy (syndrome)

HHFM high-humidity face mask

HHG hypertrophic hypersecretory gastropathy

HHH hyperornithinemia, hyperammonemia,
and homocitrullinemia (syndrome)

HHHO hypotonia, hypomentia, hypogonadism,
and obesity (syndrome)

HHM hemohydrometry
humoral hypercalcemia of malignancy

H+Hm compound hypermetropic astigmatism;
also H&Hm

H&Hm compound hypermetropic astigmatism;
also H+Hm

HHN hand-held nebulizer

HHNC hyperglycemic, hyperosmolar, nonketotic coma

HHNK hyperglycemic, hyperosmolar, nonketotic (coma)

HHNKS hyperglycemic, hyperosmolar, nonketotic syndrome

HHPC hyperoxic-hypercapnic

HHRH hereditary hypophosphatemic rickets
with hypercalciuria
hypothalamic hypophysiotropic-releasing
hormone

HHS Department of Health and Human
Services
Harris hip score
Hearing Handicap Scale
hereditary hemolytic syndrome
human hypopituitary serum
hyperkinetic heart syndrome

HHT head halter traction; also HHTx
hereditary hemolytic telangiectasia
hereditary hemorrhagic telangiectasia
heterotopic heart transplantation
hydroxyheptadecatrienoic (acid)
12-l-hydroxy-5,8,10-heptadecatrienoic acid

HHTA hypothalamo-hypophyseo-thyroidal axis

HHTx head halter traction; also HHT

HHV6 human herpesvirus 6

HI head injury
health insurance
hearing impaired
heart infusion

heat inactivated
heat input
hemagglutination inhibition; also HAI
hepatic insufficiency
hepatobiliary imaging; also HBI
high impulsiveness
histidine; also H, Hi, HIS, His, Hist, hist
homoridal ideation
hormone independent
hormone insensitive
hospital induced
hospital insurance
humoral immunity
hydriodic acid
hydroxyindole
hyperglycemic index
hypomelanosis of Ito
hypothermic ischemia

Hi histamine; also H_2, HA, Hist, hist
histidine; also H, HI, HIS, His, Hist, hist

HIA heat infusion agar
hemagglutination inhibiting antibody
hemagglutination inhibition antibody
hemagglutination inhibition assay

HIAA hydroxyindoleacetic acid

5-HIAA 5-hydroxyindoleacetic acid

HIB *Haemophilus influenzae* type b (meningitis, vaccine); also HITB, HiTb
heart infusion broth
hemolytic immune body

HIBAC Health Insurance Benefits Advisory
Council

HIC Heart Information Center

H-ICD-A hospital adaptation of International
Classification of Diseases

HICHO high carbohydrate (diet)

HiCn cyanmethemoglobin

HID headache, insomnia, and depression (syndrome)
herniated intervertebral disc; also HIVD
human infectious dose
hyperkinetic impulse disorder

HIDA hepatic 2,6-dimethyliminodiacetic acid

HIE human intestinal epithelium
hyperimmunoglobulin E
hypoxic-ischemic encephalopathy

HIES hyperimmunoglobulin E syndrome

HIF higher integrative function
higher intellectual function
histoplasma tissue inhibitory factor
Historical Information Form

HIFBS heat-inactivated fetal bovine serum

HIFC hog intrinsic factor concentrate

HIFCS heat-inactivated fetal calf serum

HIFN, hIFN human interferon; also HuIFN

hIFNa human interferon type alpha

HIG hemolysis in gel
human immunoglobulin; also HIg, hIg

HIg, hIg human immunoglobulin; also HIG

HIH hypertensive intracerebral hemorrhage

HIHA high impulsiveness, high anxiety

HiHb hemiglobin (methemoglobin); also
HbMet, Met-Hb, MHB, MHb

HII Health Industries Institute
Health Insurance Institute
hemagglutination inhibition immunoassay

HIL hypoxic-ischemic lesion

HILA high impulsiveness, low anxiety

HIM hemopoietic inductive microenvironment
hepatitis-infectious mononucleosis
hexose phosphate isomerase
Hill Interaction Matrix (psychologic test)

HIMA Health Industry Manufacturers
Association

HIMC hepatic intramitochondrial crystalloid

HIMP high-dose intravenous methylprednisolone

HIMSS Healthcare Information and
Management Systems Society

HIMT hemagglutination inhibition morphine
test

Hind II restriction endonuclease from
Haemophilus influenzae

Hind III restriction endonuclease from
Haemophilus influenzae

HINCS heat-inactivated newborn calf serum

H inf hypodermoclysis infusion

Hint Hinton (flocculation test for syphilis)

HIO hypoiodidism
hypoiodite (salt of hypoiodous acid)

HIOMT hydroxyindole-*o*-methyl transferase

HIOS high index of suspicion

HIP health illness profile
health insurance plan
hospital insurance program
hot isostatic press
humoral immunocompetence profile
hydrostatic indifference point

Hip hip amputation

hippocampus; also HC

HIPCS health insurance purchasing corpora-
tions

HiPIP high-potential iron protein

HIPO hemihypertrophy, intestinal web, preau-
ricular skin tag, and congenital corneal
opacity (syndrome)
Hospital Indicators for Physicians Orders

HiPro high protein (diet); also HiProt, Hi Prot,
HP

HiProt, Hi Prot high protein (diet); also HiPro,
HP

HIR head injury routine
high irradiance response

HIRF histamine inhibitory releasing factor

HIS Hanover Intensive Score
Haptic Intelligence Scale
health information system
Health Intention Scale
Health Interview Survey
histidine; also H, HI, Hi, His, Hist, hist
hospital information system
hyperimmune serum
hyperimmunized suppressed

His histidine; also H, HI, Hi, HIS, Hist, hist
histidinyl

HISG human immune serum globulin

HISMS How I See Myself Scale (psychologic
test)

HISSG Hospital Information Systems Sharing
Group

HIST hospital in-service training

Hist, hist histamine; also H_2, HA, Hi
histidine; also H, HI, Hi, HIS, His
histidinemia
histology; also Histo, histol
history; also H, Hx, hx, Hy

HISTLINE History of Medicine On-Line

Histo histology; also Hist, hist, histol
histoplasmin skin test

histol histologic
histologist
histology; also Hist, hist, Histo

HIT hemagglutination inhibition test
heparin-induced thrombocytopenia
histamine inhalation test
histamine ion transfer
Holtzman Inkblot Technique
home intravenous therapy
hypertrophic infiltrative tendinitis

HIT—cont'd
hypertrophied inferior turbinate

HITB, HiTb *Haemophilus influenzae* type b (meningitis vaccube); also HIB

HITES hydrocortisone, insulin, transferrin, estradiol, and selenium

HITTS heparin-induced thrombosis-thrombo-cytopenia syndrome

HIU head injury unit
hyperplasia interstitialis uteri

HIV, hIV human immunodeficiency virus

HIVAT home intravenous antibiotic therapy

HIVD herniated intervertebral disc; also HID

HIVIG HIV immunoglobulin
hyperimmune intravenous immunoglobulin

HiVit high vitamin

HJ Hebra-Jadassohn (disease)
hepatojugular (reflux)
Howell-Jolly (bodies)

HJB Howell-Jolly bodies

HJR hepatojugular reflux

HK heat-killed
heel-to-knee (test); also H-K, HTK
hexokinase
Hoffa-Kastert (syndrome)
human kidney (cell)

H-K hand to knee (test)
heel-to-knee (test); also HK, HTK

H → K hand to knee (coordination)

HK1 hexokinase 1

HKAFO hip-knee-ankle-foot orthosis

HKAO hip-knee-ankle orthosis

HKC human kidney cell

HKH hyperkinetic heart

HKLM heat-killed *Listeria monocytogenes*

HKO hip-knee orthosis (splint)

HKS heel-knee-shin (test)
hyperkinesis syndrome

HL hairline
halflife (of radioactive element)
hallux limitus
haloperidol; also HAL
harelip
hearing level
hearing loss
heart and lungs; also H&L
heavy lifting
hectoliter; also hL, hl
hemolysis; also H, HEM, Hem
heparin lock; also H/L

Hickman line
histiocytic lymphoma
histocompatibility locus
Hodgkin's lymphoma
human leukocyte
human lymphocyte
hydrophil/lipophil (number)
hygienic laboratory
hyperlipidemia
hyperlipoproteinemia; also HLP
hypermetropia, latent; also Hl
hypertrichosis lanuginosa
lateral habenular (nucleus)

H/L heart disease, low risk
heparin lock; also HL
hydrophil to lipophil (ratio)
hyperopia, latent; also Hl

H&L heart and lungs; also HL

Hl hypermetropia, latent; also HL
hyperopia, latent; also H/L

hL, hl hectoliter; also HL

HLA heart, lungs, and abdomen
histocompatibility leukocyte antigen
histocompatibility locus antigen
homologous leukocyte antibody
human leukocyte antigen
human lymphocyte antibody
human lymphocyte antigen
hypoplastic left atrium

HLA human leukocyte antigen (system)

HLA-A, HLA-B, HLA-C, HLA-D, HLA-DR varieties of human leukocyte antigens

HLALD horse liver alcohol dehydrogenase

HLA-LD human lymphocyte antigen–lympho-cyte defined

HLA-SD human lymphocyte antigen–serologi-cally defined

HLB hydrophilic-lipophilic balance
hypotonic lysis buffer

HLBI human lymphoblastoid interferon

HLC heat loss center

HLCL human lymphoblastoid cell line

HLD haloperidol decanoate; also HD, HL-D
hepatolenticular degeneration
herniated lumbar disc
hypersensitivity lung disease
von Hippel-Lindau disease

HL-D haloperidol decanoate; also HD, HLD

HLDH heat-stable lactic dehydrogenase

HLE human leukocyte elastase

HLEG hydrolysate lactalbumin Earle's glucose

HLF heat-labile factor
human lung field
human lung fluid

HLFCB horizontal laminar flow clean benches

HLH human luteinizing hormone; also hLH
hypoplastic left heart (syndrome)

hLH human luteinizing hormone; also HLH

HLHS hypoplastic left heart syndrome

HLI hemolysis inhibition
human leukocyte interferon
human lymphocyte interferon

HLK heart, liver, and kidneys; also H-L-K

H-L-K heart, liver, and kidneys; also HLK

HLN hilar lymph node
human Lesch-Nyhan (cell)
hyperplastic liver nodule

H&L OK heart and lungs normal

HLP hepatic lipoperoxidation
hind leg paralysis
hyperlipoproteinemia; also HL

HLR heart-lung resuscitation
heart-lung resuscitator

HLS Health Learning System
Hippel-Lindau syndrome

HLT heart-lung transplantation
human lipotropin
human lymphocyte transformation; also hLT

hLT human lymphocyte transformation; also HLT

hlth health

HLV herpes-like virus
hypoplastic left ventricle

HM hand motion
hand movement(s)
harmonic mean
health maintenance
heart murmur
heavily muscled
Heine-Medin (disease)
hemifacial microsomia; also HFM
hepatic metabolism
hexamethylmelamine; also Hex, HMM, Hmm, HXM
Holter monitor
Holter monitoring
hospital management
human milk
hydatidiform mole
hyperimmune mouse
hyperopia, manifest; also Hm
hypoxic-metabolic

soft corn [L. *heloma molle*]

Hm hyperopia, manifest; also HM

hm hectometer

hm^2 square hectometer

hm^3 cubic hectometer

HMA hapten-modified agent
hemorrhages and microaneurysms

HMAC Health Manpower Advisory Council

HMAS hyperimmune mouse ascites (fluid)

HMB homatropine methylbromide
Horton-Magath-Brown (syndrome)

HMBA hexamethylene bisacetamide

HMC hand-mirror cell
health maintenance cooperative
heroin, morphine, and cocaine
hospital management committee
hydroxymethyl cytosine
hyoscine-morphine-codeine

HMCCMP human mammary carcinoma cell membrane proteinase

HMD hyaline membrane disease

HMDP hydroxymethylene diphosphonate

HMDS hexamethyldisilane
hexamethyldisilazane
hexamethyldisiloxane

HME Health Media Education
heat and moisture exchanger
heat, massage, and exercise; also HMX

HMETSC heavy metal screen

HMF hydroxymethylfurfural

HMG high mobility group
human menopausal gonadotropin; also hMG
hydroxymethylglutaric acid
hydroxymethylglutaryl

hMG human menopausal gonadotropin; also HMG

HMG CoA, HMG-CoA hepatic hydroxymethylglutaryl coenzyme A

HMI healed myocardial infarction

HMIS hospital medical information system

HMK high-molecular-weight kininogen; also HMWK
homemaking

HML, hML human milk lysozyme

HM&LP hand motion and light perception

HMM heavy meromyosin (of muscle)
hexamethylmelamine; also Hex, HM, Hmm, HXM

Hmm hexamethylmelamine; also Hex, HM, HMM, HXM

HMMA 4-hydroxy-3-methoxymandelic acid

HMO Health Maintenance Organization
heart minute output
Hückel molecular orbital

HMP hexose monophosphate
hexose monophosphate pathway
hot moist packs
human menopausal
hydromotive pressure

HMPA hexamethylphosphoramide

HMPDH 2-hydroxy-4-methylpentanoic acid
dehydrogenase

HMPG 4-(hydroxy-3-methoxyphenyl)ethylene
glycol
hydroxymethoxyphenylglycol

HMPS hexose monophosphate shunt; also
HMS

HMPT hexamethylphosphoric triamide

HMR histiocytic medullary reticulosis

H-mRNA H-chain messenger ribonucleic acid

HMRTE human milk reverse transcriptase
enzyme

HMS hexose monophosphate shunt; also
HMPS
high methacholine sensitivity
hypermobility syndrome
hypothetical mean strain

HMSA hydroxymethanesulphonic acid
Medicare Health Manpower Shortage Area

HMSAS hypertrophic muscular subaortic
stenosis

HMSN hereditary motor and sensory neuropathy

HMSS Hospital Management Systems Society
(now: HIMSS, Healthcare Information and
Management Systems Society)

HMT hematocrit; also C, Crit, crit, Hc, H'crit,
HCT, Hct, hemat
hexamethylenetetramine (methenamine); also
HMTA
histamine methyltransferase
hospital management team

hMT human molar thyrotropin

HMTA hexamethylenetetramine
(methenamine); also HMT

HMU hydroxymethyl uracil

HMW high molecular weight

HMWC high-molecular-weight component

HMWGP high-molecular-weight glycoprotein

HMWK high-molecular-weight kininogen;
also HMK

HMWM heavily muscled white male

HMW-NCF high-molecular-weight neutrophil
chemotactic factor

HMX heat, massage, and exercise; also HME

HN head and neck; also H&N
head nurse
Heller-Nelson (syndrome)
hemagglutinin neuraminidase; also HANA
hematemesis neonatorum
hemorrhage of newborn
hereditary nephritis
high nitrogen
hilar node
histamine-containing neuron
home nursing
hospitalman
human nutrition
hypertrophic neuropathy

HN2, HN$_2$ mechlorethamine (nitrogen mustard)

H&N head and neck; also HN

hn tonight [L. *hac nocte*]

HNA heparin-neutralizing activity

HNB human neuroblastoma
hydroxynitrobenzylbromide

HNC hypernephroma cell
hyperosmolar nonketotic coma
hyperoxic normocapnic
hypothalamo-neurohypophyseal complex

HNKDC hyperosmolar nonketotic diabetic
coma

HNKDS hyperosmolar nonketotic diabetic
state

HNLN hospitalization no longer necessary

H&N mot head and neck motion

HNP hereditary nephritic protein
herniated nucleus pulposus
human neurophysine

hnRNA heterogeneous nuclear ribonucleic acid

hnRNP heterogeneous nuclear ribonucleoprotein

HNS head and neck surgery
head, neck, and shaft (of bone)
home nursing supervisor

HNSHA hereditary nonspherocytic hemolytic
anemia

HNTD highest nontoxic dose

HNTLA Hiskey-Nebraska Test of Learning Aptitude

HNV has not voided

HO hand orthosis
Hematology-Oncology
heterotopic ossification; also HTO
high oxygen
hip orthosis
Holt-Oram (syndrome)
house officer
hyperbaric oxygen; also HBO, HbO$_2$
hypertrophic ossification

H/O, h/o history of

Ho holmium
horse; also H

H$_2$O water

HOA hip osteoarthritis
hypertrophic osteoarthritis

Ho antigen low-frequency blood group antigen

HOAP-BLEO hydroxydaunomycin, Oncovin, Ara-C (cytarabine), prednisone, and bleomycin

HoaRhLG horse anti-rhesus lymphocyte globulin

HoaTTG horse anti-tetanus toxoid globulin

HOB head of bed

HOBDH hydroxybutyrate dehydrogenase; also HBD, HBDH

HOB UPSOB head of bed up for shortness of breath

HOC Health Officer Certificate
human ovarian cancer
hydroxycorticoid; also HC

HOCM high-osmolar contrast medium; also HOM
hypertrophic obstructive cardiomyopathy

hoc vesp this evening [L. *hoc vespere*]; also hv

HOD hereditary opalescent dentin
Hoffer-Osmond Diagnostic
hospital day; also HD
hyperbaric oxygen drenching

HOF hepatic outflow

HofF height of fundus

Hoff Hoffmann (reflex); also H

HOG halothane, oxygen, and gas (nitrous oxide)

HOGA hyperornithinemia with gyrate atrophy

HOH hard of hearing; also HH

HOI hospital onset of infection

hypoiodous acid

HoIg horse immunoglobulin

HOM hexamethylmelamine, Oncovin, and methotrexate
high-osmolar contrast medium; also HOCM

HOME Home Observation for Measurement of the Environment
Home Oriented Maternity Experience

Homeo homeopathy; also Homeop

Homeop homeopathy; also Homeo

HOMO highest occupied molecular orbital
homosexual; also H, homo, HS

homo homosexual; also H, HOMO, HS

homolat homolateral

HOOD hereditary osteo-onychodysplasia

HOODS hereditary osteo-onychodysplasia syndrome

HOOI Hall Occupational Orientation Inventory

HOP high oxygen pressure
hydroxydaunomycin (doxorubicin), Oncovin, and prednisone

HOPD hospital outpatient department

HOPE Healthcare Options Plan Entitlement
health-oriented physical education
holistic orthogonal parameter estimation

HOPI history of present illness; also HPI

HOPP hepatic occluded portal pressure

hor horizontal; also H, h, horiz

hor decub at bedtime [L. *hora decumbendi* (at the hour of lying down)]; also h, hd,

hor interm at the intermediate hours [L. *horis intermediis*]

horiz horizontal; also H, h, hor

hor som at bedtime [L. *hora somni* (hour of sleep)]; also h, HS, hs, h som

hor un spat at the end of one hour [L. *horae unius spatio*]; also hor un spatio

hor un spatio at the end of one hour [L. *horae unius spatio*]; also hor un spat

HOS human osteosarcoma

HoS horse serum; also HS

Hosp, hosp hospital; also H
hospitalization; also H, HX

HOST hypo-osmotic shock treatment

HOT human old tuberculin
hyperbaric oxygen therapy

HP Haemophilus pleuropneumonia
Haemophilus pleuropneumoniae

HP—cont'd
  halogen phosphorus
  handicapped person
  haptoglobin; also HAP, HAPTO, Hp, Hpb, Hpt
  Harding-Passey (melanoma)
  hard palate
  Harvard pump
  hastening phenomenon
  health professional
  heater probe
  heat production
  heel to patella; also H ↑ P
  hemiparesis; also hemi   hemipelvectomy
  hemiplegia; also hemi, Hp
  hemoperfusion
  heparin; also H, HEP
  highly purified
  high potency
  high-power
  high pressure
  high protein (diet); also HiPro, HiProt, Hi Prot
  Hodgen and Pearson (suspension traction); als H&P
  horizontal plane
  horsepower; also hp
  hospital participation
  hot pack(s)
  hot pad
  house physician
  human pituitary
  hybridoma product
  hydrocollator pack
  hydrogen peroxide
  hydrophilic petrolatum
  hydrophobic protein
  hydrostatic pressure
  hydroxyproline; also HYP, Hyp, hyp, hypro
  hydroxypyruvate
  hyperparathyroidism; also HPT, HPTH
  hyperphoria; also H
  hypersensitivity pneumonitis
  hypertension plus proteinuria
  hypoparathyroidism
  hypopharynx

H&P history and physical (examination); also H and P, H+P, HPE
  Hodgen and Pearson (suspension traction); also HP

H+P history and physical (examination); also H and P, H&P, HPE

H → P heel to patella; also HP

Hp haptoglobin; also HAP, HAPTO, HP, Hpb, Hpt

hematoporphyrin
hemiplegia; also hemi, HP

hp heaping
  horsepower; also HP

HPA alpha-haptoglobin
  Helix pomatia agglutinin
  hemagglutinating penicillin antibody
  Hereford Parental Attitude (survey)
  heteropolyanion
  human papilloma (virus)
  hydroxyphenylacetic acid; also HPAA
  hypothalamic-pituitary-adrenal (axis)
  hypothalamo-pituitary-adrenal (function)
  hypothalamo-pituitary-adrenocortical (system)

HPAA hydroperoxyarachidonic acid
  hydroxyphenylacetic acid; also HPA
  hypothalamic-pituitary-adrenal axis

HPAC high-performance affinity chromatography

Hpb haptoglobin; also HAP, HAPTO, HP, Hp, Hpt

HPBC hyperpolarizing bipolar cell

HPBF hepatotropic portal blood factor

HPBL human peripheral blood leukocyte

HPC hemangiopericytoma
  hippocampal pyramidal cell
  history of present complaint
  hydroxyphenylcinchoninic (acid)
  hydroxypropyl cellulose

HPD hematoporphyrin derivative
  highly probably drunk
  high protein diet
  home peritoneal dialysis

HP-D Hough-Powell digitizer

HPE hepatic portoenterostomy
  high permeability edema
  history and physical examination; also H and P, H&P, H+P
  hydrostatic pulmonary edema

HPEC hydroxypropylethylcellulose

HPETE hydroperoxyeicosatetraenoic acid

HPF heparin-precipitable fraction
  hepatic plasma flow
  high-pass filter
  high-power field (microscope); also hpf
  hypolcaloric protein feeding

hpf high power field (microscope); also HPF

HPFH hereditary persistence of fetal hemoglobin

hPFSH, HPFSH human pituitary follicle-stimulating hormone

HPG, hPG human pituitary gonadotropin
hypothalamic-pituitary-gonadal (axis)
para-hydroxyphenylglycine

HPGe high-purity germanium

HPH halothane-percent-hour

HPI hepatic perfusion index
Heston Personality Inventory (Test)
history of present illness; also HOPI
human proinsulin
human protein index

HPL human parotid lysozyme
human peripheral lymphocyte
human placental lactogen; also hPL
hyperpexia

hPL human placental lactogen; also HPL

HPLA hydroxyphenyllactic acid

HPLAC high-pressure liquid affinity chromatography

hPLAP human placental alkaline phosphatase

HPLC high-performance liquid chromatography
high-power liquid chromatography
high-pressure liquid chromatography

HPM Harding-Passey melanoma
hemiplegic migraine

HPMC human peripheral mononuclear cell
hydroxypropyl methylcellulose

HPN home parenteral nutrition
hypertension; also HT, HTN, htn, hypn

hpn our own purgative draft [L. *haustus purgans noster*]

HPNS high-pressure neurologic syndrome

HPO high-pressure oxygen
high-pressure oxygenation
hydroperoxide
hydrophilic ointment
hypertrophic pulmonary osteoarthritis
hypertrophic pulmonary osteoarthropathy

HPP hereditary pyropoikilocytosis
history of presenting problems
human pancreatic polypeptide; also hPP
hydroxyphenylpyruvate
hydroxypyrazolopyrimidine

hPP human pancreatic polypeptide; also HPP

2HPP two hours postprandial (blood sugar) [L. *post prandia* (after meals)]

HPPA hydroxyphenylpyruvic acid

HPPH hydroxyphenyl-phenylhydantoin

HPPO high partial pressure of oxygen
hydroxyphenyl pyruvate oxidase

HPPR allopurinol-1-ribonucleoside (4-hydroxypyrazolo[3,4-*d*]pyrimidine-1-ribonucleoside)

HPR hospital peer review

HPr, hPr human prolactin; also HPRL

HPRL human prolactin; also HPr, hPr

HPRP human platelet-rich plasma

HPRT hot plate reaction time
hypoxanthine phosphoribosyltransferase

HPS hematoxylin, phloxine, and saffron
Hermansky-Pudlak syndrome
high protein supplement
His-Purkinje system
human placental somatomammotropin
human platelet suspension
hypertrophic pyloric stenosis
hypothalamic pubertal syndrome

HPSL Health Professions Student Loan

HPSTI human pancreatic secretory trypsin inhibitor

HPT histamine provocation test
hot plate test
human placental thyrotropin; also hPT
hyperparathyroidism; also HP, HPTH
hypothalamic-pituitary-thyroid

Hpt haptoglobin; also HAP, HAPTO, HP, Hp, Hpb

hPT human placental thyrotropin; also HPT

HPTH hyperparathyroid hormone
hyperparathyroidism; also HP, HPT

hPTH human parathyroid hormone I_{34} (teriparatide)

HPTIN human pancreatic trypsin inhibitor

HPTM home prothrombin time monitoring

HPV *Haemophilus pertussis* vaccine
hepatic portal vein
human papilloma virus
human parvovirus
hypoxic pulmonary vasoconstriction

HPVD hypertensive pulmonary vascular disease

HPV-DE high-passage virus–duck embryo (cell)

HPV-DK high-passage virus–dog kidney (cell)

HPVG hepatic portal venous gas

HPX high peroxide-containing (cell)
hypophysectomized; also HX, hypox
partial hepatectomy

Hpx hemopexin; also Hx

HPZ high-pressure zone

H₂Q ubiquinol

HQC hydroquinone cream

HR hallux rigidus
Halstead-Reitan (battery); also HRB
Hamman-Rich (syndrome)
Harrington rod
heart rate; also HRT
hemirectococcygeus
hemorrhagic retinopathy
heterosexual relations (scale)
higher rate
high resolution
hormonal response
hormone receptor
hormone-responsive
hospital record
hospital report
hour; also H, h, hr
Howship-Romberg (syndrome)
human resources
hydroxyethylrutosides (treatment of venous disorders)
hyperimmune reaction
hypoxic responder

2HR two-hour

H&R hysterectomy and radiation

Hr blood type factor

hr hour; also H, h, HR

HRA Health Resources Administration
health risk appraisal
heart rate audiometry
high right atrial
high right atrium
histamine-releasing activity
Human Resources Administration

HRAE high right atrium electrocardiogram

HRANA histone-reactive antinuclear antibody

HRB Halstead-Reitan Battery; also HR
histamine release from basophils

HRBC horse red blood cell(s)

HRxBP heart rate x peak systolic blood pressure

HRC help-rejecting complainer
high-resolution chromatography
horse red cell
human renal carcinoma
human rights committee

HRCT high-resolution computed tomography

HRD heroin-related death

HRE high-resolution electrocardiogram
high-resolution electrocardiography
hormone-receptor enzyme

HREC hepatic reticuloendothelial cell

HREH high-renin essential hypertension

HREM high-resolution electron microscopy

HRF Harris return flow
histamine-releasing factor

HRH hypothalamic-releasing hormone

HRI Harrington rod instrumentation

HRIG, HRIg human rabies immune globulin
human rabies immunoglobulin

HRL head rotated left

HRLA human reovirus-like agent

HRLM high-resolution light microscopy

HRMS high-resolution mass spectrometry

hRNA heterogeneous ribonucleic acid

HRP high right parasternal (view)
high-risk pregnancy
histidine-rich protein
horseradish peroxidase

HRPD Hamburg Rating Scale for Psychiatric Disorders

HRR Hardy-Rand-Ritter (color vision test kit)
head rotated right
heart rate range

HRRI heart rate retardation index

HRS Hamilton Rating Scale
hepatorenal syndrome
hormone receptor site
humeroradial synostosis

HRSA Health Resources and Services Administration

HRS-D Hamilton Rating Scale for Depression

HRT half relaxation time
heart rate; also HR
hormone replacement therapy

HRTE human reverse transcriptase enzyme

HRTEM high-resolution transmission electron microscopy

HRV heart rate variability
human rhinovirus
human rotavirus

HRVL human reovirus-like

HS at bedtime [L. *hora somni* (hour of sleep)]; also h, hor som, hs, h20som
half strength
Hallervorden-Spatz (syndrome)
hamstrings; also Hams
hand surgery
Hartmann's solution
head sign
head sling
healthy subject

HS—cont'd
  heart sound(s)
  heat stable
  heavy smoker
  heel spur
  heelstick; also H
  Hegglin's syndrome
  heme synthetase
  Henoch-Schönlein (syndrome)
  heparin sulfate
  hereditary spherocytosis
  herpes simplex
  hidradenitis suppurativa
  high school
  Hollönder-Simons (disease)
  homologous serum
  homosexual; also H, HOMO, homo
  Hopelessness Scale
  horizontally selective (visual cell)
  Horner's syndrome
  horse serum; also HoS
  hospital ship
  hospital staff
  hospital stay
  hour of sleep
  House Surgeon
  human serum
  Hurler's syndrome
  hypereosinophilic syndrome
  hypersensitivity
  hypertonic saline

H/S helper to suppressor (ratio)

H → S heel to shin (test); also HTS

H&S hemorrhage and shock
  hysterectomy and sterilization

H₂S Hering's law–EOM innervation, both eyes
  Sherrington's law–EOM innervation, one eye

Hs hypochondriasis

hs at bedtime [L. *hora somni* (hour of sleep)];
  also h, HS, hor som, h som

HSA Hazardous Substances Act
  health service area
  Health Services Administration
  Health Systems Agency
  horse serum albumin
  human serum albumin; also HuSA
  hypersomnia-sleep apnea (syndrome)

HSAG HEPES (hydroxyethylpiperazine
  ethanesulfonic acid)-saline-albumin-gelatin

HSAP heat-stable alkaline phosphatase

HSAS hypertrophic subaortic stenosis; also HSS

HSBG heel-stick blood gas

HSC Hand-Schüller-Christian (disease)

health sciences center
health screening center
hemopoietic stem cell
horizontal semicircular canal
human skin collagenase

HSCA Health Sciences Communications
  Association

HSCD Hand-Schüller-Christian disease

HSCL Hopkins Symptom Checklist

HS-CoA reduced coenzyme A

HSD honest significance difference
  hydroxysteroid dehydrogenase

HSDA high single dose alternate day

HSDI Health Self-Determination Index

HSE health and safety executive
  herpes simplex encephalitis
  human serum esterase

Hse homoserine

HSF heated soybean flower
  histamine-induced suppressor factor
  histamine-sensitizing factor
  hydrazine-sensitive factor
  hypothalamic secretory factor

HSG herpes simplex genitalis
  hysterosalpingogram
  hysterosalpingography; also HSP

HSGF hematopoietic stem-cell growth factor

hSGF human skeletal growth factor

HSGP human sialoglycoprotein

HSHC hemisuccinate of hydrocortisone

HSI heat stress index
  human seminal plasma inhibitor

HSK herpes simplex keratitis

HSL herpes simplex labialis

HSLC high-speed liquid chromatography

HSM hepatosplenomegaly
  holosystolic murmur

HSMHA Health Services and Mental Health
  Administration

HSN Hansen-Street nail
  hereditary sensory neuropathy
  herpes simplex neonatorum

HSOD human superoxide dismutase

h som at bedtime [L. *hora somni* (hour of
  sleep)]; also h, hor som, HS, hs

HSP Health Systems Plan
  heat-shock protein
  hemostatic screening profile
  Henoch-Schönlein purpura
  human serum prealbumin
  human serum protein
  hysterosalpingography; also HSG

H spike His' bundle electrogram deflection

HSPM hippocampal synaptic plasma membrane

HSPQ High School Personality Questionnaire

HSQB Health Standards and Quality Bureau

HSR Harleco synthetic resin
heated serum reagent
homogeneous staining region (of chromosome)

HSRA Health Services and Resources Administration

HSRC Health Services Research Center
Human Subjects Review Committee

HSRD hypertension secondary to renal disease

HSRI Health Systems Research Institute

HSRS Health-Sickness Rating Scale
Hess School Readiness Scale

HSS Hallervorden-Spatz syndrome
hepatic stimulator substance
high-speed supernatant (fraction)
hypertrophic subaortic stenosis; also HSAS

HSSE high soap suds enema

HST health screening test(s)
Hemoccult slide test
horseshoe tear

HSTF heat-shock transcription factor
human serum thymus factor

HSTS human-specific thyroid stimulator

HSV herpes simplex virus
highly selective vagotomy

HSV 1 herpes simplex virus, type I; also HSV I

HSV 2 herpes simplex virus, type II; also HSV II

HSVE herpes simplex virus encephalitis

HSV I herpes simplex virus, type I; also HSV 1

HSV II herpes simplex virus, type II; also HSV 2

HSVtk herpes simplex virus thymidine kinase

HSyn heme synthase

HT hammertoe
Hand Test (psychologic test)
Hashimoto's thyroiditis
hearing test
hearing threshold
heart; also H, He, Ht, ht
heart test
heart tone(s); also ht
heart transplant
heart transplantation
height; also H, h, Hgt, Ht, ht

hemagglutination titer
high temperature
high tension; also ht
Histologic Technician
Histologic Technologist
histotechnology
home treatment
hospital treatment
Hubbard tank
Huhner's test
human thrombin
hydrocortisone test
hydrotherapy; also hydro
5-hydroxytryptamine (serotonin); also 5-HT, HTA
hyperopia, total; also Ht
hypertension; also HPN, HTN, htn, hypn
hyperthyroidism
hypertransfusion
hypertropia
hypodermic tablet
hypothalamus; also H, Ht, Hth, Hyp, hyp

3-HT 3-hydroxytyramine (dopamine)

^{3}HT tritiated thymidine

5-HT 5-hydroxytryptamine (serotonin); also HT, HTA

H&T hospitalization and treatment

H(T) intermittent hypertropia

Ht heart; also H, He, HT, ht
heat; also ht
height; also H, h, Hgt, HT, ht
heterozygote
hot; also H
hypermetropia, total
hyperopia, total; also HT
hypothalamus; also H, HT, Hth, Hyp, hyp

ht a draft, a drink [L. *haustus*]; also H, h, haust
heart; also H, He, HT, Ht
heart tone(s); also HT
heat; also Ht
height; also H, h, Hgt, HT, Ht
high tension; also HT

HTA heterophil transplantation antigen
human thymocyte antigen
5-hydroxytryptamine (serotonin); also HT, 5-HT
hypophysiotropic area (of hypothalamus)

HTACS human thyroid adenylcyclase stimulator

ht aer heated aerosol; also HA

HT(ASCP) Histologic Technologist (certified by the Board of Registry of the American Society of Clinical Pathologists)

HTAT human tetanus antitoxin

HTB hot tub bath
house tube (feeding)
human tumor bank

HTC hepatoma cell(s)
hepatoma tissue culture
homozygous typing cell
hypertensive crisis

HTCA human tumor colony assay

HTCVD hypertensive cardiovascular disease;
also HCVD

HTD human therapeutic dose

HTDW heterosexual development of women

HTF heterothyrotropic factor(s)
house tube feeding

HTG hypertriglyceridemia

H-TGL hepatic triglyceride lipase

HTH homeostatic thymus hormone

Hth hypothalamus; also H, HT, Ht, Hyp, hyp

HTHD hypertensive heart disease; also HHD

HTI hemisphere thrombotic infarction
human tetanus immunoglobulin; also hTIg

HTIG homologous tetanus immune globulin

hTIg human tetanus immunoglobulin; also HTI

HTK heel to knee (test); also HK, H-K

HTL hamster tumor line
hearing threshold level
histologic technologist
histotechnologist
human T-cell leukemia
human T-cell lymphoma
human thymic leukemia

HTLA high titer, low acidity
human T-lymphocyte antigen

HTL(ASCP) Histotechnologist (certified by
the Board of Registry of the American
Society of Clinical Pathologists)

HTLV human T-cell leukemia virus
human T-cell lymphoma virus
human T-cell lymphotropic virus

HTLV$_1$ human T-cell lymphotropic virus, type
1; also HTLV I

HTLV$_2$ human T-cell lymphotropic virus, type
2; also HTLV II

HTLV I human T-cell lymphotropic virus, type
1; also HTLV$_1$

HTLV II human T-cell lymphotropic virus,
type 2; also HTLV $_2$

HTLV III human T-cell lymphotropic virus,
type III

HTLV-III/LAL human T-cell lymphotropic
virus, type III/lymphadenopathy associated
virus

HTLV-MA human T-cell leukemia virus-associated membrane antigen

HTN Hantaan (virus)
hypertension; also HPN, HT, htn, hypn
hypertensive nephropathy

htn hypertension; also HPN, HT, HTN, hypn

HTO heterotopic ossification; also HO
high tibial osteotomy
hospital transfer order

HTOH hydroxytryptophol

HTP House-Tree-Person (Projective Technique
psychologic test)
hydroxytryptophan
hypothromboplastinemia

5-HTP 5-hydroxytryptophan

HTPN home total parenteral nutrition

HTR hemolytic transfusion reaction
hypermetropia, right

HTRS high-temperature reflectance spectroscopy

HTS head traumatic syndrome
heel to shin (test); also H ARROW — S
hemangioma-thrombocytopenia syndrome
human thyroid-stimulating (hormone); also
hTS
human thyroid stimulator; also hTS

hTS human thyroid-stimulating (hormone);
also HTS
human thyroid stimulator; also HTS

hTSAb human thyroid-stimulating antibody

HTSCA human tumor stem cell assay

HTSH, hTSH human thyroid-stimulating hormone

HTST high temperature–short time (pasteurization)

HTT hand thrust test

HTV herpes-type virus

HTVD hypertensive vascular disease; also
HVD

HTX hemothorax
histrionicotoxin

HU head unit
heat unit
hemagglutinating unit; also HAU
hemagglutinin unit
hemolytic unit
Hounsfield unit; also H

HU—cont'd
  human urinary
  human urine
  hydroxyurea; also HUR, HYD
  hyperemia unit
  hyperemic unit

Hu human; also H, h

HUC hypouricemia

HU-FSH human urinary follicle-stimulating
  hormone

HUI headache unit index

HUIFM human leukocyte interferon milieu

HuIFN human interferon; also HIFN, hIFN

HUIS high-dose urea in invert sugar

HUK human urinary kallikrein

HUM heat (or hot packs), ultrasound, and
  massage
  hematourimetry

hum humerus

HUMO highest unoccupied molecular orbital

HUP Hospital Utilization Project

HUR hydroxyurea; also HU, HYD

HURA health in underserved rural areas

HURT hospital utilization review team

HUS hemolytic-uremic syndrome
  hyaluronidase unit for semen

HuSA human serum albumin; also HSA

husb husband; also H

HUTHAS human thymus antiserum

HUTI human urinary trypsin inhibitor

HUV human umbilical vein

HUVEC human umbilical vein endothelial cells

HV hallux valgus
  Hantaan virus
  has voided
  heart volume
  Hemovac
  hepatic vein
  hepatic venous
  herpes virus
  high voltage
  high volume
  home visit
  hospital visit
  hyperventilation

H&V hemigastrectomy and vagotomy;
  also H and V

hv this evening [L. *hoc vespere*]; also hoc vesp

HVA homovanillic acid

HVc hyperstriatum ventrale, pars caudale

HVD hypertensive vascular disease; also HTVD
  hypoxic ventilatory drive

HVE hepatic venous effluence
  high-voltage electrophoresis

HVEM high-voltage electron microscope

HVF hepatocycle volume fraction

HVFP hepatic vein free pressure

HVG hematoxylin and van Gieson (stain)
  host versus graft (disease, response)

HVGS high-voltage galvanic stimulation (physical therapy)

HVH *Herpesvirus hominis*

HVHMA *Herpesvirus hominis* membrane antigen

HVID horizontal visible iris diameter

HVJ hemagglutinating virus of Japan

HVL, hvl half-value layer

HVLP high volume, low pressure

HVLT high-velocity lead therapy

HVM high-velocity missile
  hypothalamic ventromedial (nucleus)

HVP herpes virus Papio

HVPE high-voltage paper electrophoresis

HVPG hepatic venous pressure gradient

HVR hypervariable region
  hypoxic ventilatory response

HVS herpesvirus of Saimiri
  herpesvirus sensitivity
  hyperventilation syndrome
  hyperviscosity syndrome

H vs A home against advice (home versus
  advice)

HVSD hydrogen-detected ventricular septal
  defect

HVT half-value thickness
  herpesvirus of turkeys

HVTEM high-voltage transmission electron
  microscopy

HVUS hypocomplementemic vasculitis
  urticaria syndrome

HW Hayem-Widal (syndrome)
  healing well
  heart weight
  hemisphere width
  heparin well
  Hertwig-Weyers (syndrome)
  His-Werner (disease)
  housewife

HWB, hwb hot water bottle

HWE hot water extract

HWOK heel walking normal (OK)

HWP hepatic wedge pressure
hot wet pack
Hutchinson-Weber-Pentz (syndrome)

HWRS Habits of Work and Recreation Survey

HWS hot water soluble

HWY hundred woman years (of exposure)

HX histiocytosis X
hospitalization; also H, Hosp, hosp
hydrogen exchange
hypophysectomized; also HPX, hypox

Hx hemopexin; also Hpx
hexyl
history; also H, Hist, hist, hx, Hy
hypoxanthine; also Hyp, hyp

hx history; also H, Hist, hist, Hx, Hy

2-HxG di(hydroxyethyl)glycine

HXIS hard x-ray imaging spectrometer

HXM hexamethylmelamine; also Hex HM,
HMM, Hmm

HXR hypoxanthine riboside

HX-XO hypoxanthine-xanthine oxidase (system)

HY hypophysis; also hyp

Hy history; also H, Hist, hist, Hx, hx
hydraulic(s); also hydr
hydrostatic(s); also Hyd
hypermetropia; also H, h
hyperopia; also H, h
hypothenar
hysteria; also hy, hys, Hyst, hyst

hy hysteria; also Hy, hys, Hyst, hyst

HYD hydralazine; also HDZ
hydrated to hydration
hydroxyurea; also HU, HUR

Hyd hydrocortisone; also HC, HCT
hydrostatic(s); also Hy

hyd and tur hydration and turgor

hydr hydraulic(s); also Hy

hydrarg mercury [L. *hydrargyrum* (silver
water)]; also Hg

hydro hydrotherapy; also HT

hydrox hydroxyzine

Hyg, hyg hygiene; also H
hygienic; also H
hygienist; also H

HYL hyaline
hydroxylysine; also Hyl

Hyl hydroxylysine; also HYL
hydroxylysyl

HYNP hypersegmented neutrophil

HYP hydroxyproline; also HP, Hyp, hyp, hypro
hypnosis; also hypno

Hyp hydroxyproline; also HP, HYP, hyp, hypro
hyperresonance; also hyp
hypertrophy; also hyp
hypothalamus; also H, HT, Ht, Hth, hyp
hypoxanthine; also hyp, Hx

hyp hydroxyproline; also HP, HYP, Hyp, hypro
hypalgesia
hyperresonance; also Hyp
hypertrophy; also Hyp
hypodermic; also H, h, (H)
hypophysectomy; also HE
hypophysis; also HY
hypothalamus; also H, HT, Ht, Hth, Hyp
hypoxanthine; also Hyp, Hx

hyper A hyperactive

hyperal, hyper-al hyperalimentation; also HA,
HAL

hyper-IgE hyperimmunoglobulinemia E

hyperpara hyperparathyroidism

hypes hypesthesia

hyper T&A hypertrophy of tonsils and adenoids

hypn hypertension; also HPN, HT, HTN, htn

hypno hypnosis; also HYP

hypo hypochromasia
hypochromia
hypodermic (injection)
under [Gr. *hypo*]

hypo A hypoactive

hypox hypophysectomized; also HPX, HX

HypRF hypothalamic releasing factor

hypro hydroxyproline; also HP, HYP, Hyp, hyp

hys hysterectomy; also Hyst, hyst, Hyster, hyster
hysteria; also Hy, hy, Hyst, hyst
hysterical; also Hyst, hyst

Hyst, hyst hysterectomy; also hys, Hyster, hyster
hysteria; also Hy, hy, hys
hysterical; also hys

Hyster, hyster hysterectomy; also hys, Hyst,
hyst

HZ herpes zoster

Hz hertz

HZFO hamster zona-free ovum (test)

HZO herpes zoster ophthalmicus

HZV herpes zoster virus

I

I IOTA, UPPER CASE, ninth letter of the Greek alphabet

ι iota, lower case, ninth letter of the Greek alphabet

I antigen in the I blood group system
implantation; also IP
impression; also IMP, imp
inactive; also inac
incisor (permanent)
increased
independent; also ind, INDEP
index; also ind
indicated; also indic
induction (of labor); also Ind, ind
inhalation; also INH, inhal
inhibiting; also inhib
inhibition; also inhib
inhibitor; also inhib
initial; also int
inosine;also INO, Ino
insoluble; also i, insol
inspiration; also Insp, inspir
inspiratory (time)
inspired (gas)
insulin; also IN, In, INS
intact (bag of waters)
intake
intensity
intensity of electrical current (in amperes)
intensity of magnetism
intercalary (congenital limb absence)
intermediate; also INT, int, Intmd
intestine; also int, Intest, intest
iodide
iodine
ionic strength; also *I*
iris
isochromosome; also i
isoleucine (one-letter notation); also Ilc, ILE, Ile, Ileu, ISL
isotope
isotropic (band or disk in striated muscle fiber)
luminous intensity
moment of inertia
permanent incisor
roman numeral one
vector cardiography electrode (right midaxillary line)

¹²³I iodine 123, radioactive iodine; halflife, 13.3 hours

¹²⁵I iodine 125, radioactive iodine; halflife, 60 days

¹³⁰I iodine 130, radioactive iodine; halflife, 12.3 ± 0.1 hours

¹³¹I iodine 131, radioactive iodine; halflife, 8.07 ± 0.009 days

¹³²I iodine 132, radioactive iodine; halflife, 2.3 hours

I electric current
intensity (of radiant energy)
ionic strength; also I

Ɪ integer

i antigen in the I blood group system
archaic symbol for *meso-*
incisor (deciduous)
insoluble; also I, insol
isochromosome; also I
optically inactive (chemical)

i optically inactive by internal compensation

IA ibotenic acid; also ibo
image amplification
immune adherence
immunobiologic activity
impedance angle
inactive alcoholic
incidental appendectomy
incurred accidentally
Indian-American (Native American)
indolaminergic-accumulating (cells)
indulin agar
infantile apnea
infantile autism
infected area
inferior angle
inhibitory antigen
internal auditory
intra-alveolar
intra-amniotic; also i am
intra-aortic
intra-arterial; also ia
intra-articular
intra-atrial
intra-auricular
intrinsic activity
isonicotinic acid

I&A, I/A irrigation and aspiration

Ia immune region-associated antigen
immune response gene-associated antigen

ia intra arterial; also IA

IAA imidazoleacetic acid

indole-3-acetic acid; also I-3-AA
infectious agent, arthritis
interruption of aortic arch
iodoacetic acid

I-3-AA indole-3-acetic acid; also IAA

IAAR imidazoleacetic acid ribonucleotide

IAB Industrial Accident Board
intra-abdominal
intra-aortic balloon

IABA intra-aortic balloon assistance

IABC intra-aortic balloon catheter
intra-aortic balloon counterpulsation; also
IABCP

IABCP intra-aortic balloon counterpulsation;
also IABC

IABM idiopathic aplastic bone marrow

IABP intra-aortic balloon pump; also IBP
intra-aortic balloon pumping; also IBP

IABPA intra-aortic balloon pumping assistance

IAC ineffective airway clearance
internal auditory canal
interposed abdominal compression
intra-arterial chemotherapy
Inventory of Anger Communications

IACB intra-aortic counterpulsation balloon

IAC-CPR interposed abdominal compressions
–cardiopulmonary resuscitation

IACD implantable automatic cardioverter-
defibrillator
intra-atrial conduction defect

IACP intra-aortic counterpulsation

IACR International Association of Cancer
Registries

IAD inactivating dose
inhibiting antibiotic dose
internal absorbed dose

IADH inappropriate antidiuretic hormone

IADHS inappropriate antidiuretic hormone
syndrome

IADL instrumental activities of daily living
(scale)

IADR International Association for Dental
Research

IADS immunoadsorbent

IAds immunoadsorption

IA DSA intra-arterial digital subtraction
angiography

IAE intra-arterial electrocardiogram
intra-atrial electrocardiogram

IAEA International Atomic Energy Agency

IAET International Association for
Enterostomal Therapy

IAFI infantile amaurotic familial idiocy

IAGP International Association of Geographic
Pathology

IAGT indirect antiglobulin test; also IAT, IDAT

IAGUS International Association of Genito-
Urinary Surgeons

IAH idiopathic adrenal hyperplasia
implantable artificial heart

IAHA idiopathic autoimmune hemolytic
anemia
immune adherence hemagglutination
immune adherence hemagglutination assay

IAHD idiopathic acquired hemolytic disease

IAI intra-abdominal infection

IAM Institute of Aviation Medicine
internal acoustic meatus
internal auditory meatus

i am intra-amniotic; also IA

IAN idiopathic aseptic necrosis
intern admission note

IANC International Anatomical Nomenclature
Committee

IANC-BR International Anatomical
Nomenclature Committee, Birmingham
revision, 1933

I and O intake and output; also I&O, I/O

IAO immediately after onset
intermittent aortic occlusion

IAP immunosuppressive acidic protein
innervated antral pouch
inosinic acid pyrophosphorylase
intermittent acute porphyria
International Academy of Pathology
islet-activating protein

IAPB International Association for the
Prevention of Blindness (now: International
Agency for the Prevention of Blindness)

IAPP insulinoma amyloid polypeptide
International Association for Preventive
Pediatrics

IARC International Agency for Research on
Cancer

IAR immediate asthmatic reaction
inhibitory anal reflex
iodine-azide reaction

IARF ischemic acute renal failure

IARSA idiopathic acquired refractory sideroblastic anemia

IAS idiopathic ankylosing spondylitis
immunosuppressive acidic substance
infant apnea syndrome
interatrial septum
interatrial shunting
internal anal sphincter
intra-amniotic saline (infusion)

IASA interatrial septal aneurysm

IASD interatrial septal defect; also ISD
interauricular septal defect

IASH isolated asymmetric septal hypertrophy

IASHS Institute for Advanced Study of Human
Sexuality

IAT immunoaugmentative therapy
indirect antiglobulin test; also IAGT, IDAT
instillation abortion time
intraoperative autologous transfusion
invasive activity test
iodine-azide test
Iowa Achievement Test

IAV interactive video
intermittent assisted ventilation
intra-arterial vasopressin

IAVM intramedullary arteriovenous malformation

IB Ibrahim-Beck (disease)
ileal bypass
immune balance
immune body; also IK
inclusion body; also IncB
index of body build
infectious bronchitis
isolation bed

I-B interbody (vertebral)

ib in the same place [L. *ibidem*]; also ibid

IBA isobutyric acid

IBAR Inter-African Bureau for Animal
Resources (Nairobi, Kenya)

IBAT intravascular bronchoalveolar tumor

IBB intestinal brush border

IBBB intra-blood-brain barrier

IBBBB incomplete bilateral bundle-branch
block

IBC Institutional Biosafety Committee
iodine-binding capacity
iron-binding capacity
isobutyl cyanoacrylate; also IBCA

IBCA isobutyl cyanoacrylate; also IBC

IBD infectious bowel disease
infectious bursal disease

inflammatory bowel disease
irritable bowel disease
ischemic bowel disease

IBED Inter-African Bureau for Epizootic
Diseases (now: IBAR, Inter-African Bureau
for Animal Resources)

IB-EP immunoreactive beta-endomorphin

IBF immature brown fat (cell)
immunoglobulin-binding factor

IBG insoluble bone gelatin

IBGS intravascular blood gas system

IBI intermittent bladder irrigation
ischemic brain infarction

ibid in the same place [L. *ibidem*]; also ib

IBILI indirect bilirubin; also IDBR

IBK infectious bovine keratoconjunctivitis

IBL immunoblastic lymphadenopathy

IBM inclusion body myositis
isotonic-isometric brief maximum

IBNR incurred but not reported

ibo ibotenic acid; also IA

IBOW intact bag of waters

IBP initial boiling point
intra-aortic balloon pump; also IABP
intra-aortic balloon pumping; also IABP
iron-binding protein

IBPMS indirect blood pressure measuring
system

IBQ Illness Behavior Questionnaire

IBR infectious bovine rhinotracheitis (virus)

IBRS Inpatient Behavior Rating Scale

IBRV infectious bovine rhinotracheitis virus

IBS imidazole-buffered saline
inside bathing solution
Interpersonal Behavior Survey
irritable bowel syndrome
isobaric solution

IBSA, iBSA immunoreactive bovine serum
albumin
iodinated bovine serum albumin

IBSN infantile bilateral striatal necrosis

IBT ink blot test (Rorschach test)
isatin-beta-thiosemicarbasone

IBTR ipsilateral breast tumor recurrence

IBU ibuprofen
international benzoate unit

IBV infectious bronchitis vaccine
infectious bronchitis virus

IBW ideal body weight

IC between meals [L. *inter cibos*]; also ic,
int cib
icteric; also ICT
ileocecal
iliococcygeal
iliocostal
immune complex(es)
immune cytotoxicity
immunocompromised
immunocytochemistry; also ICC
impedance cardiogram
incomplete; also INC, inc, incomp, incompl
indirect calorimetry
indirect Coombs' (test)
individual counseling
infection control
inferior colliculus
information content
inhibitory concentration
inner canthal (distance)
inorganic carbon
inspiratory capacity
inspiratory center
institutional care
integrated circuit
integrated concentration
intensive care
intercarpal
intercostal (space)
intermediate care
intermittent catheterization; also Ic
intermittent claudication
internal capsule
internal carotid
internal cerebral
internal cholecystectomy
internal conjugate (diameter)
internal conversion
International Classification
interstitial cell(s); also ISC
interstitial change
interstitial cystitis
intracameral
intracapsular
intracardiac
intracarotid
intracavitary; also ICAV
intracellular
intracellular concentration
intracerebral; also ic
intracisternal; also ICI
intracoronary
intracranial
intracutaneous; also i cut
intrapleural catheter

irritable colon
islet cell (of pancreas)
isovolumic contraction; also IVC

I/C invalid chair

IC$_{50}$ concentration that inhibits 50%

Ic intermittent catheterization; also IC

ic between meals [L. *inter cibos*]; also IC,
int cib
intracerebral; also IC

ICA ileocolic anastomosis
Institute of Clinical Analysis
intercountry adoption
intermediate care area
internal carotid artery
intracranial anatomy
intracranial aneurysm
islet cell antibody; also ICAb

iCa ionized calcium

ICAb islet cell antibody; also ICA

ICAF internal carotid artery flow

ICAO internal carotid artery occlusion

ICAP intracisternal A particle

ICAV intracavitary; also IC

ICB intercostal nerve block
intracranial bleeding

ICBF inner cortical blood flow

ICBP intercellular binding protein
intracellular binding protein

ICBT intercostobronchial trunk

ICC immunocompetent cell
immunocytochemistry; also IC
Indian childhood cirrhosis
intensive coronary care
interchromosomal crossing-over
intermediate cell column
intermittent clean catheterization
internal conversion coefficient
Interstate Commerce Commission
islet cell carcinoma

ICCE intracapsular cataract extraction

ICCE͞cPI intracapsular cataract extraction
with peripheral iridectomy

ICCM idiopathic congestive cardiomyopathy

ICCU intensive coronary care unit

ICD immune complex disease
inclusion cell disease
induced circular dichroism
inguinal compressive device
initial claudication distance
instantaneous cardiac death
Institute for Crippled and Disabled

ICD—cont'd
intercanthal distance
internal cervical device
International Classification of Diseases (of World Health Organization)
intracervical device
intrauterine contraceptive device; also IUCD
ischemic coronary disease
isocitrate dehydrogenase; also ICDH
isolated conduction defect

ICDA International Classification of Diseases, Adapted (for use in the United States)
International Classification of Diseases and Accidents

ICDC implantable cardioverter/defibrillator catheter

ICDCD International Classification of Diseases and Causes of Death

ICD-CM International Classification of Diseases–Clinical Modification

ICDH isocitrate dehydrogenase; also ICD
isocitric acid dehydrogenase; also IDH

ICD-O International Classification of Diseases for Oncology

ICDS Integrated Child Development Scheme

ICE ice, compression, and elevation
individual career exploration
iridocorneal endothelial (syndrome)

ICES ice, compression, elevation, and support

ICET (Forty-Eight) Item Counseling Evaluation Test

ICF indirect centrifugal flotation
intensive care facility
intercellular fluorescence
interciliary fluid
intermediate care facility
intracellular fluid; also IF
intravascular coagulation and fibrinolysis (syndrome)

ICFA incomplete Freund's adjuvant; also IFA
induced complementing-fixing antigen

ICF-MR intermediate-care facility for the mentally retarded

IC fx intracapsular fracture

ICG indocyanine green
isotope cisternography

ICGN immune complex-mediated glomerulonephritis

ICH idiopathic cortical hyperostosis
immunocompromised host
infectious canine hepatitis
intracerebral hematoma; also IH

intracerebral hemorrhage
intracerebral hypertension
intracranial hemorrhage
intracranial hypertension

ICHD ischemic coronary heart disease

ICHPPC International Classification of Health Problems in Primary Care

ICI Interpersonal Communication Inventory
intracardiac injection
intracisternal; also IC

ICIDH International Classification of Impairments, Disabilities, and Handicaps

ICL intracorneal lens

ICM immune combination molecules
inner cell mass
intercostal margin
intracytoplasmic membrane
ion conductance modulator
ipsilateral competing message

ICN infection control nurse
intensive care neonatal
intensive care nursery
intermediate care nursery
International Council of Nurses

ICNC intracerebellar nuclear cell

ICNND Interdepartmental Committee on Nutrition in National Defense

ICO impedance cardiac output

i coch intracochlear

ICP incubation period; also IP
inductively coupled plasma
infection-control practitioner
infectious cell protein
intermittent catheterization protocol
intracranial pressure
intracytoplasmic

ICPMM incisors, canines, premolars, and molars (permanent dentition formula)

ICP-MS inductively coupled plasma–mass spectrometry

ICPP intubated continuous positive-pressure

ICPS Interpersonal Cognitive Problem Solving

ICR (distance between) iliac crests
Institute for Cancer Research
intermittent catheter routine
international calibrated ratio
intracardiac catheter recording
intracorneal stroma ring
intracranial reinforcement
ion cyclotron resonance

ICRD Index of Codes for Research Drugs

ICRETT International Cancer Research
Technology Transfer

ICREW International Cancer Research
Workshop

I-CRF immunoreactive corticotropin-releasing
factor

ICRP International Commission on
Radiological Protection

ICRS *Index Chemicus* Registry System

ICRU International Commission on Radiation
Units and Measurements
International Commission of Radiological
Units and Measurements (now: Inter-
national Commission on Radiation Units
and Measurements)

ICS ileocecal sphincter
immotile cilia syndrome
immunochemistry system
impulse-conducting system
intensive care, surgical
intercellular space; also IS
intercostal space; also IS
International College of Surgeons
intracranial stimulation
irritable colon syndrome

ICSA islet cell surface antibody

ICSC idiopathic central serous chorioretinopathy

ICSH International Committee for
Standardization in Hematology
interstitial cell-stimulating hormone (luteinizing hormone)

ICSP International Council of Societies of
Pathology

ICSS intracranial self-stimulating

ICT icteric; also IC
icterus; also Ict, ict
immunoglobulin consumption test
indirect Coombs' test
indirect Coombs' titer
inflammation of connective tissue
insulin coma therapy
insulin convulsive therapy
intensive conventional therapy
intermittent cervical traction; also ICTX
interstitial cell tumor
intracardiac thrombus
intracranial tumor
intradermal cancer test
intraoral cariogenicity test
isovolumic contraction time; also IVCT

Ict, ict icterus; also ICT

iCT immunoreactive calcitonin

ict ind icteric index
icterus index; also II

ICTS idiopathic carpal tunnel syndrome

ICTX intermittent cervical traction; also ICT

ICU infant care unit
intensive care unit
intermediate care unit
international chick unit

i cut intracutaneous; also IC

ICV intracellular volume
intracerebroventricular; also icv, ICVT

icv into cerebral ventricles
intracerebroventricular; also ICV, ICVT

ICVH ischemic cerebrovascular headache

ICVT intracerebroventricular; also ICV, icv

ICW intact canal wall
intensive care ward
intercellular water
intracellular water

ICX immune complex

ID identification
identify
iditol dehydrogenase
ill-defined
immunodeficiency
immunodiffusion
immunoglobulin deficiency
inappropriate disability
inclusion disease
index of discrimination
individual dose
induction delivery
infant death
infectious disease; also inf dis
infective dose
inhibitory dose
inhomogeneous deposition
initial diagnosis
initial dose
initial dyskinesia
injected dose
inside diameter
insufficient data
interdigitating (cells)
internal diameter
interstitial disease
intestinal distress
intradermal; also id
intraduodenal
isosorbide dinitrate; also ISD, ISDN

I&D incision and drainage

I-D intensity-duration (curve)

ID$_{50}$ median infective dose

Id idiotypic
India
Indian
infradentale
interdentale

id during the day [L. *in diem*]
intradermal; also ID
the same (author) [L. *idem* (the same)];
also idem

IDA image display and analysis
iminodiacetic acid
insulin-degrading activity
iron-deficiency anemia
isometheptene mucate, dichloralphenazone,
acetaminophen

id ac the same as [L. *idem ac*]; also iq

IDAMIS Integrated Dose Abuse Management
Informational Systems

IDARP Integrated Drug Abuse Reporting
Process

IDAT indirect antiglobulin test; also IAGT, IAT

IDAV immunodeficiency-associated virus

IDBR indirect bilirubin; also IBILI

IDBS infantile diffuse brain sclerosis

IDC idiopathic dilated cardiomyopathy
interdigitating cells

IDCF immunodiffusion complement fixation

IDCI intradiplochromatid interchange

IDD insulin-dependent diabetes

IDDF investigational drug data form

IDDM insulin-dependent diabetes mellitus

IDDS implantable drug delivery system
investigational drug data sheet

IDDT immuno-double diffusion test

IDE inner dental epithelium
Investigational Device Exemption

IDEAL interdisciplinary drug engineering and
assessment laboratory

ID/ED internal diameter to external diameter
(cardiac valve replacement ratio)

IDEM ischemic, drug, electrolyte, metabolic
(effect)

idem the same (author) [L. *idem* (the same)];
also id

IDF infantile digital fibromatosis

IDFC immature dead female child

IDG interdisciplinary group
intermediate-dose group

IDH isocitric acid dehydrogenase; also ICDH

IDH1 isocitrate dehydrogenase, soluble; also
IDH-S

IDH2 isocitrate dehydrogenase, mitochondrial;
also IDH-M

IDH-M isocitrate dehydrogenase, mitochondrial; also IDH2

IDH-S isocitrate dehydrogenase, soluble;
also IDH1

IDI immunologically detectable insulin
induction-delivery interval
interdentale inferius

IDIC Internal Dose Information Center

IDK internal derangement of knee (joint)

IDL Index to Dental Literature
intensity difference limen
intermediate-density lipoprotein

IDM idiopathic disease of myocardium
immune defense mechanism
indirect method
infant of a diabetic mother; also IODM
intermediate-dose methotrexate

IDMC immature dead male child
interdigestive motility complex
interdigestive motor complex

IDMEC interdigestive myoelectric complex;
also IMC

IDMS, ID-MS isotope dilution–mass spectrometry

iDNA intercalary deoxyribonucleic acid

idon vehic in a suitable vehicle [L. *idoneo
vehiculo*]

IDP imidoliphosphonate
immunodiffusion procedure(s)
initial dose period
inosine 5′-diphosphate
instantaneous diastolic pressure

IDPase inosine diphosphatase

IDPH idiopathic pulmonary hemosiderosis;
also IPH

IDPN beta-iminodipropionitrile

IDR intradermal reaction

IDS immunity deficiency state
infectious disease service
inhibitor of DNA synthesis
intraduodenal stimulation
investigational drug service

IDT immune diffusion test
instillation delivery time
interdivision time
intradermal typhoid (and paratyphoid
vaccine)

IDU idoxuridine; also IDUR, IdUrd
5-iodo-2'-deoxyuridine; also IDUR, IdUrd
Ivy dog unit

IdUA iduronic acid

IDUR idoxuridine; also IDU, IdUrd
5-iodo-2'-deoxyuridine; also IDU, IdUrd

IdUrd idoxuridine; also IDU, IDUR
5-iodo-2'-deoxyuridine; also IDU, IDUR

IDV intermittent demand ventilation

IDVC indwelling venous catheter

Idx cross-reactive idiotype

IE immediate early (gene)
immunizing unit [Ger. *Immunitäts Einheit*];
also ImmU, IU
immunoelectrophoresis; also IEP
induced emesis
infectious endocarditis
infective endocarditis
inner ear
intake energy (unit of food)
internal ear
internal elastica
international unit (European abbreviation)
intraepithelial
Introversion-Extroversion (scale)

I/E inspiratory to expiratory (ratio); also I:E

I:E inspiratory to expiratory (ratio); also I/E

I-E internal versus external (control of reinforcement scale)

I&E internal and external

ie that is [L. *id est*]

IEA immediate early antigen
immunoelectroadsorption
immunoelectrophoretic analysis
infectious equine anemia
intravascular erythrocyte aggregation

IEC injection electrode catheter
inpatient exercise center
intraepithelial carcinoma
ion-exchange chromatography

IE Ca cx intraepithelial carcinoma of cervix

IEE inner enamel epithelium

IEF isoelectric focusing

IEHMO iterative extended Hückel molecular
orbital

IEI isoelectric interval

IEL internal elastic lamina
intimal elastic lamina
intraepithelial lymphocyte

IEM immunoelectron microscopy

inborn error of metabolism

IEMG integrated electromyogram

IEMT intermediate emergency medical
technician

IEOP immunoelectro-osmophoresis

IEP immunoelectrophoresis; also IE
individualized education program
isoelectric point; also IP
isoelectric precipitation

IEPA independent electron pair approximation

IER Institute of Educational Research
(defunct)

IES ingressive-egressive sequence

IF idiopathic fibroplasia
ifosfamide; also IFOS, IFX
immersion foot
immunofixation; also IFIX
immunofluorescence; also IFL
indirect fluorescence
inferior facet
infrared; also IFR, infra, IR
inhibiting factor
initiation factor
inspiratory force
interferon; also IFN, INF, ITF
intermaxillary fixation; also IMF
intermediate filament; also IMF
intermediate frequency
internal fixation
internal friction
interstitial fluid; also ISF
intracellular fluid; also ICF
intrinsic factor
involved field (irradiation)

IFA idiopathic fibrosing alveolitis
immunofluorescent antibody
immunofluorescent assay
incomplete Freund's adjuvant; also ICFA
indirect fluorescent antibody (test)
indirect fluorescent assay

IFAT indirect fluorescent antibody test

IFC inspiratory flow cartridge
intermittent flow centrifugation
intrinsic factor concentrate

IFCC International Federation of Clinical
Chemistry

IFCL intermittent flow centrifugation leukapheresis

IFCS inactivated fetal calf serum

IFDS isolated follicle-stimulating hormone
deficiency syndrome

IFE immunofixation electrophoresis
interfollicular epidermis

IFF inner fracture face

IFGS interstitial fluids and ground substance

IFI Institutional Functioning Inventory (psychologic test)

IFIX immunofixation; also IF

IFL immunofluorescence; also IF

IFLrA recombinant human leukocyte interferon A

IFM internal fetal monitoring
intrafusal muscle

IFN immunoreactive fibronectin
interferon; also IF, INF, ITF

IFN-α (human leukocyte) interferon

IFN-β (human fibroblast) interferon

IFN-C partially pure human leukocyte interferon

if nec if necessary

IFO Institute for Fermentation

IFOS ifosfamide; also IF, IFX

IFP inflammatory fibroid polyp
insulin, Kendall compound F (hydrocortisone), and prolactin
intermediate filament protein
intrapatellar fat pad

IFR infrared; also IF, infra, IR
inspiratory flow rate

IFRA indirect fluorescent rabies antibody (test)

IFRP International Fertility Research Program
(now: FHI, Family Health International)

IFS interstitial fluid space

IFT immunofluorescence technique
immunofluorescence test
International Frequency Tables

IFU interferon unit

IFV interstitial fluid volume; also ISFV
intracellular fluid volume

IFX ifosfamide; also IF, IFOS

IG immature granule
immune globulin
immunoglobulin; also Ig
Inspector General
intragastric; also ig

I-G insulin-glucagon

Ig immunoglobulin; also IG

iG immunoreactive human gastrin

ig intragastric; also IG

IGA infantile genetic agranulocytosis

IgA immunoglobulin A

IgA1, IgA2 subclasses of immunoglobulin A

IGC intragastric cannula

IGD interglobal distance
isolated gonadotropin deficiency

IgD immunoglobulin D

IgD1, IgD2 subclasses of immunoglobulin D

IGDE idiopathic gait disorders of elderly

IGDM infant of gestational diabetic mother

IGE impaired gas exchange

IgE immunoglobulin E

IgE1 subclass of immunoglobulin E

IGF insulin-like growth factor; also ILGF

IGF-1 insulin-like growth factor 1

IGFET insulated gate field effect transistor

IgG immunoglobulin G

IgG1, IgG2, IgG3, IgG4 subclasses of
immunoglobulin G

IGH idiopathic growth hormone
immunoreactive growth hormone;
also IRGH

IGHD isolated growth hormone deficiency

IGI Institutional Goals Inventory

IGIM immune globulin, intramuscular

IGIV immune globulin, intravenous

IgM immunoglobulin M

IgM1 subclass of immunoglobulin M

IGP intestinal glycoprotein

IgQ immunoglobulin quantitation

IGR immediate generalized reaction
integrated gastrin response
intrauterine growth retardation; also IUGR

IGS inappropriate gonadotropin secretion

IgSC immunoglobulin-secreting cell; also ISC

IGT impaired glucose tolerance
interpersonal group therapy
intragastric titration

IGTN ingrown toenail

IGTT intravenous glucose tolerance test; also
IVGTT

IGV intrathoracic gas volume; also ITGV

IH idiopathic hirsutism
immediate hypersensitivity
incomplete healing
indirect hemagglutination; also IHA
industrial hygiene
infectious hepatitis
inguinal hernia
inhibiting hormone

in hospital
inner half
inpatient hospital
intermittent heparinization
intracerebral hematoma; also ICH
iron hematoxylin

IHA idiopathic hyperaldosteronism
immune hemolytic anemia
indirect hemagglutination; also IH
indirect hemagglutination antibody (test)
infusion hepatic arteriography

IHB incomplete heart block

IHBT incompatible hemolytic blood transfusion

IHBTD incompatible hemolytic blood transfusion disease

IHC idiopathic hemochromatosis
idiopathic hypercalciuria
immobilization hypercalcemia
inner hair cell (of cochlea)
intrahepatic cholestasis; also IHPC

IHCA isocapnic hyperventilation with cold air

IHCP Institute on Hospital and Community Psychiatry

IHD in-center hemodialysis
intrahepatic duct
intrahepatic ductule
ischemic heart disease

IHF integration host factor

IHG ichthyosis hystrix graviori

IHGD isolated human growth deficiency

IHH idiopathic hypogonadotropic hypogonadism
infectious human hepatitis

IHHS idiopathic hyperkinetic heart syndrome

IHMS (sodium) isonicotinylhydrazide methanesulfonate

IHO idiopathic hypertrophic osteoarthropathy

IHP idiopathic hypoparathyroidism
idiopathic hypopituitarism
interhospitalization period
inverted hand position

IHPC intrahepatic cholestasis; also IHC

IHPH intrahepatic portal hypertension

IHPP Intergovernmental Health Project Policy

IHR intrahepatic resistance
intrinsic heart rate

IHRA isocapnic hyperventilation with room air

IHS Idiopathic Headache Score
inactivated horse serum
Indian Health Service
infrahyoid strap; also IS

IHs iris hamartomas

IHSA iodinated human serum albumin

IHSC immunoreactive human skin collagenase

IHSS idiopathic hypertrophic subaortic stenosis

IHT insulin hypoglycemia test
intravenous histamine test
ipsilateral head turning

I5HT intraplatelet 5-hydroxytryptamine (intraplatelet serotonin)

IHW inner heel wedge

II icterus index; also ict ind
image intensifier
india ink
insurance index
irradiated iodine

IIA internal iliac artery

IIC integrated ion current

IICP increased intracranial pressure

IICU infant intensive care unit

IID insulin-independent diabetes

IIDM insulin-independent diabetes mellitus

IIE idiopathic ineffective erythropoiesis

IIF immune interferon
indirect immunofluorescence

IIGR ipsilateral instinctive grasp reaction

III-para tertipara

IIIVC intrahepatic interruption of inferior vena cava

III/VI moderately loud (heart murmur)

IIME Institute of International Medical Education

IIP idiopathic interstitial pneumonia
idiopathic intestinal pseudo-obstruction
indirect immunoperoxidase
Intra- and Interpersonal (relations scale)

II-para secundipara

IIS intensive immunosuppression
intermittent infusion sets
International Institute of Stress

IIT ineffective iron turnover
integrated isometric tension

II/VI quiet, but heard immediately upon placing the stethoscope on the chest (heart murmur)

IJ ileojejunal; also I-J
internal jugular (vein)
intrajejunal

I-J ileojejunal; also IJ

IJC internal jugular catheter

IJD inflammatory joint disease
IJP inhibitory junction potential
　internal jugular pressure
IJR idiojunctional rhythm
IJT idiojunctional tachycardia
IJV internal jugular vein
IK immobilized knee
　immune body [Ger. *Immune Körper*]; also IB
　immunoconglutinin
　infusoria killing (unit)
　interstitial keratitis
IKE ion kinetic energy
IKI iodine potassium iodide (Lugol's solution)
　[L. *kalium* (potassium)]
IKU infusoria killing unit
IL ileum
　iliolumbar
　immature lung(s)
　incisolingual
　independent laboratory
　insensible weight loss
　inspiratory loading
　intensity level
　interleukin
　intermediary letter
　intestinal lymphocyte
　Intralipid
　intralumbar
　intraocular lens; also IOL
IL 1 interleukin 1
IL 2 interleukin 2
I-L intensity-latency
Il illinium (promethium)
il intralesional
ILA insulin-like activity
　International Leprosy Association
ILa incisolabial
ILB infant, low birth (weight)
ILBBB incomplete left bundle-branch block
ILBW infant, low birth weight
ILC ichthyosis linearis circumflex
　incipient lethal concentration
Ilc isoleucine; also I, ILE, Ile, Ileu, ISL
ILD interstitial lung disease
　ischemic leg disease
　ischemic limb disease
　isolated lactase deficiency
ILDCSI Individual Learning Disabilities
　Classroom Screening Instrument
ILE infantile lobar emphysema
　isoleucine; also I, Ilc, Ile, Ileu, ISL

Ile isoleucine; also I, Ilc, ILE, Ileu, ISL
Ileu isoleucine; also I, Ilc, ILE, Ile, ISL
ILFC immature living female child
ILGF insulin-like growth factor; also IGF
ILL intermediate lymphocytic lymphoma
illic lag obturat let the bottle be closed at once
　[L. *illico lagona obturatur*]
ILM insulin-like material
　internal limiting membrane
ILMC immature living male child
ILMI inferolateral myocardial infarction
ILo iodine lotion
ILP inadequate luteal phase
　interstitial lymphocytic pneumonia
ILR irreversible loss rate
ILS idiopathic leucine sensitivity
　idiopathic lymphadenopathy syndrome
　increase in life span
　incremental life support
　infrared liver scanner
　intralobular sequestration
ILSS integrated life support system
　intraluminal somatostatin
ILVEN inflammatory linear verrucal
　epidermal nevus
IM idiopathic myelofibrosis; also IMF
　immunosuppression method
　Index Medicus; also Ind Med
　indomethacin; also IMT, IND, INDO
　industrial medicine; also Ind-Med
　infantile myofibromatosis
　infection medium
　infectious mononucleosis; also INFM,
　　inf mono
　inner membrane
　innocent murmur
　inspiratory muscle
　intermediate megaloblast
　intermetatarsal
　intermuscular
　internal malleolus
　internal mammary (artery)
　internal medicine; also Int Med
　internal monitor
　intestinal mesenchyme
　intramedullary
　intramuscular; also im
　intramuscularly; also im
　invasive mole
im indicates presence of >NH group
　intramuscular; also IM
　intramuscularly; also IM

IMA Industrial Medical Association (now: ACOEM, American College of Occupational and Environmental Medicine)
inferior mesenteric artery
Interchurch Medical Assistance
intermammary vein graft
internal mammary artery

IMAA iodinated macroaggregated albumin

IMAC ifosfamide, mesna uroprotection, Adriamycin, and cisplatin

IMAG internal mammary artery graft

IMAI internal mammary artery implant

IMB intermenstrual bleeding

IMBC indirect maximum breathing capacity

IMBI Institute of Medical and Biological Illustrators

IMC interdigestive migrating complex
interdigestive migrating contraction
interdigestive myoelectric complex; also IDMEC
intestinal mucosal mast cell
intramedullary catheter

IMCU intermediate medical care unit

IMD immunologically mediated disease
inherited metabolic disorder

ImD$_{50}$ median immunizing dose (immunizing dose sufficient to protect 50% of subjects)

IMDC intramedullary metatarsal decompression

IMDD idiopathic midline destructive disease

IMDM Iscove's modified Dulbecco's medium

IME independent medical examination
independent medical examiner
indirect medical education

IMEM improved minimal essential medium

IMEM-HS improved minimal essential medium, hormone supplemented

IMET isometric endurance time

IMF idiopathic myelofibrosis; also IM
ifosfamide, mesna uroprotection, methotrexate, and fluorouracil
intermaxillary fixation; also IF
intermediate filament; also IF

IMG inferior mesenteric ganglion
internal medicine group (practice)

IMH idiopathic myocardial hypertrophy
indirect microhemagglutination (test)

IMHP 1-iodomercuri-2-hydroxypropane

IMHT indirect microhemagglutination test

IMI imipramine
immunologically measurable insulin

impending myocardial infarction
indirect membrane immunofluorescence
inferior myocardial infarction
intermeal interval
intramuscular injection

IMIC International Medical Information Center

IMIG intramuscular immunoglobulin

IML internal mammary lymphoscintigraphy

IMLA intramural left anterior (descending artery)

IMLAD intramural left anterior descending (artery)

IMLC incomplete mitral leaflet closure

ImLy immune lysis

IMM inhibitor-containing minimal medium
internal medial malleolus

immat immature
immaturity

IMMC interdigestive migratory motor complex

immed immediately

immobil immobilization
immobilize

ImmU immunizing unit; also IE, IU

immun immune
immunity
immunization

Immunol immunology

IMN internal mammary lymph node

IMP idiopathic myeloid proliferation
impacted; also imp, Impx
important; also imp
impression; also I, imp
improved; also imp
incomplete male pseudohermaphroditism
individual Medicaid practitioner
inosine-5′-monophosphate (inosinic acid)
Inpatient Multidimensional Psychiatric (scale)
intramembranous particle
intramuscular compartment pressure

imp impacted; also IMP, Impx
important; also IMP
impression; also I, IMP
improved; also IMP

IMPA incisal mandibular plane angle

IMPAC Immediate Psychiatric Aid and Referral Center

imperf imperfect
imperforate

IMPEX immediate postexercise

IMPL impulse

IMPS Inpatient Multidimensional Psychiatric Scale

impvt improvement

Impx impacted; also IMP, imp

IMR individual medical record
infant mortality rate
infectious mononucleosis receptor
Institute for Medical Research
institution for the mentally retarded

IMRAD introduction, materials and methods, results, and discussion (formal structure of scientific article); also IMRD

IMRD introduction, materials and methods, results, and discussion (formal structure of scientific article); also IMRAD

IMS incurred in military service
Indian Medical Service
industrial methylated spirit
integrated medical services
international market survey

IMSS in-flight medical support system

IMT indomethacin; also IM, IND, INDO
induced muscular tension
inspiratory muscle training

ImU international milliunit

IMV inferior mesenteric vein
intermittent mandatory ventilation
intermittent mechanical ventilation
isophosphamide, methotrexate, and vincristine

IMVC indole, methyl red, Voges-Proskauer, and citrate (test); also IMViC, imvic

IMViC, imvic indole, methyl red, Voges-Proskauer, and citrate (test); also IMVC

IMVP idiopathic mitral valve prolapse

IN icterus neonatorum
impetigo neonatorum
incidence
incompatibility number
infantile nephrotic (syndrome)
infundibular nucleus
insulin; also I, In, INS
intermediate nucleus
interneuron
internist; also INT, int
interstitial nephritis
intranasal

In inch; also in
indium
inion
insulin; also I, IN, INS
inulin

in inch; also In

in² square inch

in³ cubic inch

INA infectious nucleic acid
inferior nasal artery
information not available
International Neurological Association

INAA instrumental neutron activation analysis

inac inactive; also I

INAD infantile neuroaxonal dystrophy
investigational new animal drug

INAH isoniazid acid hydrazide
isonicotinic acid hydrazide (isoniazid); also INH

INB ischemic necrosis of bone

inbr inbreeding

INC incisal
incision
incomplete; also IC, inc, incomp, incompl
inconclusive; also inc
incontinent; also inc, incont
increase; also inc, INCR, incr
inside-the-needle catheter
interstitial nucleus of Cajal

Inc including; also incl
incorporated

inc incisional
incompatibility
incomplete; also IC, INC, incomp, incompl
inconclusive; also INC
incontinent; also INC, incont
increase; also INC, INCR, incr
increment; also INCR, incr
incurred

Inc Ab incomplete abortion

INCAP Institute of Nutrition of Central America and Panama (Guatemala, Guatemala)

IncB inclusion body; also IB

INCD infantile nuclear cerebral degeneration

incid cut [L. *incide*]

incl including; also Inc

incomp incomplete; also IC, INC, inc, incompl

incompl incomplete; also IC, INC, inc, incomp

incompat incompatible

incont incontinent; also INC, inc

inc (R) increase (relative)

INCR, incr increase; also INC, inc
increment; also inc

INCS incomplete resolution, scan to follow

incur incurable
IND indapamide
   indomethacin; also IM, IMT, INDO
   induced
   industrial (medicine); also indust
   investigational new drug
Ind induction (of labor); also I, ind
ind independent; also I, INDEP
   index; also I
   indicate
   indigent
   indigo
   indirect
   induction (of labor); also I, Ind
in d daily [L. *in dies*]
   in a day
INDEP independent; also I, ind
indic indicated; also I
   indication
indig indigestion
INDIV individual
INDM infant of nondiabetic mother
Ind Med *Index Medicus*; also IM
Ind-Med industrial medicine; also IM
INDO indomethacin; also IM, IMT, IND
   intermediate neglect of differential overlap
   (method)
INDOR internuclear double resonance
INDS investigational new drug submission
indust industrial; also IND
   industry
INE infantile necrotizing encephalomyelopathy
INEX inexperienced
in extrem in the last (hours of life) [L. *in
   extremis*]
INF infant; also inf
   infantile; also inf
   infarction
   infected; also inf, infect
   infection; also inf, infect, infx
   infectious (disease)
   infective; also inf, infect
   inferior; also inf, infer
   infirmary; also inf
   information; also info
   infundibulum (of neurohypophysis)
   infused
   infusion; also inf
   interferon; also IF, IFN, ITF
   pour in [L. *infunde*]; also inf, infund
inf infancy

infant; also INF
infantile; also INF
infarct
infect
infected; also INF, infect
infection; also INF, infect, infx
infective; also INF, infect
inferior; also INF, infer
infirmary; also INF
infusion; also INF
pour in [L. *infunde*]; also INF, infund
in f at the end, finally [L. *in fine*]
inf dis infectious disease; also ID
infect infected; also INF, inf
   infection; also INF, inf, infx
   infective; also INF, inf
infer inferior; also INF, inf
INFH ischemic necrosis of femoral head
infl inflamed
   inflammation; also Inflamm
   inflammatory; also Inflamm
   influence
   influx
Inflamm inflammation; also infl
   inflammatory; also infl
infl proc inflammatory process
INFM infectious mononucleosis; also IM, inf
   mono
Inf MI inferior wall myocardial infarction; also
   IWMI
inf mono infectious mononucleosis; also IM,
   INFM
info information; also INF
infra infrared; also IF, IFR, IR
infund pour in [L. *infunde*]; also INF, inf
infx infection; also INF, inf, infect
ING inguinal; also ing
   isotope nephrogram
ing inguinal; also ING
InGP indolglycerophosphate
INH inhalation; also I, inhal
   isonicotinic acid hydrazide (isoniazid); also
   INAH
   isonicotinoylhydrazine
Inh inhaler
inhal inhalation; also I, INH
INH-G isonicotinoylhydrazone of D-glucuronic
   acid lactone (glyconiazide)
inhib inhibiting; also I
   inhibition; also I
   inhibitor; also I

INI intranasal insulin
intranuclear inclusion (agent)

inj inject
injected
injection; also inject
injured
injurious
injury

inject injection; also inj

inj enem let an enema be injected [L.
injeciatur enema]

INK injury not known

inl inlay

INN International Nonproprietary Name

innerv innervated
innervation

INO infantile nephrotic syndrome, other
(types)
inosine; also I, Ino
internuclear ophthalmoplegia

Ino inosine; also I, INO

INOC, inoc inoculate
inoculation
isonicotinoyloxycarbonyl

inop inoperable

inorg inorganic

Inox inosine, oxidized

INP idiopathic neutropenia

INPAV intermittent negative pressure-assisted
ventilation; also INPV

INPEA isopropylnitrophenylethanolamine
(beta-adrenergic blocker)

INPH iproniazid phosphate

INPRCNS information processing in central
nervous system; also INPRONS

INPRONS information processing in central
nervous system; also INPRCNS

IN-PT inpatient; also IP

in pulm in gruel [L. *in pulmento*]

INPV intermittent negative pressure-assisted
ventilation; also INPAV

INQ inferior nasal quadrant

INR international normalized ratio

INREM internal roentgen-equivalent-man
(radiation dose)

INS idiopathic nephrotic syndrome
insulin; also I, IN, In
insurance; also ins

ins insertion
insurance; also INS
insured

INS Ab insulin antibody

insem insemination

insid insidious

insol insoluble; also I, i

Insp inspect
inspection
inspiration; also I, inspir

InsP$_3$ inositol 1,4,5-triphosphate; also IP$_3$

inspir inspiration; also I, Insp
inspiratory

INSS International Staging System (for neuroblastoma)

INST instrumental (delivery)

Inst institute; also inst

inst institute; also Inst
instrument

insuf insufficiency; also insuff
insufficient; also insuff
insufflation; also insuff

insuff insufficiency; also insuf
insufficient; also insuf
insufflation; also insuf

INT intermediate; also I, int, Intmd
intermittent; also int, INTR
intermittent needle therapy
intern; also int
internal; also int, intern
internist; also IN, int
para-iodonitrotetrazolium

int initial; also I
intact; also IT
integral
interest
intermediate; also I, INT, Intmd
intermittent; also INT, INTR
intern; also INT
internal; also INT, intern
internist; also IN, INT
interval
intestinal; also Intest, intest
intestine; also I, Intest, intest
to the innermost [L. *intime*]

int cib between meals [L. *inter cibos*]; also IC, ic

INTEG integument

intern internal; also INT, int

internat international; also Intl

intertroch intertrochanteric; also IT

Intest, intest intestinal; also int
intestine; also I, int

Int/Ext internal/external (rotation)

INTH intrathecal (anesthesia injection); also IT, ITh, i-thec

int hist interval history

Intl international; also internat

Intmd intermediate; also I, INT, int

Int Med internal medicine; also IM

int noct during the night [L. *inter noctem*]

int obst intestinal obstruction; also IO

INTOX, intox intoxication

INTR intermittent; also INT, int

intracal intracalvarium

int-rot internal rotation; also IR

int trx intermittent traction; also IT

INV inferior nasal vein

inv invalid
inverse
inversion; also inver
involuntary; also invol

inver inversion; also inv
inverted

invest investigation

invet inveterate

Inv/Ev inversion/eversion

inv ins inverted insertion

invol involuntary; also inv

involv coat [L. *involve*]
involved
involvement

IO incisal opening
inferior oblique (eye muscle)
inferior olive
initial opening (pressure)
inside-out (vesicle)
intensive observation
internal os (cervix)
intestinal obstruction; also int obst
intraocular (pressure)

I&O, I/O in and out
input/output
intake and output; also I and O

Io ionium

IOA inner optic anlage

IOC in our culture

intern on call
intraoperative cholangiogram; also IOCG

IOCG intraoperative cholangiogram; also IOC

IOD injured on duty
integrated optical density
interorbital distance

IODM infant of diabetic mother; also IDM

IOEBT intraoperative electron beam therapy

IOF intraocular fluid

IOFB intraocular foreign body

IOFNA intraoperative fine needle aspiration

IOH idiopathic orthostatic hypotension

IOI intraosseous infusion

IOL intraocular lens; also IL

IOLI intraocular lens implantation

IOM Institute of Medicine

IOML infraorbitomeatal line

ION ischemic optic neuropathy

IOP intraocular pressure

IOR index of response; also IR
information outflow rate

I or I illness or injuries

IORT intraoperative radiation therapy

IOS intraoperative sonography

IOT intraocular tension
intraocular transfer
ipsilateral optic tectum

IOTA information overload testing aid

IOU intensive therapy observation unit; also ITOU
international opacity unit

IOV initial office visit
inside-out membrane vesicle

IP icterus praecox
iliopsoas (muscle)
immune precipitate
immunoblastic plasma
immunoperoxidase
immunoprecipitin
implantation; also I
inactivated pepsin
incisoproximal
incisopulpal
incontinentia pigmenti
incubation period; also ICP
individualized plan
induced potential
induction period

IP—cont'd
industrial population
infection prevention
infundibular process (of neurohypophysis)
infundibulopelvic (ligament)
infusion pump
initial pressure
inorganic phosphate
inosine phosphorylase
inpatient; also IN-PT
in plaster
instantaneous pressure
International Pharmacopoeia
interpeduncular (nucleus)
interphalangeal (joint, keratosis); also IPH
interpharyngeal
interpositus (nucleus)
interpupillary
intestinal pseudo-obstruction
intracellular proteolysis
intraperitoneal
intraperitoneally
ionization potential
isoelectric point; also IEP
isoproterenol; also IPT, IS, ISO, Iso, iso, ISP
Pasteur Institute [Fr. *Institut Pasteur*]

IP$_3$ inositol 1,4,5-triphosphate; also InsP$_3$

IPA incontinentia pigmenti achromians
independent practice association
indole, pyruvic acid
intrapulmonary artery
invasive pulmonary aspergillosis
isopropyl alcohol

IPAA International Psycho-Analytical
Association (London, England)

IPAO insulin-induced peak acid output

IPAR Institute of Personality Assessment and
Research

I-para primipara; also P, para I, primip

IPAT (Cattell's) Institute for Personality and
Ability Testing (Anxiety Scale)
Iowa Pressure Articulation Test

IPB infrapopliteal bypass

IPC interpeduncular cistern
intraperitoneal chemotherapy
ion-pair chromatography
isopropyl chlorophenyl
isopropyl phenyl carbamate (propham);
also IsoPPC

IPCD infantile polycystic disease

IPCS intrauterine progesterone contraceptive
system

IPD immediate pigment darkening
increase in pupillary diameter
incurable problem drinker
inflammatory pelvic disease
intermittent peritoneal dialysis
intermittent pigment darkening
interpupillary distance
Inventory of Psychosocial Development

IPDT inventory of Piaget's developmental
tasks

IPE infectious porcine encephalomyelitis
initial psychiatric evaluation
injury pulmonary edema
interstitial pulmonary emphysema

IPEH intravascular papillary endothelial
hyperplasia

IPF idiopathic pulmonary fibrosis
infection-potentiating factor
International Primary Factors (Test Battery)
interstitial pulmonary fibrosis

IPFD intrapartum fetal distress

IPG impedance phlebograph
impedance plethysmograph
impedance plethysmography
impedance plethysmography gradient
inspiratory phase gas

iPGE immunoreactive prostaglandin E

IPH idiopathic portal hypertension
idiopathic pulmonary hemosiderosis;
also IDPH
infant passive hand
inflammatory papillary hyperplasia
interphalangeal (joint, keratosis); also IP
intraparenchymal hemorrhage

IPHR inverted polypoid hamartoma of the
rectum

IPI Imagined Process Inventory
interphonemic interval
interpulse interval

IPIA immunoperoxidase infectivity assay

IPIP implantable programmable infusion pump

IPJ interphalangeal joint

IPK interphalangeal keratosis
intractable plantar keratosis

IPKD infantile polycystic kidney disease

IPL inner plexiform layer
interpupillary line
intrapleural

IPM impulses per minute
inches per minute
infant passive mitt

IPMI inferoposterior myocardial infarction

IPN infantile periarteritis nodosa
infectious pancreatic necrosis
interim progress note(s)
intern's progress note(s)
interpeduncular nucleus
interpenetrating polymer network

IPn interstitial pneumonitis

IPNA isopropylnoradrenaline (isoproterenol)

IPO improved pregnancy outcome
initial planning option

IPOF immediate postoperative fitting

IPOP immediate postoperative prosthesis

IPP independent practice plan
inferior point of pubic (bone)
inflatable penile prosthesis
inorganic pyrophosphate; also PPi, PP$_i$
inosine, pyruvate, and inorganic phosphate
intermittent positive pressure
intrahepatic portal pressure
intrapleural pressure

IPPA inspection, palpation, percussion, and
auscultation

IPPB intermittent positive pressure breathing

IPPB/I intermittent positive pressure breath-
ing/inspiratory

IPPB (R,V) intermittent positive pressure
breathing (respiration, ventilation)

IPPD intermittent positive pressure dialysis

IPPF immediate postoperative prosthetic fitting

IPPI interruption of pregnancy for psychiatric
indication

IPPO intermittent positive-pressure inflation
with oxygen

IPPR integrated pancreatic polypeptide
response
intermittent positive-pressure respiration

IPPT Inter-Person Perception Test

IPPUAD immediate postprandial upper abdominal distress

IPPV intermittent positive-pressure ventilation

IPQ Intermediate Personality Questionnaire
(for Indian Pupils)
intimacy potential quotient

IPR independent professional review
insulin production rate
interval patency rate
intraparenchymal resistance
iproniazid

iPr, i-Pr isopropyl (prefix denoting
L-methylethyl group)

IPRL isolated perfused rabbit lung
isolated perfused rat liver

iPrSGal isopropylthioglactoside

IPRT interpersonal reaction test

IPS idiopathic postprandial syndrome
impulse per second
inferior petrosal sinus
infundibular pulmonary stenosis
initial prognostic score
intermittent photic stimulation (electroencephalography)
Interpersonal Perception Scale
intraperitoneal shock
ischiopubic synchondrosis
isopenicillin *N*-synthetase
para-iodophenyl sulfonyl (pipsyl); also Ips

Ips *para*-iodophenyl sulfonyl (pipsyl); also IPS

ips inches per second

IPSB intrapartum stillbirth

IPSC inhibitory postsynaptic current
inventory of psychic and somatic complaints

IPSF immediate postsurgical fitting (of prosthesis)

IPSID immunoproliferative small intestinal disease

IPSP inhibitory postsynaptic potential

IPSS international pilot study of schizophrenia

IPT immunoperoxidase technique
immunoprecipatation
intermittent pelvic traction; also IPTX
interpersonal psychotherapy
ipratropium
isoproterenol; also IP, IS, ISO, Iso, iso, ISP

IPTG isopropylthiogalactoside

iPTH immunoreactive parathyroid hormone

IPTX intermittent pelvic traction; also IPT

IPU inpatient unit

IPV inactivated poliovirus vaccine
incompetent perforator vein
infectious pustular vaginitis
infectious pustular vulvovaginitis (of cattle)
intrapulmonary vein

IPVC interpolated premature ventricular
contraction

IPVD index of pulmonary vascular disease

IPW interphalangeal width

IPZ insulin-protamine zinc

IQ intelligence quotient

iq the same as [L. *idem quod*]; also id ac

IQ&S iron, quinine, and strychnine

IR ileal resection
immune response (genes); also Ir
immunization rate
immunologic response
immunoreactive; also ir
immunoreagent
index of response; also IOR
individual reaction
inferior rectus (muscle)
infrared; also IF, IFR, infra
inside radius
insoluble residue
inspiratory reserve
inspiratory resistance
insulin receptor
insulin requirement
insulin resistance
insulin response
integer ratio
intelligence ratio
internal reduction
internal resistance
internal rotation; also int-rot
inversion recovery
inverted repeats
irritant reaction
isotope ratio
isovolumetric relaxation (wave)

I-R Ito-Reenstierna (reaction, test)

I&R insertion and removal

Ir immune response (genes); also IR
iridium

ir immunoreactive; also IR
intrarectal
intrarenal

IRA ileorectal anastomosis
immunoradioassay
immunoregulatory alpha-globulin
inactive renin activity

IR-ACTH immunoreactive adrenocorticotropic
hormone

IRA-EEA ileorectal anastomosis with end-to-
end anastomosis

IRB institutional review board

IRBBB incomplete right bundle-branch block

IRBC immature red blood cell; also iRBC
infected red blood cell

iRBC immature red blood cell; also IRBC

IRBP interphotoreceptor retinoid-binding
protein

IRC indirect radionuclide cystography
infrared coagulator

inspiratory reserve capacity
instantaneous resonance curve
International Red Cross

IRCA intravascular red cell aggregation

IRCS International Research Communications
System

IRCU intensive respiratory care unit

IRD isorythmic dissociation

IRDS idiopathic respiratory distress syndrome
infant respiratory distress syndrome

IRE internal rotation in extension

IRF idiopathic retroperitoneal fibrosis
internal rotation in flexion

IRG immunoreactive gastrin
immunoreactive glucagon; also IRGl
immunoreactive glucose

IRGH immunoreactive growth hormone;
also IGH

IRGl immunoreactive glucagon; also IRG

IRH Institute for Research in Hypnosis (now:
IRHP, Institute for Research in Hypnosis
and Psychotherapy)
Institute of Religion and Health
intraretinal hemorrhage

IRHC immunoradioassayable human chorionic
(somatomammotropin)

IRhCG immunoreactive human chorionic
gonadotropin

IRHCS immunoradioassayable human chorionic somatomammotropin

IRhCS immunoreactive human chorionic
somatomammotropin

IRhGH immunoreactive human growth
hormone

IRHP Institute for Research in Hypnosis and
Psychotherapy

IRhPL immunoreactive human placental
lactogen

IRI immunoreactive insulin
insulin radioimmunoassay
insulin resistance index

IRIA indirect radioimmunoassay

irid iridescent

IRI/G ratio of immunoreactive insulin to serum
or plasma glucose

IRIg insulin-reactive immunoglobulin

IRIS interleukin regulation of immune system
International Research Information Service

IRM inherited releasing mechanism
innate releasing mechanism

IRMA immunoradiometric assay
intraretinal microangiopathy
intraretinal microvascular abnormalities

iRNA immune ribonucleic acid
informational ribonucleic acid

IROS ipsilateral routing of signal

IRP immunoreactive plasma
immunoreactive proinsulin
incus replacement prosthesis
inhibitor of radical process
insulin-releasing polypeptide
International Reference Preparation

IRR infrared refractometry
intra-renal reflux
irritation; also Irr, irr

Irr, irr irradiation
irritation; also IRR

irreg irregular
irregularity

IRRIG, irrig irrigate; also IRRG
irrigation; also IRRG

IRRG irrigate; also IRRIG, irrig
irrigation; also IRRIG, irrig

IRS immunoreactive secretin
infrared spectrophotometry
insulin receptor species

IRSA idiopathic refractory sideroblastic
anemia
iodinated rat serum albumin

IRT immunoreactive trypsin
immunoreactive trypsinogen
instrument retrieval container
interresponse time
isometric relaxation time
item response theory (psychologic testing)

IRTO immunoreactive trypsin output

IRTU integrating regulatory transcription unit

IRU industrial rehabilitation unit
interferon reference unit

IRV inferior radicular vein
inspiratory reserve volume
inverse-ratio ventilation

IS ilial segment
immediate sensitivity
immune serum
immunology status
immunosuppression
incentive spirometer
index of saponification
index of sexuality
induced sputum
infant size

information system
infrahyoid strap; also IHS
initial segment
in original place [L. *in situ*]; also is
insertion sequence
insulin secretion
intercellular space; also ICS
intercostal space; also ICS
interictal spike (in electroencephalography)
internal standard
intersegmental (nerve)
interspace; also is, ISP
interstitial space
interventricular septum; also IVS
intracardial shunt
intraspinal; also ISP
intrasplenic
intrastriatal
invalided from service
inventory of systems
Ionescu-Shiley (artificial cardiac valve);
also I-S
ipecac syrup
Irvine's syndrome
ischemic score
island; also is
isoproterenol; also IP, IPT, ISO, Iso, iso, ISP

I-S Ionescu-Shiley (artificial cardiac valve);
also IS

I-10-S invert sugar (10%) in saline

is in original place [L. *in situ*]; also IS
interspace; also IS, ISP
island; also IS
islet
isolation; also isol, isoln

ISA intrinsic stimulating activity
intrinsic sympathomimetic activity
iodinated serum albumin
irregular spiking activity (in electroencephalography)

ISA₅ internal surface area of lung at volume of
five liters

ISADH inappropriate secretion of antidiuretic
hormone

IS and R information storage and retrieval;
also ISR

ISB incentive spirometry breathing

ISC immunoglobulin-secreting cell; also IgSC
insoluble collagen
intensive supportive care
International Statistical Classification
intershift coordination
interstitial cell(s); also IC

ISC—cont'd
  intersystem crossing
  irreversibly sickled cell(s); also ISCs
  Isolette servo control
ISCA ionization spectroscopy for chemical
  analysis
ISCCO intersternocostoclavicular ossification
ISCF interstitial cell fluid
ISCLT International Society for Clinical
  Laboratory Technology
ISCN International System for Human
  Cytogenetic Nomenclature
ISCOMS immunity-stimulating complexes
ISCP infection surveillance and control
  program
  International Society of Comparative
  Pathology
ISCs irreversibly sickled cells; also ISC
ISCV International Society for Cardiovascular
  Surgery
ISD immunosuppressive drug
  inhibited sexual desire
  initial sleep disturbance
  intensity of service, severity of illness, dis-
  charge screens
  interatrial septal defect; also IASD
  interventricular septal defect; also IVSD
  isosorbide dinitrate; also ID, ISDN
ISDB indirect self-destructive behavior
ISDN isosorbide dinitrate; also ID, ISD
ISE inhibited sexual excitement
  integrated square error
  ion-selective electrode
ISED Interview Schedule for Events and
  Difficulties
ISF interstitial fluid; also IF
ISFET ion-specific field effect transducer
ISFV interstitial fluid volume; also IFV
ISG immune serum globulin
ISGE International Society of
  Gastroenterology
ISH icteric serum hepatitis
  International Society of Hematology
  isolated systolic hypertension
ISI infarct size index
  initial slope index
  injury severity index
  International Sensitivity Index
  International Slope Index
  interstimulus interval
ISIH interspike interval histogram

ISL interscapular line
  interspinous ligament
  isoleucine; also I, Ilc, ILE, Ile, Ileu
ISM International Society of Microbiologists
  intersegmental muscle
ISMA infantile spinal muscular atrophy
ISMO isosorbide-5-mononitrate
ISN intussusception
ISO International Organization for
  Standardization
  isoproterenol; also IP, IPT, IS, Iso, iso, ISP
  isotropic; also Iso, iso
Iso, iso isoproterenol; also IP, IPT, IS, ISO, ISP
  isotropic; also ISO
Is of Lang islets of Langerhans
Isol Isolette
isol isolated
  isolation; also is, isoln
isoln isolation; also is, isol
isom isometric
  isometrophic
IsoPPC isopropyl phenyl carbamate (propham);
  also IPC
IsoRAS isorenin-angiotensin system
isox isoxsuprine
ISP distance between iliac spines
  immunoreactive substance P
  International Streptomyces Project
  interspace; also IS, is
  interspinal
  intraspinal; also IS
  isoproterenol; also IP, IPT, IS, ISO, Iso, iso
ISPT interspecies ovum penetration test
ISPX Ionescu-Shiley pericardial xenograft
isq unchanged [L. *in statu quo*]
ISR information storage and retrieval; also
  IS and R
  Institute for Sex Research
  Institute of Surgical Research
  insulin secretion rate
ISS Injury Severity Scale
  ion-scattering spectroscopy
  ion surface scattering
ISSN international standard serial number
IST in situ transcription
  insulin sensitivity test
  insulin shock therapy
  interstitiospinal tract
  ischemic ST-segment depression
  isometric systolic tension
ISTD insulin standard

ISU International Society of Urology

I-sub inhibitor substance

ISW interstitial water

ISWI incisional surgical wound infection

ISY intrasynovial

IT iliotibial
immunity test
immunologic test
immunotherapy
implantation test
individual therapy
inferior temporal
inferior turbinate
information technology
inhalation test
inhalation therapist
inhalation therapy
inspiratory time
insulin treatment
intact; also int
intensive therapy
intentional tremor
intermittent traction; also int trx
internal thoracic
interstitial tissue
intertrochanteric; also intertroch
intertuberous (pelvic diameter)
intimal thickening
intolerance and toxicity
intracellular tachyzoite
intradermal test
intratesticular
intrathecal (anesthesia injection); also INTH,
ITh, i-thec
intrathoracic
intratracheal; also ITR
intratracheal tube
intratumoral; also i-tumor
ischial tuberosity
isometric transition (of radioactive isotopes)

I/T intensity/time (duration of contractions)

ITA individual treatment assessment
inferior temporal artery
International Tuberculosis Association
itaconic acid

ITAG internal thoracic artery graft

ITB iliotibial band

ITC imidazolyl-thioguanine chemotherapy
incontinence treatment center
Interagency Testing Committee

ITc International Table calorie

ITCP idiopathic thrombocytopenia purpura;
also ITP

ITCU intensive thoracic cardiovascular unit

ITCVD ischemic thrombotic cerebrovascular
disease

ITD insulin-treated diabetic

ITE insufficient therapeutic effect
in the ear (hearing aid)
intrapulmonary interstitial emphysema

ITET isotonic endurance test

ITF interferon; also IF, IFN, INF

ITFF intertrochanteric femoral fracture

ITFS iliotibial tract friction syndrome
incomplete testicular feminization syndrome

ITGV intrathoracic gas volume; also IGV

ITh intrathecal (anesthesia injection); also
INTH, IT, i-thec

i-thec intrathecal (anesthesia injection); also
INTH, IT, ITh

ITI inter-alpha-trypsin inhibitor; also I αTI
interatrial interval

IαTI inter-alpha-trypsin inhibitor; also ITI

ITLC instant thin-layer chromatography

ITLC-SG instant thin-layer
chromatography–silica gel

ITM improved Thayer-Martin (medium)
intrathecal methotrexate
Israel turkey meningoencephalitis

ITOU intensive therapy observation unit;
also IOU

ITP idiopathic thrombocytopenic purpura;
also ITCP
immunogenic thrombocytopenic purpura
inosine 5′-triphosphate
interim treatment plan
islet-cell tumor of the pancreas
isotachophoresis

ITPA Illinois Test of Psycholinguistic Abilities
inosine triphosphatase; also ITPase

ITPase inosine triphosphatase; also ITPA

ITQ Infant Temperament Questionnaire
inferior temporal quadrant

ITR intraocular tension recorder
intratracheal; also IT

ITSC It Scale for Children (psychologic test)

ITSHD isolated thyroid-stimulating hormone
deficiency

ITT identical twins raised together
iliotibial tract
insulin tolerance test
internal tibial torsion
iron tolerance test

ITU intensive therapy unit

i-tumor intratumoral; also IT

ITV inferior temporal vein

ITVAD indwelling transcutaneous vascular access device

ITX intertriginous xanthoma

ITyr monoiodotyrosine

IU immunizing unit; also IE, ImmU
indouracil
International Unit
intrauterine
in utero

[I]U concentration of insulin in urine

iu infectious unit

IUA intrauterine adhesion

IUB International Union of Biochemistry

IUC idiopathic ulcerative colitis
International Union of Chemistry
intrauterine catheter

IUCD intrauterine contraceptive device; also ICD

IUD intrauterine death
intrauterine device

IUF isolated ultrafiltration

IUFB intrauterine foreign body

IUFD intrauterine fetal death
intrauterine fetal demise
intrauterine fetal distress

IUFGR intrauterine fetal growth retardation

IUG infusion urogram
intrauterine gestation
intrauterine growth

IUGR intrauterine growth rate
intrauterine growth retardation; also IGR

IUI intrauterine insemination

IU/L International Unit per liter

IUM internal urethral meatus
intrauterine fetally malnourished
intrauterine malnourishment
intrauterine membrane

IU/min International Unit per minute

IUP intrauterine pregnancy
intrauterine pressure

IUPAC International Union of Pure and Applied Chemistry (Oxford, England)

IUPC intrauterine pressure catheter

IUPD intrauterine pregnancy, delivered

IUP,TBCS intrauterine pregnancy, term birth, cesarean section

IUP,TBLC intrauterine pregnancy, term birth, living child

IUP,TBLI intrauterine pregnancy, term birth, living infant

IUR intrauterine retardation

IUT intrauterine transfusion

IV class 4 controlled substances
ichthyosis vulgaris
interventricular
intervertebral
intravascular
intravenous
intravenously
intraventricular; also I-V, IVT
intravertebral
invasive
in vitro
in vivo
iodine value; also iv

I-V intraventricular; also IV, IVT

iv iodine value; also IV

IVAC intravenous accurate control (device)

IVAD implantable vascular access device

IVag intravaginal

IVAP in vivo adhesive platelet

IVAR insulin variable

IVB intraventricular block
intravitreal blood

IVBAT intravascular bronchioalveolar tumor

IVBC intravascular blood coagulation

IVC individually viable cell
inferior vena cava
inferior venacavagram; also IVCV
inferior venacavography; also IVCV
inspiratory vital capacity
inspired vital capacity
integrated vector control
intravascular coagulation
intravenous cholangiogram; also IVCh
intravenous cholangiography; also IVCh
intraventricular catheter
isovolumic contraction; also IC

IVCC intravascular consumption coagulopathy

IVCD intraventricular conduction defect
intraventricular conduction delay

IVCh intravenous cholangiogram; also IVC
intravenous cholangiography; also IVC

IVCP inferior vena cava pressure

IVCT inferior vena cava thrombosis
intravenously enhanced computed tomography
isovolumic contraction time; also ICT

IVCV inferior venacavagram; also IVC
inferior venacavography; also IVC

IVD intervertebral disk
intravenous drip

IVDA intravenous drug abuse
intravenous drug abuser

IVDSA intravenous digital subtraction angiography

IVDU intravenous drug use
intravenous drug user

IVF interventricular foramen
intravascular fluid
intravenous fluid
in vitro fertilization
in vivo fertilization

IVFE intravenous fat emulsion

IVF-ET in vitro fertilization–embryo transfer

IVFT intravenous fetal transfusion

IVG isotopic ventriculogram

IVGG intravenous gamma-globulin

IVGT intravenous glucose tolerance

IVGTT intravenous glucose tolerance test; also IGTT

IVH intravenous hyperalimentation
intraventricular hemorrhage

IVI In Vitro International, Inc (culture collection)

I/VI may not be heard in all positions, heard only after listener has "tuned in" (heart murmur)

IVIG intravenous immune globulin
intravenous immunoglobulin

IVJC intervertebral joint complex

IVL intravenous lock

IVLBW infant of very low birth weight

IVM immediate visual memory
intravascular mass

IVMP intravenous methylprednisolone

IVN intravenous nutrition

IVNF intravitreal neovascular frond

IVOX intravascular oxygenator

IVP intravenous push (dose); also IVp, IVPU
intravenous pyelogram
intravenous pyelography

intraventricular pressure
intravesical pressure

IVp intravenous push (dose); also IVP, IVPU

IVPB intravenous piggyback (drug administration)

IVPD in vitro protein digestibility

IVPF isovolume pressure flow (curve)

IVPU intravenous push (dose); also IVP, IVp

IVR idioventricular rhythm
internal visual reference
intravaginal ring
isolated volume responder
isovolumic relaxation (time)

IVRT isovolumic relaxation time

IVS inappropriate vasopressin secretion
intact ventricular septum
intervening sequence (DNA)
interventricular septum; also IS
intervillous space
irritable voiding syndrome

IVSD interventricular septal defect; also ISD

IVSE interventricular septal excursion

IVT index of vertical transmission
intravenous transfusion
intraventricular; also IV, I-V
isovolumic time

IVTTT intravenous tolbutamide tolerance test

IVU intravenous urogram
intravenous urography

IVV influenza virus vaccine
intravenous vasopressin

IV/VI loud (heart murmur)

IW inner wall

I-5-W invert sugar (5%) in water

IWI inferior wall infarction
interwave interval

IWL insensible water loss

IWMI inferior wall myocardial infarction; also Inf MI

IWML idiopathic white matter lesion

IWS Index of Work Satisfaction

IYS inverted Y-suspensor

IZ infarction zone
ischemic

IZS insulin zinc suspension

J

J dynamic movement of inertia
electric current density
Jewish
joint; also jnt, jt
joule
Joule's equivalent
journal; also jour, jrl, jrnl
juice; also j, jc
juvenile; also juv
juxtapulmonary capillary (receptor)
magnetic polarization
polypeptide chain in polymeric immuno-
globulins
reference point following QRS complex, at
beginning of ST segment
sound intensity

J flux (density)

J1, J2, J3, etc Jaeger test type number 1, 2, 3,
etc

j jaundice; also jaund, JD
juice; also J, jc

JA juvenile atrophy
juxta-articular

JAI juvenile amaurotic idiocy

jam now [L. *jam*]

JAMA *Journal of the American Medical
Association*

JAMG juvenile autoimmune myasthenia gravis

JAS Jenkins Activity Survey (psychologic test)
Job Attitude Scale

jaund jaundice; also j, JD

JBC Jesness Behavior Checklist

JBE Japanese B encephalitis

JBJS *Journal of Bone and Joint Surgery*

JC Jakob-Creutzfeldt (syndrome)
Jamestown Canyon (virus)
joint contracture
junior clinician (medical student)

J/C joules per coulomb

jc juice; also J, j

JCA juvenile chronic arthritis

JCAE Joint Committee on Atomic Energy

JCAH Joint Commission on Accreditation of
Hospitals (now: JCAHO, Joint Commission
on Accreditation of Healthcare
Organizations)

JCAHO Joint Commission on Accreditation of
Healthcare Organizations

JCAHPO Joint Commission on Allied Health
Personnel in Ophthalmology

JCI Journal of Clinical Investigation

JCF juvenile calcaneal fracture

JCL job control language (computers)

JCML juvenile chronic myelocytic leukemia
juvenile chronic myelogenous leukemia

JCP juvenile chronic polyarthritis

jct junction; also junct, Jx

JCV Jamestown Canyon virus

JD Janet's disease
jaundice; also j, jaund
jejunal diverticulitis
jugulodigastric (node)
juvenile delinquent
juvenile-onset diabetes; also JOD

JDM juvenile-onset diabetes mellitus; also JODM

JDMS juvenile dermatomyositis

JE Japanese encephalitis
junctional escape

JEE Japanese equine encephalitis

JEJ, Jej, jej jejunum

JEM *Journal of Experimental Medicine*

JEMBEC agar plates for transporting cultures
of gonococci

jentac breakfast [L. *jentaculum*]

JEPI Junior Eysenck Personality Inventory

JER Japanese erection ring
junctional escape rhythm

jerry geriatric(s)

JEV Japanese encephalitis virus

JF joint fluid
jugular foramen
junctional fold

JFET junction field-effect transistor

JFS Jewish Family Service
jugular foramen syndrome

JG June grass (test)
juxtaglomerular; also jg, j-g

jg, j-g juxtaglomerular; also JG

JGA juxtaglomerular apparatus

JGC juxtaglomerular cell

JGCT juxtaglomerular cell tumor

JGI jejunogastric intussusception
  juxtaglomerular granulation index
  juxtaglomerular index
JGP juvenile general paralysis
JH heavy-chain joining (segment)
  juvenile hormone (of insects)
j_H heat transfer factor
JHA juvenile hormone analog
JHMO Junior Hospital Medical Officer
JHMV J Howard Mueller virus
JHR Jarisch-Herxheimer reaction
JI jejunal intestinal
  jejunoileal (bypass)
  jejunoileitis
  jejunoileostomy
JIB jejunoileal bypass
JIH joint interval histogram
JIS juvenile idiopathic scoliosis
JJ jaw jerk
  jejunojejunostomy
Jk^a antigen in the Kidd blood group system
Jk^b antigen in the Kidd blood group system
JKD Junius-Kuhnt disease
J/kg joules per kilogram
JKST Johnson-Kenney Screening Test (psychologic test)
JL Jadassohn-Lewandowsky (syndrome)
  Jaffe-Lichtenstein (disease, syndrome)
  Jaksch-Luzet (disease)
JLP juvenile laryngeal papilloma
JM josamycin
  jugomaxillary
j_M mass transfer factor (in heat transfer)
JMD juvenile macular degeneration
JMH John Milton Hagen (antibody)
JMR Jones-Mote reactivity
JMS junior medical student
JNA Jena Nomina Anatomica, 1935
JND just noticeable difference
jnt joint; also J, jt
JOD juvenile-onset diabetes; also JD
JODM juvenile-onset diabetes mellitus; also JDM
JOMAC judgement, orientation, memory, abstraction, and calculation
JOMACI judgement, orientation, memory, abstraction, and calculation intact
jour journal; also J, jrl, jrnl

JP Jackson-Pratt (drain)
  Jobst pump
  joint protection; also JTP
  juvenile periodontitis
JPB junctional premature beat
JPC junctional premature contraction
JPD juvenile plantar dermatosis
JPET *Journal of Pharmacology and Experimental Therapeutics*
JPI Jackson Personality Inventory
JPS joint position sense
JPSA Joint Program for the Study of Abortions
JR Jolly's reaction
  junctional rhythm
JRA juvenile rheumatoid arthritis
jrl journal; also J, jour, jrnl
JRAN junior resident admission note
Jr BF junior baby food
JRC joint replacement center
J receptor juxtapulmonary-capillary receptor
jrnl journal; also J, jour, jrl
JS jejunal segment
  Job syndrome
  junctional slowing
  Junkman-Schoeller (unit of thyrotropin)
J/s joules per second
Js^a antigen in the Sutter blood group system
JSI Jansky Screening Index (psychologic test)
JSU Junkman-Schoeller unit (of thyrotropin)
JSV Jerry-Slough virus
JT jejunostomy tube
  joint
  junctional tachycardia
J/T joules per tesla
jt joint; also J, jnt
jt asp joint aspiration
JTF jejunostomy tube feeding
JTP joint protection; also JP
JTPS juvenile tropical pancreatitis syndrome
Jts joints
Ju jugale
jug jugular
jug comp jugular compression (test)
junct junction; also jct, Jx
juscul soup or broth [L. *jusculum*]
juv juvenile; also J
juxt near [L. *juxta*]

JV jugular vein
  jugular venous (pressure, pulse)
JVC jugular venous catheter
JVD jugular venous distention
JVIS Jackson Vocational Interest Survey
JVP jugular vein pulse
  jugular venous pressure
  jugular venous pulse
JVPT jugular venous pulse tracing
JW Jehovah's Witness
  jump walker
Jx junction; also jct, junct
JXG juvenile xanthogranuloma

K

K KAPPA,UPPER CASE, tenth letter of the Greek alphabet

κ kappa, lower case, tenth letter of the Greek alphabet

magnetic susceptibility; also *k*

one of two types of immunoglobulin light chains

𝗑 kappa, lower case, tenth letter of the Greek alphabet, variant

K 1024 (number of bytes in a kilobyte)

absolute zero

antigen in the Kell blood group system

burst of diphasic slow waves in response to stimuli during sleep (in electroencephalo-graphy)

calix [Gr. *kalyx* (cup)]

capsular antigen [Ger. *Kapsel* (capsule)]

carrying capacity (genetics)

cathodal [Ger. *Kathoden*]; also Ka

cathode [Ger. *Kathode*]; also Ka

coefficient of heat transfer

coefficient of scleral rigidity

cretaceous

dissociation constant; also K, K_d, K_d

electron capture

electrostatic capacity

equilibrium constant; also K, K_{eq}

ionization constant

kallikrein-inhibiting unit; also KIU

kanamycin; also KM

kappa-carageenan (agar)

Kelvin (SI fundamental unit of temperature)

Kelvin (temperature scale)

keratometer

kerma

ketotifen

kidney

killer (cell)

kilo- (10^3); also k

kilopermeability coefficient

kinetic energy; also KE

knee; also KN, Kn, kn

lysine (one-letter notation); also LYS, Lys

modulus of compression

motor coordinator (in General Aptitude Test Battery)

one thousand [Fr. *kilo*]; also k, kilo

phylloquinone (vitamin K_1); also K-1, K_1

potassium [L. *kalium*]; also Kal

ratio of curvature of flattest meridian of apical cornea (in fitting of contact lens)

time

K dissociation constant; also K, K_d, K_d

empirical factor

equilibrium constant; also K, K_{eq}

°K degree on the Kelvin scale (obsolete, now K)

K-1, K_1 phylloquinone (vitamin K_1); also K

K-10 gastric tube

K_3 menadione (vitamin $K_{3(0)}$)

K-4, K_4 menadiol diacetate (vitamin K_4)

17K, 17-K 17-ketosteroids; also 17-Keto, 17-KS

^{40}K potassium 40, radioactive potassium [L. *kalium* (potassium)]; halflife 1.28×10^9 years

^{42}K potassium 42, radioactive potassium [L. *kalium* (potassium)]; halflife 12.4 hours

^{43}K potassium 43, radioactive potassium [L. *kalium* (potassium)]; halflife 22.4 hours

K_3 menadione

K-4, K_4 menadiol sodium diphosphate

K34 hexachlorophene

k antigen in the Kell blood group system

Boltzmann's constant; also *k*

constant

kilo- (10^3); also K

one thousand [Fr. *kilo*]; also K, kilo

rate of velocity constant

reaction rate constant

κ Boltzmann's constant; also k

glass electrode constant

magnetic susceptibility; also κ

rate constant

KA kainic acid

keratoacanthoma

keto acid

ketoacidosis

King-Armstrong (unit); also K-A

kynurenic acid

K/A ketogenic to antiketogenic (ratio)

K-A King-Armstrong (unit); also KA

Ka cathodal [Ger. *Kathoden*]; also K

cathode [Ger. *Kathode*]; also K

kallikrein

K_a, K_a acid dissociation constant

kA kiloampere

KAAD kerosene, alcohol, acetic acid, and dioxane (mixture)

KAB knowledge, attitude, and behavior

KABC Kaufman Assessment Battery for Children

KABINS knowledge, attitude, behavior, and improvement in nutritional status

KAF conglutinogen-activating factor
killer-assisting factor
kinase-activating factor

KAFO knee-ankle-foot orthosis

KAHRP knob-associated histidine-rich protein

Kal potassium [L. *kalium*]; also K

KAO knee-ankle orthosis

KAP knowledge, aptitudes, and practices (fertility)

KAS Katz Adjustment Scales (psychologic test)

KASH knowledge, abilities, skills, and habits

KAST Kindergarten Auditory Screening Test

KAT kanamycin acetyltransferase

kat katal (enzyme unit of measurement)

kat/L katals per liter

KAU King-Armstrong unit

KB human oral epidermoid carcinoma cells
Kashin-Bek (disease)
ketone bodies
kilobyte
knee brace
knuckle-bender (splint)

K-B Kleihauer-Betke (test); also KL-BET

K/B knee bearing (prosthesis)

K$_b$, *K*$_b$ dissociation constant of a base

Kb, kb kilobase (1000 base pairs)

kbp kilobase pair(s) (nucleic acid molecules)

kBq kilobecquerel

KBS Klüver-Bucy syndrome

KC cathodal closing [Ger. *Kathoden* (cathodal)]
keratoconjunctivitis
keratoconus
keratoma climacterium
knees to chest
knuckle cracking
Kupffer's cell

kC kilocoulomb

kc kilocycle

K Cal, Kcal, kcal kilocalorie

KCC cathodal closing contraction [Ger. *Kathoden* (cathodal)] as in KCT, KCTe and others; also KSC, KSK
Kulchitsky's cell carcinoma

KCCT kaolin-cephalin clotting time

KCG kinetocardiogram

kCi kilocurie

KCM keratinocyte-conditioned medium

K complex slow waves related to sleep arousal (in electroencephalography)

kcps kilocycles per second; also kc/sec, kc/s

KCS keratoconjunctivitis sicca

kc/sec kilocycles per second; also kcps, kc/s

kc/s kilocycles per second; also kcps, kc/sec

KCT cathodal closing tetanus [Ger. *Kathoden* (cathodal)]; also KCTe, KST

KCTe cathodal closing tetanus [Ger. *Kathoden* (cathodal)]; also KCT, KST

KD cathodal duration [Ger. *Kathoden* (cathodal)]
Kawasaki disease
kidney donor
killed
kilodalton; also kd, kdal
knee disarticulation
knitted Dacron

K$_d$, *K*$_d$ dissociation constant; also K, *K*
distribution coefficient
partition coefficient

kd kilodalton; also KD, kdal

KDA known drug allergies

kdal kilodalton; also KD, kd

KDC cathodal duration contraction [Ger. *Kathoden* (cathodal)]
independent kidney disease treatment center

KDO ketodeoxyoctonate
ketodeoxyoctonic acid

KDP potassium dihydrogen phosphate [L. *kalium* (potassium)]

KDS Kaufman Development Scale

KDSM keratinizing desquamative squamous metaplasia

KDT cathodal duration tetanus [Ger. *Kathoden* (cathodal)]; also KDTe

KDTe cathodal duration tetanus [Ger. *Kathoden* (cathodal)]; also KDT

kdyn kilodyne

KE Kendall's compound E (cortisone)
kinetic energy; also K

Ke antigenic marker distinguishing human immunoglobulin lambda (λ) light chain subtypes

K$_e$ exchangeable body potassium [L. *kalium* (potassium)]

KED Kendrick extrication device

K-el phyllochromenol

Kemo Tx chemotherapy

K_{eq} equilibrium constant; also K, K

Kera keratitis

KERV Kentucky equine respiratory virus

keto 17-ketosteroid (test)

17-Keto 17-ketosteroids; also 17K, 17-K, 17-KS

kev, keV kiloelectron volt

KF Kenner-fecal (medium)
kidney function
Klippel-Feil (syndrome)

kf flocculation rate in antigen-antibody reaction

KFAB kidney-fixing antibody

K factor gamma-ray dose (roentgens per hour at 1 cm from 1-mCi point source of radiation)

KFAO knee-foot-ankle orthosis

KFD Kinetic Family Drawing
Kyasanur Forest disease

KFR Kayser-Fleischer ring

KFS Klippel-Feil syndrome

KG ketoglutarate

α**KG** alpha-ketoglutarate

Kg conglutinin
kilogram; also kg, kilo

kG kilogauss

kg kilogram; also Kg, kilo

KG-1 Koeffler Golde-1 (cell line)

KGC Keflin (cephalothin), gentamicin, and carbenicillin

kg-cal kilogram-calorie (large calorie)

KGHT kidney Goldblatt hypertension

kg/cm² kilograms per square centimeter

KGDHC ketoglutarate dehydrogenase complex

kgf kilogram-force

kg/L kilograms per liter

kg-m kilogram-meter

kg-m/s² kilogram-meter per second squared (Newton)

Kgn kininogen

kgps kilograms per second; also kg/s

KGS ketogenic steroid

17-KGS 17-ketogenic steroid

kg/s kilograms per second; also kgps

Kg Sp conglutinin solid phase

KH Krebs-Henseleit (buffer, cycle)

K24H potassium in 24-hour urine [L. *kalium* (potassium)]

KHB Krebs-Henseleit bicarbonate

KHb potassium hemoglobinate [L. *kalium* (potassium)]; also K hgb

KHC kinetic hemolysis curve

KHD kinky hair disease

KHF Korean hemorrhagic fever

K hgb potassium hemoglobinate [L. *kalium* (potassium)]; also KHb

KHM keratoderma hereditaria mutilans

KHN Knoop hardness number (of solids)

KHS kinky hair syndrome
Krebs-Henseleit solution

kHz kilohertz

KI karyopyknotic index; also KPI
knee immobilizer
Krönig's isthmus

K_i dissociation of enzyme-inhibitor complex
inhibition constant

KIA Kliger's iron agar (medium)

KIC ketoisocaproate
ketoisocaproic acid

KICB killed intracellular bacteria

KID keratitis, ichthyosis, and deafness (syndrome)

KIDS Kent Infant Development Scale

kilo kilogram; also Kg, kg
kilometer; also km
one thousand [Fr. *kilo*]; also K, k

KIMSA Kirsten murine sarcoma

KIMSV, Ki-MSV Kirsten murine sarcoma virus

KIP key intermediary protein

KIS Krankenhaus Information System

KISS key integrative social system
kidney internal splint/stent
potassium iodide, saturated solution [L. *kalium* (potassium)]

KIT Kahn intelligence test

KIU kallikrein-inactivation unit
kallikrein-inhibiting unit; also K

KJ kilojoule; also kJ
knee jerk; also kj

kj knee jerk; also KJ

kJ kilojoule; also KJ

KK kallikrein
knee kick; also kk

kk knee kick; also KK

kkat kilokatal

KL kidney lobe
Klebs-Löffler (agar, bacillus)
Kleine-Levin (syndrome)

kL kiloliter; also kl

kl kiloliter; also kL
musical overtone (ringing, in acoustics) [Ger.
Klang (sound, tone)]

KL bac Klebs-Löffler bacillus

KL-BET Kleihauer-Betke (test); also K-B

Kleb *Klebsiella* species

K level lowest level (of x-rays)

KLH keyhole limpet hemocyanin

KLS kidney(s), liver, and spleen
Kreuzbein lipomatous syndrome

KLST Kindergarten Language Screening Test

KM kanamycin; also K
kappa-immunoglobulin (light chain)
Kraepelin-Morel (disease)

Km, K_m, K_M, K_m, K_m Michaelis' constant (in
enzyme assays)
Michaelis-Menten dissociation constant

km kilometer; also kilo

km² square kilometer

km³ cubic kilometer

kMc kilomegacycle

K-MCM potassium-containing minimal-capac-
itation medium [L. *kalium* (potassium)]

kMcps kilomegacycles per second; also kMc/s

kMc/s kilomegacycles per second; also kMcps

KMDAT Key Math Diagnostic Arithmetic Test

KMEF keratin, myosin, epidermis, and fibrin
(class of proteins)

kmps kilometers per second; also km/s

km/s kilometers per second; also kmps

KMSV Kirsten murine sarcoma virus

KMV killed measles virus (vaccine)

KN knee; also K, Kn, kn

Kn knee; also K, KN, kn
know
knowledge
Knudsen number (low-pressure gas flow)

kN kilonewton

kn knee; also K, KN, Kn

K nail Küntscher's nail

KNO keep needle open

knork knife and fork (physiatry)

KNRK Kirsten sarcoma virus in normal rat
kidney (cell)

KO keep on (continue); also K/O
keep open; also K/O
killed organism
knee orthosis
knocked out; also KO'd

K/O keep on (continue); also KO
keep open; also KO

KOC cathodal opening contraction [Ger.
Kathoden (cathodal)]

KO'd knocked out; also KO

KOH potassium hydroxide (test)

KOIS Kuder Occupational Interest Survey

kΩ kilohm

KOT Knowledge of Occupations Test

KP Kaufmann-Peterson (base)
keratitic precipitate
keratitis punctata
keratoprecipitate
keratotic patch
kidney protein
kidney punch (trauma)
killed parenteral (vaccine)
Klebsiella pneumoniae

K-P Kaiser-Permanente

KPA kidney plasminogen activator (prourokinase)

kPa kilopascal

kPa·s/L kilopascal-seconds per liter; also
kPa-s/L

kPa-s/L kilopascal-seconds per liter; also
kPa·s/L

KPB ketophenylbutazone (kebuzone)
potassium phosphate buffer [L. *kalium* (potassium)]

KPBS potassium phosphate buffer saline [L.
kalium (potassium)]

KPE Kelman phacoemulsification

KPI karyopyknotic index; also KI

KPM kilo-pound-meters

KPR key pulse rate
Kuder Preference Record

KPR-V Kuder Preference Record–Vocational

KPT kidney punch test (physical exam)
Kuder Performance Test

KPTI Kunitz pancreatic trypsin inhibitor

KPTT kaolin partial thromboplastin time

KPV killed parenteral vaccine
killed polio vaccine

KR knowledge of results
Kopper Reppart (medium)

Kr krypton

kR kiloroentgen

KRA Klinefelter-Reifenstein-Albright (syndrome)

KRB Krebs-Ringer bicarbonate buffer; also KRBB

KRBB Krebs-Ringer bicarbonate buffer; also KRB

KRBG Krebs-Ringer bicarbonate buffer with glucose

KRBS Krebs-Ringer bicarbonate solution

KRH HEPES (see HEPES)-buffered Krebs-Ringer saline

KRP Kolmer's test with Reiter protein antigen
Krebs-Ringer phosphate

KRPS Krebs-Ringer phosphate buffer solution

KRRS kinetic resonance Raman spectroscopy

KS Kaposi's sarcoma
Kartagener's syndrome
Kawasaki syndrome
keratin sulfate
ketosteroid
Klinefelter's syndrome
Kochleffel's syndrome
Korsakoff's syndrome
Kugel-Stoloff (syndrome)
Kveim-Siltzbach (test)

17-KS 17-ketosteroids; also 17K, 17-K, 17-Keto

ks kilosecond

KSA knowledge, skills and abilities

KSC cathodal closing contraction [Ger. *Kathodenschließungs* (cathodal closing)]; also KCC, KSK

KSK cathodal closing contraction [Ger. *Kathodenschließungs-Kontraktion*]; also KCC, KSC

KS/OI Kaposi's sarcoma and opportunistic infections

KSP kidney-specific protein

K$_{sp}$ potassium solubility product

K$_{sp}$ solubility product constant

KSS Kearns-Sayre syndrome

KST cathodal closing tetanus [Ger. *Kathodenschließungs-Tetanus*]; also KCT, KCTe

KSU Kent State University (Speech Discrimination Test)

KT kidney transplant
kidney transplantation
kidney treatment
Klippel-Trenaunay (syndrome)

KTI kallikrein-trypsin inhibitor
Kunitz' trypsin inhibitor

KTS kethoxal thiosemicarbazone

KTSA Kahn Test of Symbol Arrangement

KTVS Keystone Telebinocular Visual Survey

KTWS Klippel-Trenaunay-Weber syndrome

KU kallikrein unit
Karmen unit
Kimbel unit
Kimbrel unit

Ku kurchatovium

KUB kidney and urinary bladder
kidneys, ureter, and bladder (x-ray examination)

KUS kidney(s), ureter(s), and spleen

KV kanamycin-vancomycin
killed vaccine

kV, kv kilovolt

kVA, kVa kilovolt-ampere

KVBA kanamycin-vancomycin blood agar

kVcp, kvcp kilovolt constant potential

KVE Kaposi's varicelliform eruption

KVLBA kanamycin-vancomycin laked blood agar

KVO keep vein open (IV lines)

KVO C D5W keep vein open with 5% dextrose in water [L. *cum* (with)]

kVp, kvp kilovolt peak

KW Keith-Wagener (retinopathy)
Kimmelstiel-Wilson (syndrome)
Kugelberg-Welander (disease)

K$_w$, K_W dissociation constant of water

kW, kw kilowatt

KWB Keith-Wagener-Barker (classification of eyeground findings)

kWh kilowatt-hour; also kW-hr, kw-hr

kW-hr, kw-hr kilowatt-hour; also kWh

KWIC keyword in context (computers)

K wire Kirschner's wire

KWOC keyword out of context (computers)

kx crystallography unit

kyph kyphosis

KZ Kaplan-Zuelzer (syndrome)

L

Λ LAMBDA, UPPER CASE, eleventh letter of the Greek alphabet

λ lambda, lower case, eleventh letter of the Greek alphabet
craniometric point
decay constant
homosexuality
junction of lambdoid and sagittal sutures (craniotomy)
mean free path
microliter (now μl)
one of two forms of immunoglobulin light chain
thermal conductivity; also TC
wavelength; also WL

L angular momentum
Avogadro's constant or number
book [L. *liber*]
boundary [L. *limes* (boundary or limit)]; also LIM
coefficient of induction
diffusion length
inductance (in henries)
Lactobacillus species; also L
lambert (unit of luminance); also La
latent heat
latex; also LX, Lx
Latin; also Lat
left; also (L), l, laev, lf, LT, lt
length; also l, *l*
Lente insulin
lesser
lethal (Ehrlich's symbol for fatal); also l
leucine (one-letter notation); also LEU, Leu, leu
levo- (to the left, counterclockwise); also l-, *l-*
levorotary (rotated to the left or counterclockwise); also l-, *l-*
lewisite
licensed (to practice)
lidocaine; also LIDO
ligament; also l, Lgt, lgt, lig
ligamentum [L. *ligamentum* (ligament)]; also l, Lgt, lgt, lig
light; also LT, lt
light (chain of protein molecules)
light sense
lilac (indicator color)
limes [L. *limes* (boundary or limit)]
lincomycin; also LM

lingual; also ling
liquor; also LIQ, Liq, liq
liter; also l, ℓ
liver; also LIV
living; also liv
longitudinal (section)
low; also LO
lower; also LO
lowest; also LO
lumbar; also lum, lumb
lumen; also lm
luminance; also *L*
lung; also LU, Lu
lymph; also LYM
lymphocyte; also LY, lym, lymph
lymphogranuloma
lysosome; also LYS, Lys
pound [L. *libra*]; also lb, lib
radiance
self-inductance; also *L*
syphilis [L. *lues* (pestilence, plague)]
threshold [L. *limen*]

L *Lactobacillus* species; also L
Leishmania species
luminance; also L
self-inductance; also L

$\mathcal{L}$ laplace transform

(L) left; also L, l, laev, lf, LT, lt
lunch

L0, L$_0$ limes null (neutralized toxin-antitoxin mixture) [L. *limes nullus* (no path)]

L+, L$_+$ limes tod (toxin-antitoxin mixture that contains one fatal dose in excess) [L. *limes* (boundary or limit), Ger. *tod* (death)]

L-I first stage of syphilis [L. *lues* (plague)]; also Lues I

L-II second stage of syphilis [L. *lues* (plague)]; also Lues II

L-III third stage of syphilis [L. *lues* (plague)]; also Lues III

L1 - L5, L$_1$ - L$_5$ first through fifth lumbar vertebrae or lumbar nerves

L/3 lower third (of leg bone)

L- sterically related to L-glyceraldehyde

l left; also L, (L), laev, lf, LT, lt
length; also L, *l*
lethal; also L
ligament; also L, Lgt, lgt, lig

ligamentum [L. *ligamentum* (ligament)]; also L, Lgt, lgt, lig

line

liter; also L, ℓ

long; also lg

longitudinal; also long

lyxose; also Lyx

radioactive constant

specific latent heat

l- levo- (to the left, counterclockwise); also L, *l-*

levorotary (rotated to the left or counterclockwise); also L, *l-*

l length; also L, l

ℓ liter; also L, l

l- levo- (to the left, counterclockwise); also L, l-

levorotatory (rotated to the left or counterclockwise); also L, l-

LA lactic acid

language age

large amount

late abortion

late antigen

latex agglutination

Latin American

left angle

left angulation

left anterior; also L ANT

left arm

left atrial (pressure)

left atrium (echocardiography image)

left auricle

leucine aminopeptidase; also LAP

leukemia antigen

leukoagglutinating

levator ani (muscle)

lichen amyloidosis

Lightwood-Albright (syndrome)

linguoaxial

linoleic acid

lobuloalveolar

local anesthesia

long-acting (drug)

long-arm (cast)

low anxiety

Ludwig angina

lupus anticoagulant

lymphocyte antibody

L&A light and accommodation (reaction of pupils); also L+A, l&a

living and active (family history); also L+A, l&a

L+A light and accommodation (reaction of pupils); also L&A, l&a

living and active (family history); also L&A, l&a

LA50 lethal area (total body surface area of burn that will kill 50% of patients)

La labial

lambert (unit of luminance); also L

lanthanum

la according to the art [L. *lege artis*]

l&a light and accommodation (reaction of pupils); also L&A, L+A

living and active (family history); also L&A, L+A

LAA left atrial abnormality

left atrial appendage

left auricular appendage

leukemia-associated antigen

leukocyte ascorbic acid

LAAO L-amino acid oxidase

LAARD long-acting antirheumatic drug

LAB Leisure Activities Blank (psychology)

laboratory; also lab, LB

lab laboratory; also LAB, LB

rennet [Ger. *Lab* (rennet)]

LABS Laboratory Admission Baseline Studies

LABVT left atrial ball-valve thrombus

LAC laceration; also lac

La Crosse (arbovirus)

lactose; also Lac

left atrial contraction

linguoaxiocervical

long-arm cast

low amplitude contraction

lung adenocarcinoma cell

LaC labiocervical

Lac lactose; also LAC

lac laceration; also LAC

lactate; also lact

lactating; also lact

lactation; also lact

lac & cont lacerations and contusions

LACN local area communications network

lacr lacrimal

LACT Lindamood Auditory Conceptualization Test (psychology)

LAC T lactose tolerance

lact lactate; also lac

lactating; also lac

lactation; also lac

lactic

LACT-ART lactate arterial

lact hyd lactalbumin hydrolysate; also LAH

LAD lactic acid dehydrogenase; also LADH, LD, LDG, LDH
language acquisition device
left anterior descending (coronary artery)
left axis deviation
linoleic acid depression
lipoamide dehydrogenase
lymphocyte-activating determinant

LADA laboratory animal dander allergy
left acromiodorso-anterior (fetal position)

LADCA left anterior descending coronary artery

LADD lacrimoauriculodentodigital (syndrome)
left anterior descending diagonal (branch of coronary artery)

LADH lactic acid dehydrogenase; also LAD, LD, LDG, LDH
liver alcohol dehydrogenase

LADME liberation, absorption, distribution, metabolism, and excretion

LAD-MIN left axis deviation, minimal

LADP left acromiodorso-posterior (fetal position)

LADu lobuloalveolar-ductal

LAE left atrial enlargement
long above-elbow (cast)

LAEDV left atrial end-diastolic volume

LAEI left atrial emptying index

LAESV left atrial end-systolic volume

laev left [L. *laevus*]; also L, (L), l, lf, LT, lt

LAF laminar air flow; also LAM
Latin American female
leukocyte-activating factor
low animal fat
lymphocyte-activating factor

LAFB left anterior fascicular block

LAFR laminar air flow room

LAFU laminar air flow unit

LAG labiogingival; also LaG
linguoaxiogingival
lymphangiogram
lymphangiography

LaG labiogingival; also LAG

lag a flask [L. *lagona*]

LAH lactalbumin hydrolysate; also lact hyd
left anterior hemiblock; also LAHB
left atrial hypertrophy
lithium-aluminum hydride

LAHB left anterior hemiblock; also LAH

LAHV leukocyte-associated herpesvirus

LAI labioincisal; also LaI
latex particle agglutination inhibition
left atrial involvement
leukocyte adherence inhibition (assay)
location-activity inventory

LaI labioincisal; also LAI

LAIF leukocyte adherence inhibition factor

LAIT latex agglutination-inhibition test

LAK lymphokine-activated killer (cell)

LAL left axillary line
Limulus amebocyte lysate
low air loss

LaL labiolingual

L-Ala L-alanine

LALI lymphocyte antibody lymphocytolytic interaction

LALLS low-angle laser-light scattering interaction

LAM lactation amenorrhea method
laminar air flow; also LAF
laminectomy; also Lam, lam
L-asparaginase and methotrexate
late ambulatory monitoring
Latin American male
left anterior measurement
left atrial myxoma
lymphangioleiomyomatosis

Lam, lam lamina
laminectomy; also LAM
laminogram

LA-MAX maximal left atrial (dimension)

LAMB lentigines, atrial myxoma, mucocutaneous myxomas, and blue nevi

lam & fus laminectomy and fusion

lami laminotomy

LAMMA laser microprobe mass analyzer

LAN long-acting neuroleptic
lymphadenopathy

Lan lanthionine

LANC long-arm navicular cast

Lang, lang language

L ANT left anterior; also LA

LANV left atrial neovascularization

LAO lateral anterior oblique
left anterior oblique
left anterior occipital
left atrial overloading

LAP laparoscopy; also lap
laparotomy; also lap
left atrial pressure

leucine aminopeptidase; also LA
leukocyte alkaline phosphatase; also
    LEUKAP
low atmospheric pressure
lyophilized anterior pituitary (tissue)

lap laparoscopy; also LAP
laparotomy; also LAP

LAPA leukocyte alkaline phosphatase activity

LAPF low-affinity platelet factor

lapid stony [L. *lapideum*]

LAPMS long-arm posterior-molded splint

LAPOCA L-asparaginase, prednisone,
    Oncovin, cytarabine, and Adriamycin

LAPSE long-term ambulatory physiologic
    surveillance (vital sign monitor)

LAPW left atrial posterior wall

LAR laryngology; also Laryngol
late asthmatic response
left arm, reclining (blood pressure, pulse
    measurement)
left arm, recumbent (blood pressure, pulse
    measurement)

lar larynx; also lx

LARC leukocyte automatic recognition com-
    puter

LARS Language-Structured Auditory
    Retention Span (Test)

laryn laryngeal
laryngitis
laryngoscopy

Laryngol laryngology; also LAR

LAS laboratory automation system
lateral amyotrophic sclerosis
laxative abuse syndrome
left anterior-superior
left arm, sitting (blood pressure, pulse
    measurement)
leucine acetylsalicylate
linear alkyl sulfonate
local adaption syndrome
long-arm splint
lower abdominal surgery
lymphadenopathy syndrome
lymphangioscintigraphy

LASER, laser light amplification by stimulated
    emission of radiation

LASFB left anterior-superior fascicular block

LASH left anterior-superior hemiblock

L-ASP L-asparaginase

LASS labile aggregation-stimulating substance
Linguistic Analysis of Speech Samples

LAST leukocyte-antigen sensitivity testing

LAT latent
lateral; also lat
latex agglutination test
left anterior thigh

Lat Latin; also L

lat lateral; also LAT
latissimus (dorsi)
latitude

LAT-A latrunculin A

lat admov let it be applied to the side [L. *lateri
    admoveatur*]

LAT-B latrunculin B

LATCH literature attached to charts

lat dol to the painful side [L. *lateri dolenti*]

lat & loc lateralizing and localizing

l·atm liter-atmosphere; also l-atm

l-atm liter-atmosphere; also l·atm

lat men lateral meniscectomy

LATP left atrial transmural pressure

lat Rin lactated Ringer's (injection, solution);
    also LR

LATS long-acting thyroid-stimulating (hor-
    mone)
long-acting thyroid stimulator
long-acting transmural stimulator

LATS-P, LATS-p long-acting thyroid stimula-
    tor protector

LATu lobuloalveolar tumor

LAV lymphadenopathy-associated virus

lav lavatory

LAW left atrial wall

lax laxative
laxity

LB laboratory; also LAB, lab
lamellar body
large bowel
lateral bending
Lederer-Brill (syndrome)
left breast
left bundle
left buttock
leiomyoblastoma; also LMB
lipid body
live birth
liver biopsy
Living Bank
loose body
low back (pain)
low breakage
lung biopsy

L-B Liebermann-Burchardt (test for cholesterol)

L&B left and below

Lb pound force; also lbf

lb pound [L. *libra*]; also L, lib

LBA left basal artery

lb ap apothecary pound [L. *libra apothecary*]

lb av avoirdupois pound [L. *libra avoirdupois*]

LBB left breast biopsy
left bundle-branch
low back bend

LBBB left bundle-branch block

LBBsB left bundle-branch system block

LBBX left breast biopsy examination

LBC lidocaine blood concentration

LBCD left border cardiac dullness

LBCF Laboratory Branch Complement Fixation (test)

LBD large bile duct
left border dullness (of heart to percussion)

LBDQ Leader Behavior Description Questionnaire

LBE long below-elbow (cast)

LBF *Lactobacillus bulgaricus* factor (pantetheine)
limb blood flow
liver blood flow

lbf pound force; also Lb

lbf-ft pound force foot

lb-ft pound-feet

LBH length, breadth, height

LBI low serum-bound iron

lb/in^2 pounds per square inch; also PSI, psi

LBL labeled lymphoblast
lymphoblastic lymphoma; also LL

LBM last bowel movement
lean body mass
loose bowel movement
lung basement membrane

LBNP lower-body negative pressure

LBO large bowel obstruction

LBP low back pain
low blood pressure

LBPQ Low Back Pain Questionnaire

LBRF louse-borne relapsing fever

LBS lactobacillus selector (agar)
low back syndrome

lbs pounds [L. *librae*]

LBSA lipid-bound sialic acid; also LSA

LBT low back tenderness
low back trouble
lupus band test

lb t pound troy [L. *libra troy*]; also lb tr

LBTI lima bean trypsin inhibitor

lb tr pound troy [L. *libra troy*]; also lb t

LBV left brachial vein
lung blood volume

LBW lean body weight
low birth weight

LBWI low birth weight infant

LBWR lung-body weight ratio

LC lactation consultant
Laennec's cirrhosis
lamina cortex
Langerhan's cell
Lannois-Cleret (syndrome)
large chromophobe
large cleaved (cell)
late clamped (umbilical cord)
lecithin cholesterol (acyltransferase)
left circumflex (coronary artery); also LCF, LCX, LCx
left ear, cold stimulus
leisure counseling
lethal concentration
Library of Congress
life care
light chain
light coagulation
linguocervical
lining cell
lipid cytosome(s)
liquid chromatography
liquid crystal
lithocholic (acid)
live clinic
liver cirrhosis
liver clinic
living children
locus ceruleus
long-chain (triglycerides)
longus capitis (muscle)
low calorie; also lo cal
lung cancer
lung cell
lymph capillary
lymphocyte count
lymphocytotoxin; also LCT, LT
lymphoma culture

LC$_{50}$ median lethal concentration

lc in the place cited [L. *loco citato*]; also loc cit

LCA Leber's congenital amaurosis

left circumflex artery
left coronary artery
leukocyte common antigen
light contact assist
lithocholic acid
lymphocyte chemoattractant activity
lymphocytotoxic antibody; also LCTA

LCAO linear combination of atomic orbitals

LCAO-MO linear combination of atomic orbital–molecular orbital

LCAR late cutaneous anaphylactic reaction

LCAT lecithin-cholesterol acyltransferase

LCB Laboratory of Cancer Biology
left costal border

LCBF local cerebral blood flow

LCC lactose coliform count
left coronary cusp
liver cell carcinoma

LCCA late cortical cerebellar atrophy
left circumflex coronary artery
left common carotid artery
leukoclastic angiitis
leukocytoclastic angiitis

LCCME Liaison Committee on Continuing
Medical Education (now: ACCME,
Accreditation Council for Continuing
Medical Education)

LCCP limited channel-capacity process

LCCS low cervical cesarean section

LCCSCT large-cell calcifying Sertoli cell
tumor

LCD liquid-crystal display
liquor carbonis detergens (coal tar solution)
localized collagen dystrophy
low calcium diet
lowest common denominator

LCDD light-chain deposition disease

LCED liquid chromatography with electrochemical detection

LCF least common factor
left circumflex (coronary artery); also LC,
LCX, LCx
linear correction factor
low-frequency current field
lymphocyte culture fluid

LCFA long-chain fatty acid

LCFAO long-chain fatty acid oxidation

LCFC linear combination of fragment configuration

LCFM left circumflex marginal

LCFU leukocyte colony-forming unit

LCG Langerhan's cell granule

LCGME Liaison Committee on Graduate
Medical Education

LCGU local cerebral glucose utilization

LCH local city hospital

LCh Licentiate in Surgery [L. *Licentiate
Chirurgiae*]; also LS

LCI length complexity index
lung clearance index

LCIS lobular carcinoma in situ

LCL large cell lymphoma
lateral collateral ligament
Levinthal-Coles-Lillie (cytoplasmic inclusion
body)
lower confidence limit
lymphoblastoid cell line
lymphocytic leukemia; also LL
lymphocytic lymphosarcoma
lymphoid cell line

LCLC large-cell lung carcinoma

LCLo lethal concentration low

LCM latent cardiomyopathy
left costal margin
leukocyte-conditioned medium
lower costal margin
lowest common multiple
lymphatic choriomeningitis
lymphocytic choriomeningitis

LCME Liaison Committee on Medical
Education

LCMG long-chain monoglyceride

l/cm H₂O liters per centimeter of water

LCMR local cerebral metabolic rate

LCMV lymphocytic choriomeningitis virus;
also LCV

LCN lateral cervical nucleus
left caudate nucleus

LCO low cardiac output

LCOS low cardiac output syndrome; also LOS

LCP Legg-Calvé-Perthes (disease)
long-chain polysaturated (fatty acid)

LCPD Legg-Calvé-Perthes disease

LCPS Licentiate of the College of Physicians
and Surgeons

LCQG left caudal quarter ganglion

LCR late cortical response
late cutaneous reaction
leurocristine (vincristine)

LCS left coronary sinus
Leydig cell stimulation
lichen chronicus simplex

LCS—cont'd
life care service
liquor cerebrospinalis
low continuous suction

LCSG Lung Cancer Study Group

LCSW Licensed Clinical Social Worker

LCT liquid crystal thermogram
liquid crystal thermography
liver cell tumor
long-chain triglyceride
low cervical transverse
lung capillary time
Luscher Color Test
lymphocyte cytotoxic test
lymphocytotoxicity test
lymphocytotoxin; also LC, LT

LCTA lymphocytotoxic antibody; also LCA

LCTD low calcium test diet

LCU life change unit

LCV lecithovitellin; also LV
leucovorin; also LEU, LV, Lv, LVR
low cervical vertical (incision)
lymphocytic choriomeningitis virus; also
LCMV

LCX, LCx left circumflex (coronary artery);
also LC, LCF

LD labor and delivery; also L&D
laboratory data
labyrinthine defect
lactate dehydrogenase; also LDG, LDH
lactic acid dehydrogenase; also LAD, LADH,
LDG, LDH
last dose
L-DOPA
learning disability
learning disabled
learning disorder
left deltoid
Legionnaires' disease
Leishman-Donovan (bodies); also L-D
Leishmania donovani
lethal dose
levodopa; also L-DOPA, L-dopa, L-DOPA
light-dark
light difference (perception of)
light differentiation
light duty
limited disease
linear dichroism
linguodistal
lipodystrophy
lithium diluent

lithium discontinuation
liver disease
living donor
loading dose
Lombard-Dowell (agar)
longitudinal diameter (of heart)
long time dialysis
low density
low dosage
lung destruction
lymphocyte-defined (antigen)
lymphocyte-depleted (Hodgkin's disease)
lymphocyte depletion
lymphocytically determined

L-D Leishman-Donovan (bodies); also LD

L/D light to dark (ratio)

L&D labor and delivery; also LD
light and distance (in ophthalmology)

LD$_1$–LD$_5$ lactate dehydrogenase, fractions 1
through 5; also LDH$_1$–LDH$_5$

LD$_{50}$ median lethal dose (lethal dose for 50%
of test subjects)

LD$_{50}$ time median lethal time

LD$_{50/30}$ lethal dose for 50% of test subjects
within 30 days

LD100, LD$_{100}$ lethal dose in all exposed subjects

LDA laser Doppler anemometry
left descending artery
left dorso-anterior (fetal position)
linear discriminant analysis
linear displacement analysis
lymphocyte-dependent antibody

LDAR latex direct agglutination reaction

LDB lamb dysentery bacillus
Legionnaires' disease bacillus

LDC leukocyte differential count
lymphoid dendritic cell

LDCC lectin-dependent cellular cytotoxicity

LDCT late distal cortical tubule

LDCV large dense-core vesicle

LDD late dedifferentiation
light-dark discrimination

LDDS local dentist

LDE lauric diethamide (*N, N*-diethyllauramide)

LD-EYA Lombard-Dowell egg yolk agar

LDF limit dilution factor

LDG lactate dehydrogenase; also LD, LDH
lactic acid dehydrogenase; also LAD, LADH,
LD, LDH

lingual developmental groove
long-distance group
low-dose group

LDH lactate dehydrogenase; also LD, LDG
lactic acid dehydrogenase; also LAD, LADH, LD, LDG
low-dose heparin

LDH₁–LDH₅ lactate dehydrogenase, fractions 1 through 5; also LD₁–LD₅

LDHA lactate dehydrogenase A

LDHB lactate dehydrogenase B

LDHI lactate dehydrogenase isoenzyme; also LDISO

LDIH left direct inguinal hernia

LDISO lactate dehydrogenase isoenzyme; also LDHI

LDL loudness discomfort level
low-density lipoprotein; also LDLP
low-density lymphocyte

LDLC, LDL-C low-density lipoprotein cholesterol

LDLo lethal dose low

LDLP low-density lipoprotein; also LDL

LDM lactate dehydrogenase, muscle

LDMS laser desorption mass spectrometry

LD-NEYA Lombard-Dowell neomycin egg yolk agar

L-DOPA, L-dopa, L-DOPA levodopa; also LD

L doses limes doses (toxin/antitoxin combining power) [L. *limes* (boundary or limit)]

LDP left dorsoposterior (fetal position)
lumbodorsal pain

LDRP labor, delivery, recovery, postpartum

LDS Licentiate in Dental Surgery
ligating and dividing stapler

LDT left dorsotransverse (fetal position)

LDU long double upright (brace)

LDUB long double upright brace

LDV lactic dehydrogenase virus
large dense-cored vesicle
laser Doppler velocimetry
lateral distant view

LE left ear
left eye
lens extraction
leukocyte elastase
leukocyte esterase; also LKESTR
leukoerythrogenic
live embryo

Long Evans (rat)
lower extremity; also L ext, l/ext, lx
lupus erythematosus

Le Leonard (cathode ray unit)
Lewis (blood group system, number)

LEA language experience approach
left ear advantage
lower extremity amputation
lower extremity arterial
lumbar epidural anesthesia

Leᵃ antigen in the Lewis blood group system

LEADS Leadership Evaluation and Development Scale

LEB lateral efferent bundle
lupus erythematosus body

Leᵇ antigen in the Lewis blood group system

LEC leukoencephalitis
ligand exchange chromatography
low-energy charged (particle)

LECP low-energy charged particle

LED light-emitting diode
lowest effective dose
lupus erythematosus disseminatus

LEED low-energy electron diffraction

LEEDS low-energy electron diffraction spectroscopy

LEEP left end-expiratory pressure
loop electrosurgical excision (of the cervix)

LEER lower extremity equipment related

LEE W Lee-White (clotting time); also LW, L&W, L/W

LEF leukokinesis-enhancing factor
lupus erythematosus factor

Leg leg amputation

leg legal
legislation
legislative

leg com legal commitment
legally committed

LEHPZ lower esophageal high-pressure zone; also LHPZ

LeIF leukocyte interferon

leio leiomyoma

LEIS low-energy ion scattering

LEJ ligation of esophagogastric junction

LEL lowest effect level (of toxicity)

LEM lateral eye movement
Leibovitz-Emory medium; also LEV
leukocyte endogenous mediator
light electron microscope

LEMO lowest empty molecular orbital

LEMS Lambert-Eaton myasthenic syndrome

lenit gently [L. *leniter*]
lenitive

LEOPARD lentigines (multiple), electrocardiographic conduction abnormalities, ocular hypertelorism, pulmonary stenosis, abnormal genitalia, retardation of growth, and sensorineural deafness (syndrome)

LEP leptospirosis
lethal effective phase
lipoprotein electrophoresis; also LPE
low egg passage (strain of virus)
lower esophageal pressure
lower esophagus

L$_{EPN}$ effective perceived noise level

LE PREP, LE$_{PREP}$ lupus erythematosus preparation

LEPT leptocyte

LEPTOS leptospirosis agglutinins

Leq loudness equivalent

LER life-elongation ratio
lysosomal enzyme release

LERG local electroretinogram

L-ERX leukoerythroblastic reaction

LES Lawrence Experimental Station (agar)
Life Experience Survey
local excitatory state; also les
Locke's egg serum (medium)
lower esophageal segment
lower esophageal sphincter
lower esophageal stricture
lupus erythematosus, systemic

les lesion
local excitatory state; also LES
low excitatory state

LESA liposomally entrapped second antibody

LESP lower esophageal sphincter pressure

LESS lateral electrical spine stimulation

LET language enrichment therapy
linear energy transfer
low energy transfer

LETD lowest effective toxic dose

LETS large, external transformation-sensitive (fibronectin)

LEU leucine; also L, Leu, leu
leucovorin; also LCV, LV, Lv, LVR
leukocyte equivalent unit

Leu, leu leucine; also L, LEU

Leu-CAM leukocyte adhesion molecule

leuk leukemia
leukocyte; also leuko, Lkc

leuko leukocyte; also leuk, Lkc

LEUKAP leukocyte alkaline phosphatase; also LAP

LEV Leibovitz-Emory medium; also LEM
lower extremity venous

lev levator (muscle)
light [L. *levis*]

levit lightly [L. *leviter*]

LEW Lewis (rat)

LEX lactate extraction

L ext, l/ext lower extremity; also LE, lx

LF labile factor
laryngofissure
Lassa fever
latex fixation
lavage fluid
leaflet
left foot
leucine flux
limit of flocculation; also Lf
low fat (diet)
low forceps (delivery)
low frequency; also lf

Lf limes flocculation (type of diphtheria dose); also L$_f$
limit of flocculation; also LF

L$_f$ limes flocculation (type of diphtheria dose); also Lf

lf left; also L, (L), l, laev, LT, lt
low frequency; also LF

LFA left femoral artery
left forearm
left fronto-anterior (fetal position)
leukotactic factor activity
low friction arthroplasty
lymphocyte function antigen
lymphocyte function associated (glycoprotein)

LFB lingual-facial-buccal
liver, iron, and B complex [L. *ferrum* (iron)]

LFC left frontal craniotomy
living female child
low fat and cholesterol (diet)

LFD lactose-free diet
large for date
late fetal death
lateral facial dysplasia
least fatal dose
low-fat diet

low-fiber diet
low forceps delivery
LFECT loose fibroelastic connective tissue
LFER linear free-energy relationship
LFH left femoral hernia
LFL left frontolateral (fetal position)
leukocyte feeder layer
LFN lactoferrin
LFOV large field of view
LFP left frontoposterior (fetal position)
LFPPV low-frequency positive pressure ventilation
LFPS Licentiate of the Faculty of Physicians and Surgeons
LFR lymphoid follicular reticulosis
LF-RF local-regional failure
LFS limbic forebrain structure
liver function series
LFT latex fixation test
latex flocculation test
left frontotransverse (fetal position)
liver function test(s)
low-frequency tetanic (stimulation)
low-frequency tetanus
low-frequency transduction (lysate)
low-frequency transfer (sex factor)
LFTSW left foot switch
LFU limit flocculation unit
lipid fluidity unit
LFV Lassa fever virus
low-frequency ventilation
L fx linear fracture
LG lactoglobulin
lamellar granule
large; also lg, lge
laryngectomy
left gluteal
left gluteus
leucylglycine
linguogingival
lipoglycopeptide
liver graft
low glucose
lymph gland
lymphography
L$_g$-, L$_g$- sterically related to L-glyceraldehyde (denotes that rules of carbohydrate nomenclature are being employed; the subscript refers to the standard substance glyceraldehyde)

lg large; also LG, lge
leg
long; also l
LGA large for gestational age
left gastric artery
LGB Landry-Guillain-Barré (syndrome)
lateral geniculate body
LGBS Landry-Guillain-Barré-Strohl
Landry-Guillain-Barré syndrome
LGC left giant cell
LGD Leaderless Group Discussion (situational test)
LGd dorsal lateral geniculate (nucleus)
lge large; also LG, lg
LGF lateral giant fiber
LGH lactogenic hormone; also LTH
little growth hormone
LGI large glucagon immunoreactivity
lower gastrointestinal
LGL large granular leukocyte
large granular lymphocyte
lobular glomerulonephritis
Lown-Ganong-Levine (syndrome)
LGM left gluteus maximus
LGMD limb-girdle muscular dystrophy
LGMG lipid and glycopeptide (moieties)
LGN lateral geniculate nucleus
lobular glomerulonephritis
LGP labioglossopharyngeal
LGS large green soft (stool)
limb-girdle syndrome
LGT Langat encephalitis
late generalized tuberculosis
Lgt, lgt ligament; also L, l, lig
ligamentum [L. *ligamentum* (ligament)]; also L, l, lig
LGV large granular vesicle
lymphogranuloma venereum
LGVHD lethal graft-versus-host disease
LgX lymphogranulomatosis X
LH late healed
lateral hypothalamic (syndrome)
lateral hypothalamus
left hand
left hemisphere
left hyperphoria
liver homogenate
lower half
lues hereditaria (hereditary syphilis)

LH—cont'd
lung homogenate
luteinizing hormone
luteotropic hormone; also LTH

LHA lateral hypothalamic area
left hepatic artery

LHb lateral habenular

LHBV left heart blood volume

LHC left heart catheterization
left hypochondrium

LHCG luteinizing hormone–chorionic
gonadotropin (hormone)

LHCP light-harvesting chlorophyll *a/b*-binding
protein

LHF left heart failure
ligament of head of femur

LHFA lung Hageman factor activator

LH/FSH-RF luteinizing hormone/follicle-stim-
ulating hormone-releasing factor

LHG left-hand grip
localized hemolysis in gel

LHH left homonymous hemianopia

LHI lipid hydrocarbon inclusion

LHL left hemisphere lesion
left hepatic lobe

LHLN left hilar lymph node

LHM lisuride hydrogen maleate

LHMP Life Health Monitoring Program

LHN lateral hypothalamic nucleus

LHO left heel off

LHON Leber's hereditary optic neuropathy

LHP left hemiparesis
left hemiplegia

LHPZ lower esophageal high-pressure zone;
also LEHPZ

LHR leukocyte histamine release (test)
liquid holding recovery

l-hr lumen-hour

LHRF, LH-RF luteinizing hormone-releasing
factor; also LRF
luteotropin hormone-releasing factor

LHRH, LH-RH luteinizing hormone-releasing
hormone; also LRH

LHS left-hand side
left heart strain
left heel strike
lymphatic and hematopoietic system

LHT left hypertropia

LHV lymphotropic human herpesvirus

LI labeling index
lactose intolerance
lamellar ichthyosis
large intestine
learning impaired
left injured
left involved
Leptospirosis icterohemorrhagica
life island
linguoincisal
lithogenic index
low impulsiveness

L&I liver and iron

Li labrale inferius
lithium

LIA Laser Institute of America
left iliac artery
leukemia-associated inhibitory activity
lock-in amplifier
lymphocyte-induced angiogenesis
lysine-iron agar

LIAC light-induced absorbance change

LIAF lymphocyte-induced angiogenesis factor

LIAFI late infantile amaurotic familial idiocy

LIB left in bottle

lib pound [L. *libra*]; also L, lb

LIBC latent iron-binding capacity

LIBR Librium

LIC left iliac crest
left internal carotid
leisure-interest class
limiting isorrheic concentration

LICA left internal carotid artery

LICC lectin-induced cellular cytotoxicity

LICD lower intestinal Crohn's disease

LICM left intercostal margin

Lic Med Licentiate in Medicine

LICNR lysine-iron-cystine-neutral red (broth)

LICS left intercostal space; also LIS

LID late immunoglobulin deficiency
lymphocytic infiltrative disease

LIDC low-intensity direct current

LIDO lidocaine; also L

LIF laser-induced fluorescence
left iliac fossa
left index finger
leukemia inhibitory factor
leukocyte infiltration factor
leukocyte inhibitory factor
leukocytosis-inducing factor
liver migration inhibitory factor

LIFE Longitudinal Interval Follow-up Evaluation

LIFO last in, first out (computer data)

LIFT lymphocyte immunofluorescence test

lig ligament; also L, l, Lgt, lgt
ligamentum [L. *ligamentum* (ligament)]; also L, l, Lgt, lgt
ligate
ligation
ligature; also ligg

ligg ligamenta
ligaments
ligature; also lig

LIH left inguinal hernia

LIHA low impulsiveness, high anxiety

LII Leisure Interest Inventory

LIJ left internal jugular (catheter, vein)

LILA low impulsiveness, low anxiety

LIM boundary [L. *limes* (boundary or limit)]; also L

lim limit
limitation

LIMA left internal mammary artery

LiMB Listing of Molecular Biology Databases

lin linear
liniment; also Linim

LINAC linear accelerator

ling lingual; also L
lingular

Linim liniment; also lin

LIO left inferior oblique (muscle)

LIP lithium-induced polydipsia
lymphocytic interstitial pneumonia

Lip lipoate (lipoic acid)

LIPA lysosomal acid lipase A

LIPB lysosomal acid lipase B

LIPHE Life Interpersonal History Enquiry

lipoMM lipomyelomeningocele

LIP P lipid profile

LIPS Leiter International Performance Scale

LIQ liquid; also Liq, liq
liquor; also L, Liq, liq
lower inner quadrant

Liq, liq liquid; also LIQ
liquor; also L, LIQ

liq dr liquid dram

liq oz liquid ounce

liq pt liquid pint

liq qt liquid quart

LIR left iliac region
left inferior rectus

LIRBM liver, iron, red bone marrow

LIS laboratory information system
lateral intercellular space
left intercostal space; also LICS
lithium salicylate
lobular in situ (carcinoma)
low intermittent suction
low ionic strength

LISP List Processing Language

LISS low ionic strength saline
low ionic strength solution (medium test)

litho lithotripsy

LIV law of initial value
left innominate vein
liver; also L

liv live
livin lso L

LIV-Bl ieucine, isoleucine, and valine-binding protein

LIVC left inferior vena cava

LIVEN linear inflammatory verrucous epidermal nevus

LIVIM lethal intestinal virus of infant mice

LIVPRO liver profile

LJ Larsen-Johansson (syndrome)
Löwenstein-Jensen (medium)

LJL lateral joint line

LJM limited joint mobility
Löwenstein-Jensen medium

LK lamellar keratoplasty; also LKP
Landry-Kussmaul (syndrome)
left kidney; also LKID
lichenoid keratosis
Löhr-Kindberg (syndrome)

LK+ low potassium ion [L. *kalium* (potassium)]

LKA Lazare-Klerman-Armour (personality inventory)

Lkc leukocyte; also leuk, leuko

Lkcs leukocytes

LKESTR leukocyte esterase; also LE

LKID left kidney; also LK

LKKS liver, kidneys, and spleen; also LKS

LKM liver-kidney microsome

LKP lamellar keratoplasty; also LK

LKPD Lillehei-Kaster pivoting disk

LKQCPI Licentiate of the King and Queen's College of Physicians of Ireland

LKS liver, kidneys, and spleen; also LKKS
LKSB liver, kidneys, spleen, and bladder
LKS non pal liver, kidneys, and spleen not palpable
LKV laked kanamycin vancomycin (agar)
Lengyeh-Kerman-Vargar (rating)
LL large local
large lymphocyte
lateral lemniscus
left lateral; also LLAT, L lat, lt lat
left leg
left lower
left lung
lepromatous leprosy
Lewandowsky-Lutz (disease)
lid lag
limb lead
lines
lingual lipase
lipoprotein lipase; also LPL
long leg
loudness level
lower eyelid
lower limb
lower lip
lower lobe
lumbar length
lung length
lymphoblastic lymphoma; also LBL
lymphocytic leukemia; also LCL
lymphocytic lymphoma
lymphoid leukemia
lysolecithin; also LLT
L&L lids and lashes
LLA lids, lashes, and adnexa
Limulus lysate assay
lupus-like anticoagulant
L lam lumbar laminectomy
LLAT left lateral; also LL, L lat, lt lat
lysolecithin acyltransferase
L lat left lateral; also LL, LLAT, lt lat
LLB left lateral bending
left lateral border
left lower border
long-leg brace
lower lobe bronchus
LLBCD left lower border cardiac dullness
LLBP long-leg brace with pelvic (band)
LLC Lewis lung carcinoma
liquid-liquid chromatography
long-leg cast

lower level of care
lymphocytic leukemia, chronic
LLCC long-leg cylinder cast
LLD *Lactobacillus lactis,* Dorner
left lateral decubitus (muscle)
leg-length discrepancy
liquid liquid distribution
long-lasting depolarization
LLDF *Lactobacillus lactis,* Dorner factor (vitamin B_{12})
LLDH liver lactate dehydrogenase
liver lactic acid dehydrogenase
LLE left lower extremity; also LLX
LLF Laki-Lorand factor (factor XIII)
left lateral femoral (site of injection)
left lateral flexion
LL-GXT low-level graded exercise test
LLL left liver lobe
left long-leg (brace); also L LL
left lower eyelid
left lower leg
left lower limb
left lower lobe (of lung)
left lower lung
L LL left long-leg (brace); also LLL
LLLE lower lid, left eye; also LLOS
LLLM low liquid level monitor
LLLNR left lower lobe, no rales
LLM localized leukocyte mobilization
LLO Legionella-like organism
LLOD lower lid, right eye also LLRE
LLOS lower lid, left eye [L. *oculus sinister* (left eye)]; also LLLE
LLP late luteal phase
long-lasting potentiation
long-leg plaster (cast)
LLPMS long-leg posterior molded splint
LLQ left lower quadrant (of abdomen)
LLR large local reaction
left lateral rectus (eye muscle)
left lumbar region
LLRE lower lid, right eye; also LLOD
LLRW low-level radioactive waste
LLS lateral loop suspensor
lazy leukocyte syndrome
linear least squares (method)
long-leg splint
LLSB left lower scapular border
left lower sternal border

LLT left lateral thigh
lysolecithin; also LL

LLV lymphatic leukemia virus
lymphoid leukosis virus

LLV-F lymphatic leukemia virus, Friend (virus associated)

LLVP left lateral ventricular pre-excitation

LLW low-level waste

LLWC long-leg walking cast

LLX left lower extremity; also LLE

LM labiomental
lactic acid mineral (medium)
lactose malabsorption
laryngeal muscle
lateral malleolus
left main
left median
legal medicine
lemniscus medialis
Licentiate in Medicine; also Lic Med
Licentiate in Midwifery
light microscope
light microscopy
light minimum
lincomycin; also L
lingual margin
linguomesial
lipid mobilization
lipid-mobilizing (hormone)
liquid membrane
Listeria monocytogenes
longitudinal muscle
Looser-Milkman (syndrome)
lower motor (neuron)

L/M liters per minute; also L/min, LPM, lpm

lm lumen; also L

LMA left mento-anterior (fetal position)
limbic midbrain area
liver cell membrane autoantibody
liver membrane antibody

LMB Laurence-Moon-Biedl (syndrome)
left main-stem bronchus
leiomyoblastoma; also LB

LMBB Laurence-Moon-Bardet-Biedl (syndrome)

LMBS Laurence-Moon-Biedl syndrome

LMC large motile cell
lateral motor column (motor neuron)
left main coronary (artery)
left middle cerebral (artery)
living male child

lymphocyte-mediated cytolysis
lymphocyte-mediated cytotoxicity
lymphocyte microcytotoxicity
lymphomyeloid complex

LMCA left main coronary artery
left middle cerebral artery

LMCAD left main coronary artery disease

LMCAT left middle cerebral artery thrombosis

LMCL left midclavicular line

LMCT ligand-to-metal charge transfer

LMD left main disease (cardiology)
lipid-moiety modified derivative
local medical doctor
low-molecular-weight dextran; also LMDX, LMWD

LMDF lupus miliaris disseminatus faciei

LMDX low-molecular-weight dextran; also LMD, LMWD

LME left mediolateral episiotomy; also LMLE
leukocyte migration enhancement

LMEE left middle ear exploration

LMF left middle finger
Leukeran (chlorambucil), methotrexate, and fluorouracil
leukocyte mitogenic factor
lymphocyte mitogenic factor

LMFBR liquid metal fast-breeder reactor

lm/ft² lumens per square foot

LMG lethal midline granuloma
low-mobility group

LMH lipid-mobilizing hormone

lm·h lumen-hour

LMI leukocyte migration inhibition (assay)

LMIF leukocyte migration inhibition factor

L/min liters per minute; also L/M, LPM, lpm

L/min/m² liters per minute per square meter

LMIR leukocyte migration inhibition reaction

LMIT leukocyte migration inhibition test

LML large and medium lymphocytes
left mediolateral (episiotomy)
left middle lobe (of lung)
lower midline

LMLE left mediolateral episiotomy; also LME

LML scar w/h lower midline scar with hernia

LMM Lactobacillus maintenance medium
lentigo maligna melanoma
light-molecular-weight meromyosin

lm/m² lumens per square meter

LMN lower motor neuron

LMNL lower motor neuron lesion

LMO localized molecular orbital

LMP last menstrual period
left mentoposterior (fetal position)
lumbar puncture; also LP

LMR left medial rectus (eye muscle)
linguomandibular reflex
localized magnetic resonance
log magnitude ratio

LMRCP Licentiate in Midwifery of the Royal College of Physicians

LMS lateral medullary syndrome
leiomyosarcoma; also LS
Licentiate in Medicine and Surgery
lymphocyte mitogen stimulation

lm·s lumen-second; also lm-s

lm-s lumen-second; also lm·s

LMSSA Licentiate in Medicine and Surgery of the Society of Apothecaries

LMSV left maximal spatial voltage

LMT left main trunk
left mentotransverse (fetal position)
leukocyte migration technique
Lowenfeld mosaic test
luteomammotrophic (hormone)

LMTA Language Modalities Test for Aphasia

LMV larva migrans visceralis

LMW low molecular weight

lm/W lumens per watt; also lpw

LMWD low-molecular-weight dextran; also LMD, LMDX

LMWH low-molecular-weight heparin

LN labionasal
later onset nephrotic (syndrome)
Lesch-Nyhan (syndrome)
lipoid nephrosis
lobular neoplasia
lupus nephritis
lymph node

L/N letter/numerical (system)

LN$_2$ liquid nitrogen

ln natural logarithm

LNAA large neutral amino acid

LNB lymph node biopsy

LNC lymph node cell

LND Lesch-Nyhan disease
light-near dissociation
lymph node dissection

LNE lymph node enlargement

LNG liquified natural gas

LNH large number hypothesis

LNI logarithm neutralization index

LNL lower normal limit
lymph node lymphocyte

LNLS linear-nonlinear least squares (method)

LNMP last normal menstrual period

LNNB Luria-Nebraska Neuropsychological Battery

LNP large neuronal polypeptide

LNPF lymph node permeability factor

LNR lymph node region

LNS lateral nuclear stratum
Lesch-Nyhan syndrome
lymph-node seeking (equivalent)

LO lateral oblique (x-ray view)
leucine oxidation
linguo-occlusal
low; also L
lower; also L
lowest; also L
lumbar orthosis

LOA leave of absence
Leber's optic atrophy
left occipito-anterior (fetal position)
looseness of associations
lysis of adhesions

LOC laxative of choice; also LXC
level of care
level of consciousness
liquid organic compound
local; also loc
location; also loc
locus of control
loss of consciousness

loc local; also LOC
localized
location; also LOC

LoCa low calcium (diet); also lo calc

lo cal low calorie (diet); also LC

lo calc low calcium (diet); also LoCa

LOC-C Locus of Control–Chance

loc cit in the place cited [L. *loco citato*]; also lc

loc dol to the painful spot [L. *loco dolenti*]

LOC-E Locus of Control–External

LoCHO low carbohydrate (diet)

LoChol low cholesterol (diet)

LOC-I Locus of Control–Internal

LOCM low osmolar contrast medium; also LOM

LOC-PO Locus of Control–Powerful Others

LOCS lens opacities classification system

LOD line of duty
logarithm of odds (method of genetics linkage analysis); also lod

lod logarithm of odds (method of genetics linkage analysis); also LOD

log common logarithm

LOH loop of Henle

LOI level of incompetence
level of injury
Leyton Obsessive Inventory
limit of impurities; also loi

loi limit of impurities; also LOI

LOIH left oblique inguinal hernia

LoK low potassium [L. *kalium* (potassium)]

LOL left occipitolateral (fetal position)
little old lady

LOM left otitis media
limitation of motion
limitation of movement
loss of motion
loss of movement
low osmolar contrast medium; also LOCM

LOMPT Lincoln-Oseretsky Motor Performance Test

LOMSA left otitis media, suppurative, acute

LOMSC left otitis media, suppurative, chronic; also LOMSCH, LOMSCh

LOMSCH, LOMSCh left otitis media, suppurative, chronic; also LOMSC

LoNa low sodium (diet) [L. *natrium* (sodium)]; also LS

long longitudinal; also l

LOP leave on pass
left occipitoposterior (fetal position)

LOPP chlorambucil, Oncovin, procarbazine, prednisone

LoPro low protein (diet); also LP

LOPS length of patient stay

LOQ Leadership Opinion Questionnaire
lower outer quadrant

LOR license of right
long open reading (frame in genomes)
lorazepam; also LRZ
lorcainide

lord lordosis
lordotic

LORS-1 Level of Rehabilitation Scale 1

LOS length of stay; also LS

loss of sight
low cardiac output syndrome; also LCOS
lower (o)esophageal sphincter

LOSP lower (o)esophageal sphincter pressure

LOT lateral olfactory tract
left occipitotransverse (fetal position)
lengthened off time

Lot, lot lotion

LOV large opaque vesicle
loss of vision

LOWBI low-birth-weight infant

lox liquid oxygen

LOZ lozenge

LP labile peptide
labile protein
laboratory procedure
lactoperoxidase
lamina propria
laryngopharyngeal
latent period
lateral plantar
lateral pylorus
latex particle
leading pole
leukocyte poor
leukocytic pyrogen
levator palatini (muscle)
lichen planus
ligamentum patella
lightly padded
light perception; also LPerc
linear programming
linguopulpal
lipoprotein
lost privileges
low potency
low power (microscopy)
low pressure
low protein (diet); also LoPro
lumbar puncture; also LMP
lumboperitoneal
lung parenchyma
lymphocyte-predominant (Hodgkin's disease)
lymphoid plasma
lymphoid predominance
lymphomatoid papulosis
(nucleus) lateralis posterior

L/P lactate to pyruvate (ratio)
liver to plasma (concentration ratio)
lymphocyte to polymorphonuclear (ratio)
lymph to plasma (ratio)

LPA larval photoreceptor axon
latex particle agglutination
left pulmonary artery

Lp(a) lipoprotein little A antigen

LPAM, L-PAM L-phenylalanine mustard
  (melphalan)

LPB lipoprotein B
  low-profile bioprosthesis; also LPBP

LPBP low-profile bioprosthesis; also LBP

LPC laser photocoagulation
  late positive component
  leukocyte-poor cell
  Liberman plasma cell
  lysophosphatidyl choline

LPc̄P light perception with projection

LPCM low-placed conus medullaris

LPCT late proximal cortical tubule

LPD low protein diet
  luteal phase defect

LPDF lipoprotein-deficient fraction

LPE lipoprotein electrophoresis; also LEP

LPerc light perception; also LP

LPF leukocytosis-promoting factor
  leukopenia factor
  lipopolysaccharide factor
  liver plasma flow
  localized plaque formation
  low-power field; also lpf
  lymphocytosis-promoting factor

lpf low-power field; also LPF

LPFB left posterior fascicular block

LPFN low-pass-filtered noise

LPFS low-pass-filtered signal

LPG liquiefied petroleum gas

LPH left posterior hemiblock; also LPHB
  lipotropic pituitary hormone (lipotropin)

LPHB left posterior hemiblock; also LPH

LPI laser peripheral iridectomy
  left posterior-inferior
  long process of incus

LPICA left posterior internal carotid artery

LPIFB left posterior-inferior fascicular block

LPIH left posterior-inferior hemiblock

LPK liver pyruvate kinase

LPL lamina propria lymphocyte
  lichen planus-like lesion
  lipoprotein lipase; also LL

LPLA lipoprotein lipase activity

LPLE leukocyte pepsin-like enzyme

LPM lateral pterygoid muscle
  left posterior measurement
  liters per minute; also L/M, L/min, lpm

liver plasma membrane
localized pretibial myxedema
lymphoproliferative malignancy

lpm lines printed per minute
  liters per minute; also L/M, L/min, LPM

LPN Licensed Practical Nurse

LPO lateral preoptic (area)
  left posterior oblique (radiologic view)
  light perception only
  lobus parolfactorius

LPOA lateral preoptic area

L POST left posterior

LPP lateral pterygoid plate

LP&P light perception and projection

LPPH late postpartum hemorrhage

LPR lactate-pyruvate ratio
  late-phase response

LPRBC leukocyte-poor red blood cell

LProj light projection

LPS last Pap smear
  levator palpebrae superioris (muscle)
  linear profile scan
  lipase
  lipopolysaccharide
  London Psychogeriatric Scale

lps liters per second

LPSR lipopolysaccharide receptor

LPT lipotropin
  lymphocyte transfer (reaction)

LPV left portal view
  left pulmonary vein(s)
  lymphopathia venereum
  lymphotropic papovavirus

LPVP left posterior ventricular pre-excitation

LPW lateral pharyngeal wall

lpw lumens per watt; also lm/W

LPX, Lp-X lipoprotein-X

LQ longevity quotient
  lordosis quotient
  lower quadrant
  lowest quadrant

LQTS long QT syndrome

LQV *Leiurus quinquestriatus* venom

LR labeled release (experiment)
  laboratory reference
  laboratory report
  labor room
  lactated Ringer's (injection, solution);
    also lat Rin
  large reticulocyte

latency reaction
latency relaxation
lateral rectus (eye muscle)
left rotation
ligand receptor
light reaction
light reflex
light resistant
limit of reaction
lymphocyte recruitment

L/R left to right (ratio)

L&R left and right

L-R, L → R, L R left to right

Lr lawrencium; also Lw
limes reacting (type of diphtheria toxin
dose); also L_r

L_r limes reacting (type of diphtheria toxin
dose); also Lr

LRA left renal artery
low right atrium

LRAS leucyl-transfer ribonucleic acid
synthetase

LRC locomotor-respiratory coupling
lower rib cage

LRCP Licentiate of the Royal College of
Physicians

LRCPE, LRCP(E) Licentiate of the Royal
College of Physicians (Edinburgh)

LRCPI, LRCP(I) Licentiate of the Royal
College of Physicians (Ireland)

LRCP&SI Licentiate of the Royal College of
Physicians and Surgeons, Ireland

LRCS Licentiate of the Royal College of
Surgeons

LRCSE, LRCS(E) Licentiate of the Royal
College of Surgeons (Edinburgh)

LRCSI, LRCS(I) Licentiate of the Royal
College of Surgeons (Ireland)

LRD living related donor
living renal donor
local regional disease

LRDT living related donor transplant

LRE least restrictive environment
leukemic reticuloendotheliosis
lymphoreticuloendothelial

LREH low renin essential hypertension

LRF latex and resorcinol formaldehyde
left rectus femoris
liver residue factor

luteinizing hormone-releasing factor; also
LHRF, LH-RF

LRFPS Licentiate of the Royal Faculty of
Physicians and Surgeons (a Scottish institution)

LRH luteinizing hormone-releasing hormone;
also LHRH, LH-RH

LRI lower respiratory illness
lower respiratory infection
lymphocyte reactivity index

LRM left radical mastectomy

LRMP last regular menstrual period

LRN lateral reticular nucleus

LRNA low renin, normal aldosterone

LRND left radical neck dissection

LROP lower radicular obstetrical paralysis

LRP lichen ruber planus
long-range planning

LRQ lower right quadrant (of abdomen)

LRQG left rostral quarter ganglion

LRR labyrinthine righting reflex
lymphatic return rate

LRS lactated Ringer's solution
lateral recess syndrome

LRSF lactating rat serum factor
liver regenerating serum factor

LR-SH left-right shunt

LRSP long-range systems planning

LRSS late respiratory systemic syndrome

LRT local radiation therapy
lower respiratory tract

LRTI lower respiratory tract illness
lower respiratory tract infection

LRV left renal vein

LRZ lorazepam; also LOR

LS lateral septal
lateral suspensor (ligament)
left sacrum
left septum
left side
legally separated
leiomyosarcoma; also LMS
length of stay; also LOS
lesser sac
Letterer-Siwe (disease)
Libman-Sacks (disease)
Licentiate in Surgery; also LCh
life science
light sensitive

LS—cont'd
light sensitivity
light sleep
liminal sensation
liminal sensitivity
linear scleroderma
lipid synthesis
liver and spleen; also L&S
liver scan
lower segment
low sodium (diet); also LoNa
lumbar spine; also L-sp
lumbosacral; also L/S
lung strip
lymphosarcoma; also LSA, Lyp

L-S lipid-saccharide
lecithin to sphingomyelin (ratio, in amniotic fluid); also L/S

L/S lactase to sucrase (ratio)
lecithin to sphingomyelin (ratio, in amniotic fluid); also L-S
liver to spleen (ratio)
lumbosacral; also LS

L&S liver and spleen; also LS

L$_s$-, L$_s$- sterically related to L-glyceraldehyde (used in amino acid nomenclature to avoid confusion with carbohydrate nomenclature; the subscript refers to the standard substance serine)

LSA Language Sampling Analysis
left sacro-anterior (fetal position)
left subclavian artery
leukocyte-specific activity
Licentiate of the Society of Apothecaries
lichen sclerosis et atrophicus
lipid-bound sialic acid; also LBSA
lymphosarcoma; also LS, Lyp

LSA$_2$-L$_2$ cyclophosphamide, vincristine, prednisone, daunorubicin, methotrexate, cytarabine, thioguanine, colaspase, hydroxyurea, carmustine

LSANA leukocyte-specific antinuclear antibody

LSAR lymphosarcoma cell

LSA/RCS lymphosarcoma-reticulum cell sarcoma

LSB least significant bit (binary numbers)
left scapular border
left sternal border
local standby
long spike burst
lumbar sympathetic block

LS BPS laparoscopic bilateral partial salpingectomy

LSC late systolic click
left-sided colon (cancer)
left subclavian (artery)
lichen simplex chronicus
liquid scintillation counting
liquid-solid chromatography
lower-segment cesarean (section)

LSCA, LScA left scapulo-anterior (fetal position)

LSCL lymphosarcoma cell leukemia; also LSL

LSCP, LScP left scapuloposterior (fetal position)

LSCS lower-segment cesarean section

LSCV left subclavian vein; also LSV

LSD least significant difference
least significant digit (computers)
Letterer-Siwe disease
low-salt diet
low-sodium diet
lumpy skin disease (virus)
D-lysergic acid diethylamide [Ger. *lysergsäure Diethylamid*]; also LSD-25

LSD-25 D-lysergic acid diethylamide [Ger. *lysergsäure Diethylamid*]; also LSD

LSE left sternal edge
local side effect

LSEP left somatosensory evoked potential

LSF low saturated fat
lymphocyte-stimulating factor

LSG labial salivary gland

LSH lutein-stimulating hormone
lymphocyte-stimulating hormone

LSI large-scale integration
Life Satisfaction Index
light-scattering index
lumbar spine index

LSK liver, spleen, and kidneys

LSKM liver-spleen-kidney megaly

LSL left sacrolateral (fetal position)
left short-leg (brace)
lymphosarcoma cell leukemia; also LSCL

LSM late systolic murmur
lymphocyte separation medium
lysergic acid morpholide

LSN left substantia nigra
left sympathetic nerve

LSO lateral superior olive (of brain)
left salpingo-oophorectomy

left superior oblique (muscle)
lumbosacral orthosis

LSP left sacroposterior (fetal position)
liver-specific protein

LSp left span
life span

L-sp lumbar spine; also LS

L-Spar asparaginase (Elspar); also Aase,
ASP, Asp

LSQ least square

LSR lanthanide shift reagent (in magnetic
resonance imaging)
left superior rectus (muscle)

LSRA low-septal right atrium

LSS Life Span Study
Life Study Sample
life support station
liver-spleen scan
lumbosacral spine

LSSA lipid-soluble secondary antioxidant

LST lateral sinus thrombophlebitis
lateral spinothalamic tract
left sacrotransverse (fetal position)

LSTC laparoscopic tubal cautery
laparoscopic tubal coagulation

LSTL laparoscopic tubal ligation; also LTL

L's & T's lines and tubes

LSU lactose-saccharose-urea (agar)
life support unit

LSV lateral sacral vein
left subclavian vein; also LSCV

LSVC left superior vena cava

LSW left-sided weakness

LSWA large-amplitude, slow-wave activity (in
electroencephalography)

LT heat-labile toxin
laminar tomography
left; also L, (L), l, laev, lf, lt
left thigh
left triceps
less than
lethal time
leukotriene
Levin tube
levothyroxine
light; also L, lt
light touch
long term
low temperature
low transverse
L-tryptophan; also LTP

lues test
lumbar traction
lung transplantation
lymphocyte transformation
lymphocyte transitional
lymphocytic thyroiditis
lymphocytotoxin; also LC, LCT
lymphotoxin

lt left; also L, (L), l, laev, lf, LT
light; also L, LT
low tension

LTA leukotriene A
lipoate transacetylase
lipoteichoic acid
local tracheal anesthesia
lymphocyte-transforming activity

LTAF local tissue-advancement flap

LTAS lead tetra-acetate Schiff

LTB laparoscopic tubal banding
laryngotracheobronchitis
leukotriene B

LTC large transformed cell
left to count
leukotriene C
lidocaine tissue concentration
long-term care
lysed tumor cell

LTCF long-term care facility

LTCP L-tryptophan-containing product

LTCS low transverse cervical cesarean section

LTD largest tumor dimension
Laron-type dwarfism
leukotriene D
limited; also ltd
long-term disability

ltd limited; also LTD

LTDQ limited quantity (test performed on
small specimen)

LTE laryngotracheoesophageal
leukotriene E

LT-ECG long-term electrocardiography

LTF lipotropic factor
lymphocyte-transforming factor

LTG long-term goal

LTGA left transposition of great artery

LTH lactogenic hormone; also LGH
local tumor hyperthermia
low-temperature holding (pasteurization)
luteotropic hormone; also LH

LtH left-handed

LTI low temperature isotropic
   lupus-type inclusion

LTL laparoscopic tubal ligation; also LSTL

lt lat left lateral; also LL, LLAT, L lat

LTM long-term memory

LTOT long-term oxygen therapy

LTP laboratory test profile
   leukocyte thromboplastin
   long-term potentiation
   L-tryptophan; also LT

LTPP lipothiamide pyrophosphate

LTR long terminal repeat (unit)
   lymphocyte transfer reaction

LTS laparoscopic tubal sterilization
   long-term storage
   long-term surviving
   long tract sign (neurology)
   low-threshold spike

LTT lactose tolerance test
   leucine tolerance test
   limited treadmill test
   lymphoblastic transformation test
   lymphocyte transformation test

LTUI low transverse uterine incision

LTV Lucké tumor virus
   lung thermal volume

lt vent BBB left ventricular bundle-branch
   block

LTW Leydig-cell tumor in Wistar (rat)

LTX lophotoxin

LU left uninjured
   left uninvolved
   left upper
   living unit
   loudness unit
   lung; also L, Lu
   lytic unit

L&U lower and upper (extremities)

Lu lung; also L, LU
   lutetium
   Lutheran blood group system

LUA left upper arm

Lu^a antigen in the Lutheran blood group
   system

Lu^b antigen in the Lutheran blood group
   system

LUC large unstained cell

luc prim at daybreak [L. *luce prima*]

LUE left upper extremity; also LUX

Lues I primary syphilis [L. *lues* (plague)];
   also L-I

Lues II secondary syphilis [L. *lues* (plague)];
   also L-II

Lues III tertiary syphilis [L. *lues* (plague)];
   also L-III

LUF luteinized unruptured follicle

LUFS luteinized unruptured follicle syndrome

LUIS low-dose urea in invert sugar

LUL left upper (eye) lid
   left upper limb
   left upper lobe (of lung)
   left upper lung

lum lumbar; also L, lumb

lumb lumbar; also L, lum

LUMO lowest unoccupied molecular orbital

LUO left ureteral orifice

LUOB left upper outer buttock

LUOQ left upper outer quadrant

LUP left ureteropelvic (junction)

LUQ left upper quadrant

LURD living unrelated donor

LUS lower uterine segment

LUSB left upper scapular border
   left upper sternal border

lut yellow [L. *luteus*]

LUTT lower urinary tract tumor

LUV large unilamellar vesicle

LUX left upper extremity; also LUE

LV lacto-ovo-vegetarian
   laryngeal vestibule
   lateral ventricle (brain)
   lecithovitellin; also LCV
   left ventricle
   left ventricular
   leucovorin; also LCV, LEU, Lv, LVR
   leukemia virus
   live vaccine
   live virus
   low vertical
   low volume
   lumbar vertebra
   lung volume

Lv leucovorin; also LCV, LEU, LV, LVR

lv leave

LVA left ventricular aneurysm
   left ventricular aneurysmectomy
   left vertebral artery
   low vision aid

LVAD left ventricular assist device

L-VAM leuprolide acetate, vinblastine,
   Adriamycin, and mitomycin

LVAS left ventricular assist system

LVAT left ventricular activation time

LVB lomustine, vindesine, and bleomycin sulfate

LVBP left ventricle bypass pump

LVCS low vertical cesarean section

LVD left ventricular dimension; also LVDI left ventricular dysfunction

LV$_D$, LVd left ventricular end-diastolic (pressure)

LVDd left ventricular dimension in end-diastole

LVDI left ventricular dimension; also LVD

LVDP left ventricular diastolic pressure

LVDT linear variable differential transformer

LVDV left ventricular diastolic volume

LVE left ventricular ejection left ventricular enlargement

LVED left ventricular end-diastolic

LVEDC left ventricular end-diastolic circumference

LVEDD left ventricular end-diastolic diameter left ventricular end-diastolic dimension

LVEDP left ventricular end-diastolic pressure; also LVEP

LVEDV left ventricular end-diastolic volume

LVEF left ventricular ejection fraction

LVEndo left ventricular endocardial half

LVEP left ventricular end-diastolic pressure; also LVEDP

LVESD left ventricular end-systolic dimension

LVESV left ventricular end-systolic volume

LVESVI left ventricular end-systolic volume index

LVET left ventricular ejection time

LVETI left ventricular ejection time index

LVF left ventricular failure left ventricular function left visual field low-voltage fast low-voltage foci

LVFP left ventricular filling pressure

LVFT$_1$ left ventricular fast filling time

LVFT$_2$ left ventricular slow filling time

LVG left ventrogluteal

LVH large vessel hematocrit left ventricular hypertrophy

LVI left ventricular insufficiency left ventricular ischemia

LVID left ventricular internal diastolic left ventricular internal dimension

LVIDd left ventricular internal dimension diastole

LVID(ed) left ventricular internal diameter (end diastole)

LVID(es) left ventricular internal diameter (end systole)

LVIDP left ventricular initial diastolic pressure

LVIDs left ventricular internal dimension systole

LVIV left ventricular infarct volume

LVL left vastus lateralis (muscle)

LVLG left ventrolateral gluteal (injection site)

LVM lateral ventromedial (nucleus) left ventricular mass

LVMF left ventricular minute flow

LVMM left ventricular muscle mass

LVN lateral ventricular nerve lateral vestibular nucleus Licensed Visiting Nurse Licensed Vocational Nurse limiting viscosity number

LVO left ventricular outflow left ventricular overactivity; also LVOA

LVOA left ventricular overactivity; also LVO

LVOT left ventricular outflow tract

LVP large volume parenteral (infusion) left ventricular pressure levator veli palatini (muscle) lysine-vasopressin

LVPEP left ventricular pre-ejection period

LVPFR left ventricular peak filling rate

LVPSP left ventricular peak systolic pressure

LVPW left ventricular posterior wall

LVPWT left ventricular posterior wall thickness

LVR leucovorin; also LCV, LEU, LV, Lv limb vascular resistance

L$_1$VR, L$_2$VR, etc first lumbar ventral nerve root, second lumbar ventral nerve root, etc

LVRE liver fraction elevated

LVS left ventricular strain

LVs (mean) left ventricular systolic (pressure)

LVSEMI left ventricular subendocardial myocardial ischemia

LVSI left ventricular systolic index

LVSO left ventricular systolic output

LVSP left ventricular systolic pressure

LVST lateral vestibulospinal tract

LVSV left ventricular stroke volume

LVSW left ventricular septal wall
left ventricular stroke work

LVSWI left ventricular stroke work index

LVT left ventricular tension
lysine vasotonin

LVV left ventricular volume
live varicella vaccine

LVW lateral vaginal wall
lateral ventricular width
left ventricular wall
left ventricular work

LVW/HW lateral ventricular width to hemispheric width

LVWI left ventricular work index

LVWM left ventricular wall motion

LVWMA left ventricular wall motion abnormality

LVWMI left ventricular wall motion index

LVWT left ventricular wall thickness

LW lacerating wound
lateral wall
Lee-White (clotting time); also LEE W, L&W, L/W
left ear, warm stimulus
Léri-Weill (syndrome)
lung weight
lung width

L&W Lee-White (clotting time); also LEE W, LW, L/W

L/W Lee-White (clotting time); also LEE W, LW, L&W
living and well

L-10-W levulose (10%) in water

Lw lawrencium; also Lr

LWBS left without being seen

LWC leave without consent

LWCT Lachar-Wrobel Critical Items
Lee-White clotting time

LWD living with disease

LWK large white kidney

LWP large whirlpool
lateral wall pressure

LX, Lx latex; also L
local irradiation
lux; also lx

lx larynx; also lar
lower extremity; also LE, L ext, l/ext
lux; also LX, Lx

LXC laxative of choice; also LOC

LXT left exotropia

LY lymphocyte; also L, lym, lymph
lymphocytic; also lym, lymph
lyophilization

LYDMA lymphocyte-detected membrane antigen

LYCD live yeast cell derivative

LYDIEA lymphocyte-detected immunoglobulin E antigen

LYEL lost years of expected life

LYG lymphomatoid granulomatosis

LyHIF lymphoblast human interferon

LYM lymph; also L

lym lymphocyte; also L, LY, lymph
lymphocytic; also LY, lymph

lymph lymphocyte; also L, LY, lym
lymphocytic; also LY, lym

lymphs lymphocytes

LyNeF lytic nephritic factor

LYMPH% percentage of lymphocytes (in differential count)

lyo lyophilized

LYP lactose, yeast, and peptone (agar)
lower yield point

Lyp lymphosarcoma; also LS, LSA

LYS, Lys lysine; also K
lysosome; also L

LySLk lymphoma syndrome leukemia

LYTES, lytes electrolytes; also Elecs, elytes

Lyx lyxose; also l

LZM, lzm lysozyme

M

M MU, UPPER CASE, twelfth letter of the Greek alphabet

μ mu, lower case, twelfth letter of the Greek alphabet
chemical potential
dynamic viscosity
electrophoretic mobility
heavy chain of immunoglobulin M
linear attenuation coefficient
magnetic moment; also m
mass absorption coefficient
mean; also M, m, $\bar{X}$
micro- (10^{-6}); also mu
micrometer (micron); also mu, μm
mutation rate
permeability
population mean (statistics)

μ₀ permeability of vacuum

μA microampere

μb microbar; also μbar

μβ Bohr's magneton

μbar microbar; also μb

μC microcoulomb; also μcoul

μc microcurie; also μCi

μch microcurie-hour; also μC-hr, μCi-hr

μC-hr microcurie-hour; also μch, μCi-hr

μCi microcurie; also μc

μCi-hr microcurie-hour; also μch, μC-hr

μcoul microcoulomb; also μC

μ Eq microequivalent

μF, μf microfarad

μg microgram; also mcg

μγ microgamma (picogram)

μGy microgray

μH microhenry

μHg micrometer of mercury; also μmHg

μin microinch

μIU one millionth International Unit

μkat microkatal

μL, μl microliter

μM micromolar; also μmol/L

μm micrometer (micron); also mu, μ
micromilli- (nano, 10^{-9})

μm² square micrometer

μm³ cubic micrometer; also cum

μmg micromilligram (nanogram)

μmHg micrometers of mercury; also μHg

μmm micromillimeter (nanometer); also mmm

μmμ meson

μmol micromole; also mcmol

μmol/L micromolar; also μM

μΩ microhm

μOsm micro-osmolar

μR, μr microroentgen

μ/ρ mass attenuation coefficient

μs microsecond; also μsec

μsec microsecond; also μs

μU microunit; also McU

μV, μv microvolt; also mcv

μW, μw microwatt

μμ micromicro- (10^{-12}, replaced by pico)
micromicron (picometer)

μμC micromicrocurie (picocurie);
also μμCi

μμCi micromicrocurie (picocurie); also μμC

μμF micromicrofarad (picofarad)

μμg micromicrogram (picogram)

M a handful [L. *manipulus*]; also m, man, manip
antigen in the MNS blood group system
chin [L. *mentum*]; also m
concentration in moles per liter
death [L. *mors*]
dullness (of sound) [L. *mutitas*]
dumbness [L. *mutitas*]
macerate; also m, Mac, mac
macerated; also m
macroglobulin
macroglobulinemia; also MC
magnetization
main group elements (periodic table)
male
malignant; also MAL, mal, malig
mannose (broth)
manual
marital
married
masculine; also masc
mass; also m, *m*
massage; also mass, MSS, mss
maternal contribution
matrix; also MX
matt (dull, slightly granular, bacterial colonies)
mature; also MAT, Mat, mat
maximal
maximum; also max

M —cont'd
  mean; also m, μ, X̄
  meatus
  mechlorethamine hydrochloride
  media
  median; also m, md, mdn, Med, med
  mediator (chemical released in the tissues)
  medical; also MED, Med, med
  medicine; also MED, Med, med
  medium; also MED, Med, med
  mega- (10^6)
  megohm; also MΩ
  melts at; also m
  membrane; also memb
  memory (associative)
  mental
  mesial; also m
  meta-; also m, m-, *m*-
  metabolite
  metal
  metastasis; also MET, metas, met
  meter; also m
  methionine (one-letter notation); also MET,
    Met
  method
  methotrexate; also MTRX, MTX, Mtx, MXT
  mexiletine; also MEX
  Micrococcus species; also *M*
  Microsporum species; also *M*
  mil [L. *mille* (thousand)]; also m
  milli- (10^{-3}) [L. *mille* (thousand)]; also m
  million
  minim; also m, min
  minimum; also MIN, min
  minute(s); also m, MIN, min
  mitochondria
  mitosis
  mitral; also mit
  mix; also m, misce
  mixed
  mixture; also m, mix, mixt
  molal; also *m*
  molality; also m, molal
  molar (permanent tooth)
  molar (solution)
  molarity
  mole; also mol
  molecular; also mol
  molecular weight; also mol wt, MW, MWt
  moment of force
  Monday; also Mon
  monkey; also Mk
  monocyte; also mon, mono
  month; also MO, Mo, mo, mon

morgan (unit of gene separation)
morphine; also m, MOR, morph
mother; also MO, Mo, mo
motile; also m
mouse
mouth; also Mo
movement response to human figure
mucoid; also m
mucous (adjective)
mucus (noun)
multipara; also multip
murmur; also m, (m), mm
muscarinic (receptor)
muscle(s); also m, musc
muscular response to electrical stimulation of
  motor nerve
Mycobacterium species; also *M*
Mycoplasma species; also *M*
myelocyte; also Myel
myeloma (component)
myopia; also My, my, myop
myopic
myosin
noon [L. *meridies*]; also m
soften [L. *macerare*]; also ma, mac
strength of pole
thousand [L. *mille*]

$\alpha_2 M$ alpha$_2$-macroglobulin

M1 left mastoid
  matrix protein 1

M_1 mitral first sound (slight dullness)
  myeloblast (first stage of myelocyte maturation)

M2 matrix protein 2
  right mastoid

M-2 vincristine, carmustine, cyclophosphamide, melphalan, and prednisone

M^2 square meter; also m^2

M_2 mitral second sound (marked dullness)
  promyelocyte (second stage of myelocyte
  maturation)

3-M syndrome Miller, McKusic, and Malvaux
  (those who first described the syndrome)

M/3 middle third (of long bones); also mid/3

M_3 mitral third sound (absolute dullness)
  myelocyte at third stage of maturation

M_4 myelocyte at fourth stage of maturation

M_5 metamyelocyte (fifth stage of myelocyte
  maturation); also ME, MET, META

M_6 band form (sixth stage of myelocyte maturation)

M₇ polymorphonuclear neutrophil (seventh stage of myelocyte maturation); also PMN, PMNN

M/10 tenth molar solution

M/100 hundredth molar solution

M *Micrococcus* species; also M
  Microsporum species; also M
  molar concentration; also molc
  molar mass
  mutual inductance
  Mycobacterium species; also M
  Mycoplasma species; also M

m a handful [L. *manipulus*]; also M, man, manip
  by mouth; also (m)
  chin [L. *mentum*]; also M
  electromagnetic moment
  electron rest mass
  in the morning [L. *mane*]; also matut
  macerate; also M, Mac, mac
  macerated; also M
  Mach
  magnetic moment; also μ
  magnetic quantum number
  mass; also M, *m*
  mean; also M, μ, $\bar{X}$
  median; also M, md, mdn, Med, med
  melts at; also M
  mesial; also M
  meta-; also M, m-, *m*-
  meter; also M
  mil [L. *mille* (thousand)]; also M
  milli- (10^{-3}) [L. *mille* (thousand)]; also M
  minim; also M, min
  minute(s); also M, MIN, min
  mix; also M, misce
  mixture; also M, mix, mixt
  modulus
  molality; also M, molal
  molar (deciduous tooth)
  morphine; also M, MOR, morph
  motile; also M
  mucoid; also M
  murmur; also M, (m), mm
  muscle(s); also M, musc
  noon [L. *meridies*]; also M
  sample mean
  send [L. *mitte*]; also mit

m mass; also M, m
  molal; also M

m-, *m*- meta; also M, m

(m) by mouth; also m
  murmur; also M, m, mm

m² square meter; also M₂

m³ cubic meter; also cu m

m₈ spin quantum number

MA machine
  mafenide acetate
  main arterial (blood pressure)
  mammary adenocarcinoma
  mandelic acid
  manifest achievement
  Martin-Albright (syndrome)
  masseter
  Master of Arts
  maternal aunt
  mean arterial (blood pressure)
  medical abbreviation
  medical assistance
  medical assistant
  medical audit
  medical authorization
  mega-ampere
  megaloblastic anemia
  megestrol antigen
  membrane antigen; also MAg
  menstrual age
  mental age
  mentoanterior (fetal position)
  metatarsus adductus
  meter-angle; also mA, ma
  Mexican American
  microagglutination
  microaneurysm
  microcytotoxicity assay
  microscopic agglutination
  Miller-Abbott (tube)
  milliampere; also mA, ma
  mitochondrial antibody
  mitogen activation
  mitotic apparatus
  mixed agglutination
  moderately advanced
  monoamine
  monoclonal antibody; also MAB, MAb, mAB, mAb, MCA, MCAB, MC-Ab MOAB, MoAb
  motorcycle accident; also MCA
  multiple action
  muscle activity
  mutagenic activity
  myelinated axon

M/A male, altered (animal); also MALT
  mood and/or affect

MA1, MA-1 mechanically assisted (Bennett brand of respirator)

Ma mass of atom
  masurium (technetium)

mA meter-angle; also MA, ma
  milliamperage; also ma
  milliampere; also MA, ma

mÅ milliangstrom

ma meter-angle; also MA, mA
  milliamperage; also mA
  milliampere; also MA, mA
  soften [L. *macerare*]; also M, mac

MAA macroaggregated albumin; also MIAA
  Medical Assistance for the Aged
  melanoma-associated antigen
  monoarticular arthritis

MAAAP macroaggregated albumin arterial
  perfusion

MAAC Medical Assistants Advisory Council

MAACL Multiple Affect Adjective Check List

MAB Metropolitan Asylums Board (British)
  monoclonal antibody; also MA, MAb, mAB,
  mAb, MCA, MCAB, MC-Ab, MOAB,
  MoAb

MAb, mAB, mAb monoclonal antibody; also
  MA, MAB, MCA, MCAB, MC-Ab,
  MOAB, MoAb

MABI Mother's Assessment of the Behavior of
  Her Infant

MABOP Mustargen (nitrogen mustard),
  Adriamycin, bleomycin, Oncovin, and
  prednisone

MABP mean arterial blood pressure

MAC MacConkey (agar)
  MacIntosh (laryngoscope blade)
  macrocytic erythrocyte
  macula; also Mac
  malignancy-associated change
  maximal acid concentration
  maximal allowable concentration
  maximal allowable cost
  medical alert center
  membrane attack complex
  methotrexate, actinomycin D, and chlorambucil
  methotrexate, actinomycin D, and
  cyclophosphamide
  midarm circumference
  minimum alveolar concentration
  minimum anesthetic concentration
  minimum antibiotic concentration
  mitral annular calcium
  modulator of adenylate cyclase
  monitored anesthesia care

  multidimensional actuarial classification
  Mycobacterium avium complex

Mac macerate; also M, m, mac
  macula; also MAC

mac macerate; also M, m, Mac
  maceration; also macer
  soften [L. *macerare*]; also M, ma

MAC AWAKE minimum alveolar anesthetic
  concentration (patient recovering from general anesthesia able to respond to instructions)

Mac blade MacIntosh (laryngoscope) blade

MACC macro-ovalocyte
  methotrexate, Adriamycin, cyclophosphamide, and CCNU (lomustine)

m accur mix very accurately [L. *misce accu-
  ratissime*]

MACDP Metropolitan Atlanta Congenital
  Defects Program

MACE methylchloroform chloroacetophenone

macer maceration; also mac

mAChR muscarinic acetylcholine receptor

MAC INH membrane attack complex inhibitor

MACOP-B methotrexate, Adriamycin,
  cyclophosphamide, Oncovin, prednisone,
  and bleomycin

MACP Master of the American College of
  Physicians

MACR macrocytosis
  mean axillary count rate

macro macrocyte
  macrocytic
  macroscopic

MAD maximal allowable dose
  MeCCNU and Adriamycin
  methandriol
  methylandrostenediol
  mind-altering drug
  minimal average dose
  myoadenylate deaminase

mAD muscle adenylate deaminase; also
  MADA

MADA muscle adenylate deaminase; also
  mAD

MADD Mothers Against Drunk Driving
  multiple acyl-CoA dehydrogenation deficiency

MADRS Montgomery-Asberg Depression
  Rating Scale

MAE medical air evacuation
  moves all extremities

Multilingual Aphasia Examination

MAEW moves all extremities well

MAF macrophage activating factor
macrophage-agglutinating factor
minimal audible field
mouse amniotic fluid
movement aftereffect

MAFA midarm fat area

MAFAs movement-associated fetal heart rate accelerations

MAFH macroaggregated ferrous hydroxide

MAG myelin-associated glycoprotein

MAg membrane antigen; also MA

Mag magnesium; also Mg

mag large [L. *magnus*]; also magn
magnification; also magn
magnify; also magn

mag cit magnesium citrate

MAGE mean amplitude of glycerine excursion

MAGF male accessory gland fluid

MAggF macrophage agglutination factor

MAGIC microprobe analysis generalized intensity correction

magn large [L. *magnus*]; also mag
magnification; also mag
magnify; also mag

MAGS Multidimensional Assessment of Gains in School (psychologic test)

mag sulf magnesium sulfate

mAH millampere-hours

MAHA microangiopathic hemolytic anemia; also MHA

MAHH malignancy-associated humoral hyper-calcemia

MAI maximal aggregation index
microscopic aggregation index
minor acute illness
morbid anxiety inventory
movement assessment of infants
Mycobacterium avium intracellular

MAIA magnetic antibody immunoassay

MAID mesna, Adriamycin, ifosfamide, and dacarbazine

MAII Milwaukee Academic Interest Inventory

MAKA major karyotypic abnormality

MAL malfunction; also Mal
malignant; also M, mal, malig
midaxillary line

Mal ill [L. *malum*]; also mal
malate

malfunction; also MAL

mal by blistering [L. *malanandro*]
ill [L. *malum*]; also Mal
malignant; also M, MAL, malig

MALA malarial parasites

MALAR malaria

Mal-BSA maleated bovine serum albumin

MALG Minnesota antilymphoblast globulin

malig malignant; also M, MAL, mal

MALIMET Master List of Medical Indexing Terms

MALS rabbit antiserum to mouse lymphocytes

MALT male, altered (animal); also M/A
mucosa-associated lymphoid tissue

MAM methylazoxymethanol

mam milliampere-minute; also MA min, ma-min

M+Am compound myopic astigmatism

MAMA midarm muscle area
monoclonal antimalignin antibody

MAM Ac methylazoxymethanol acetate

MAMC mean arm muscle circumference
midarm muscle circumference

MAmg medical amygdaloid (nucleus)

MA min, ma-min milliampere-minute; also mam

mammo mammography

m-AMSA amsacrine

MAN magnocellular nucleus (of anterior neostriatum)
mannose

man a handful [L. *manipulus*]; also M, m, manip
manipulate
morning [L. *mane*]; also mng

mand mandible
mandibular; also MD

manifest manifestation

manip a handful [L. *manipulus*]; also M, m, man
manipulation

MANOVA multivariate analysis of variance

MAN-6-P mannose-6-phosphate

man pr early in the morning [L. *mane primo*]; also mp

manu manufacture; also mfr

MAO maximum acid output
medical ankle orthosis
monoamine oxidase

MAOI monoamine oxidase inhibitor

MAP maximal aerobic power
mean airway pressure
mean aortic pressure
mean arterial pressure
Medical Audit Program
megaloblastic anemia of pregnancy
mercapturic acid pathway
methyl acceptor protein
methylacetoxyprogesterone
methylacetylenic putrescine
methylaminopurine
microlithiasis alveolaris pulmonum
microtubule-associated protein
minimal audible pressure
mitomycin, Adriamycin, and Platinol
monophasic action potential
mouse antibody production (test)
muscle-action potential
Musical Aptitude Profile

MAPA muscle adenosine phosphoric acid

MAPC migrating action potential complex

MAPE Multidimensional Assessment of Philosophy of Education

MAPF microatomized protein food

MAPI microbial alkaline protease inhibitor
Millon Adolescent Personality Inventory

MAPS Make A Picture Story (test)

MAPTAM 1,2-bis-5-methylaminophenoxy-ethane-N,N,N', N'-tetraacetoxymethyl acetate

MAR Main Admitting Room
marasmus
marrow
maximal aggregation ratio
medication administration record
microanalytical reagent
minimal angle resolution
mixed antiglobulin reaction
monoclonal antibody to rat

mar margin; also marg, MG
marker (chromosome)

MARC multifocal and recurrent choroidopathy

MARG acute marginal (branch of left circumflex artery)

marg margin; also mar, MG

MARIA macroaggregated radio-iodinated albumin

MARS Mathematics Anxiety Rating Scale
mouse antirat serum

MARS-A Mathematics Anxiety Rating Scale–Adolescents

MARTI mobile advanced real-time image

MAS Management Appraisal Survey
Manifest Anxiety Scale
meconium aspiration syndrome
medical advisory service
mesoatrial shunt
milk-alkali syndrome
milliampere-second; also MaS, Mas, mAs, mas, mA-s
minor axis shortening (of left ventricle)
mobile arm support
monoclonal antibodies
Morgagni-Adams-Stokes (syndrome)
motion analysis system

MaS, Mas, mAs, mas milliampere-second; also MAS, mA-s

mA-s milliampere-second; also MAS, MaS, Mas, mAs, mas

masc masculine; also M
mass concentration; also massc

MASER microwave amplification by stimulated emission of radiation
molecular application by stimulated emission of radiation

MASF Melcher acid-soluble fraction

MASH Mobile Army Surgical Hospital
multiple automated sample harvester

mas pil pill mass [L. *massa pilularum*]

mass massage; also M, MSS, mss
massive

massfr mass fraction

massc mass concentration; also masc

mass spec mass spectrometry; also MS

MAST medical antishock trousers
Michigan Alcoholism Screening Test
military antishock trousers

mAST mitochondrial aspartate aminotransferase

mast mastectomy; also mx
mastoid

MAT mammary ascites tumor
Manipulative Aptitude Test
manual arts therapist
maternal; also Mat, mat
maternity; also Mat, mat
mature; also M, Mat, mat
mean absorption time
medication administration team
methionine adenosyltransferase
Metropolitan Achievement Tests
microagglutination test
Miller Analogies Test

motivation analysis test
multifocal atrial tachycardia;
　also MFAT, MFT
multiple agent therapy

Mat, mat material
maternal; also MAT
maternity; also MAT
mature; also M, MAT

MATE Maternal Attitudes Evaluation

MATSA Marek associated tumor-specific
antigen

matut in the morning [L. *matutinus*]; also m

MAU Meyenburg-Altherr-Uehlinger (syndrome)

MAV mechanical auxiliary ventricle
minimal apparent viscosity
minute alveolar volume
movement arm vector
myeloblastosis-associated virus

MAVA multiple abstract variance analysis

MAVIS mobile artery and vein imaging system

MAVR mitral and aortic valve replacement

max maxilla
maxillary; also mx
maximum; also M

max EP maximal esophageal pressure

MB Bachelor of Medicine [L. *Medicinae
Baccalaureus*]
isoenzyme of creatine kinase (containing
M and B subunits)
Mallory's body
mamillary body
margin, buccal
Marie-Bamberger (disease)
Marsh-Bendall (factor)
mercury bougie
mesiobuccal
methyl bromide
methylene blue; also MBl, MEB, MeB
microbiologic assay
muscle balance
myocardial band

6MB six-meal bland (diet)

M&B May & Baker, Ltd. (used with numbers
to designate specific products of the company before they have been given chemical
or registered names)

Mb mandible body
mouse brain
myoglobin; also MG, MYO, MYOGLB

mb millibar; also mbar
mix well [L. *misce bene*]

MBA methylbenzyl alcohol
methyl bisacrylamide
methylbis(chloroethyl)amine (nitrogen mustard)
methylbovine albumin

M-BACOD methotrexate, bleomycin,
Adriamycin, cyclophosphamide, Oncovin,
dexamethasone, and leucovorin calcium

m-BACOS methotrexate, bleomycin,
Adriamycin, cyclophosphamide, Oncovin,
and leucovorin calcium

MBAG 1,1′-(methylethanediylidene)dinitrilo-
bis(3-aminoguanidine)

MBAR myocardial beta-adrenergic receptor

mbar millibar; also mb

MBAS methylene blue active substance

MBB modified barbital buffer

MBC male breast cancer
maximum breathing capacity
maximum bladder capacity
methotrexate, bleomycin, and cisplatin
methylthymol blue complex
microcrystalline bovine collagen
minimal bacteriocidal concentration

MB-CK creatine kinase isoenzyme (containing
M and B subunits)

MbCO myoglobin combined with carbon
monoxide

MBCU metallic bead-chain urethrocystograph

MBD maximal bactericidal dilution
methotrexate, bleomycin, and *cis*-
diamminedichloroplatinum (cisplatin)
methylene blue dye
minimal brain damage
minimal brain dysfunction
Morquio-Brailsford disease

MBDG mesiobuccal developmental groove

MBE may be elevated
medium below-elbow (cast)

MBEST modulus blipped echo-planar
single-pulse technique

MBF meat base formula
medullary blood flow
muscle blood flow
myocardial blood flow

MBFC medial brachial fascial compartment

MBFLB monaural bifrequency loudness
balance

MBG mean blood glucose

MBGS Morphine-Benzedrine Group Scale

MBH maximal benefit from hospitalization
medial basal hypothalamus

MBH$_2$ methylene blue, reduced; also MBR
MBHI Million Behavioral Health Inventory
MBI methylene blue instillation
MBK methyl butyl ketone
MBL medium brown loose (stool)
  menstrual blood loss
  minimal bactericidal level
MBl methylene blue; also MB, MEB, MeB
MBLA methylbenzyl linoleic acid
  mouse-specific bone marrow-derived lympho-
    cyte antigen
MBM mineral basal medium
  mother's breast milk
MBNW multiple-breath nitrogen washout
MBO mesiobucco-occlusal
MbO$_2$ oxymyoglobin (myoglobin combined
  with oxygen)
MBP major basic protein
  maltose-binding protein
  mean blood pressure
  melitensis, bovine, porcine (antigen prepared
    from *Brucella melitensis, B. bovis* and *B.*
    suis)
  mesiobuccopulpal
  myelin basic protein
MBPS multigated cardiac blood pool scanning
MBq megabecquerel
MBR methylene blue, reduced; also MBH$_2$
MBRT methylene blue reduction time
MBS methionyl bovine somatotropin
MBSA methylated bovine serum albumin; also
  MeBSA
MBSD maple bark stripper disease
MBT mercaptobenzothiazole
  mixed bacterial toxin
MBTFA methyl-bis(trifluoroacetamide)
MBTI Myers-Briggs Type Indicator (psycho-
  logic test)
MC macroglobulinemia; also M
  mass casualty
  mast cell
  Master of Surgery [L. *Magister Chirurgiae*];
    also MCh, MS
  maximal concentration
  Medical Center
  Medical Clinic
  Medical Corps
  medium-chain (triglyceride)
  medullary cavity
  medullary cystic (disease)
  megacoulomb

  megacurie; also Mc, MCi
  megacycle; also Mc, meg
  melanoma cell
  meningeal carcinomatosis
  Merkel's cell
  mesenteric collateral
  mesiocervical
  mesocaval (shunt)
  metacarpal; also MCP, meta
  metacarpal amputation
  metatarsocuneiform
  methyl cellulose
  methylcholanthrene; also MCA
  microcephaly
  microciliary clearance
  microcirculation
  microcrystalline cellulose
  midcapillary
  midcarpal
  mineralocorticoid; also M-C
  minimal-change
  Minkowski-Chauffard (syndrome)
  mitomycin C; also Mit-C, MITO-C, MMC,
    MMC C, Mmc C, MTC
  mitotic cycle
  mitoxantrone and cytarabine
  mitral commissurotomy
  mixed cellularity (Hodgkin's disease)
  mixed cryoglobulinemia
  molluscum contagiosum
  monkey cell
  mononuclear cell; also MNC
  mouth care
  mycelial phase (of fungi)
  myocarditis
MC540 merocyanide 540
M-C Magovern-Cromie (prosthesis)
  mineralocorticoid; also MC
M/C male, castrated (animal)
M&C morphine and cocaine; also m + c
Mc mandible coronoid
  megacurie; also MC, MCi
  megacycle; also MC, meg
mC millicoulomb; also mcoul
mc millicurie (older abbreviation, now mCi);
  also mCi
m+c morphine and cocaine; also M&C
MCA major coronary artery
  Manufacturing Chemists Association (now:
    CMA, Chemical Manufacturers
    Association)
  medical care administration
  megestrol, cyclophosphamide, and
    Adriamycin

methylcholanthrene; also MC
microcentrifugal analyzer
middle cerebral aneurysm
middle cerebral artery
monocarboxylic acid
monoclonal antibody; also MA, MAB,
   MAb, mAB, mAb, MCAB, MC-Ab,
   MOAB, MoAb
motorcycle accident; also MA
multichannel analyzer
multiple congenital abnormalities
multiple congenital anomalies

MCAB, MC-Ab monoclonal antibody; also
MA, MAB, MAb, mAB, mAb, MCA,
MOAB, MoAb

MCAD medium chain acyl-coenzyme A
dehydrogenase

MCA/MR multiple congenital anomalies/mental retardation (syndrome)

MCAR mixed cell agglutination reaction

MCAS middle cerebral artery syndrome

MCAT Medical College Admission Test
middle cerebral artery thrombosis

m caute mix with caution [L. *misce caute*]

MCB membranous cytoplasmic body
monochlorobenzidine

McB McBurney's (point)

mCBF mean cerebral blood flow

MCBM muscle capillary basement membrane

MCBMT muscle capillary basement membrane thickening

MCBP melphalan, cyclophosphamide, BCNU
(bischloroethylnitrosourea), and prednisone

MCBR minimal concentration of bilirubin

MCC marked cocontraction
mean corpuscular hemoglobin concentration;
   also MCHbC, MCHC
medial cell column
metacarpal-carpal (joints)
metacerebral cell
metastatic cord compression
microcrystalline collagen
midstream clean catch (urine)
minimum complete-killing concentration
mucocutaneous candidiasis

McC McCarthy (panendoscope)
McCoy (antibody)

MCCD minimal cumulative cardiotoxic dose

MCCNU methylchloroethylcyclohexyl-
nitrosourea (semustine); also MeCCNU,
MeCcnu, methyl-CCNU

MCCU mobile coronary care unit

MCD magnetic circular dichroism
margin crease distance
mast-cell degranulation
mean cell diameter
mean corpuscular diameter
mean of consecutive differences
medullary cystic disease
metabolic coronary dilation
metacarpal cortical density
minimal-cerebral dysfunction
minimal change disease
multicystic disease
multiple carboxylase deficiency
muscle carnitine deficiency

mcD millicuries destroyed; also mCid

MCDI Minnesota Child Development
Inventory

MCDK multiseptic dysplastic kidney

MCDP mast cell degranulating peptide

MCDT mast cell degranulation test
multiple choice discrimination test

MCDV maize chlorotic dwarf virus

MCE medical-care evaluation
Medicare Code Editor
multicystic encephalopathy

MCES multiple cholesterol emboli syndrome

MCF African malignant catarrhal fever
macrophage chemotactic factor
macrophage cytotoxicity factor
median cleft face
medium corpuscular fragility
microcomplement fixation
mink cell focus (inducing virus)
mitoxantrone, cyclophosphamide, and
   fluorouracil
mononuclear cell factor
most comfortable frequency
myocardial contractile force

MCFA medium-chain fatty acid
miniature centrifugal fast analyzer

MCFP mean circulating filling pressure

MCG magnetocardiogram
membrane coating granule
mesangiocapillary glomerulonephritis; also
   MCGN
mesencephalic central gray
Minkowski-Chauffard-Gäusslen
monoclonal gammopathy; also MG

Mcg an immunoglobulin λ-light chain antigenic marker

mcg microgram; also μg

MCGC metacerebral giant cell

MCGF mast cell growth factor

MCGN mesangiocapillary glomerulonephritis; also MCG
minimal-change glomerulonephritis
mixed cryoglobulinemia with glomerulo-nephritis

MCH Maternal and Child Health
mean corpuscular hemoglobin; also MCHb, MCHg
methacholine
microfibrillar collagen hemostat
muscle contraction headache

MCh Master of Surgery [L. *Magister Chirurgiae*]; also MC, MS

mch, mc-h millicurie-hour; also mchr, mc-hr, mCi-hr

MCHB Maternal and Child Health Bureau

MCHb mean corpuscular hemoglobin; also MCH, MCHg

MCHbC mean corpuscular hemoglobin concentration; also MCC, MCHC

MCHC maternal and child health care
mean corpuscular hemoglobin concentration; also MCC, MCHbC

MCHg mean corpuscular hemoglobin; also MCH, MCHb

MCHR Medical Committee on Human Rights

mchr, mc-hr millicurie-hour; also mch, mc-h, mCi-hr

MCHS Maternal and Child Health Service

MCI mean cardiac index
methicillin; also METH

MCi megacurie; also MC, Mc

mCi millicurie; also mc

mCid millicuries destroyed; also mcD

mCi-hr millicurie-hour; also mch, mc-h, mchr, mc-hr

MCINS minimal change idiopathic nephrotic syndrome

MCK M-type creatine kinase
multicystic kidney

MCKD multicystic kidney disease

MCL maximal comfort level
maximal containment laboratory
medial collateral ligament
midclavian line
midclavicular line
midcostal line
minimal-change lesion
mixed culture, leukocyte

modified chest lead
most comfortable listening (level)
most comfortable loudness (level)

MCLD *Mycobacterium chelonei*-like organism

MCLL most comfortable listening level
most comfortable loudness level

MCLNS mucocutaneous lymph node syndrome; also MCLS, MLNS

MCLS mucocutaneous lymph node syndrome; also MCLNS, MLNS

MCMI Millon Clinical Multiaxial Inventory (psychiatric battery)

mcmol micromole; also μmol

MCMV mouse cytomegalovirus
murine cytomegalovirus

MCN minimal-change nephropathy

MC-N mixed cell nodular (lymphoma)

MCNS minimal-change nephrotic syndrome

MCO medical care organization

M colony mucoid colony

mcoul millicoulomb; also mC

MCP maximal closure pressure
melanosis circumscripta precancerosa
melphalan, cyclophosphamide, and prednisone
metacarpal; also MC, meta
metacarpophalangeal; also MCPH, MP
metaclopramide
methyl-accepting chemotaxis protein
2-methyl-4-chlorophenoxy-acetic acid; also MCPA
mitotic-control protein
mucin clot-prevention (test)

MCPA 2-methyl-4-chlorophenoxy-acetic acid; also MCP

MCPH metacarpophalangeal; also MCP, MP

MCPJ metacarpal phalangeal joint

MCPS Missouri Children's Picture Series (psychologic test)

Mcps, mcps megacycles per second; also mc/s

MCQ multiple choice question

MCR Medical Corps Reserve
message competition ratio
metabolic clearance rate

MCS malignant carcinoid syndrome
Marlowe-Crown Social Desirability Scale; also MCSDS
mesocaval shunt
methylcholanthrene-induced sarcoma
microculture and sensitivity; also M&S
moisture control system

multiple combined sclerosis
myocardial contractile state

mc/s megacycles per second; also Mcps, mcps

MCSA minimal cross-sectional area
Moloney cell surface antigen

M-CSF macrophage colony-stimulating factor

MCSDS Marlowe-Crown Social Desirability
Scale; also MCS

MCSP Member of the Chartered Society of
Physiotherapists (British)

MCT manual cervical traction
mean cell thickness
mean cell threshold
mean circulation time
mean corpuscular thickness
medium-chain triglyceride
medullary carcinoma of the thyroid
medullary collecting tubule
microtoxicity test
monocrotaline
multiple compressed tablet

MCTC metrizamide computed tomographic
cisternography

MCTD mixed connective tissue disease

MCTF mononuclear cell tissue factor

MCU malaria control unit
maximal care unit
micturating cystourethrography
motor cortex unit

McU microunit; also μU

MCUS millicuries

MCV mean cell volume
mean clinical value
mean corpuscular volume
molluscum contagiosum virus
motor conduction velocity

mcv microvolt; also μV, μv

MCZ miconazole

MD Doctor of Medicine [L. *Medicinae Doctor*]
macula degeneration
macula densa
magnesium deficiency
main duct
maintenance dialysis
maintenance dose
major depression
malate dehydrogenase; also MDH
malic dehydrogenase; also MDH
malrotation of the duodenum
mammary dysplasia
mandibular; also mand
manic-depression

manic-depressive
Mantoux's diameter
Marek's disease
maternal deprivation
maximal dose
mean deviation
mean diastolic
measurable disease
Meckel's diverticulum
mediastinal disease
medical department
medical doctor
mediodorsal
medium dosage
megadalton
mental deficiency
mental depression
mentally deficient
mentally depressed
mesiodistal
Minamata disease
minimal dosage
mitral disease
mixed diet
moderate disability
monocular deprivation
movement disorder
multiple deficiency
muscular dystrophy
myeloproliferative disease; also MPD
myocardial damage
myocardial disease
(nucleus) medialis dorsalis

Md mendelevium; also Mv

md as directed [L. *more dicto*]; also m dict,
MP, mp
median; also M, m, mdn, Med, med

MDA malondialdehyde
manual dilatation of anus
M.D. Anderson Hospital and Tumor Institute
monodehydroascorbate
motor discriminative acuity
multivariant discriminant analysis
Muscular Dystrophy Association
right mentoanterior (fetal position) [L.
mento-dextra anterior]

MDAD mineral dust airway disease

MDAP Machover Draw-A-Person (test)

MDBDF March of Dimes Birth Defect
Foundation

MDBK Madin-Darby bovine kidney (cell)

MDBSS Mischell-Dutton balanced salt
solution

MDC major diagnostic category
  medial dorsal cutaneous (nerve)
  minimal detectable concentration

MDCK Madin-Darby canine kidney (cell)

MDD major depressive disorder
  manic-depressive disorder
  mean daily dose

MDDA Minnesota Differential Diagnosis of
  Aphasia

MDE major depressive episode

MDEBP mean daily erect blood pressure

MDF mean dominant frequency
  myocardial depressant factor

MDG mean diastolic gradient

MDGF macrophage-derived growth factor

MDH malate dehydrogenase; also MD
  malic dehydrogenase; also MD
  medullary dorsal horn

MDHM malate dehydrogenase, mitochondrial

MDHR maximum determined heart rate

MDHS malate dehydrogenase, soluble

MDHV Marek's disease herpesvirus

MDI manic-depressive illness
  metered dose inhaler
  multiple daily injection
  multiple dosage insulin
  Multiscore Depression Inventory

MDIA Mental Development Index, Adjusted

m dict as directed [L. *more dicto*]; also md,
  MP, mp

MDII multiple daily insulin injection

MDIT mean disintegration time

MDL Master Drug List

MDM mid-diastolic murmur
  minor determinant mixture (of penicillin)

MDMV maize dwarf mosaic virus

mdn median; also M, m, md, Med, med

MDNB mean daily nitrogen balance
  meta-dinitrobenzene

MDO membrane-derived oligosaccharide

MDP mandibular dysostosis and peromelia
  manic-depressive psychosis
  methylene diphosphate
  muramyl dipeptide
  muscular dystrophy, progressive
  right mentoposterior (fetal position) [L.
    mento-dextra posterior]

MDPI maximum daily permissible intake

MDQ memory deviation quotient
  minimal detectable quantity

MDR mammalian diving response
  median duration of response
  minimum daily requirement

MDRH multidisciplinary rehabilitation hospital

MDRS Mattis Dementia Rating Scale

MDS Master of Dental Surgery
  maternal deprivation syndrome
  medical data screen
  medical data system
  microdilution system
  microsurgical drill system
  mild drinker's syndrome
  Miller-Dieker syndrome
  multidimensional scaling
  multiple deficiency syndrome
  myelodysplasia
  myelodysplastic syndrome
  myocardial depressant substance

MDSBP mean daily supine blood pressure

MDSO mentally disordered sex offender

MDT mast cell degeneration test
  mean dissolution time
  median detection threshold
  multidisciplinary team
  right mentotransverse (fetal position) [L.
    mento-dextra transversa]

MDTA McDonald Deep Test of Articulation

MDTP multidisciplinary treatment plan

MDTR mean diameter-thickness ratio

MDUO myocardial disease of unknown origin

MDV Marek's disease virus
  mucosal disease virus
  multiple dose vial

MDY month, day, year

Mdyn megadyne

ME Mache unit [Ger. *Mache Einheit*]; also
  MU, Mu, mu
  macular edema
  magnitude estimation
  male equivalent
  malic enzyme
  manic episode
  maximal effort
  median eminence
  medical education
  medical engineering
  Medical Examiner
  meningoencephalitis
  mercaptoethanol
  metabolic and electrolyte (disorder)
  metabolic energy
  metabolism; also metab
  metabolizable energy

metamyelocyte; also M_5, MET, META
methyleugenol
microembolization
middle ear
mouse embryo
mouse epithelial (cell)
muscle examination
myoepithelial (cells)

M/E myeloid to erythroid (ratio); also M:E

M:E myeloid to erythroid (ratio); also M/E

ME$_{50}$ 50% maximal effect

2ME 2-mercaptoethanol

Me menton
methyl; also meth

MEA Malic enzyme A
mercaptoethylamine
multiple endocrine abnormalities
multiple endocrine adenomatosis

MEA-I multiple endocrine adenomatosis, type I

meas measurement

MEB malic enzyme B
medial efferent bundle
Medical Evaluation Board
methylene blue; also MB, MBl, MeB

MeB methylene blue; also MB, MBl, MEB

ME-BH medial eminence-basal hypothalamus

MeBSA methylated bovine serum albumin; also MBSA

MEC mecillinam
meconium; also Mec, mec
median effective concentration
middle ear canal
middle ear cell
minimum effective concentration
myoepithelial cell

Mec, mec meconium; also MEC

MeCbl methylcobalamin

MeCCNU, MeCcnu methylchloroethylcyclo-hexylnitrosourea (semustine); also MCCNU, methyl-CCNU

MECG maternal electrocardiogram
mixed essential cryoglobulinemia

MECIF monocyte-derived endothelial cell inhibitory factor

Me$_2$CO acetone

MeCP methyl-CCNU (semustine), cyclophos-phamide, and prednisone

MECT maximal extrapolated clotting time

MECTA mobile electroconvulsive therapy apparatus

MECY methotrexate and cyclophosphamide

MED Meckeren-Ehlers-Danlos (syndrome)
medial; also Med, med
median erythrocyte diameter
medical; also M, Med, med
medication; also Med, med
medicine; also M, Med, med
medium; also M, Med, med
minimum effective dose
minimum erythema dose
multiple epiphyseal dysplasia

Med, med medial; also MED
median; also M, m, md, mdn
medical; also M, MED
medication; also MED
medicine; also M, MED
medium; also M, MED

MEDAC multiple endocrine deficiency, Addi-son's disease, and candidiasis (syndrome)
multiple endocrine deficiency-autoimmune candidiasis

MED-ART Medical Automated Records Technology

MEDEX, Medex extension of physician (physician assistant program using former military medical corpsmen) [L. *medicus extensus*]

medic military medical corpsman [L. *medicus*]

MEDICO Medical International Cooperation Organization

MEDIHC Military Experience Directed into Health Careers

MEDLARS Medical Literature Analysis and Retrieval System

MEDLINE MEDLARS On-Line

med men medial meniscus
medial meniscectomy

MEDPAR Medical Provider Analysis and Review

MEdREP Medical Education Reinforcement and Enrichment Program

MEDs, meds medications

MEDScD Doctor of Medical Science

MedSurg medicine and surgery

Med Tech Medical Technician
Medical Technologist; also MT
Medical Technology

MEE measured energy expenditure
methyl ethyl ether
middle ear effusion

MEET Multistage Exercise Electrocardiographics Test

MEF maximal expiratory flow
middle ear fluid
midexpiratory flow
migration enhancement factor
mouse embryo fibroblast

MEF$_{50}$ mean maximal expiratory flow

MEFA methyl-CCNU (semustine), fluoro-uracil, and Adriamycin

MEFR maximal expiratory flow rate

MEFSR maximal expiratory flow–static recoil (curve)

MEFV maximal expiratory flow volume

MEFVC maximal expiratory flow volume curve
mechanical expiratory flow volume curve

MEG magnetoencephalogram
magnetoencephalograph
magnetoencephalography
megakaryocyte(s); also meg
megestrol acetate; also Meg
mercaptoethylguanidine
multifocal eosinophilic granuloma

Meg megestrol acetate; also MEG

meg megacycle; also MC, Mc
megakaryocytes(s); also MEG

mega- one million (10^6)

mEGF mouse epidermal growth factor

Meg-CSF megakaryocytic colony-stimulating factor

MEGS male electronic genital stimulator

MEGX monoethylglycinexylidide

MEK methyl ethyl ketone

MEI Medicare Economic Index

MEL metabolic equivalent level
mouse erythroleukemia
murine erythroleukemia

mel melena

MELAN melanin

MELC murine erythroleukemia cell

MELDOS melioidosis

MELI met-enkephalin-like immunoreactivity

MEM macrophage electrophoretic mobility (test)
malic enzyme, mitochondrial; also MEm
minimal essential medium

MEm malic enzyme, mitochondrial; also MEM

MEMA methyl methacrylate; also MMA

memb membrane; also M

MEMR multiple exostoses–mental retardation (syndrome)

MEN methylethylnitrosamine
multiple endocrine neoplasia

multiple endocrine neoplasms

men meningeal
meninges
meningitis; also mgtis

MEND Medical Education for National Defense

menst menstrual
menstruate
menstruating

MEO malignant external otitis

MeOH methyl alcohol

MEOS microsomal ethanol-oxidizing system

MEP maximal expiratory pressure
mean effective pressure
meperidine; also mep
molecular electrostatic potential
motor end-plate
motor-evoked potential
multimodality-evoked potential

mep meperidine; also MEP

MEPC miniature end-plate current

MEPH mephobarbital

MEPP miniature end-plate potential

MePr methylprednisolone

mEQ, mEq, meq milliequivalent

mEq/L milliequivalents per liter

MER mandatory experience regulation
mean ejection rate
mersalyl acid
methanol extraction residue (of bacille Calmette-Guérin)
methanol-extruded residue
molar esterification rate
multimodality evoked response

MER-25 ethamoxytriphetol

MER-29 triparanol

MERB Medical Examination and Review Board
met-enkephalin receptor binding

MERG macular electroretinogram

MES maintenance electrolyte solution
maximal electroshock
maximal electroshock seizure
mesial
Metrazol-electroshock seizure
morpholinoethanesulfonic acid
muscle in elongated state
myoelectric signal

Mes mesencephalic
mesencephalon

Mesc mescaline

MESCH Multi-Environment Scheme

MESGN mesangial glomerulonephritis

MeSH Medical Subject Headings (in MEDLARS)

MesPGN mesangial proliferative glomerulo-nephritis; also MSPGN

MET medical emergency treatment
metabolic; also metab
metabolic equivalent of task
metabolic equivalent test
metamyelocyte; also M_5, ME, META
metastasis; also M, metas, met
metastasize; also metas, met
metastasizing; also metas, met
metastatic; also metas, met
methionine; also M, Met
metoprolol
midexpiratory time
multistage exercise test; also MSET

Met methionine; also M, MET

met metallic (chest sounds)
metastasis; also M, MET, metas
metastasize; also MET, metas
metastasizing; also MET, metas
metastatic; also MET, metas

META metamyelocyte; also M_5, ME, MET

meta metacarpal; also MC, MCP
metatarsal; also MT

metab metabolic; also MET
metabolism; also ME
metabolites

metas metastasis; also M, MET, met
metastasize; also MET, met
metastasizing; also MET, met
metastatic; also MET, met

METH methicillin; also MCI

Meth methedrine

meth methyl; also Me

MetHb, Met-Hb methemoglobin; also HbMet, HiHb, MHB, MHb

MeTHF methyltetrahydrofolic acid

methyl-CCNU methylchloroethylcyclohexyl-nitrosourea (semustine); also MCCNU, MeCCNU, MeCcnu

methyl-GAG methylglyoxal bis(guanyl-hydrazone) dihydrochloride

MetMb metmyoglobin

m et n morning and night [L. *mane et nocte*]; also M&N

METS metabolic equivalents (multiples of rest-ing oxygen consumption)
metastases; also Mets

Mets metastases; also METS

m et sig mix and write a label [L. *misce et signa*]

METT maximal exercise tolerance test

m et v morning and evening [L. *mane et vespere*]

MEV maximal exercise ventilation
million electron volts; also mev
murine erythroblastosis virus

MeV, Mev megaelectron volt; also mev

meV millielectron volt

mev megaelectron volt; also MeV, Mev
million electron volts; also MEV

MEX Mexican
mexiletine; also M

MF masculinity/femininity
mass fragmentography
meat free
medium frequency
megafarad
melamine formaldehyde
merthiolate-formaldehyde (solution)
methanol formaldehyde
methotrexate, fluorouracil, and calcium leucovorin
methoxyflurane; also MOF
5-methyltetrahydrofolate
microfibril
microfilament
microfilaria; also Mf, *Mf*, mf
microscopic factor
midcavity forceps
Miller-Fischer (syndrome)
mitogenic factor
mitomycin and fluorouracil
mitotic figure
mossy fiber
mucosal fluid
multifactorial
multiplication factor
multiplying factor
mutation frequency
mycosis fungoides
myelin figures
myelofibrosis
myocardial fibrosis
myofibrillar

M/F male to female (ratio)

M&F male and female
mother and father

Mf maxillofrontal
microfilaria; also MF, *Mf*, mf

Mf *microfilaria*; also MF, Mf, mf

mF millifarad

mf microfilaria; also MF, Mf, *Mf*

MFA methyl fluoroacetate
monofluoroacetate
multifocal functional autonomy
multifunctional acrylic
multiple factor analysis

MFAT multifocal atrial tachycardia; also MAT, MFT

MFB mammal fibroblast
medial forebrain bundle
metallic foreign body

MFC mean frequency of compensation
microfibrillated cellulose
minimal fungicidal concentration

m-FC membrane focal coli (broth)

MFD mandibulofacial dysostosis
Memory for Designs
midforceps delivery
milk-free diet
minimal fatal dose

MFEM maximal forced expiratory maneuver

MFG modified heat-degraded gelatin

mfg manufacturing

MFH malignant fibrous histiocytoma
membrane-free hemolysate

MFID multielectrode flame ionization detector

m flac pars flaccida membranae tympani (Shrapnell's membrane) [L. *membrana flaccida*]

MFM millipore filter method

MFMD monofluoromethylDOPA

MFMH monofluoromethylhistidine

MFO mixed function oxidase

MFP monofluorophosphate
myofascial pain

MFPVC multifocal premature ventricular contraction

MFR mean flow rate
midforceps rotation
mucus flow rate

mfr manufacture; also manu

MFRL maximal force at rest length

MFS medical fee schedule
merthiolate-formaldehyde solution; also MF sol
Minnesota Follow-up Study

MF sol merthiolate-formaldehyde solution; also MFS

MFSS Medical Field Service School

MFST Medical Field Service Technician

MFT multifocal atrial tachycardia; also MAT, MFAT
muscle function test

m ft let a mixture be made [L. *mixtura fiat*]

MFU medical follow-up

MFVD midforceps vaginal delivery

MFVNS middle fossa vestibular nerve section

MFVPT Motor-Free Visual Perception Test; also MVPT

MFW multiple fragment wounds

MG Marcus Gunn (pupil); also M-G
margin; also mar, marg
medial gastrocnemius (muscle)
membranous glomerulonephritis; also MGN
membranous glomerulopathy
menopausal gonadotropin
mesiogingival
methylglucoside
methylguanidine
Michaelis-Gutmann (bodies)
Millard-Gubler (syndrome)
minigastrin
monoclonal gammopathy; also MCG
monoglyceride
mucigen granule
mucous granule
muscle group
myasthenia gravis; also MyG
Mycoplasma gallisepticum
myoglobin; also Mb, MYO, MYOGLB

M-G Marcus Gunn (pupil); also MG

Mg magnesium; also Mag
megagram

mg milligram; also mgm, mgr

mg% milligrams per deciliter; also mg/dL, mg/dl
milligrams per 100 cubic centimeters or per 100 grams
milligrams per 100 milliliters
milligrams percent

MGA medical gas analyzer
melengestrol acetate

mγ milligamma (nanogram)
millimicrogram (nanogram); also mμg

MGB medical geniculate body
Michaelis-Gutmann bodies

MGBG methylglyoxal bis(guanylhydrazone); also MGGH

MGC minimal glomerular change

MgC magnocellular neuroendocrine cell

MGD maximal glucose disposal
mixed gonadal dysgenesis

mg/dL, mg/dl milligrams per deciliter; also mg%

mg-el milligram-element

MGES multiple gated equilibrium scintigraphy

MGF macrophage growth factor
maternal grandfather

MGG May-Grünwald-Giemsa (stain)
molecular and general genetics
mouse gamma globulin

MGGH methylglyoxal bis(guanylhydrazone); also MGBG

MGH monoglyceride hydrolase

mgh milligram-hour; also mg-hr

mg-hr milligram-hour; also mgh

MGI macrophage and granulocyte inducer

mg/kg milligrams per kilogram; also mpk

MGL minor glomerular lesion

mg/L milligrams per liter

MGM maternal grandmother

mgm milligram; also mg, mgr

MGN membranous glomerulonephritis; also MG

MGP Marcus Gunn pupil
marginal granulocyte pool
marginated granulocyte pool
membranous glomerulonephropathy
methyl green pyronin (dye)
mucin glycoprotein
mucous glycoprotein

MGR modified gain ratio
multiple gas rebreathing
murmurs, gallops, or rubs

mgr milligram; also mg, mgm

MGS metric gravitational system

MGSA melanoma growth-stimulating activity

MGSD mean gestational sac diameter

mgtis meningitis; also men

MGUS monoclonal gammopathy of undetermined significance

MGW magnesium sulfate, glycerine, and water (enema)

MGXT multistage graded exercise test

mGy milligray

MH maleic hydrazide
malignant histiocytosis
malignant hyperpyrexia
malignant hypertension
malignant hyperthermia
mammotropic hormone
mannoheptulose
marital history
medial hypothalamus
medical history; also MHx
melanophore-stimulating hormone; also MSH
menstrual history
mental health
mental hygiene
moist heat
monosymptomatic hypochondriasis
multiple handicapped
murine hepatitis
mutant hybrid
mylohyoid

M/H microcytic hypochromic (anemia)

M-H Mueller-Hinton (agar)

Mh mandible head

mH millihenry

MHA May-Hegglin anomaly
Mental Health Association
methemalbumin
microangiopathic hemolytic anemia; also MAHA
microhemagglutination
middle hepatic artery
mixed hemadsorption
Mueller-Hinton agar

MHATP, MHA-TP microhemagglutination assay–*Treponema pallidum*

MHB maximal hospital benefit
mental health assistance benefit
methemoglobin; also HbMet, HiHb, MetHb, Met-Hb, MHb

MHb medial habenular
methemoglobin; also HbMet, HiHb, MetHb, Met-Hb, MHB
myohemoglobin

MHBSS modified Hank's balanced salt solution

MHC major histocompatibility complex
mental health care
mental health center
mental health counselor
multiphasic health check-up
myosin heavy chain

mhcp mean horizontal candle-power

MHCS Mental Hygiene Consultation Service

MHCT modified human calcitonin

m/hct microhematocrit

MHCU mental health care unit

MHD magnetohydrodynamics
maintenance hemodialysis
maximal human dose

MHD—cont'd
mean hemolytic dose
mental health department
minimal hemolytic dilution
minimal hemolytic dose

mHg millimeters of mercury; also mmHg

MHI malignant histiocytosis of the intestine
Mental Health Index (information)
Mental Health Institute

MHLC Multidimensional Health Locus of Control

MHLS metabolic heat load stimulator

MH/MR mental health and mental retardation

MHN massive hepatic necrosis
Mohs hardness number
morbus haemolyticus neonatorum

MHNTG multiheteronodular toxic goiter

MHO microsomal heme oxygenase

mho reciprocal ohm (unit of conductance [ohm spelled backward])
Siemens unit

MHP maternal health program
1-mercuri-2-hydroxypropane
methoxyhydroxypropane
monosymptomatic hypochondriacal psychosis

MHPA mild hyperphenylalaninemia
Minnesota-Hartford Personality Assay

MHPG methoxyhydroxyphenylglycol

MHR major histocompatibility region
malignant hyperthermia resistance
maximal heart rate
methemoglobin reductase; also MR, MR-E

MHRI Mental Health Research Institute

MHS major histocompatibility system
malignant hypothermia susceptibility
multiple health screening

MHSA microaggregated human serum albumin

MHST multiphasic health screen test

MHT multiphasic health testing

MHTI minor hypertensive infant

MHTS Multiphasic Health Testing Services

MHV magnetic heart vector
Mill Hill virus
minimal height velocity
mouse hepatitis virus
murine hepatitis virus

MHVD Marek's herpesvirus disease

MHW medial heel wedge
mental health worker

MHx medical history; also MH

MHz, mHz megahertz

MI massa intermedia
maturation index
medical inspection
melanophore index
membrane intact
menstruation induction
mental illness
mental institution
mercaptoimidazole
mesioincisal
metabolic index
metaproterenol inhaler
methyl indole
migration index
migration inhibition
mild irritant
mitotic index
mitral incompetence
mitral insufficiency; also MIS, mit insuf
mononucleosis infectiosa
morphology index
motility index
myocardial infarction
myocardial ischemia
myoinositol

M&I maternal and infant (care)

Mi mitomycin; also MIT

mi mile

mi² square mile

mi³ cubic mile

MIA medically indigent adult
missing in action
multi-institutional arrangement

MIAA microaggregated albumin; also MAA

MIAP modified innervated antral pouch

MIB Medical Impairment Bureau

MIBG, mIBG meta-iodobenzylguanidine

MIBI sestamibi

MIBK methyl isobutyl ketone

MIBT methylisatin-beta-thiosemicarbasone

MIC maternal and infant care
Maternity and Infant Care
medical intensive care
Medical Interfraternity Conference
methacholine inhalation challenge
methyl isocyanate
microcytic; also micro
microscope
microscopic; also micro
minimum inhibitory concentration
minimum isorrheic concentration

mobile intensive care
model immune complex

MiC minocycline; also MNO

MICC mitogen-induced cellular cytotoxicity

MICG macromolecular insoluble cold globulin

MICN mobile intensive care nurse

mic pan bread crumb [L. *mica panis*]

MICR methacholine inhalation challenge
response

micro microcyte
microcytic; also MIC
microscopic; also MIC

micro- one-millionth (10^{-6})

microbiol microbiological
microbiology

microcryst microcrystalline

MICU medical intensive care unit
mobile intensive care unit

MID maximum inhibiting dilution
mesioincisodistal
midazolam
minimal infective dose
minimal inhibitory dilution
minimal inhibitory dose
minimal irradiation dose
multi-infarct dementia
multiple ion detection

mid middle

mid/3 middle third (of long bones); also M/3

Mid I middle insomnia

midnoc midnight [mid + L. *nocte* (night)];
also MN, M/N, Mn, mn

MIDS Management Information Decision
System

midsag midsagittal

MIE medical improvement expected
methylisoeugenol

MIF macrophage-inhibiting factor
macrophage-inhibitory factor
melanocyte-inhibiting factor
melanocyte-stimulating hormone inhibiting
factor
membrane immunofluorescence
merthiolate-iodine-formaldehyde (method)
merthiolate-iodine-formalin (solution)
methylene-iodine-formalin
microimmunofluorescence
mid-inspiratory flow
migration-inhibition factor
mixed immunofluorescence
müllerian inhibiting factor

MIFA mitomycin-C, fluorouracil, and
Adriamycin

MIFC merthiolate-iodine-formaldehyde
concentration

MIFR maximal inspiratory flow rate
mid-inspiratory flow rate

MIFT merthiolate-iodine-formaldehyde
technique

MIG measles immune globulin

MIg malaria immunoglobulin
measles immunoglobulin
membrane immunoglobulin

MIGW maximal increment in growth and
weight

MIH melanocyte-stimulating hormone
inhibitory hormone
methylhydrazine methylisopropylbenzamide
(procarbazine)
migraine with interparoxysmal headache
minimal intermittent dosage of heparin
monoiodohistidine

MIKA minor karyotype abnormality

MIKE mass-analyzed ion kinetic energy

MIL military
mother-in-law; also M/L
motility-indole-lysine (medium)

mil 0.001 [L. *mille* (thousand)]

milli- one-thousandth (10^{-3}) [L. *mille*
(thousand)]

MILP mitogen-induced lymphocyte
proliferation

MILS medication information leaflet for
seniors

MiLv mink endogenous virus

MIME mean indices of meal excursions
methyl GAG, ifosfamide, methotrexate,
and etoposide

MIMNG National Collection of Agricultural
and Industrial Microorganisms (Budapest)

MIMR minimal inhibitor molar ratio

MIMS Medical Information Management
System
Medical Inventory Management System
Monthly Index of Medical Specialties

MIN medial interlaminar nucleus
mineral; also min
minimal; also min
minimum; also M, min
minor; also min
minute(s); also M, m, min

min mineral; also MIN
  minim; also M, m
  minimal; also MIN
  minimum; also M, MIN
  minor; also MIN
  minute(s); also M, m, MIN

MINA monoisonitrosoacetone

MINDO modified intermediate neglect of differential overlap (method)

MINE medical improvement not expected
  mesna uroprotection, ifosfamide, Novantrone, and etoposide

MINIA monkey intranuclear inclusion agent

MIO minimum identifiable odor
  motility, indole production, ornithine decarboxylase activity (medium)

MIP maximum inspiratory pressure
  mean intravascular pressure
  medical improvement possible
  metacarpointerphalangeal
  minimal inspiratory pressure

MIPS Martinsreid Institute for Protein Sequence
  myocardial isotopic perfusion scan

MIR main immunogenic region
  multiple isomorphous replacement

MIRD medical internal radiation dose

MIRF macrophage immunogenic antigen-recruiting factor

MIRP myocardial infarction rehabilitation program

MIRU myocardial infarction research unit

MIS management information system
  Medical Information Service
  meiosis-inducing substance
  minimal intervention surgery
  mitral insufficiency; also MI, mit insuf
  müllerian inhibiting substance

misc miscarriage
  miscellaneous
  miscible

misce mix [L. *misce*]; also M, m

MISG modified immune serum globulin

MISO misonidazole

MISS modified injury severity score (scale)

MISSGP mercury in Silastic strain gauge plethysmography

MIST Medical Information Service by Telephone

MIT Makari intradermal test
  Male Impotence Test

  marrow iron turnover
  meconium in trachea
  melodic intonation therapy
  metabolism inhibition test
  migration inhibition test
  miracidial immobilization test
  mitomycin; also Mi
  monoiodotyrosine

mit mitral; also M
  send [L. *mitte*]; also m

Mit-C mitomycin C; also MC, MITO-C, MMC, MMC C, Mmc C, MTC

Mith mithramycin

mit insuf mitral insufficiency; also MI, MIS

MITO-C mitomycin C; also MC, Mit-C, MMC, MMC C, Mmc C, MTC

mit sang bleed [L. *mitte sanguinem* (let go the blood)]; also mitt sang
  blood-letting procedure [L. *mitte sanguinem* (let go the blood)]; also mitt sang

mitt sang bleed [L. *mitte sanguinem* (let go the blood)]; also mit sang
  blood-letting procedure [L. *mitte sanguinem* (let go the blood)]; also mit sang

mitt tal send such [L. *mitte tales*]

MIU, mIU milli-International unit

mix mixture; also M, m, mixt

Mix Astig mixed astigmatism

mix mon mixed monitor

mixt mixture; also M, m, mix

MJ marijuana
  megajoule

MJA mechanical joint apparatus

MJL medial joint line

MJT Mead Johnson tube
  Mowlem-Jackson technique

MK main kitchen
  marked
  menaquinones (vitamin(s) K_2)
  monkey kidney; also MkK
  monkey lung (cell culture)
  Morel-Kraepelin (disease)
  Mounier-Kuhn (syndrome)
  myokinase

MK6, MK$_6$, MK-6 menaquinone-6 (vitamin $K_{2(30)}$)

MK-7 menaquinone-7 (vitamin $K_{2(35)}$)

Mk monkey; also M

MKAB may keep at bedside

mkat millikatal

mkat/L millikatals per liter

MKB megakaryoblast

MKC mammal kidney cell
monkey kidney cell

MK-CSF megakaryocyte colony-stimulating
factor

mkg meter-kilogram

MkK monkey kidney; also MK

MKP monobasic potassium phosphate

MKS, mks meter-kilogram-second

MKSAP Medical Knowledge Self-Assessment
Program

MKTC monkey kidney tissue culture

MKV killed measles vaccine

ML Licentiate in Medicine
Licentiate in Midwifery
malignant lymphoma
Marie-Léri (syndrome)
marked latency
maximal left
maximum likelihood (method)
meningeal leukemia
mesiolingual
middle lobe
midline; also ml
molecular layer; also MOL
motor latency
mucolipidosis
multiple lentiginosis
muscular layer
myeloid leukemia

M:L maltase to lactase (ratio)
monocyte to lymphocyte (ratio); also M/L

M-L Martin-Lewis (medium)

M/L monocyte to lymphocyte (ratio); also M:L
mother-in-law; also MIL

M$_L$, M$_L$ left electrode

Ml megaliter

mL millilambert; also mLa
milliliter; also ml

ml midline; also ML
milliliter; also mL

MLA left mentoanterior (fetal position) [L.
mento-laeva anterior]
marker-labelled antigen
Medical Library Association
medium long-acting
mesiolabial; also MLa
monocytic leukemia, acute
multilanguage aphasia

MLa mesiolabial; also MLA

mLa millilambert; also mL

MLAB Multilingual Aphasia Battery

MLAI, MLaI mesiolabioincisal

MLAP mean left atrial pressure

MLaP mesiolabiopulpal

MLB monaural loudness balance

MLb macrolymphoblast

MLBP mechanic low back pain

MLBW moderately low birth weight

MLC Marginal Line Calculus (Index)
minimal lethal concentration
mixed leukocyte concentration
mixed leukocyte culture
mixed ligand chelate
mixed lymphocyte concentration
mixed lymphocyte culture
morphine-like compound
multilamellar cytosome
multilevel care
multilumen catheter
myelomonocytic leukemia, chronic

MLCK myosin light-chain kinase

MLCN multilocular cystic nephroma

MLCP myosin light-chain phosphatase

MLCR mixed lymphocyte culture reaction

MLCT metal-to-ligand charge transfer

ML-CVP multilumen central venous pressure

MLCW mixed lymphocyte culture, weak

MLD masking level difference
median lethal dose; also MLD$_{50}$
mesencephalicus lateralis dorsalis
metachromatic leukodystrophy
minimal lesion disease
minimal lethal dose

MLD$_{50}$ median lethal dose; also MLD

mL/dL milliliters per deciliter

MLE maximal likelihood estimation
mediolateral episiotomy; also MLEpis
midline episiotomy; also MLEpis

MLEpis mediolateral episiotomy; also MLE
midline episiotomy; also MLE

MLF medial longitudinal fasciculus
median longitudinal fasciculus
monocyte leukotactic factor
morphine-like factor

MLG mesiolingual groove
mitochondria lipid glycogen

MLGN minimal lesion glomerulonephritis

ML-H malignant lymphoma, histiocytic

MLI mesiolinguoincisal
mixed lymphocyte interaction
motilin-like immunoreactivity

MLL malignant lymphoma, lymphoblastic

mL/L milliliters per liter

MLMV Medical Lake macaque virus

MLN membranous lupus nephropathy
mesenteric lymph node

MLNS mucocutaneous lymph node syndrome;
also MCLNS, MCLS

MLO mesiolinguo-occlusal
mycoplasma-like organism

MLP left mentoposterior (fetal position) [L.
mento-laeva posterior]
mesiolinguopulpal
microsomal lipoprotein

ML-PDL malignant lymphoma, poorly
differentiated lymphocytic

MLR middle latency response
mixed leukocyte reaction
mixed leukocyte response
mixed lymphocyte reaction
mixed lymphocyte response

MLS mean life span
median longitudinal section
myelomonocytic leukemia, subacute

MLT left mentotransverse (fetal position) [L.
mento-laeva transversa]
mean latency time
median lethal time
Medical Laboratory Technician

MLT(ASCP) Medical Laboratory Technician
(certified by the American Society of
Clinical Pathologists)

MLTC mixed leukocyte-trophoblast culture

MLTF major late transcription factor

MLTI mixed lymphocyte target interaction

MLU mean length of utterance

MLV Moloney's leukemogenic virus
monitored live voice
mouse leukemia virus
multilamellar large vesicle
multilamellar lipid vesicle
multilaminar vesicle
murine leukemia virus; also MuLV, MuLv

MLVDP maximal left ventricular developed
pressure

mlx millilux

MM macromolecule
major medical (insurance)
malignant melanoma
manubrium of malleus
Marshall-Marchetti (procedure)
medial malleolus
megamitochondria

melanoma metastasis
melanotic melanoma
meningococcic meningitis
mercaptopurine and methotrexate
metastatic melanoma
methadone maintenance
middle molecule
milk and molasses; also M&M
morbidity and mortality; also M&M
Morel-Morgagni (syndrome)
motor meal
mucous membrane(s); also mm
Müller's maneuver
multiple myeloma; also MYEL
muscles; also mm
muscularis mucosae
myeloid metaplasia
myelomeningocele

M&M milk and molasses; also MM
morbidity and mortality; also MM

Mm mandible mentum
megameter

Mm² square megameter

Mm³ cubic megameter

mM millimolar
millimole; also mmol

mm methylmalonyl
millimeter
mucous membrane(s): also MM
murmur; also M, m, (m)
muscles; also MM

mm² square millimeter

mm³ cubic millimeter; also cmm, c mm, cu mm

mμ millimicro- (10^{-9}, replaced by nano)
millimicron (replaced by nanometer)

MMA mastitis-metritis-agalactia (syndrome)
medical materials account
methylmalonic acid
methylmercuric acetate
methyl methacrylate; also MEMA
monocyte monolayer assay

MMAA mini-microaggregated albumin colloid

MMAD mass median aerodynamic diameter

MMAO monomethylamine oxidase

MMATP methadone maintenance and aftercare
treatment program

MMC migrating motor complex
migrating myoelectric complex
minimal medullary concentration
mitomycin C; also MC, Mit-C, MITO-C,
MMC C, Mmc C, MTC
mucosal mast cell

mμc millimicrocurie (nanocurie); also mμCi

MMC C, Mmc C mitomycin C; also MC, Mit-C, MITO-C, MMC, MTC

mμCi millimicrocurie (nanocurie); also mμc

MMD mass median diameter (of particles)
mean marrow dose
minimal morbidostatic dose
myotonic muscular dystrophy; also MYD, MyD, MyMD

MMDA methoxymethylene dioxyamphetamine

MMDDS mucous membrane drug delivery system

MME M-mode echocardiography
mouse mammary epithelium

MMECT multiple monitored electroconvulsive therapy

MMEF maximal midexpiratory flow; also MMF

MMEFR maximal midexpiratory flow rate; also MMFR

MMF magnetomotive force
maximal midexpiratory flow; also MMEF
mean maximal flow

MMFG mouse milk fat globule

MMFR maximal midexpiratory flow rate; also MMEFR
maximum midflow rate

MMFV maximal midexpiratory flow volume

MMG mean maternal glucose

mμg millimicrogram (nanogram); also mγ

MMH monomethylhydrazine

mmHg millimeters of mercury; also mHg

mmH₂O millimeters of water

MMI macrophage migration index
macrophage migration inhibition
methylmercaptoimidazole (methimazole)

MMIHS megacystis-microcolon-intestinal hypoperistalsis syndrome

MMIS Medicaid Management Information System

MMK Marshall-Marchetti-Krantz (cystourethroplexy)

MML Moloney murine leukemia (virus)
monomethyllysine
myelomonocytic leukemia

mM/L, mM/l millimoles per liter; also mmol/L

MMLV Moloney murine leukemia virus; also MMuLV

MMM microsome-mediated mutagenesis
Montana myotis meningoencephalitis

myelofibrosis with myeloid metaplasia
myeloid metaplasia with myelofibrosis
myelosclerosis with myeloid metaplasia

mmm micromillimeter (nanometer); also μmm

MMMF man-made mineral fiber

MMMS Merck molecular modelling system

MMMT malignant mixed müllerian tumor
metastatic mixed müllerian tumor

MMN morbus maculosus neonatorum

MMNC marrow mononuclear cell

MMO methane mono-oxygenase

MMOA maxillary mandibular odontectomy alveolectomy

MMoL myelomonoblastic leukemia

mmol millimole; also mM

mmol/L millimoles per liter; also mM/L, mM/l

mmp mixture melting point

MMPI McGill-Melzack Pain Index
Minnesota Multiphasic Personality Inventory

MMPI-D Minnesota Multiphasic Personality Inventory Depression Scale

MMPNC Medical Maternal Program for Nuclear Casualties

mmpp millimeters partial pressure

MMPR methylmercaptopurine riboside

mm-PTH mid-molecule parathyroid hormone

MMR mass miniature radiography
mass miniature roentgenography
maternal mortality rate
measles, mumps, and rubella (vaccine)
midline malignant reticulosis
mild mental retardation
mobile mass x-ray
monomethylorutin
myocardial metabolic rate

MMRV measles, mumps, rubella, and varicella

MMS Massachusetts Medical Society
methyl methanesulfonate
Mini-Mental State (examination)

mμs millimicrosecond (nanosecond)

MMSc Master of Medical Science

MMSE Mini-Mental State Examination

mm st muscle strength

MMSV mouse Moloney sarcoma and leukemia virus

MMT manual muscle test
Mini-Mental Test
mouse mammary tumor

MMTA methyl-meta-tyramine

MMTP methadone maintenance treatment program

MMTV mouse mammary tumor virus

MMU medical maintenance unit
mercaptomethyl uracil

mmu millimass unit

MMuLV Moloney murine leukemia virus; also MMLV

MMV mandatory minute ventilation
mandatory minute volume

MMWR *Morbidity and Mortality Weekly Report*

MN antigens M and N in MNS blood group system
malignant nephrosclerosis
meganewton
melena neonatorum
melanocytic nevus
membranous neuropathy
mesenteric node
metanephrine
midnight; also M/N, Mn, mn
mononuclear
motor neuron
mucosal neurolysis
multinodular
myoneural

M/N macrocytic/normochromic (anemia)
microcytic/normochromic (anemia)
midnight; also midnoc, MN, Mn, mn

M&N morning and night

Mn manganese
midnight; also midnoc, MN, M/N, mn

mN micronewton
millinormal

mn midnight; also midnoc, MN, M/N, Mn

MNA maximum noise area

MNAP mixed nerve action potential

MNB murine neuroblastoma

MNC mononuclear cell; also MC
mononuclear leukocyte; also MNL

MNCV motor nerve conduction velocity

MND minimal necrosing dose
minor neurologic dysfunction
modified neck dissection
motor neuron disease

MNDO modified neglect of diatomic overlap

MNG multinodular goiter

mng morning; also man

MNI minimum number of individuals

MNJ myoneural junction

MNL maximal number of lamellae
mononuclear leukocyte; also MNC

MN/m² meganewton per square meter

MNMK maximal number of microbes killed

MNMS myonephropathic metabolic syndrome

MNNG *N*-methyl-*N′*-nitro-*N*-nitrosoguanidine

MNO minocycline; also MiC

MNP mononuclear phagocyte; also MP

MNPA methoxy-naphthyl propionic acid

MnPO median preoptic area

MnPV *Mastomys natalensis* papillomavirus

MNR marrow neutrophil reserve

MNS antigens in the MNSs blood group system
medial nuclear stratum
Melnick-Needles syndrome

MNSER mean normalized systolic ejection rate

Mn-SOD manganese-superoxide dismutase

MNSs antigens in the MNSs blood group system

MnSSEP median nerve somatosensory-evoked potential

MNTB medial nucleus of trapezoid body

MNU methylnitrosourea

MNZ metronidazole; also MTR

MO manually operated
medial oblique (x-ray view)
Medical Officer
mesio-occlusal
metastases 0 (zero) (no evidence of distant metastases)
mineral oil
Minor-Oppenheim (syndrome)
minute output
mitral orifice
molecular orbital
mono-oxygenase
month; also M, Mo, mo, mon
months old; also mo
morbidly obese
mother; also M, Mo, mo

MO₂ myocardial oxygen consumption

Mo mode; also mo
Moloney (strain)
molybdenum
monoclonal
month; also M, MO, mo, mon
mother; also M, MO, mo
mouth; also M

mo mode; also Mo

month; also M, MO, Mo, mon
months old; also MO
mother; also M, MO, Mo
motor

MΩ megohm; also M

MOA mechanism of action
Medical Office Assistant

MOAB, MoAb monoclonal antibody; also MA, MAB, MAb, mAB, mAb, MCA, MCAB, MC-Ab

MOAD methotrexate, Oncovin, L-asparaginase, and dexamethasone

MOB mechlorethamine, Oncovin, and bleomycin
medical office building

mob mobility; also mobil
mobilization; also mobil

mobil mobility; also mob
mobilization; also mob

MOB-PT mitomycin C, Oncovin, bleomycin, and Platinol

MOC maximal oxygen consumption
mother of child

MOCA methotrexate, Oncovin, Cytoxan (cyclophosphamide), and Adriamycin

MoCM molybdenum-conditioned medium

MOD maturity-onset diabetes
Medical Officer of the Day
medical, osteopathic, and dental
mesio-occlusodistal
moderate; also mod

mod moderate; also MOD
moderation
modification
modulation
module

modem modulator/demodulator

MODM maturity-onset diabetes mellitus

mod praesc in the way directed [L. *modo prae-scripto*]

MODY maturity-onset diabetes of youth

MOF marine oxidation/fermentation
methotrexate, Oncovin, and fluorouracil
methoxyflurane; also MF
multiple organ failure

MOFS multiple organ failure syndrome

MOH Medical Officer of Health

MOI maximal oxygen intake
multiplicity of infection

MOJAC mood, orientation, judgment, affect, and content

MOL molecular layer; also ML

mol mole; also M
molecular; also M
molecule

molal molality; also M, m

molc molar concentration; also *M*

molfr mole fraction

mol/kg moles per kilogram

moll soft [L. *mollis*]

mol/L, mol/l moles per liter

mol/m³ moles per cubic meter

mol/s moles per second

mol wt molecular weight; also M, MW, MWt

MOM milk of magnesia
mucoid otitis media

MoM multiples of the median

MOMA methylhydroxymandelic acid

mΩ milliohm

MOMP major outer membrane protein

MoMSV Moloney murine sarcoma virus

MON mongolian (gerbil)
monitor

Mon Monday, also M

mon monocyte; also M, mono
month; also M, MO, Mo, mo

Monatsh Monthly Notebooks for Chemistry [Ger. *Monatshefte für Chemie*]

MONO, Mono mononucleosis; also mono

mono monocyte; also M, mon
mononucleosis; also MONO, Mono
monospot (test)

monos monocytes

MOOW Medical Officer of the Watch

MOP major organ profile
mechlorethamine (nitrogen mustard), Oncovin, and procarbazine
medical outpatient
medical outpatient program
methotrexate, Oncovin, and prednisone

8-MOP 8-methoxypsoralen

MOP-BAP Mustargen (mechlorethamine), Oncovin, prednisone, bleomycin, Adriamycin, and procarbazine

MOPEG 3-methoxy-4-hydroxyphenylglycol

MOPP mechlorethamine, Oncovin, procarbazine, prednisone

MOPP-ABVD mechlorethamine, Oncovin, procarbazine, prednisone, Adriamycin, bleomycin, vinblastine, and dacarbazine

MOPS 4-morpholinepropanesulphonic acid

MOPV monovalent oral poliovirus vaccine

MOR Medical Officer Report
morphine; also M, m, morph

MORA mandibular orthopedic repositioning
appliance

MORC Medical Officers Reserve Corps

MORD magnetic optical rotatory dispersion

mor dict in the manner directed [L. *more dicto*]

morph morphine; also M, m, MOR
morphological; also morphol
morphology; also morphol

morphol morphological; also morph
morphology; also morph

mor sol in the usual way [L. *more solito*]

mortal mortality

MOS medial orbital sulcus
mirror optical system
months; also mos
myelofibrosis osteosclerosis

mOs milliosmolal

mos months; also MOS

MOSFET metal oxide semiconductor field
effect transistor

mOsm, MOsm milliosmole; also mOsmol

mOsm/kg milliosmoles per kilogram

mOsmol milliosmole; also mOsm, MOsm

MOT mini-object test
motility examination
mouse ovarian tumor

MOTT mycobacteria other than tubercle
(bacillus)

MotV motor nucleus of the trigeminal nerve
(fifth cranial nerve)

MOU memorandum of understanding

MOUS multiple occurrence of unexplained
symptoms

MOV multiple oral vitamin

MOVC membranous obstruction of inferior
vena cava

MOX moxalactam

MP as directed [L. *modo prescripto*]; also md,
m dict, mp
macrophage
matrix protein
mean pressure
mechanical percussion
mechanical percussor
medial plantar
melphalan and prednisone

melting point; also mp
membrane potential
menstrual period
mentoposterior (fetal position)
mentum posterior
mercaptopurine
Merzbacher-Pelizaeus (disease)
mesial pit
mesiopulpal
metacarpophalangeal; also MCP, MCPH
metaphalangeal (joint)
methylprednisolone; also MPS
modulator protein
moist pack
mononuclear phagocyte; also MNP
monophosphate
mouthpiece
mouth pressure
mucopolysaccharide; also MPS
multiparous; also multip
muscle potential
mycoplasmal pneumonia

4MP4 methylpyrazole

6-MP 6-mercaptopurine; also Mp

Mp 6-mercaptopurine; also 6-MP

mp as directed [L. *modo praescripto*]; also md,
m dict, MP
early in the morning [L. *mane primo*]; also
man pr
melting point; also MP
millipond

MPA main pulmonary artery
medial preoptic area; also MPOA
Medical Procurement Agency
medroxyprogesterone acetate
methylprednisolone acetate
micropattern analyzer
minor physical anomaly
mycophenolic acid

MPa, mPa megapascal

MPAP mean pulmonary arterial pressure

MPAQ McGill Pain Assessment Questionnaire

MPAS mantle-paraaortic-splenic (irradiation);
also MPS

MPB male pattern baldness

MPC marine protein concentrate
maximal permissible concentration
meperidine, promethazine, and chlorpromazine
metallophthalocyanine
minimal mycoplasmacidal concentration
minimal protozoacidal concentration
morphine-positive control

mucopurulent cervicitis
myeloblast-promyelocyte compartment

MPCD minimal perceptible color difference

MPCN microscopically positive, culturally negative

MPCU maximum permissible concentration of unidentified (radionuclides)

MPCUR maximum permissible concentration of unidentified radionuclides

MPCWP mean pulmonary capillary wedge pressure

MPD main pancreatic duct
maximum permissible dose
mean population doubling
membrane potential difference
minimal perceptible difference
minimal phototoxic dose
minimal popular dose
minimal port diameter
Minnesota Percepto-Diagnostic (test); also MPDT
multiplanar display
multiple personality disorder
myeloproliferative disease; also MD
myofascial pain dysfunction

MPDS mandibular pain dysfunction syndrome
myofascial pain dysfunction syndrome

MPDT Minnesota Percepto-Diagnostic Test; also MPDT

MPDW mean percentage of desirable weight

MPE maximal possible effect
maximal possible error

MPEC monopolar electrocoagulation

MPED minimal phototoxic erythema dose

MPEH methylphenylethylhydantoin

MPF maturation-promoting factor
mean power frequency

m-PFL methotrexate, Platinol, fluorouracil, and leucovorin calcium

MPFM mini-Wright peak flow meter

MPG magnetopneumography

MPGM monophosphoglycerate mutase

MPGN membranoproliferative glomerulo-nephritis
mesangioproliferative glomerulonephritis

MPH male pseudohermaphroditism
Master of Public Health
milk protein hydrolysate

mph miles per hour

M phase phase of mitosis in cell growth cycle

MPHD multiple pituitary hormone deficiencies

MPHR maximum predicted heart rate

MPhysA Member of Physiotherapists' Association (British)

MPI mannose phosphate isomerase
Maudsley Personality Inventory
maximum permitted intake
maximal point of impulse
Multiphasic Personality Inventory
multiphoton ionization
Multivariate Personality Inventory
myocardial perfusion imaging

MPJ metacarpophalangeal joint
metatarsophalangeal joint; also MTPJ

mpk milligrams per kilogram; also mg/kg

MPL maximum permissible level
melphalan
mesiopulpolabial; also MPLa
mesiopulpolingual
monophosphoryl lipid

MPLa mesiopulpolabial; also MPL

MPM malignant papillary mesothelioma
medial pterygoid muscle
monoclonal paratypic molecule
Mortality Prediction Model
multiple primary malignancy
multipurpose meal

MPMT Murphy punch maneuver test

MPMV Mason-Pfizer monkey virus

MPN most probable number

MPO maximal power output
minimal perceptible odor
myeloperoxidase

MPOA medial preoptic area; also MPA

MPOS myeloperoxidase system

MPP massive periretinal proliferation
maximal perfusion pressure
maximal print position
medial pterygoid plate
medical personnel pool
mercaptopyrazine pyrimidine
metacarpophalangeal profile
1-methyl-4-phenyl-1,2,3,6-tetrahydropyridine; also MPTP

mppcf millions of particles per cubic foot

MPPG microphotoelectric plethysmography

MPPN malignant persistent positional nystagmus

MPPP 1-methyl-4-phenyl-4-propionoxy-piperidine

MPPT methylprednisolone pulse therapy

MPR marrow production rate
massive preretinal retraction
maximal pulse rate

MPR—cont'd
mercaptopurine riboside
myeloproliferative reaction

MPRE minimal pure radium equivalent

MPS mantle-paraaortic-splenic (irradiation);
also MPAS
Medical Publishing Standard
methylprednisolone; also MP
microbial profile system
mononuclear phagocyte system
Montreal platelet syndrome
movement-produced stimulus
mucopolysaccharide; also MP
mucopolysaccharidosis
multiphasic screening
myocardial perfusion scintigraphy

MPSMT Merrill-Palmer Scale of Mental Tests

MPSRT matched pairs signed rank test

MPSS methylprednisolone sodium succinate

MPSV myeloproliferative sarcomavirus

MPT maximal predicted phonation time
Michigan Picture Test

MPTAH Mallory phosphotungstic acid hematoxylin

MPTP 1-methyl-4-phenyl-1,2,3,6-tetra-
hydropyridine; also MPP

MPTR motor, pain, touch, reflex (deficit)

MPT-R Michigan Picture Test, Revised

MPU Medical Practitioners Union (British)

MPV mean plasma volume
mean platelet volume
metatarsus primus varus

mpz millipiéze

MQ memory quotient
menaquinone (former abbreviation)

MQC microbiologic quality control

MR Maddox's rod
magnetic resonance
mandibular reflex
mannose-resistant
maximal right
may repeat
measles-rubella (vaccine)
medial rectus (muscle)
median raphe
medical record
medical rehabilitation
medical report
medication responder
medium range
megaroentgen
Melkersson-Rosenthal (syndrome)

menstrual regulation
mentally retarded
mental retardation
mesencephalic raphe
metabolic rate
methemoglobin reductase; also MHR, MR-E
methyl red
milk ring (test)
milliroentgen; also mR, mr
mitral reflux
mitral regurgitation
mixed respiratory
moderate resistance
modulation rate
mortality rate
mortality ratio
motivation research
motor retardation
multicentric reticulohistiocytosis
multiplication rate
multiplicity reactivation
muscle receptor
muscle relaxant
myotactic reflex

M$_R$ right electrode

M$_r$ molecular-weight ratio
relative molecular mass; also M_r
relative molecular weight

M_r relative molecular mass; also M$_r$

M&R measure and record

MRx1 may repeat one time

Mr mandible ramus

mR, mr milliroentgen; also MR

MRA main renal artery
marrow repopulation activity
Medical Records Administrator
mid-right atrium
multivariate regression analysis

MRACP Member of the Royal Australasian
College of Physicians

mrad millirad

MRAN medical resident admitting note

MRAP maximal resting anal pressure
medial right atrial pressure

MRAS main renal artery stenosis
mean renal artery stenosis

MRBC monkey red blood cell
mouse red blood cell

MRBF mean renal blood flow

MRC maximal recycling capacity
Medical Registration Council
Medical Research Council (of Great Britain)

Medical Reserve Corps
methylrosaniline chloride (gentian violet, crystal violet)
Müller-Ribbing-Clement (syndrome)

MRCP Member of the Royal College of Physicians

MRCPE Member of the Royal College of Physicians of Edinburgh

MRCP (Glasg) Member of the Royal College of Physicians and Surgeons of Glasgow

MRCPI Member of the Royal College of Physicians of Ireland

MRCS Member of the Royal College of Surgeons

MRCSE Member of the Royal College of Surgeons of Edinburgh

MRCSI Member of the Royal College of Surgeons of Ireland

MRCVS Member of the Royal College of Veterinary Surgeons

MRD margin reflex distance
medical records department
method of rapid determination
minimal reacting dose; also mrd
minimal renal disease
minimal residual disease

mrd millirutherford
minimal reacting dose; also MRD

MRDM malnutrition-related diabetes mellitus

MRE maximal restrictive exercise
maximal risk estimate
meals ready to eat
metal regulatory element

MR-E methemoglobin reductase; also MHR, MR

mrem millirem
milliroentgen equivalent, man

mrep milliroentgen equivalent, physical

MRF medical record file
melanocyte-releasing factor
melanocyte-stimulating hormone-releasing factor
mesencephalic reticular formation
midbrain reticular formation
mitral regurgitant flow
moderate renal failure
monoclonal rheumatoid factor; also mRF
müllerian regression factor

mRF monoclonal rheumatoid factor; also MRF

MRFC mouse rosette-forming cell

MRFIT Multiple Risk Factor Intervention Trial

MRFT modified rapid fermentation test

MRG murmurs, rubs, and gallops

MRH Maddox's rod hyperphoria
melanocyte-stimulating hormone-releasing hormone

MRHA mannose-resistant hemagglutination

MRHD maximal recommended human dose

mrhm milliroentgens per hour at one meter

MRHT modified rhyme hearing test

MRI machine-readable identifier
magnetic resonance imaging
medical records information
Medical Research Institute
moderate renal insufficiency

MRIF melanocyte-stimulating hormone release-inhibiting factor

MRIH melanocyte-stimulating hormone release-inhibiting hormone

MRK Mayer-Rokitansky-Kuster (syndrome)

MRL Medical Record Librarian
Medical Research Laboratory
minimal response level

MRM modified radical mastectomy

MRN malignant renal neoplasm

mRNA messenger ribonucleic acid

mRNP messenger ribonucleoprotein

MRO minimal recognizable odor
muscle receptor organ

MROD Medical Research and Operations Directorate

MRP maximal reimbursement point
mean resting potential
medical reimbursement plan

MRPAH mixed reverse passive antiglobulin hemagglutination

MRPN medical resident progress notes

MRR marrow release rate
maximal relation rate
maximal relaxation rate
maximum rate of rise

MRS magnetic resonance spectroscopy
malignant neuroleptic syndrome
mania rating scale
median range score
medical receiving station
Melkersson-Rosenthal syndrome
methicillin-resistant *Staphylococcus (aureus)*

MRSA methicillin-resistant *Staphylococcus aureus*

MRT major role therapy
mean residence time
median reaction time
median recognition threshold
median relapse time
Medical Records Technician
milk ring test
modified rhyme test
muscle response test

MRU mass radiography unit
measure of resource use
minimal reproductive unit

MRUS maximal rate of urea synthesis

MRV minute respiratory volume
mixed respiratory vaccine

MRVP mean right ventricular pressure
methyl red, Voges-Proskauer (medium)

MS main scale
maladjustment score
manic state
mannose-sensitive
Marie-Sée (syndrome)
Marie-Strümpell (disease)
mass spectrometry; also mass spec
Master of Science; also MSc
Master of Surgery; also MC, MCh
mean score
mechanical stimulation
Meckel's syndrome
medical services
medical student
medical supplies
medical-surgical
medical survey
menopausal syndrome
mental status
metaproterenol sulfate
microbial susceptibility
microscope slide
Mikulicz's syndrome
milkshake
minimal support
mitral sound
mitral stenosis
mobile surgical (unit)
modal sensitivity
molar solution
molar substitution
mongolian spot
morning stiffness
morphine sulfate; also ms
Morquio-Silverskiöld (syndrome)
motile sperm
mucosubstance

multilaminated structure
multiple sclerosis
Murphy-Sturm (lymphosarcoma)
muscle shortening
muscle strength
musculoskeletal; also Ms, MSK

MS-1 magic spot 1 (guanosine 3′,5′-diphosphate)

MS-222 tricaine

M&S microculture and sensitivity; also MCS

Ms murmurs
musculoskeletal; also MS, MSK

ms manuscript
millisecond; also msec
morphine sulfate; also MS

m/s meters per second; also m/sec

m/s² meters per second squared

MSA major serologic antigen
male-specific antigen
mannitol salt agar
Medical Services Administration
membrane stabilizing action
midsystolic click
mouse serum albumin
multichannel signed averager
Multidimensional Scalogram Analysis
multiple-system atrophy
multiplication-stimulating activity
muscle sympathetic activity

MSAA multiple sclerosis-associated agent

MSAF meconium-stained amniotic fluid

MSAFP maternal serum alpha-fetoprotein

MSAL mammal serum albumin

MSAP mean systemic arterial pressure

MSB Martius scarlet blue
mid-small bowel
most significant bit

MSBC maximal specific binding capacity

MSBLA mouse-specific B-lymphocyte antigen

MSBOS maximal surgical blood order schedule

MSC Medical Service Corps
multiple sib case

MSc Master of Science; also MS

MSCA McCarthy Scales of Children's Abilities

MSCLC mouse stem cell-like cell

MSCP, mscp mean spherical candle-power

MSCU medical special care unit

MSCWP musculoskeletal chest wall pain

MSD Master of Science in Dentistry

mean square deviation
Merck Sharp & Dohme, Inc.
metabolic screening disorder
microsurgical diskectomy
midsleep disturbance
mild sickle-cell disease
minimal steric difference
most significant digit
multiple sulfatase deficiency

MSDS material safety data sheet

MSE medical support equipment
mental status examination
muscle-specific enolase

mse mean square error

msec millisecond; also ms

m/sec meters per second; also m/s

MSEL myasthenic syndrome of Eaton-Lambert

MSER mean systolic ejection rate
Mental Status Examination Record

MSES medical school environmental stress

MSET multistage exercise test; also MET

MSF macrophage slowing factor
macrophage spreading factor
meconium-stained fluid
Mediterranean spotted fever
megakaryocyte-stimulating factor
migration-stimulating factor
modified sham feeding

MSG methysergide
monosodium glutamate

MSGV mouse salivary gland virus

MSH medical self-help
melanocyte-stimulating hormone
melanophore-stimulating hormone; also MH

MSHA mannose-sensitive hemagglutination

MSH-IF melanocyte-stimulating hormone-inhibiting factor

MSH-RF melanocyte-stimulating hormone-releasing factor

MSI medium-scale integration
microbiological safety index

MSIII third-year medical student

MSIR morphine sulfate immediate-release (tablet)

MSIS multistate information system

MSK medullary sponge kidney
musculoskeletal; also MS, Ms

MSKP Medical Sciences Knowledge Profile

MSL Memorial Sloan-Kettering Cancer Center
midsternal line
multiple symmetric lipomatosis

MSLA mouse-specific lymphocyte antigen
multisample Luer adapter

MSLR mixed skin cell–leukocyte reaction

MSLT multiple sleep latency test

MSM medial superior olive
mineral salts medium

MSN Master of Science in Nursing
medial septal nucleus
mildly subnormal

MSO Medical Management Services Organization

MSOF multiple systems organ failure

MSP microspectrophotometry

MSPGN mesangial proliferative glomerulonephritis; also MesPGN

MSPN medical student progress note

MSPS myocardial stress perfusion scintigraphy

MSPU medical short procedure unit

MSR mitral stenoregurgitation
monosynaptic reflex
muscle stretch reflex

MSRPP Multidimensional Scale for Rating Psychiatric Patients

MSRT Minnesota Spatial Relations Test

MSS Marital Satisfaction Scale
massage; also M, mass, mss
Medicare Statistical System
mental status schedule
Metabolic Support Service
minor surgery suite
motion sickness susceptibility
mucus-stimulating substance
multiple sclerosis susceptibility
muscular subaortic stenosis

mss massage; also M, mass, MSS

MSSA methicillin-susceptible *Staphylococcus aureus*

MSSG multiple sclerosis susceptibility gene

MSSU midstream specimen of urine

MSSVD Medical Society for the Study of Venereal Diseases

MST mean survival time
mean swell time (botulism test)
median survival time

MSTA mumps skin test antigen

MSTh, MsTh mesothorium

MsTh$_1$ mesothorium-1

MsTh$_2$ mesothorium-2

MSTI multiple soft tissue injuries

MSU maple syrup urine
 medical studies unit
 midstream urine (specimen)
 monosodium urate
 myocardial substrate uptake

MSUA midstream urinalysis

MSUD maple syrup urine disease

MSUM monosodium urate monohydrate

MSV maize streak virus
 maximal sustained level of ventilation
 mean scale value
 Moloney's sarcoma virus
 murine sarcoma virus

MSVC maximal sustained ventilatory capacity

MSVL maximal spatial vector to left

MSW Master of Social Work
 Medical Social Worker
 multiple stab wounds

MSWYE modified sea water yeast extract
 (agar)

MT empty
 malaria therapy
 malignant teratoma
 mammary tumor
 Martin-Thayer (plate, medium)
 mastoid tip
 maximal therapy
 medial thalamus
 medial thickening
 mediastinal tube
 Medical Technologist; also Med Tech
 Medical Transcriptionist
 medical treatment
 melatonin
 membrane thickness
 mesangial thickening
 mesangial thickness
 metallothionein
 metatarsal; also meta
 metatarsal amputation
 methoxytyramine
 methyltyrosine
 microtome
 microtubule
 middle temporal
 midtrachea
 minimal threshold
 mitotic time
 Monroe tidal (drainage)
 more than
 moxalactam and ticarcillin
 multiple tics
 multitest (plate)

 muscles and tendons
 muscle test
 music therapy
 tympanic membrane [L. *membrana tympani*]

M-T macroglobulin-trypsin

M/T masses of tenderness
 myringotomy and tubes; also M&T

M&T Monilia and Trichomonas
 myringotomy and tubes; also M/T

3-MT 3-methoxytyramine

MT6 mercaptomerin (thiomerin)

Mt megatonne

mt send of such [L. *mitte talis*]

MTA 5′-deoxy-5′-methylthioadenosine
 malignant teratoma, anaplastic
 mammary tumor agent
 Medical Technical Assistant
 metatarsus adductus; also MA
 myoclonic twitch activity

MTAC mass transfer-area coefficient

MTAD tympanic membrane of right ear [L.
 membrana tympani auris dextrae]

MTAL medullary thick ascending limb

MTAS tympanic membrane of left ear [L.
 membrana tympani auris sinistrae]

MT(ASCP) Medical Technologist (certified by
 American Society of Clinical Pathologists)

MTAU tympanic membranes of both ears [L.
 membranae tympanorum aures unitae]

MTB methylthymol blue
 Mycobacterium tuberculosis

MTBE meningeal tick-borne encephalitis
 methyl *tert*-butyl ether

MTBF mean time between (or before) failures

MTC mass transfer coefficient
 maximal tolerated concentration
 medical test cabinet
 medical training center
 medullary thyroid carcinoma
 metoclopramide
 minimum toxic concentration
 mitomycin C; also MC, Mit-C, MITO-C,
 MMC, MMC C, Mmc C

MTCA 1-methyl-1,2,3,4-tetrahydro-beta-
 carboline-3-carboxylic acid

MTD maximum tolerated dose
 mean total dose
 metastatic trophoblastic disease
 Monroe tidal drainage
 multiple tic disorder
 send such doses [L. *mitte tales dotes*]; also mtd

mtd send such doses [L. *mitte tales dotes*]; also MTD

MTDDA Minnesota Test for Differential Diagnosis of Aphasia

MTDI maximal tolerable daily intake

MT-DN multitest, dermatophytes and *Nocardia* (plate)

mtDNA mitochondrial deoxyribonucleic acid

MTDT modified tone decay test

MTE medical toxic environment

MTET modified treadmill exercise testing

MTF maximum terminal flow
medical treatment facility
modulation transfer factor
modulation transfer function

MTG midthigh girth

MTg mouse thyroglobulin

MTH methylthiohydantoin

MTHF methyl tetrahydrofolic acid

MTHHF methyltetrahydrohomofolate

MTI malignant teratoma, intermediate
minimal time interval
Moi-tout-idéal (test)

MTJ midtarsal joint

MTLP metabolic toxemia of late pregnancy

MTM modified Thayer-Martin (agar)

MT-M multitest, mycology (plate)

MT-NMR magnetic transfer nuclear magnetic resonance

MTO Medical Transport Officer

MTOC microtubule organizing center
mitotic organizing center

MTP master treatment plan
maximal tolerated pressure
medial tibial plateau
medical termination of pregnancy
metatarsophalangeal (joint)
microtubule protein
muramyl tripeptide

MTPJ metatarsophalangeal joint; also MPJ

MTQ methaqualone

MTR mass, tenderness, rebound (abdominal examination)
mean total reactivity
Meinicke's turbidity reaction
mental treatment rules
5-methylthioribose
metronidazole; also MNZ

MTR-0 no masses, tenderness, or rebound (abdominal examination)

MTRX methotrexate; also M, MTX, Mtx, MXT

MTS moderate tactile stimulus
multicellular tumor spheroid

MTSH maximum TSH response

MTSO medical transcription service organization

MTST maximal treadmill stress test

MTT malignant teratoma, trophoblastic
maximal treadmill testing
meal tolerance test
mean transit time
monotetrazolium

MT&T myringotomy and insertion of tubes

MTU malignant teratoma, undifferentiated
methylthiouracil

MTV mammary tumor virus (of mice)
metatarsus varus

MTW mean tumor weight

MTX, Mtx methotrexate; also M, MTRX, MXT

MTX-CHOP methotrexate, cyclophosphamide, hydroxydaunomycin, Oncovin, and prednisone

MT-Y multitest yeast (plate)

MTZ mitoxantrone

MU Mache unit; also ME, Mu, mu
maternal uncle
megaunit
mescaline unit
million units
Montevideo unit
motor unit
mouse unit; also mu

Mu Mache unit; also ME, MU, mu

mU milliunit

mu Mache unit; also ME, MU, Mu
micro (10^{-6}); also μ
micrometer (micron); also μ, μm
micron (micrometer)
mouse unit; also MU
twelfth letter of the Greek alphabet

MUA middle uterine artery
multiple unit activity

MUAC middle upper-arm circumference

MUAP motor unit action potential

MUC maximum urinary concentration

muc mucilage

MUD minimal urticarial dose

MUE motor unit estimate

MUG MUMPS (Massachusetts General Hospital Utility Multi-Programming System) Users' Group

MUGA multigated angiogram
multiple gated acquisition (blood pool image)

MU-GAL methylumbelliferyl-beta-galactosidase

MUGEx multigated (blood pool image during) exercise; also MUGX

MUGR multigated (blood pool image at) rest

MUGX multigated (blood pool image during) exercise; also MUGEx

mult multiple; also mx
multiplication

multip multipara; also M
multiparous; also M

multivits multivitamins

MuLV, MuLv murine leukemia virus; also MLV

MUMPS Massachusetts General Hospital Utility Multi-Programming System

MuMTv murine mammary tumor virus

MUN(WI) Munich Wistar (rat); also MW

MUO metastasis of unknown origin
myocardiopathy of unknown origin

MUP major urinary protein
maximal urethral pressure
motor unit potential

Mur muramic acid

MURC measurable undesirable respiratory contaminants

MurNAc N-acetylmuramate

musc muscle(s); also M, m
muscular
musculature

mus-lig musculoligamentous

MUST medical unit, self-contained, and transportable
Mustargen (mechlorethamine hydrochloride); also Must

Must Mustargen (mechlorethamine hydrochloride); also MUST

MUU mouse uterine unit(s)

MUWU mouse uterine weight unit

MV malignant rabbit fibroma virus
measles virus
mechanical ventilation
megavolt
microvilli
millivolt; also mV, mv

minute ventilation
minute volume
mitoxantrone and Vepesid
mitral valve
mixed venous
multivesicular
multivessel
Veterinary Physician [L. *Medicus Veterinarius*]

Mv mendelevium; also Md

mV, mv millivolt; also MV

MVA malignant ventricular arrhythmia
mechanical ventricular assistance
mevalonic acid
mitral valve area
modified vaccine virus, Ankara
motor vehicle accident

MV·A megavolt-ampere; also MV-A

MV-A megavolt-ampere; also MV·A

mV·A millivolt-ampere; also mV-A

mV-A millivolt-ampere; also mV·A

M-VAC methotrexate, vinblastine, Adriamycin, and cisplatin

MVAT metacyclic-variant antigen type

MVB mixed venous blood
multivesicular body

MVC maximal vital capacity
maximal voluntary contraction
myocardial vascular capacity

MVD Doctor of Veterinary Medicine
Marburg's virus disease
microvascular decompression
mitral valve disease
mouse vas deferens
multivessel coronary disease

MVE mitral valve echo
mitral valve leaflet excursion
Murray Valley encephalitis

MV grad, MVgrad mitral valve gradient

MVH massive variceal hemorrhage
massive vitreous hemorrhage
methotrexate, Vepesid, and hexamethylmelamine

MVI multiple vitamin injection
multivalvular involvement
multivitamin infusion

MVLS mandibular vestibulolingual sulcoplasty
Mecham Verbal Language Scale

MVM microvillose membrane
minute virus of mice

MVMT movement

MVN medial ventromedial nucleus

MVO maximal venous outflow

MVO2, MVO$_2$ maximal venous oxygen consumption
myocardial oxygen demand
myocardial ventilation, oxygen (rate)
oxygen content of mixed venous blood

mVO$_2$ minimal venous oxygen consumption

MVOA mitral valve orifice area

MVOS mixed venous oxygen saturation

MVP mean venous pressure
microvascular pressure
mitral valve prolapse

MVPP mechlorethamine, vinblastine, procarbazine, and prednisone

MVPS mitral valve prolapse syndrome

MVPT Motor-Free Visual Perception Test; also MFVPT

MVR massive vitreous retraction
massive vitreous retractor (blade)
minimal vascular resistance
mitral valve regurgitation
mitral valve replacement

MVRI mixed vaccine, respiratory infection
mixed virus respiratory infection

MVS mitral valve stenosis
motor, vascular, and sensory

mV·s millivolt-second; also mV-sec

mV-sec millivolt-second; also mV· s

MVT maximal ventilation time

MVV maximal ventilatory volume; also MVV$_1$
maximal voluntary ventilation

MVV$_1$ maximal ventilatory volume; also MVV

MVVPP Mustargen (nitrogen mustard), vincristine, vinblastine, procarbazine, and prednisone

MVW Minot-von Willebrand (syndrome)

MW Mallory-Weiss (syndrome); also M-W
mean weight
megawatt
microwave; also mw
molecular weight; also M, mol wt, MWt
Munich Wistar (rat); also MUN(WI)

M-W Mallory-Weiss syndrome; also MW
men and women

mW milliwatt

μW microwatt

mw microwave; also MW

MWB minimal weight bearing

mWb milliweber

MWCB manufacturer's working cell bank

MWC Monod-Wyman-Changeux (model)

MWD microwave diathermy
molecular weight distribution

MWI Medical Walk-In (clinic)

MWLT Modified Word Learning Test

MWMT Monotic Word Memory Test

MWP mean wedge pressure

MWPC multiwire proportional chamber

MWS Marden-Walker syndrome
Mickety-Wilson syndrome
Moersch-Woltmann syndrome

MWT malpositioned wisdom teeth

MWt molecular weight; also M, mol wt, MW

MX matrix; also M

Mx maxwell; also mx
MEDEX (extension of physician [L. *medicus extensus*], a physician assistant program using former military medical corpsmen); also mx

mx management
mastectomy; also mast
maxillary; also max
maxwell; also Mx
MEDEX (extension of physician [L. *medicus extensus*], a physician assistant program using former military medical corpsmen); also Mx
metastases
multiple; also mult
myringotomy

MXT methotrexate; also M, MTRX, MTX, Mtx

M$_{xy}$ transverse magnetization

My myopia; also M, my, myop
myria (10^4); also my
myxedematous

my mayer (unit of heat capacity)
myopia; also M, My, myop
myria (10^4); also My

Mycol mycologist
mycology

MYD mydriatic
myotonic muscular dystrophy; also MMD, MyD, MyMD

MyD myotonic muscular dystrophy; also MMD, MYD, MyMD

MYEL multiple myeloma; also MM

Myel myelocyte; also M

myel myelin
  myelinated
Myelo myelogram
  myelography
MyG myasthenia gravis; also MG
Myg myriagram
MyL, Myl myrialiter
Mym myriameter
MyMD myotonic muscular dystrophy; also
  MMD, MYD, MyD
MYO myoglobin; also Mb, MG, MYOGLB
myo myocardial
  myocardium
MYOGLB myoglobin; also Mg, MG, MYO

myop myopia; also M, My, my
MYS myasthenia syndrome
MYTGC Miller-Yoder Test of Grammatical
  Comprehension
MZ mantle zone
  mezlocillin
  monozygotic
M_z longitudinal magnetization
MZA monozygotic twins raised apart
MZL marginal zone lymphocyte
m/z mass-to-charge ratio
MZT monozygotic twins raised together

N

N NU, UPPER CASE, thirteenth letter of the
   Greek alphabet
ν nu, lower case, thirteenth letter of the Greek
   alphabet
   frequency
   kinematic viscosity
   neutrino
   number of degrees of freedom
N antigenic determinant of erythrocytes
   antigen in the MNS blood group system
   asparagine (one-letter notation); also ASN,
     Asn
   Avogadro's number; also N, N_A, Na
   loudness
   nasal; also n, NAS
   nasion
   nausea; also n
   negative; also neg
   Negro
   Neisseria species; also N
   neomycin; also NE, neo, NM
   neper (unit for comparing magnitude of two
     powers, usually electrical or accoustic);
     also Np
   nerve; also n
   neural
   neuraminidase; also NA
   neurologic; also neur, neuro, neurol
   neurological; also neur, neuro, neurol
   neurologist; also neur, neuro, neurol
   neurology; also neur, neuro, neurol
   neuropathy
   neutron; also n
   neutrophil; also neut
   newton
   nicotinamide; also NA
   nitrogen
   no
   Nocardia species; also N
   nodal
   node
   nodule
   none
   nonmalignant; also NM
   Nonne (globulin test)
   noon
   normal; n, NL, Nl, nl, NOR, norm, NR
   normal (solution, as pertains to concentration)
   normality (equivalents per liter)
   not
   noun

NPH insulin
   nucleoside; also Nuc
   nucleus; also Nu
   number; also N, n, NO, No, no
   number density (number of moles of sub-
     stance per unit of volume)
   number in sample
   number of atoms
   number of molecules
   number of neutrons in an atomic nucleus
   number of observations (in statistics)
   numerical aptitude (General Aptitude Test
     Battery)
   population size; also N
   radiance
   refractive index; also n, n, N_D, n_D
   sample size; also n, n
   spin density
   unit of neutron dosage
N Avogadro's number; also N, N_A, Na
   Neisseria species; also N
   neutron number
   Nocardia species; also N
   normal (as pertains to chemical structure);
     also n-
   number; also N, n, NO, No, no
   population size; also N
ℕ natural number
N-I thru N-XII first through twelfth cranial
   nerves
0.02N fiftieth-normal (solution); also N/50
0.1N tenth-normal (solution); also N/10
0.5N half-normal (solution); also N/2
2N 2 normal (solution)
5′-N 5′-nucleotidase
N/2 half-normal (solution); also 0.5N
N/10 tenth-normal (solution); also 0.1N
N/50 fiftieth-normal (solution); also 0.02N
n amounts of substance expressed in moles
   born [L. *natus*]
   haploid chromosome number; also n
   nano- (10^{-9})
   nasal; also N, NAS
   nausea; also N
   nerve; also N
   neuter; also neut
   neutron; also N
   neutron dosage (unit of)
   neutron number density
   night; also nt

n—con'd
normal; also N, NL, Nl, nl, NOR, norm, NR
nostril
number; also N, *N*, NO, No, no
number of density of molecule
number of observations
principle quantum number
refractive index; also N, *n,* N_D, n_D
rotational frequency
sample size; also N, *n*

n haploid chromosome number; also n
refractive index; also N, n, N_D, n_D
sample size; also N, n

n! *n* factorial

n- normal (as pertains to chemical structure);
also *N*

n̄ mean value of n for a number of observations
(in statistics)

2n diploid chromosome number

3n triploid chromosome number

4n tetraploid chromosome number

NA nalidixic acid
Narcotics Anonymous
Native American
network administrator
neuraminidase; also N
neurologic age
neutralizing antibody
neutrophil antibody
nicotinamide; also N
nicotinic acid
nitric acid
no abnormality
Nomina Anatomica [L. (anatomical name)]
nonadherent
non-A (hepatitis)
nonalcoholic
non-amnionic
nonmyelinated axon
noradrenaline
not admitted
not antagonized
not applicable; also N/A
not attempted
not available
nuclear antibody
nuclear antigen
nucleic acid
nucleus accombens
nucleus ambiguus
numerical aperture
nurse anesthetist
nurse's aid

nursing action
nursing assistant

N_A Avogadro's number; also N, *N*, Na

N/A no alternative
not applicable; also NA

N&A normal and active

Na Avogadro's number; also N, *N*, N_A
noise rating number (in acoustics)
sodium [L. *natrium*]; also natr

nA nanoampere

²⁴Na sodium 24, radioactive sodium;
halflife, 15.0 hours

NAA naphthaleneacetic acid
neutral amino acid
neutron activation analysis
neutrophil aggregation activity
nicotinic acid amide
no apparent abnormalities

NAAC no apparent anesthetic complication

NAACLS National Accrediting Agency for
Clinical Laboratory Sciences

NAACOG NAACOG: The Organization for
Obstetric, Gynecologic, and Neonatal
Nurses
Nurses Association of the American College
of Obstetrics and Gynecology (now:
NAACOG: The Organization for Obstetric,
Gynecologic, and Neonatal Nurses)

NAACP neoplasia, allergy, Addison's disease,
collagen vascular disease, and parasites

NAAP *N*-acetyl-4-aminophenazone

NAB novarsenobenzene

NABR National Association for Biomedical
Research

NABS normoactive bowel sounds

NABX needle aspiration biopsy

NAC accessory nucleus (Monakow's nucleus)
N-acetyl-L-cysteine
nitrogen mustard, Adriamycin, and CCNU
(lomustine)
nonadherent cell

NACA National Advisory Council on Aging

NACD not acidified

NAC-EDTA *N*-acetyl-L-cysteine ethylenediaminetetraacetic acid

n-Ach achievement need (psychology)

NACI National Advisory Committee on
Immunization

NAcneu *N*-acetylneuraminic acid; also NAN,
NANA

NACOR National Advisory Committee on Radiation

NACT National Alliance of Cardiovascular Technologists (now: NSCT/NSPT, National Society for Cardiovascular Technology/National Society for Pulmonary Technology)

NAD new antigenic determinant
nicotinamide adenine dinucleotide
nicotinic acid dehydrogenase
no abnormal discovery
no abnormality demonstrable
no abnormality detected
no active disease
no acute disease
no acute distress
no apparent disease
no apparent distress
no appreciable disease
normal axis deviation
nothing abnormal detected
nothing abnormal discovered

NAD⁺ oxidized form of nicotinamide adenine dinucleotide

NaD sodium dialysate [L. *natrium* (sodium)]

NADA New Animal Drug Application

NADABA *N*-adenosyldiaminobutyric acid

NADG nicotinamide adenine dinucleotide glycohydrolase

NADH reduced form of nicotinamide adenine dinucleotide

NADL National Association of Dental Laboratories

NaDodSO₄ sodium dodecyl sulfate [L. *natrium* (sodium)]; also SDS

NADONA/LTC National Association of Directors of Nursing Administration in Long Term Care

NADP nicotinamide adenine dinucleotide phosphate

NADP⁺ oxidized form of nicotinamide adenine dinucleotide phosphate

NADPH reduced form of nicotinamide adenine dinucleotide phosphate

NADSIC no apparent disease seen in chest

NAE net acid excretion

Na_e exchangeable body sodium [L. *natrium* (sodium)]

NAEMT National Association of Emergency Medical Technicians

NAF nafcillin; also NF
net acid flux

NAG *N*-acetylglucosaminidase
narrow angle glaucoma
non-agglutinable (vibrios)
non-agglutinating

NAGA *N*-acetyl-beta-glucosaminidase

NAGO neuraminidase and galactose oxidase

NAHC National Association for Home Care

NAHI National Athletic Health Institute

NAHOD *N*-acetylhexosamine oxidase

NAHSA National Association for Hearing and Speech Action

NAHST National Association of Human Services Technologies (defunct)

NAI net acid input (urinary)
neuraminidase inhibition; also NI
no acute inflammation
non-accidental injury
non-adherence index

NAIR non-adrenergic inhibitory response

NaI(T) thallium-activated sodium iodide crystal (in gamma-ray detectors) [L. *natrium* (sodium)]; also NaI(Tl)

NaI(Tl) thallium-activated sodium iodide crystal (in gamma-ray detectors) [L. *natrium* (sodium)]; also NaI(T)

NaK ATPase sodium and potassium-activated adenosine triphosphate [L. *natrium* (sodium), *kalium* (potassium)]

Na&K sodium and potassium [L. *natrium* (sodium), *kalium* (potassium)]

Na&KSP sodium and potassium spot (urine test) [L. *natrium* (sodium), *kalium* (potassium)]

NAL nonadherent leukocyte

NALD neonatal adrenoleukodystrophy

NALL null cell line of acute lymphocytic leukemia

NALP neuroadenolysis of pituitary

NAM natural actomyosin

NAMCS National Ambulatory Medical Care Survey

NAME National Association of Medical Examiners
nevi, atrial myxoma, myxoid neurofibromas, ephelides (syndrome)

NAMH National Association for Mental Health (now: NMHA, National Mental Health Association)

NAMN nicotinic acid mononucleotide

NAMRU Navy Medical Reserve Unit

NAMT National Association for Music Therapy

NAN *N*-acetylneuraminic acid; also NAcneu, NANA

NANA *N*-acetylneuraminic acid; also NAcneu, NAN

NANB non-A, non-B (hepatitis)

NANBH non-A, non-B hepatitis

NANBV non-A, non-B hepatitis virus

NAND not-and (result is false only if all arguments are true—otherwise, result is true)

NANDA North American Nursing Diagnosis Association

NANPRH National Association of Nurse Practitioners in Reproductive Health

NANSAIDS non-aspirin, nonsteroidal, anti-inflammatory drugs

N ant/post anterior and posterior "zones" (nerve cell groups—nuclei) of hypothalamus

NAP narrative, assessment, and plan
nasion, point A, pogonion (angle of convexity in craniometrics)
nerve action potential
neutrophil alkaline phosphatase
Nomina Anatomica Parisiensia
non-acute profile
nucleic acid phosphatase
nucleic acid phosphorus

NAPA *N*-acetylated procainamide
N-acetyl-*p*-aminophenol
N-acetylprocainamide

NAPD no active pulmonary disease

Na Pent Pentothal Sodium [L. *natrium* (sodium)]

NaPG sodium pregnanediol glucuronide [L. *natrium* (sodium)]

NAPH naphthyl

NAPNES National Association for Practical Nurse Education and Service

NAR nagasa analbuminemic rat
nasal airway resistance
no action required
not at risk

NARA Narcotics Addict Rehabilitation Act

NARC, narc narcotic; also narco
narcotics (hospital, officer, treatment center); also narco
slang for narcotics officer

Narc nucleus arcuatus

narco narcotic; also NARC, narc
narcotics (hospital, officer, treatment center); also NARC, narc
slang for narcotic addict or narcotics officer

NARF National Association of Rehabilitation Facilities

NARMC Naval Aerospace and Regional Medical Center

NAS nasal; also N, n
National Academy of Sciences
neonatal abstinence syndrome
neonatal air leak syndrome
neuroallergic syndrome
no added salt
normalized alignment score

NASE National Association for the Study of Epilepsy

Na-Spt sodium spot (urine test) [L. *natrium* (sodium)]

NAS-NRC National Academy of Sciences–National Research Council

NASW National Association of Social Workers

NAT *N*-acetyltransferase
natal
nature; also nat
neonatal alloimmune thrombocytopenia
no action taken
non-accidental trauma

Nat native; also nat
natural; also nat

nat national
native; also Nat
natural; also Nat
nature; also NAT

NATB Nonreading Aptitude Test Battery

NATM sodium aurothiomalate [L. *natrium* (sodium)]

NATP neonatal autoimmune thrombocytopenic purpura

natr sodium [L. *natrium*]; also Na

NATTS National Association of Trade and Technical Schools (now: CCA, Career College Association)

NAW nasal antrum windows

NB nail bed
needle biopsy
Negri bodies
nervus buccalis
neurometric test battery
newborn; also nb

nitrogen balance
nitrous oxidebarbiturate
non-B (hepatitis)
normoblast; also nbl
note well [L. *nota bene*]; also nb
novobiocin; also Nov
nuclear bag (certain intrafusal muscle fiber
nuclei of a neuromuscular spindle)
nutrient broth

N/B neopterin to biopterin (ratio)

Nb niobium

95Nb niobium 95, radioactive niobium;
halflife, 35.15 ± 0.03 days

nb newborn; also NB
note well [L. *nota bene*]; also NB

NBC non-battle casualty
non-bed care
nuclear, biologic, chemical

NBCC nevoid basal cell carcinoma

NBCCGA National Bladder Cancer
Collaborative Group A

NBCCS nevoid basal cell carcinoma
syndrome; also NBS

NBD neurogenic bladder dysfunction
neurologic bladder dysfunction
no brain damage

NBE northern bean extract

NBEI non-butanol-extractable iodine
(syndrome)

NBF not breast fed

NBI neutrophil bactericidal index
no bone injury
non-battle injury

NBICU newborn intensive care unit; also
NICU

NBIL neonatal bilirubin

NB Int newborn intensive (care unit)

nbl normoblast; also NB

NBM no bowel movement
normal bone marrow
normal bowel movement
nothing by mouth; also NPO
nucleus basalis magnocellularis
nucleus basalis of Meynert

nbM newborn mouse

nbMb newborn mouse brain

NBME National Board of Medical Examiners
normal bone marrow extract

NBN narrow band noise
newborn nursery

NBO non-bed occupancy

NBP needle biopsy of prostate
neomycin, bacitracin, polymyxin B
neoplastic brachial plexopathy
non-invasive blood pressure

NBQC narrow base quad cane

NBS National Bureau of Standards
Neri-Barré syndrome
nevoid basal cell carcinoma syndrome; also
NBCCS
newborn screen
Nijmegen breakage syndrome
no bacteria seen
normal blood serum
normal bowel sounds
normal brain stem
normal burro serum
nystagmus blockage syndrome

NBT nitroblue tetrazolium
normal breast tissue

NBTE non-bacterial thrombotic endocarditis

NBTG nitrobenzylthioguanosine

NBTNF newborn, term, normal, female

NBTNM newborn, term, normal, male

NBTS National Blood Transfusion Service

NBW normal birth weight

NC nabothian cyst
nasal cannula
nasal clearance
natural cytotoxicity
neck complaint
neonatal cholestasis
nerve conduction
neural crest
neurologic check
neurologic control
nevus comedonicus
nitrocellulose
nitrosocarbazole
no casualty
no change; also N/C
no charge
no complaints; als N/C
noise criterion
non-cirrhotic
noncontributory
normal control
normocephalic
noseclip
nose cone
not classified
not completed

NC—cont'd
not cultured
nucleocapsid
Nurse Corps
nursing coordination

N:C nuclear to cytoplasmic (ratio); also N/C

N/C nerves and circulation; also N&C
neurocirculatory
no change; also NC
no complaints; also NC
nuclear to cytoplasmic (ratio); also N:C

N&C nerves and circulation; also N/C

nC nanocoulomb

nc nanocurie; also nCi

NCA National Council on Alcoholism (now:
NCADD, National Council on Alcoholism
and Drug Dependence)
neurocirculatory asthenia
neutrophil chemotactic activity
no congenital abnormalities
nodulocystic acne
noncontractile area
nonspecific cross-reacting antigen
nuclear cerebral angiogram

NCACC National Collection of Animal Cell
Cultures (United Kingdom)

NCADD National Council on Alcoholism and
Drug Dependence

NCAIM National Collection of Agricultural
and Industrial Microorganisms (Budapest)

N-CAM nerve cell adhesion molecule

NCAMLP National Certification Agency for
Medical Lab Personnel

NcAMP nephrogenous cyclic adenosine
monophosphate

NCAS neocarzinostatin (zinostatin); also NCS

NCAT normal cephalic and atraumatic; also
NC/AT

NC/AT normal cephalic and atraumatic; also
NCAT

NCB no code blue

NCBI National Center for Biotechnology
Information

NCC no concentrated carbohydrates
non-coronary cusp
nucleus caudalis centralis
nursing care continuity

NCCLS National Committee for Clinical
Laboratory Standards

NCCNHR National Citizen's Coalition for
Nursing Home Reform

NCCTG North Central Cancer Treatment
Group

NCCU newborn convalescent care unit

NCD neurocirculatory dystonia
nitrogen clearance delay
no congenital deformities
normal childhood diseases
normal childhood disorders
not considered disabling

NCDC National Communicable Disease Center

NCDV Nebraska calf diarrhea virus

NCE negative contrast echocardiography
new chemical entity
non-convulsive epilepsy

NCEHPHP National Council on the Education
of Health Professionals in Health
Promotion

NCF night care facility
no cold fluids
polymorphonuclear neutrophil chemotactic
factor

NCF(C) neutrophil chemotactic factor (complement)

NCGL nucleus corporis geniculati lateralis

NCHCA National Commission for Health
Certifying Agencies (now: NOCA,
National Organization for Competency
Assurance)

NCHLS National Council on Health
Laboratory Services

NCHS National Center for Health Statistics

NCI naphthalene creosote, iodoform
National Cancer Institute
nuclear contour index
nucleus colliculi inferioris
nursing care integration

nCi nanocurie; also nc

NCIB National Collection of Industrial
Bacteria

NCJ needle catheter jejunostomy

NCL neuronal ceroid lipofuscinosis
nuclear cardiology laboratory

NCLEX-RN National Council Licensure
Examination for Registered Nurses

NCM nailfold capillary microscope

N/cm² newtons per square centimeter

NCMC natural cell-mediated cytotoxicity

NCME Network for Continuing Medical Education

NCMH National Committee for Mental Hygiene (now: NMHA, National Mental Health Association)

NCMHI National Clearinghouse for Mental Health Information

NCN National Council of Nurses

NCNC normochromic normocytic (erythrocyte)

NCNCA normochromic normocytic anemia; also NNA

NCO no complaints offered

NCP no caffeine or pepper
non-clonogenic proliferating (cells)
non-collagen protein
nursing care plan

n-CPAP nasal continuous positive airway pressure

NCPE non-cardiogenic pulmonary edema

NCPR no cardiopulmonary resuscitation

NCR neurologic, circulatory, range of motion
neutrophil chemotactic response
nitrogen consumption rate
normotensive control
nuclear to cytoplasmic ratio

NCRC non-child-resistant container

NCRE National Council on Rehabilitation Education

NCRND National Committee for Research in Neurological Disorders

NCRPM National Council on Radiation Protection and Measurements

NCS neocarzinostatin (zinostatin); also NCAS
nerve conduction study
newborn calf serum
no concentrated sweets
non-circumferential stenosis
non-coronary sinus
non-cured sarcoidosis
non-current serum

NCT neural crest tumor
neutron capture therapy
non-contact tonometry
number connection test

NCTC National Cancer Tissue Culture
National Collection of Type Cultures

NCV nerve conduction velocity (study)
no commercial value
non-cholera vibrios

NCVS nerve conduction velocity studies

NCYC National Collection of Yeast Cultures

ND Doctor of Naturopathy
nasal deformity
nasolacrimal duct; also NLD
natural death
Naval Dispensary
neonatal death; also NND
neoplastic disease
nervous debility
neurologic development
neuropsychologic deficit
neurotic depression
neutral density
Newcastle disease
new drug
nifedipine; also NIF
no data
no date
no disease
non-detectable
non-determined
nondiabetic
non-disabling
none detectable
normal delivery
normal deposition
normal development
normal dose
nose drops
not detectable
not detected
not determined
not diagnosed
not done; also nd
nothing done
nucleus of Darkschewitsch
nurse's diagnosis
nutritionally deprived

N/D no defects

N&D nodular and diffuse (lymphoma)

N$_D$, n$_D$ refractive index; also N, n, n

Nd neodymium
number of dissimilar (matches)

nd not done; also ND

NDA National Dental Association
new drug application
no data available
no demonstrable antibodies
no detectable activity
no detectable antibody

NDC National Data Communications
National Drug Code
Naval Dental Clinic
non-differentiated cell
nuclear dehydrogenating clostridia

NDCD National Drug Code Directory

NDD no-dialysis days

NDDG National Diabetes Data Group

NDE near-death experience
nondiabetic extremity

NDEA no deviation of electrical axis

NDELA *N*-nitrosodiethanolamine

NDF neutral detergent fiber
neutrophil diffraction factor
new dosage form
Nicolas-Durand-Favre (disease)
no disease found

NDGA nordihydroguaiaretic acid

NDI naphthalene diisocyanate
nephrogenic diabetes insipidus

NDIR non-dispersive infrared (analyzer)

NDMA nitrosodimethylamine
nitrosodimethylaniline

NDMS National Disaster Medical System

N dm/vm nucleus dorsomedialis-ventro-
medialis

nDNA native deoxyribonucleic acid

ND/NT non-distended/non-tender

NDP net dietary protein
nucleoside 5′-phosphate

NDR neonatal death rate
neurotic depressive reaction
normal detrusor reflex
nucleus dorsalis raphe

NDS Naval Dental School
New Drug Submission
normal dog serum

NDSB Narcotic Drugs Supervisory Board

NDT neurodevelopmental treatment
(physical therapy)
noise detection threshold
nondestructive testing

NDTI National Disease and Therapeutic Index

NDV Newcastle disease virus

NDx non-diagnostic

Nd:YAG neodymium: yttrium-aluminum-
garnet (surgical laser)

NE national emergency
necrotic enteritis
neomycin; also N, neo, NM
nephropathia epidemica
nerve ending
nerve excitability (test)
neural excitation
neuroendocrine
neuroepithelium
neurologic examination
neutrophil elastase
never exposed
no ectopia
no effect
no enlargement
nonelastic
non-endogenous
norepinephrine; also NOR-EPI
not elevated
not enlarged
not equal
not evaluated
not examined
nutcracker esophagus

Ne neon

NEA neoplasm embryonic antigen
no evidence of abnormality

NEB neuroendocrine body

nebul a spray [L. *nebula*]

NEC necrotizing enterocolitis
neuroendocrine cell
no essential change
non-esterified cholesterol
not elsewhere classifiable
not elsewhere classified
not elsewhere coded
not enough cells

nec necessary

NECHI Northeastern Consortium for Health
Information

NECT non-enhanced computed tomography

NED no evidence of disease
no expiration date
normal equivalent deviation

NEEE Near East equine encephalomyelitis

NEEP negative end-expiratory pressure

NEF negative expiratory force
nephritic factor; also NF

NEFA non-esterified fatty acid

NEFG normal external female genitalia

NEG neglect

neg negative; also N

NEHA National Environmental Health Association

NEI National Eye Institute

NEISS National Electronic Injury Surveillance System

NEJ neuroeffector junction

NEM *N*-ethylmaleimide
no evidence of malignancy
nonspecific esophageal motility (disorder)

nem nutritional milk unit [Ger. *Nährungs Einheit Milch*]

NEMA National Eclectic Medical Association (defunct)

nema nematode (threadworm)

Nemb Nembutal

NEMD nonspecific esophageal motility disorder
nonspecific esophageal motor dysfunction

neo neoarsphenamine
neomycin; also N, NE, NM
neonatal; also neonat, NN
neovascularity

NEOH neonatal/high (risk)

NEOM neonatal/medium (risk)

neonat neonatal; also neo, NN

NEP negative expiratory pressure
nephrology; also NEPH
no evidence of pathology
noise equivalent power

nep nephrectomy; also NX, Nx

NEPD no evidence of pulmonary disease

NEPH nephrology; also NEP

neph nephritis

NEPHGE non-equilibrium pH gradient gel electrophoresis

NEPHRO nephrogram

NER no evidence of recurrence
non-ionizing electromagnetic radiation

ner nervous; also nerv
nervousness; also nerv

NERD no evidence of recurrent disease

NERO non-invasive evaluation of radiation output

NERS neurotic/endogenous rating scale

nerv nervous; also ner
nervousness; also ner

NES not elsewhere specified

NET nasoendotracheal tube
nerve excitability test
netilmicin
norethisterone

net Network

NETEN norethisterone enanthate

n et m night and morning [L. *nocte et mane*]; also NM, nm, N&M

ne tr s num do not deliver unless paid [L. *ne tradas sine nummo*]

NETT nasal endotracheal tube

neu neuraminic acid
neurilemma; also nu

neur neurologic; also N, neuro, neurol
neurological; also N, neuro, neurol
neurologist; also N, neuro, neurol
neurology; also N, neuro, neurol

neuro neurologic; also N, neur, neurol
neurological; also N, neur, neurol
neurologist; also N, neur, neurol
neurology; also N, neur, neurol

neurol neurologic; also N, neur, neuro
neurological; also N, neur, neuro
neurologist; also N, neur, neuro
neurology; also N, neur, neuro

neuropath neuropathology; also NP

neurosurg neurosurgeon; also NS, Nsurg
neurosurgery; also NS, Nsurg

neut neuter; also n
neutral
neutralize
neutrophil; also N

NEX nose to ear to xiphoid

NEY neomycin egg yolk (agar)

NEYA neomycin egg yolk agar

NF nafcillin; also NAF
nasopharyngeal fibroma
National Formulary
nephritic factor; also NEF
neurofibromatosis
neurofilament
neutral fraction
noise factor
none found
non-filtered
nonfluent
non-front
non-function
Nonne-Froin (syndrome)
nonwhite female
normal flow

NF—cont'd
  not felt; also nf
  not filtered
  not found
  nuclear factor
  nursed fair
  nylon fiber

nF nanofarad

nf not felt; also NF

NFAR no further action required

NFB National Foundation for the Blind
  non-fermenting bacteria

NFC not favorably considered

NFCC neighborhood family care center

NFD neurofibrillary degeneration
  no family doctor

NFDR neurofacial-digitorenal (syndrome)

NFE nonferrous extract

NFH non-familial hematuria

NFL nerve fiber layer

NFLD nerve-fiber-layer defect

NFLPN National Federation of Licensed
  Practical Nurses

NFM northern fowl mite

NFN Nordisk Farmakopenaevn

NFP natural family planning
  neurofilament protein
  no family physician

NFS National Fertility Study
  non-fire setter

NFT neurofibrillary tangle
  Nitrazine fern test

NFTD normal, full-term delivery

NFTSD normal, full-term, spontaneous
  delivery

NFTT nonorganic failure to thrive

NFW nursed fairly well

NG nasogastric; also N-G
  new growth
  nitroglycerin; also Nitro, NTG, NTZ
  nodose ganglion
  no good
  no growth
  non-genetic
  non-groupable

N-G nasogastric; also NG

ng nanogram; also ngm

NGA nutrient gelatin agar

NGB neurogenic bladder

NGC nucleus reticularis gigantocellularis; also
  NRGC

N-Ger neurologic geriatrics

NGF nerve growth factor

NG fdgs nasogastric feedings

NGGR non-glucogenic to glucogenic ratio

NGI nuclear globulin inclusion
  nurse's global impressions

n giv not given

ngm nanogram; also ng

ng/mL nanograms per mL

NGR narrow gauze roll
  nasogastric replacement

NGS normal goat serum

NGSA nerve growth stimulating activity

NGSF non-genital skin fibroblast

NGT nasogastric tube
  normal glucose tolerance

NGU non-gonococcal urethritis

NH natriuretic hormone
  Naval Hospital
  neonatal hepatitis
  neurologically handicapped
  nodular histiocytic (lymphoma)
  nonhuman
  Novikoff's hepatoma
  nursing home

NHA nonspecific hepatocellular abnormality

NHAIS Naylor-Harwood Adult Intelligence
  Scale

NHANES National Health and Nutritional
  Examination Survey

NHANES-I National Health and Nutritional
  Examination Survey I

NHBE normal human bronchial epithelial
  (cells)

NHC National Health Council
  neighborhood health center
  neohemocyte
  neonatal hypocalcemia
  nonhistone chromatin
  nonhistone chromosomal (protein)
  nursing home care

NHCP nonhistone chromosomal protein

NHCU nursing home care unit

NHD normal hair distribution

NHDF normal human diploid fibroblast

NHDL non-high-density lipoprotein

NHDS National Hospital Discharge Survey

NHEFS NHANES Epidemiologic Followup Study

NHG normal human globulin

NHGJ normal human gastric juice

NHH neurohypophyseal hormone

NHI National Health Insurance
National Heart Institute

NHIS National Health Interview Survey

NHK normal human kidney

NHL nodular histiocytic lymphoma
non-Hodgkin's lymphoma

nHL normalized hearing level

NHLBI National Heart, Lung & Blood Institute

NHLI National Heart and Lung Institute

NHM no heroic measures

NHML non-Hodgkin's malignant lymphoma

NHMRC National Health and Medical Research Council

NHP non-hemoglobin protein
nonhistone protein
normal human pooled plasma; also NHPP
nursing home placement

NHPF National Health Policy Forum

NHPP normal human pooled plasma; also NHP

NHPPN National Health Professions Placement Network

NHR net histocompatibility ratio

NHS National Health Service (England)
normal horse serum
normal human serum

NHSR National Hospital Service Reserve

NHV nursing home visit

NHWM normal human white matter

NI neuraminidase inhibition; also NAI
neurologic improvement
neutralization index
nitroxoline
no information
noise index
not identified
not isolated
nucleus intercalatus

N-I thru N-XII first through twelfth cranial nerves

Ni nickel

NIA National Institute on Aging
nephelometric inhibition assay

neutrophil-inducing activity
niacin
no information available

NIAAA National Institute on Alcohol Abuse & Alcoholism

NIAID National Institute of Allergy and Infectious Diseases

NIAL not in active labor

NIAMD National Institute of Arthritis and Metabolic Diseases

NIAMSD National Institute of Arthritis and Musculoskeletal and Skin Diseases

NIB non-involved bone

NIBS nearly ideal binary solvent

NIC neurogenic intermittent claudication
non-invasive carotid (study)
Normarsky interference contrast

Nic nicotinyl alcohol

NICC neonatal intensive care center

NICE non-invasive carotid examination

NICHHD National Institute of Child Health and Human Development

NICU neonatal intensive care unit
neurologic intensive care unit
neurosurgical intensive care unit
newborn intensive care unit; also NBICU
non-immunologic contact urticaria

NIDA National Institute on Drug Abuse

NIDD non-insulin-dependent diabetes

NIDDKD National Institute for Diabetes and Digestive and Kidney Diseases

NIDDM non-insulin-dependent diabetes mellitus

NIDR National Institute of Dental Research

NIDS nonionic detergent soluble

NIEHS National Institute of Environmental Health Sciences

NIF negative inspiratory force; also Nif
neutrophil immobilizing factor
neutrophil migration inhibition factor
nifedipine; also ND
nifuroquine
non-intestinal fibroblast
not in file

Nif negative inspiratory force; also NIF

nif nitrogen fixation (genes)

NIG non-immunoglobulin; also Nig
NSAIA (nonsteroidal anti-inflammatory agent)-induced gastropathy

Nig non-immunoglobulin; also NIG

nig black [L. *niger*]

NIGMS National Institute of General Medical Sciences

NIH National Institutes of Health (of the US Public Health Service)

NIH 204 antimalarial drug

NIHD noise-induced hearing damage

NIHL noise-induced hearing loss

NIIC National Injury Information Clearinghouse

NIIP National Institute of Industrial Psychology

NIL noise interference level
nothing in light
not in labor

nil nothing [L. *nihil*]

NIMH National Institute of Mental Health

NIMH-DIS National Institute of Mental Health Diagnostic Interview Schedule

NIMR National Institute for Medical Research

NINCDS National Institute of Neurological and Communicative Disorders and Stroke

NINDB National Institute of Neurological Diseases and Blindness

NINDS National Institute of Neurological Diseases and Stroke

NINR National Institute for Nursing Research

NINU neurointermediate nursing unit

NINVS non-invasive neurovascular studies

NIOSH National Institute for Occupational Safety and Health

NIP National Inpatient Profile
nipple
nitroiodophenyl
no infection present
no inflammation present

NIPS non-involved psoriatic skin

NIPTS noise-induced permanent threshold shift

NIR near infrared
near infrared reflectance

NIRA nitrite reductase

NIRD non-immune renal disease

NIRMP National Intern and Resident Matching Program (now: NRMP, National Resident Matching Program)

NIRNS National Institute for Research in Nuclear Science

NIRR non-insulin-requiring remission

NIRS normal inactivated rabbit serum

NIS no inflammatory signs
non-immune sheep (serum)

NIT nasointestinal tube
National Intelligence Test
neonatal isoimmune thrombocytopenia

NITD non-insulin-treated disease

nit ox nitrous oxide; also NO

nitro nitroglycerin; also NG, NTG, NTZ

NITTS noise-induced temporary threshold shift

NIV nodule-inducing virus

NJ nasojejunal

NK Committee on Nomenclature of the German Anatomical Society (Ger. *Nomenklatur Kommission*]
natural killer (cell)
normal keratinocyte
normal killer (cell)
not known; also N/K

N/K not known; also NK

NKA no known allergies

nkat nanokatal

NKC non-ketotic coma

NKDA no known drug allergies

NKFA no known food allergies

NKH non-ketotic hyperglycemia; also NKHG
non-ketotic hyperosmolar
non-ketotic hyperosmotic

NKHA non-ketotic hyperosmolar acidosis

NKHG non-ketotic hyperglycemia; also NKH

NKHS non-ketotic hyperosmolar syndrome
normal Krebs-Henseleit solution

NKMA no known medication allergies

NKR normal rat kidney; also NRK

NKTS natural killer target structure

NL nasolacrimal
neural lobe
neutral lipid
nodular lymphoma
normal; also N, n, Nl, nl, NOR, norm, NR
normal libido
normal limits; also nl
normolipemic
Nyhan-Lesch (syndrome)

Nl normal; also N, n, NL, nl, NOR, norm, NR

nL nanoliter; also nl

nl it is not clear [L. *non liquet*]
it is not permitted [L. *non licet*]

nanoliter; also nL
normal; also N, n, NL, Nl, NOR, norm, NR
normal limits; also NL

NLA neuroleptanalgesia
neuroleptoanesthesia
normal lactase activity

NLAA naphthoxylactic acid

NLAL nodule-like alveolar lesion

NLB needle liver biopsy

NLC&C normal libido, coitus, and climax;
also NL C/Cl

NL C/Cl normal libido, coitus, and climax;
also NLC&C

NLD nasolacrimal duct; also ND
necrobiosis lipoidica diabeticorum

NLDL normal low-density lipoprotein

NLE neonatal lupus erythematosus
nurse's late entry

Nle norleucine; also norleu

NLF nasolabial fold
neonatal lung fibroblast
non-lactose fermentation

NLM National Library of Medicine
noise level monitor

NLMC nocturnal leg muscle cramp

NLN National League for Nursing
no longer needed

NLNE National League of Nursing Education
(now: NLN, National League for Nursing)

NLP neurolinguistic program
neurolinguistic programming
nodular liquefying panniculitis
no light perception
normal light perception
normal luteal phase

NLPD nodular lymphocytic, poorly differentiated

NLS neonatal lupus syndrome
nonlinear least squares (method)
normal lymphocyte supernatant

NLSD normal life-span for dogs

NLT Names Learning Test
normal lymphocyte transfer (test)
not later than; also nlt
not less than; also nlt
nucleus lateralis tuberis

nlt not later than; also NLT
not less than; also NLT

NLX naloxone; also NX, Nx

NM neomycin; also N, NE, neo
neuromedical
neuromuscular
nictitating membrane [L. *nictāre* (to wink)]
night and morning; also n et m, N&M, nm
nitrogen mustard
nodular melanoma
nodular mixed (lymphocytic-histiocytic)
nonmalignant; also N
nonmotile (bacteria)
nonwhite male
normetadrenaline
normetanephrine; also NMN, normet
not measurable
not measured
not mentioned
not motile
nuclear medicine; also NUC
nuclear membrane

N/M newtons per meter

N&M nerves and muscles
night and morning; also n et m, NM, nm

Nm newton-meter; also N·m, N x m
nutmeg [L. *nux moschata*]; also nm

N·m newton-meter; also Nm, N x m

N x m newton-meter; also Nm, N·m

N/m² newtons per square meter

nM nanomolar

nm nanometer
night and morning; also n et m, NM, N&M
nonmetallic
nutmeg [L. *nux moschata*]; also Nm

nm² square nanometer

nm³ cubic nanometer

NMA National Malaria Association
National Medical Association
neurogenic muscular atrophy
N-methylaspartate

NMAC National Medical Audio-Visual Center

NM(ASCP) Technologist in Nuclear Medicine
(certified by American Society of Clinical
Pathologists)

NMATWT New Mexico Attitude Toward Work
Test

NMBA nitrosomethylbenzylamine

NMC National Medical Care
neuromuscular control
nodular, mixed-cell (lymphoma)
nucleus reticularis magnocellularis; also
NRM
nurse-managed center

NMCC non-myeloid cell content

NMCD nephrophthisis-medullary cystic disease

NWCPT New Mexico Career Planning Test

NMCUES National Medical Care Utilization and Expenditure Survey

NMD normal muscle development

NMDA N-methyl-D-aspartate

NME new molecular entity

NMF non-migrating fraction (of spermatozoa)

NMFI National Master Facility Inventory

NMHA National Mental Health Association

NMI no mental illness
no middle initial
normal male infant

NMJ neuromuscular junction

NMJAPT New Mexico Job Application Procedures Test

NMKOT New Mexico Knowledge of Occupations Test

NML National Medical Library
nodular mixed histiocytic-lymphocytic lymphoma

NMM nodular malignant melanoma
Nonne-Milroy-Meige (syndrome)

NMN nicotinamide mononucleotide
no middle name
normetanephrine; also NM, normet

NMN⁺ nicotinamide mononucleotide (oxidized form)

NMNRU National Medical Neuropsychiatric Research Unit

NMO nitrogen mustard oxide

nmol nanomole

nmol/L millimicromolar
nanomoles per liter

NMOS N-type metal oxide semiconductor

NMP neutral metallopeptidase
normal menstrual period
nucleoside 5′-monophosphate

NMPCA non-metric principal component analysis

NMR Neill-Mooser reaction
neonatal mortality rate
nictitating membrane response
nuclear magnetic resonance

NMRDC Naval Medical Research and Development Command

NMRI Naval Medical Research Institute
nuclear magnetic resonance imaging

NMRL Naval Medical Research Laboratory

NMRU Naval Medical Research Unit

NMS Naval Medical School
neuroleptic malignant syndrome
neuromuscular spindle
normal mouse serum

N·m/s newton-meters per second

NMSIDS near-miss sudden infant death syndrome

NMSR normalized mean square root

NMSS National Multiple Sclerosis Society

NMT nebulized mist treatment
neuromuscular tension
neuromuscular transmission
N-methyltransferase
no more than
nuclear medicine technology

NMTB neuromuscular transmission blockade

NMTD non-metastatic trophoblastic disease

NMTS neuromuscular tension state

NMU neuromuscular unit

NMUT nitrosomethylurethane

NN neonatal; also neo, neonat
nevocellular nevus
normally nourished
normal nursery
nurse's notes; also N/N

N/N negative/negative
nurse's notes; also NN

N:N indicates presence of azo group (chemical group with two nitrogen atoms)

N-N nurse to nurse (orders)

nn nerves; also NS, Ns
new name [L. *nomen novum*]; also n nov, nom nov, nov n

NNA normochromic normocytic anemia; also NCNCA

NNAS neonatal narcotic abstinence syndrome

NNBA National Nurses in Business Association

NNC National Nutrition Consortium (defunct)

NND neonatal death; also ND
New and Nonofficial Drugs
nonspecific non-erosive duodenitis

NNDC National Naval Dental Center

NNDO neglect of non-bonded differential overlap

NNE neonatal necrotizing enterocolitis
non-neuronal enolase

NNG nonspecific non-erosive gastritis

NNHL nodular non-Hodgkin's lymphoma

NNHS National Nursing Home Survey

NNI noise and number index

NNL no new laboratory (test orders)

NNM neonatal mortality
Nicolle-Novy-MacNeal (medium); also NNN

NNMC National Naval Medical Center

NNN Nicolle-Novy-MacNeal (medium); also
NNM
nitrosonornicotine

NNO no new orders

n nov new name [L. *nomen novum*]; also nn,
nom nov, nov n

NNP neonatal nurse practitioner
nerve net pulse

NNR New and Nonofficial Remedies
not necessary to return

NNS National Natality Survey
neonatal screen
nonneoplastic syndrome
non-nutritive sucking
non-nutritive sweetener

NNT neonatally tolerant
nuclei nervi trigemini

NNU net nitrogen utilization

NNWI Neonatal Narcotic Withdrawal Index

NO narcotics officer
nasal oxygen
nitric oxide
nitrol ointment
nitroso-
nitrous oxide; also nit ox
none obtained
non-obese
number [Old French. *nombre*, fr. L. *numerus*];
also N, *N*, n, No, no
nursing office

No nobelium
number; also [Old French. *nombre*, fr. L.
numerus] N, *N*, n, NO, no

no number; also [Old French. *nombre*, fr. L.
numerus] N, *N*, n, NO, No

NOA nurse obstetric assistant

NOAEL no observed adverse effect level

NOBS nursing observation of behavior
syndromes

NOBT nonoperative biopsy technique

noc at night [L. *nocte*]; also noct
nocturia; also noct
nocturnal [L. *noctis* (of the night)]; also noct

NOCA National Organization for Competency
Assurance

NO-CCE no clubbing, cyanosis, or edema

noc maneq at night and in the morning [L.
nocte maneque]; also noct maneq

NOCT National Occupational Competency
Testing (Program)

noct at night [L. *nocte*]; also noc
nocturia; also noc
nocturnal [L. *noctis* (of the night)]; also noc

noct maneq at night and in the morning [L.
nocte maneque]; also noc maneq

NOD nodular (melanoma)
non-definitive (pattern)
non-obese diabetic
normalized absorbance of the entire chromosome
notify of death

NOE Nuclear Overhauser effect
Nuclear Overhauser enhancement

NOEL no observed effect level (of toxin)

no ess abn no essential abnormalities

NOESY Nuclear Overhauser enhancement
spectroscopy

NOFT nonorganic failure to thrive

NOGM no gammopathy (detected)

NOII non-occlusive intestinal ischemia

NOK next of kin

NOM nonsuppurative otitis media
normal extraocular movements

nom dub a doubtful name [L. *nomen dubium*]

NOMI non-occlusive mesenteric infarction

nom nov new name [L. *nomen novum*]; also
nn, n nov, nov n

nom nud name without designation [L. *nomen
nudum*]

NOND none detected

NONF non-fasting

non pal non-palpable; also NP

non reb non-rebreathing; also NR

non-REM non-rapid eye movement (sleep);
also NREM

non rep do not repeat, no refills [L. *non
repetatur*]; also non repetat, NR, nr

non repetat do not repeat, no refills [L. *non
repetatur*]; also non rep, NR, nr

NONS nonspecific; also NS

nonsegs nonsegmented (neutrophils)

nonvis non-visualized; also nonviz

nonviz non-visualized; also nonvis

NOOB not out of bed

NOP national outpatient profile
not otherwise provided (for); also NP

NOPHN National Organization for Public
Health Nursing (now: NLN, National
League for Nursing)

NOR noradrenaline; also Noradr
normal; also N, n, NL, Nl, nl, norm, NR
nortriptyline; also NT
nucleolar organizing region (cytogenetics)

nor- Nitrogen Ohne Radikal [Ger. *ohne* (without), *Radikal* (radical)]

Noradr noradrenaline; also NOR

NORC normal curve

NOR-EPI norepinephrine; also NE

norleu norleucine; also Nle

norm normal; also N, n, NL, Nl, nl, NOR, NR

normet normetanephrine; also NM, NMN

NOS network operating system
not on staff
not otherwise specified

nos numbers [L. *numeros*]

NOSAC nonsteroidal anti-inflammatory compound

NOSIE Nurse's Observation Scale for Inpatient
Evaluation

NOSM (bed) nucleus of stria medullaris

NOST (bed) nucleus of stria terminalis

NOSTA Naval Ophthalmic Support and
Training Activity

NOT nocturnal oxygen therapy
nucleus of optic tract

NOTB National Ophthalmic Treatment Board
(British)

NOTT nocturnal oxygen therapy trial

Nov novobiocin; also NB

nov new [L. *novum*]

nov n new name [L. *novum nomen*]; also nn, n
nov, nom nov

NOVS National Office of Vital Statistics

nov sp new species [L. *novum species*]

NOW negotiable order of withdrawal

NP nasal prongs
nasopharyngeal
nasopharyngoscopy
nasopharynx; also NPhx
near point (ophthalmology)
neonatal perinatal
nerve palsy
neuritic plaque
neuropathology; also neuropath
neuropeptide
neurophysine; also Np
neuropsychiatric
neuropsychiatry
newly presented
new patient
Niemann-Pick (disease)
nitrogen-phosphorus (detector in gas chromatography)
nitrophenide
nitrophenol
nitroprusside
non-palpable; also non pal
non-pathologic
nonpaying
non-phagocytic
non-practicing
non-producer (cell)
no pain
no phone
no progression
normal plasma
normal pressure
not otherwise provided (for); also NOP
not perceptible
not performed
not practiced
not pregnant
not present
nuclear pharmacist
nuclear pharmacy
nucleoplasmic (index)
nucleoprotein
nucleoside phosphorylase
nucleotide phosphorylase
nursed poorly
Nurse Practitioner
nursing practice
nursing procedure
proper name [L. *nomen proprium*]; also np

N-P need-persistence

Np neper (unit for comparing magnitude of
two powers, usually electrical or
acoustic); also N
neptunium
neurophysine; also NP

np nucleotide pair
proper name [L. *nomen proprium*]; also NP

NPA nasal pharyngeal airway
National Perinatal Association
near-point of accommodation
no previous admission
nucleus of pretectal area

NPa nail patella

Np-AVP neurophysine associated with vaso-pressin

NPAT non-paroxysmal atrial tachycardia

NPB nodal premature beat
non-protein bound

NPBF non-placental blood flow

NPC nasopharyngeal cancer
nasopharyngeal carcinoma; also NPCa
near point of convergence
nodal premature complex
nodal premature contractions
non-parenchymal liver cell
non-patient contract
nonproductive cough
nonprotein calorie
no prenatal care; also NPNC
no previous complaint
nucleus of posterior commissure

NPCa nasopharyngeal carcinoma; also NPC

NPCP National Prostatic Cancer Project

NPD narcissistic personality disorder
natriuretic plasma dialysate
negative pressure device
Niemann-Pick disease
nitrogen-phosphorus detector
nonprescription drugs
no pathologic diagnosis

NPDB National Practitioner Data Bank

NPDL nodular, poorly differentiated lympho-cytes
nodular, poorly differentiated lymphocytic
(lymphoma)

NPDR non-proliferative diabetic retinopathy

NPE neurogenic pulmonary edema
neuropsychologic examination
no palpable enlargement
normal pelvic examination

N periv nuclei periventriculares

NPEV non-polio enterovirus

NPF nasopharyngeal fiberscope
no predisposing factor

NPFT Neurotic Personality Factor Test

NPG nonpregnant

NPGS neopentyl glycol succinate

NPH neutral protamine Hagedorn (insulin)
no previous history
normal pressure hydrocephalus
nucleus pulposus herniation

NPHI neutral protamine Hagedorn insulin

NPhx nasopharynx; also NP

NPI Narcissistic Personality Inventory
neonatal perception inventory
Neuropsychiatric Institute
no present illness
nucleoplasmic index

NPIC neurogenic peripheral intermittent
claudication

NPII Neonatal Pulmonary Insufficiency
Index

NPJT non-paroxysmal atrioventricular
junctional tachycardia

NPL neoproteolipid
nodular poorly differentiated lymphoma

NPM nothing per mouth

NPN nonprotein nitrogen
nurse's progress note(s)

NPNC no prenatal care; also NPC

NPO nothing by mouth [L. *nulla per os*];
also NBM
nucleus preopticus

NPO/HS nothing by mouth at bedtime [L.
nulla per os hora somni]

NPOS nitrite positive

Np-OT oxytocin-associated neurophysine

NPP nitrophenylphosphate
normal pool plasma
normal postpartum

4-NPP 4-nitrophenylphosphate

NPPase nitrophenylphosphatase

NPPD nitrophenylpentadiene

NPPNG non-penicillinase-producing
Neisseria gonorrhoeae

NP polio nonparalytic poliomyelitis

NPR net protein ratio
normal pulse rate
nothing per rectum
nucleoside phosphoribosyl

NPRM notice of proposed rule-making

NPS, Nps *N-o*-nitrophenylsulfenyl

NPSA non-physician surgical assistant
normal pilosebaceous apparatus

NPSG nocturnal polysomnogram

NPSH nonprotein sulfhydryl (group)

NPT neomycin phosphotransferase
neoprecipitin test
nocturnal penile tumescence
normal pressure and temperature
nucleoside phosphotransferase

NPU net protein utilization

NPV negative pressure ventilation
nuclear polyhidrosis virus
nucleus paraventricularis

NPX norpropoxyphene

NPYLI neuropeptide Y-like immunoreactivity

NQA nursing quality assurance

NQMI non-Q wave myocardial infarction

NQR nuclear quadruple resonance

NR do not repeat [L. *non repetatur*]; also
non rep, non repetat, nr
nerve root
neural retina
neutral red
noise reduction
nonreactive
non-rebreathing; also non reb
nonreimbursable
no radiation
no reaction
no recurrence
no refills; also nr
no rehearsal
no report
no response
no return
normal; also N, n, NL, Nl, nl, NOR, norm
normal range
normal reaction
normal record
normotensive rat; also NTR
not reached
not readable
not recorded
not reported
not resolved
nurse
nutrition ratio
nutritive ratio
Reynold's number; also N$_R$

N$_R$ Reynold's number; also NR

N/R not remarkable

nr do not repeat [L. *non repetatur*]; also
non rep, non repetat, NR
near
no refills; also NR

NRA nitrate reductase
nucleus raphe alatus
nucleus retroambigualis

NRAF non-rheumatic atrial fibrillation

NRB non-rejoining DNA strand break

NRBC normal red blood cell
nucleated red blood cell; also NRbc

NRbc nucleated red blood cell; also NRBC

NRBS non-rebreathing system

NRC National Research Council
noise reduction coefficient
normal retinal correspondence
not routine care
Nuclear Regulatory Commission

NRCA National Rehabilitation Counseling
Association

NRCC National Registry in Clinical Chemistry

NRCL non-renal clearance

NRD non-renal death

NRDC National Research Development
Corporation

NREH normal renin essential hypertension

NREM non-rapid eye movement (sleep); also
non-REM

NREMS non-rapid eye movement sleep

NREMT National Registry of Emergency
Medical Technicians

NRF normal renal function

NRFC non-rosette-forming cell

NRGC nucleus reticularis gigantocellularis;
also NGC

NRH nodular regenerative hyperplasia (of
liver)

NRI nerve root involvement
nerve root irritation
neutral regular insulin
non-respiratory infection

NRK normal rat kidney: also NKR

NRL nucleus reticularis lateralis

NRM National Registry of Microbiologists
normal range of motion; also NROM
normal retinal movement
nucleus raphe magnus
nucleus reticularis magnocellularis; also
NMC

NRMP National Resident Matching Program

NRN no return necessary

nRNA nuclear ribonucleic acid

nRNP nuclear ribonucleoprotein

NROM normal range of motion; also NRM
NRP nucleus reticularis parvocellularis
NRPAT net revenue, patient
NRPC nucleus reticularis pontis caudalis
NRPG nucleus reticularis paragigantocellularis
NRR net reproduction rate
Noise Reduction Rating
note, record, report
NRRL Northern Regional Research Laboratory
NRS non-immunized rabbit serum
normal rabbit serum
normal reference serum
numerical rating scale
NRSCC National Reference System in Clinical Chemistry
NRSFPS National Reporting System for Family Planning Services
nrsng nursing; also NSG, nsg
NRT neuromuscular re-education technique
NRTOT net revenue, total
NRV nucleus reticularis ventralis
NS natural science
needle shower
nephrosclerosis
nephrotic syndrome
nerves; also nn, Ns
nervous system
neurologic sign
neurologic surgery
neurologic survey
neurosecretory
neurosurgeon; also neurosurg, NSurg
neurosurgery; also neurosurg, NSurg
neurosyphilis
neurotic score
nipple stimulation
nodular sclerosis
nonsmoker; also NSM
non-snorer
nonspecific; also NONS
nonstimulating
non-stimulation
nonstructural (protein)
non-stutter
non-symptomatic
Noonan's syndrome
normal saline; also N/S, ns
normal serum
normal sodium (diet)
normal study
Norwegian scabies
no sample
no sequelae; also ns
no specimen; also ns, NSPE
not seen
not significant; also ns
not specified; also NSP
not stated
not symptomatic
not sufficient
nuclear sclerosis
nursing services
nylon suture; also ns
N/S normal saline; also NS, ns
NS1 nonstructural protein 1
NS2 nonstructural protein 2
Ns nasospinale
nerves; also nn, NS
ns nanosecond; also nsec
normal saline; also NS, N/S
no sequelae; also NS
no specimen; also NS, NSPE
not significant; also NS
nylon suture; also NS
NSA Neurological Society of America
normal serum albumin
no salt added; also nsa
no serious abnormality
no significant abnormality
no significant anomaly
nutritional status assessment
nsa no salt added; also NSA
NSABP National Surgical Adjuvant Breast and Bowel Project
NSAD no signs of acute disease
NSAE non-supported arm exercise
NSAI nonsteroidal anti-inflammatory
NSAIA nonsteroidal anti-inflammatory agent
nonsteroidal anti-inflammatory analgesic
NSAID nonsteroidal anti-inflammatory drug
NSB nonspecific binding
NSC National Service Center (number)
neurosecretory cell
non-service-connected (disability)
nonspecific suppressor cell
no significant change
not service-connected
NSCC National Society for Crippled Children
NSCD non-service-connected disability
NSCLC non-small-cell lung cancer

NSCPT National Society for Cardiopulmonary Technology (now: NSCT/NSPT, National Society for Cardiovascular Technology/National Society for Pulmonary Technology)

NSCT/NSPT National Society for Cardio-vascular Technology/National Society for Pulmonary Technology

NSD Nairobi sheep disease
neonatal staphylococcal disease
night sleep deprivation
nitrogen-specific detector
nominal single dose
nominal standard dose (radiation)
normal spontaneous delivery
no significant defect
no significant deficiency
no significant deviation
no significant difference
no significant disease

NSDA non-steroid-dependent asthmatic

NSDP National Society of Denture Prosthetists (now: ADP, Academy of Denture Prosthetics)

NSE neuron-specific enolase
nonspecific esterase
normal saline enema

NSĒ nausea without emesis [Fr. *sans*, L. *sine* (without)]

nsec nanosecond; also ns

NSED nonsurgical, emergency department

NSF National Science Foundation
nodular subepidermal fibrosis
no significant findings

NSFP natural suppressor factor protein

NSFTD normal spontaneous full-term delivery

NSG neurosecretory granule
nursing; also nrsng, nsg

nsg nursing; also nrsng, NSG

NSGCT non-seminomatous germ cell tumor

NSG STA nursing station

NSGCTT non-seminomatous germ cell testicular tumor

NSH National Society for Histotechnology

NSHD nodular sclerosing Hodgkin's disease

NSI negative self-image
no sign of infection
no sign of inflammation

NSIDS near sudden infant death syndrome

NSILA non-suppressible insulin-like activity

NSILP non-suppressible insulin-like protein

NSL non-salt loser

NSLF normal sheep lung fibroblast

NSM neurosecretory material
neurosecretory motor (neuron)
non-antigenic specific mediator
nonsmoker; also NS
nutrient sporulation medium

N·s/m² newton-seconds per square meter

NSMR National Society for Medical Research (now: NABR, National Association for Biomedical Research)

NSN nephrotoxic serum nephritis
nicotine-stimulated neurophysine
number of similar negatives

NSNA National Student Nurses' Association

NSND non-symptomatic, non-disabling

NSO Neosporin ointment
nucleus supraopticus

NSol nerve to soleus

NSP neck and shoulder pain
neuron-specific protein
not specified; also NS
N-succinylperimycin
number of similar positives

NSPB National Society for the Prevention of Blindness (now: National Society to Prevent Blindness)
National Society to Prevent Blindness

NSPE no specimen; also NS, Ns

NSPVT non-sustained polymorphic ventricular tachycardia

NSQ Neuroticism Scale Questionnaire
not sufficient quantity

NSR nasoseptal reconstruction
nasoseptal repair
nonspecific reaction
non-systemic reaction
normal sinus rhythm
not seen regularly

nSRBC normal sheep red blood cell

NSS normal saline solution
normal size and shape
not statistically significant
nutritional support service

NSSC normal size, shape, and consistency

NSSL normal size, shape, and location

NSSP normal size, shape, and position

NSSPAVAF normal size, shape, and position, anteverted and anteflexed (uterus)

NSST nonspecific ST (wave segment changes on electroencephalogram); also NS-ST
Northwestern Syntax Screening Test

NS-ST nonspecific ST (wave segment changes on electroencephalogram); also NSST

NSSTT, NS-ST-T nonspecific ST segment and T (wave)

NST neospinothalamic (tract)
non-shivering thermogenesis
non-stress test (fetal monitoring)
not sooner than
nuclear spin tomography
nutritional status type
nutritional support team

NS-T nonspecific T (wave)

NSTT non-seminomatous testicular tumor

NSU neurosurgical unit
nonspecific urethritis

NSurg neurosurgeon; also neurosurg, NS
neurosurgery; also neurosurg, NS

NSV nonspecific vaginitis

NSVD normal spontaneous vaginal delivery

NSVT non-sustained ventricular tachycardia

NSX neurosurgical examination

NSY nursery

NT nasotracheal
neotetrazolium
neurotensin
neutralization technique
neutralization test
neutralizing
nicotine tartrate
nodal tachycardia
non-tumorous
non-typeable
normal temperature
normal tissue
normotensive
nortriptyline; also NOR
no test
not tender
not tested
nourishment taken
nucleotidase

N&T nose and throat; also N+T

N+T nose and throat; also N&T

5'-NT 5'-nucleotidase; also NTD

Nt amino terminal

nt night; also n

NTA National Tuberculosis Association (now: ALA, American Lung Association)
natural thymocytotoxic autoantibody
nitrilotriacetic acid
Nurse Training Act

NTAB nephrotoxic antibody

N/TBC non-tuberculous

NTBR not to be resuscitated

NTC neurotrauma center

NTD neural tube defect
nitroblue tetrazolium dye
noise tone difference
5'-nucleotidase; also 5'-NT

NTE neurotoxic esterase
non-test ear
not to exceed
nuclear track emulsion

NTF normal throat flora

NTG nitroglycerin; also NG, Nitro, NTZ
nontoxic goiter
non-treatment group
normal triglyceridemia
normal triglyceridemic (subject)

NTGO nitroglycerin ointment

NTHH non-tumorous hypergastrinemic hyperchlorhydria

NTI non-thyroid illness
non-thyroid index
no treatment indicated

NTIS National Technical Information Service

NTLI neurotensin-like immunoreactivity

NTM Neuman-Tytell medium
nocturnal tumescence monitor
non-tuberculous mycobacteria; also NTMB

NTMB non-tuberculous mycobacteria; also NTM

NTMI non-transmural myocardial infarction

NTMNG nontoxic multinodular goiter

NTN nephrotoxic nephritis

NTND not tender, not distended (abdomen)

NTP National Toxicology Program
nitropaste
normal temperature and pressure
nucleoside triphosphatase
nucleoside 5'-triphosphate
sodium nitroprusside

NTR negative therapeutic reaction
normotensive rat; also NR
nutrition

NTRS National Therapeutic Recreation Society

NTS nasotracheal suction
nephrotoxic serum
non-turning against self (psychology)
nucleus tractus solitarii

NTT nasotracheal tube

NTV nervous tissue vaccine

NTX naltrexone

NTZ nitroglycerin; also NG, Nitro, NTG
normal transformation zone (colposcopy)

NU name unknown

Nu nucleolus
nucleus; also N

nU nanounit; also nu

nu nanounit; also nU
neurilemma; also neu
nude (mouse)

NUC nuclear; also nucl
nuclear medicine; also NM
sodium urate crystal [L. *natrium* (sodium)]

Nuc nucleoside; also N

nuc nucleated

nucl nuclear; also NUC

NUD non-ulcer dyspepsia

NUG necrotizing ulcerative gingivitis

NUI number user identification

nullip nulliparous

num numerator

numc number concentration

numfr number fraction

NUN non-urea nitrogen

nunc now [L. *nunc*]

Nur nitrosourea

NURB Neville upper reservoir buffer

NUV near-ultraviolet

NV naked vision; also Nv
nausea and vomiting; also N/V, N&V, N,V
near vision
negative variation
neurovascular
new vessel
next visit
non-vegetarian
non-veteran
normal value
normal volunteer
norverapamil
not vaccinated
not venereal
not verified
not volatile

N/V nausea and vomiting; also NV, N&V, N,V

N&V nausea and vomiting; also NV, N/V, N,V

N,V nausea and vomiting; also NV, N/V, N&V

Nv naked vision; also NV

nv nonvolatile

NVA near visual acuity
normal visual acuity

NVAF non-valvular atrial fibrillation

Nval norvaline

NVB neurovascular bundle

NVC non-valved conduit

NVD nausea, vomiting, and diarrhea
neck vein distention
neovascularization of optic disc
neurovesicle dysfunction
Newcastle virus disease
non-valvular heart disease
no venereal disease
no venous distention
number of vessels diseased

NVE neovascularization elsewhere
new vessels elsewhere

NVF nasal visual field

NVG neovascular glaucoma
neoviridogrisein
non-ventilated group

NVL neurovascular laboratory

NVM nonvolatile matter

NVS neurologic vital signs
non-vaccine serotype

NVSS normal variant short stature

NVWSC nonvolatile whole-smoke condensate

NW naked weight
nasal wash
non-withdrawn
Norman-Wood (disease)
not weighed

NWB non-weight-bearing
no weight bearing

NWC number of words chosen

NWD neuroleptic withdrawal

NWDL nodular well-differentiated lympho-cytic lymphoma

NWF new working formulation

NWm nitrogen washout, multiple (breath)

NWR normotensive Wistar rat

NWs nitrogen washout, single (breath)

NWSN Nocardia water-soluble nitrogen

NWTSG National Wilms' Tumor Study Group

NX, Nx naloxone; also NLX
nephrectomy; also nep

NY nystatin

NYC New York City (medium)

NYD not yet diagnosed
not yet discovered

NYHA New York Heart Association (classification)

NYP not yet published

nyst nystagmus

NZ non-ischemic
normal zone

NZB New Zealand black (mouse)
New Zealand bred (mice)

NZO New Zealand obese (mouse)

NZR New Zealand red (rabbit)

NZW New Zealand white (mouse)

O

Ω OMEGA, UPPER CASE, twenty-fourth and last letter of the Greek alphabet
ohm

ω omega, lower case, twenty-fourth and last letter of the Greek alphabet
angular frequency
angular velocity
carbon atom farthest from principal functioning group

Z omega, lower case, twenty-fourth and last letter of the Greek alphabet, variant

O OMICRON, UPPER CASE, fifteenth letter of the Greek alphabet

o omicron, lower case, fifteenth letter of the Greek alphabet

O absence of sex chromosome
blood type in ABO blood group system
degree of
electrical reaction (in formulas)
eye [L. *oculus*]
negative; also $\emptyset$, ō
nil; also $\emptyset$
no; also $\emptyset$
none; also $\emptyset$, ō
nonmotile microorganisms and their somatic antigens, antibodies, and agglutinative reactions [Ger. *ohne Hauch* (without breath)]; also *O*
no special preparation necessary (for test)
obese; also OB, ob
objective (findings); also Obj, obj
observation; also OBS, Obs
observed; also OBS, Obs, obs, obsd
obstetrics; also OB, OBS, Obs, obs, Obst, obst, obstet
obvious
occipital; also Occ, occ, occip
occiput; also Occ, occ, occip
occlusal
office
often
old
open; also o
opening; also o, opg
operator; also OP, op
operon (genetics)
opium
oral; also (O)
orally; also (O)
orange (indicator color)
orbit

orderly; also ord
Oriental
orotidine; also Ord
orthopedic; also OR, Orth, ortho
osteocyte
other; also OTH
output
oxidative
oxygen; also O2, O_2, Ox, OXY, oxy
pint [L. *octarius*]; also Ō, oct, P, p, PT, pt
respirations (on anesthesia chart)
suture size (zero)
vincristine (Oncovin)
without; also $\emptyset$, ō, s̄

O denoting attachment to oxygen
nonmotile microorganisms and their somatic antigens, antibodies, and agglutinative reactions [Ger. *ohne Hauch* (without breath)]; also O
observed frequency in a contingency table

$\emptyset$ negative; also O, ō
nil; also O
no; also O
none; also O, ō
without; also O, ō, s̄

Ō pint [L. *octarius*]; also O, oct, P, p, PT, pt

(O) oral; also O
orally; also O

O2, O_2 both eyes [L. *oculus* (eye)]
oxygen (symbol for the diatomic gas); also O, Ox, OXY, oxy

O_3 ozone

o open; also O
opening; also O, opg
ovary transplant

ō negative; also O, $\emptyset$
none; also O, $\emptyset$
without; also O, $\emptyset$, s̄

o-, *o*- ortho- (chemical symbol)

OA object assembly (psychology)
obstructive apnea
occipital artery
occipito-anterior (fetal position)
occipito-atlantal
ocular albinism
old age
oleic acid
opiate analgesia
opsonic activity
optic atrophy

oral airway; also OAW
oral alimentation
orotic acid; also ORO, Oro
orthopedic assistant
osteoarthritis; also osteo
ovalbumin; also OVA, OV
overall assessment
oxalic acid
oxolinic acid

O-A Objective-Analytic (Anxiety Battery)

O&A observation and assessment
odontectomy and alveoloplasty

O₂a oxygen availability

OA1 ocular albinism type 1

OA2 ocular albinism type 2

OAA Old Age Assistance
Opticians Association of America
oxaloacetate
oxaloacetic acid

OAAD ovarian ascorbic acid depletion (test)

OAB old age benefits

OABP organic anion-binding protein

OAC oral anticoagulant
overaction

OAD obstructive airway disease
occlusive arterial disease
organic anionic dye

OADC oleic acid, albumin, dextrose, and
catalase (medium)

OADMT Oliphant Auditory Discrimination
Memory Test

OAE otacoustic emission

OAF open air factor
osteoclast-activating factor

OAG open-angle glaucoma

OAH ovarian androgenic hyperfunction

OAJ open apophyseal joint

OALF organic acid-labile fluoride

OALL ossification of anterior longitudinal
ligament

o alt hor every other hour [L. *omnibus
alternis horis*]

OAM outer acrosomal membrane
oxyacetate malonate

OAP old age pension
old age pensioner
Oncovin, Ara-C, and prednisone
ophthalmic artery pressure
osteoarthropathy
oxygen at atmospheric pressure

OAPs Occupational Ability Patterns (psychologic test)

OAR orientation/alertness remediation
other administrative reasons

OARSA oxacillin aminoglycoside-resistant
Staphylococcus aureus

OAS old age security
osmotically active substance

OASDHI Old Age, Survivors, Disability, and
Health Insurance

OASDI Old Age, Survivors, and Disability
Insurance

OASI Old Age and Survivors Insurance

OASO overactive superior oblique

OASP organic acid-soluble phosphorus

OASR overactive superior rectus

OAST Oliphant Auditory Synthesizing Test

OAT ornithine aminotransferase
oxoacid aminotransferase

OAV oculoauriculovertebral (dysplasia,
syndrome)

OAW oral airway; also OA

OAWO opening abductory wedge osteotomy

OB he/she died [L. *obiit*]; also ob
obese; also O, ob
objective benefit
obstetrician; also OBS, Obs, Obst, obst
obstetrics; also O, OBS, Obs, obs, Obst,
obst, obstet
occult bleeding
occult blood
olfactory bulb; also OLB

OB+ occult blood positive

O&B opium and belladonna

ob he/she died [L. *obiit*]; also OB
obese; also O, OB

OBB own bed bath

OBD organic brain disease

OBE out-of-body experience

OBF organ blood flow

OBG, ObG obstetrician-gynecologist; also
OB/GYN, OB-GYN, ObGyn, OG, O&G
obstetrics and gynecology; also OB/GYN,
OB-GYN, ObGyn, OG, O&G

OBGS obstetric and gynecologic surgery

OB-GYN, OB/GYN, ObGyn obstetrician-
gynecologist; also OBG, ObG, OG, O&G
obstetrics and gynecology; also OBG, ObG,
OG, O&G

Obj objective; also O, obj

obj object
objective; also O, Obj

obl oblique

OBP odorant-binding protein
ova, blood and parasites (stool exam)

OBRA Omnibus Budget Reconciliation
Act (of 1989)

OBRR obstetric recovery room

OBS observation; also O, Obs
observed; also O, Obs, obs, obsd
obstetrical service
obstetrician; also OB, Obs, Obst, obst
obstetrics; also O, OB, Obs, obs, Obst, obst,
obstet
organic brain syndrome

Obs observation; also O, OBS
observed; also O, OBS, obs, obsd
obsolete; also obs
obstetrician; also OB, OBS, Obst, obst
obstetrics; also O, OB, OBS, obs, Obst, obst,
obstet

obs observed; also O, OBS, Obs, obsd
obsolete; also Obs
obstetrics; also O, OB, OBS, Obs, Obst, obst,
obstet

obsd observed; also O, OBS, Obs, obs

Obst obstetrician; also OB, OBS, Obs, obst
obstetrics; also O, OB, OBS, Obs, obs, obst,
obstet

obst obstetrician; also OB, OBS, Obs, Obst
obstetrics; also O, OB, OBS, Obs, obs, Obst,
obstet
obstipation
obstructed
obstruction

obstet obstetrics; also O, OB, OBS, Obs, obs,
Obst, obst

obt obtained

OB-US obstetrical ultrasound

OBzL benzyl ester

OC obstetrical conjugate
occlusocervical
office call
on call
only child
optic chiasma; also OX
oral care
oral cavity
oral contraceptive
organ culture

original claim
osteochondritis
outer canthal (distance)
ovarian cancer
oxygen consumed

O&C onset and course (of disease);
lso O+C

O+C onset and course (of disease); also O&C

Oc ochre (suppressor)
octyl

OC-6 octahedral

OCA oculocutaneous albinism
olivopontocerebellar atrophy; also OPCA
open care area
operant conditioning audiometry
oral contraceptive agent

OCAD occlusive carotid artery disease

O₂ cap oxygen capacity

OCBF outer cortical blood flow

Occ occasional; also occ, occas
occipital; also O, occ, occip
occiput; also O, occ, occip
occlusion; also occl
occlusive; also occl

occ occasional; also Occ, occas
occasionally; also occas
occipital; also O, Occ, occip
occiput; also O, Occ, occip
occupation; also occup
occupational; also occup
occurrence

occas occasional; also Occ, occ
occasionally; also occ

OCCC open-chest cardiac compression

occip occipital; also O, Occ, occ
occiput; also O, Occ, occ

occip F occipitofrontal; also OF

occip-F HA occipitofrontal headache;
also O-FHA, OF-HA

occl occlusion; also Occ
occlusive; also Occ

OCCPR open-chest cardiopulmonary resuscitation

OccTh occupational therapist; also Occup
Rx, OT
occupational therapy; also Occup Rx, OT

occup occupation; also occ
occupational; also occ
occupies
occupying

Occup Rx occupational therapist; also
    OccTh, OT
    occupational therapy; also OccTh, OT

OCD obsessive-compulsive disorder
    Office of Child Development
    Office of Civil Defense
    osteochondritis dissecans
    ovarian cholesterol depletion (test)

OCF-7 octahedral-faced monocapped

OCG omnicardiogram
    oral cholangiogram
    oral cholecystogram

OCH oral contraceptive hormone

OCHS Office of Cooperative Health Statistics

OCIS Oncology Center Information System

OCL Occupational Check List (psychologic
    test)
    oral colonic lavage

OCM oral contraceptive medication

OCN oculomotor nucleus; also OMN
    Oncology Certified Nurse

OCP octacalcium phosphate
    oral contraceptive pill
    ova, cysts, and parasites (stool exam)

OCR ocular counterrolling
    ocular countertorsion reflex
    oculocardiac reflex
    oculocerebrorenal
    optical character recognition

oCRF ovine corticotropin-releasing factor

OCRS oculocerebrorenal syndrome

OCS open canalicular system (of platelets)
    oral contraceptive steroid
    outpatient clinic substation
    oxycorticosteroid

OCT Object Classification Test
    optimal cutting temperature (medium)
    oral contraceptive therapy
    ornithine carbamyltransferase
    oxytocin challenge test

O₂CT oxygen content
O$_2$CT oxygen content

oct pint [L. *octarius*]; also O, Ō, P, p, PT, pt

OCT-8 octahedral transbicapped

OCTD ornithine carbamoyltransferase defi-
    ciency

octup eightfold [L. *octuplus*]

OCU observation care unit

OCV ordinary conversational voice

OCVM occult vascular malformation

OD Doctor of Optometry
    in the right eye [L. *oculo dextro*]
    occipital dysplasia
    occupational dermatitis
    occupational disease
    ocular dominance
    once daily
    on duty
    open drop (anesthesia)
    open duct
    optical density
    optic disk
    optimal dose
    organization development
    originally derived
    outdoor
    out-of-date
    outside diameter
    overdose (drug)
    right eye [L. *oculus dexter*]

O-D obstacle-dominance
    original-derived

od every day, daily [L. *omni die*]

ODA osmotic driving agent
    right occipito-anterior (fetal position)
    [L. *occipitodextra anterior*]

ODAC on-demand analgesia computer

ODAP Oncovin, dianhydrogalactitol,
    Adriamycin, and Platinol

ODAT one day at a time

ODB opiate-directed behavior

ODC oligodendrocyte; also OG, OLG
    ornithine decarboxylase
    orotidine 5-phosphate decarboxylase
    orotidylate decarboxylase (deficiency)
    outpatient diagnostic center
    oxygen dissociation curve

ODCH ordinary diseases of childhood

ODD oculodentodigital (dysplasia, syndrome)

OD'd overdosed (drug)

ODE *o*-desmethylencainide

ODGF osteosarcoma-derived growth factor

ODM, ODm ophthalmodynamometer
    ophthalmodynamometry

ODOD oculodento-osseous dysplasia

Odont odontology

odont odontogenic

odoram perfume [L. *odoramentum*]

odorat odorous, smelling, perfuming
    [L. *odoratus*]

ODP offspring of diabetic parents
right occipitoposterior (fetal position) [L. *occipitodextra posterior*]

ODQ on direct questioning
opponens digiti quinti (muscle)

ODSG ophthalmic Doppler sonogram

ODT oculodynamic test
right occipitotransverse (fetal position) [L. *occipitodextra transversa*]

ODTS organic dust toxic syndrome

ODU optical density unit

OE on examination; also O/E
orthopedic examination; also OX
otitis externa

O/E observed to expected (ratio)
on examination; also OE

O&E observation and examination

Oe oersted (centimeter-gram-second unit of magnetic field strength)

OeAB Austrian Pharmacopeia [Ger. *Oesterreichisches Arzneibuch*]

OEC outer ear canal
oxygen equilibrium curve

OEE osmotic erythrocyte enrichment
outer enamel epithelium

OEF oil emersion field
oxygen extraction fraction

OEM open-end marriage
opposite ear masked
original equipment manufacturer (computers)

OEMO one-electron molecular orbital (theory)

OER osmotic erythrocyte (enrichment)
oxygen enhancement ratio

O₂ER oxygen extraction ratio

OES optical emission spectroscopy
oral esophageal stethoscope

oesoph (o)esophagus; also E, ES, ESO, esoph

OESP orthopedic examination, special

OET oral endotracheal tube; also OETT
oral esophageal tube

OETT oral endotracheal tube; also OET

OF occipitofrontal; also occip F
optic fundi
orbitofrontal
osmotic fragility (test)
osteitis fibrosa
Ostrum-Furst (syndrome)
other medical/surgical facility
Ovenstone factor

oxidation-fermentation (medium); also O-F, O/F

O-F oxidation-fermentation (medium); also OF, O/F

O/F oxidation-fermentation (medium); also OF, O-F

Of official; also Off, off

OFA oncofetal antigen

OFAGE orthogonal-field-alternation gel electrophoresis

OFBM oxidation-fermentation basal medium

OFC occipitofrontal circumference
orbitofacial cleft
osteitis fibrosa cystica

ofc office; also off

OFD object-film distance (radiology); also ofd
occipitofrontal diameter
oral-facial-digital (dysostosis, syndrome)
orofaciodigital (dysostosis, syndrome)

ofd object-film distance (radiology); also OFD

OFE osteogenic factor extract

Off official; also Of, off

off office; also ofc
official; also Of, Off

O-FHA, OF-HA occipitofrontal headache; also occip-F HA

OFM orofacial malformation

OFPF optic fundi and peripheral fields

OF rad occipitofrontal radiation

OFTT organic failure to thrive

OG obstetrics and gynecology; also OBG, ObG, OB/GYN, OB-GYN, ObGyn, O&G
obstetrician-gynecologist; also OBG, ObG, OB/GYN, OB-GYN, ObGyn, O&G
occlusogingival
octyl glucoside
oligodendrocyte; also ODC, OLG
optic ganglion
orange green (stain)
orogastric (feeding)

O&G obstetrician-gynecologist; also OBG, ObG, OB/GYN, OB-GYN, ObGyn, OG
obstetrics and gynecology; also OBG, ObG, OB/GYN, OB-GYN, ObGyn, OG

OGA orogastric gonococcal aspirate

OGD old granulomatous disease

OGF ovarian growth factor
oxygen gain factor

OGH ovine growth hormone

OGM outgrowth medium

OGS oxygenic steroid

OGT oral glucose tolerance

OGTT oral glucose tolerance test

OGU orogenital ulceration

OGYE oxytetracycline-glucose-yeast extract (agar)

OH hydroxycorticosteroids; also HCS, OHCS
hydroxyl group
hydroxyl radical
obstructive hypopnea
occipital horn
occupational health
occupational history
on hand
open-heart (surgery)
oral hygiene
orthostatic hypotension
osteopathic hospital
out of hospital
outpatient hospital

oh every hour [L. *omni hora*]; also omn hor

OHA oral hypoglycemic agent

OHB$_{12}$ hydroxocobalamin (vitamin B$_{12}$); also OH-Cbl

O$_2$Hb oxyhemoglobin

OHC hydroxycholecalciferol (the synthetic analog of calcitriol, the hormonal form of Vitamin D$_3$); also OHD
occupational health center
outer hair cell

OH-Cbl hydroxocobalamin (vitamin B$_{12}$); also OHB$_{12}$

OHCS hydroxycorticosteroids; also HCS, OH

17-OHCS 17-hydroxycorticosteroid

OHD hydroxycholecalciferol (the synthetic analog of calcitriol, the hormonal form of Vitamin D$_3$); also OHC
organic heart disease

OHDA hydroxydopamine; also HD, HDA

OH-DOC hydroxydesoxycorticosterone

OHF Omsk hemorrhagic fever
overhead frame

OHFA hydroxy fatty acid

OHFT overhead frame trapeze

OHG oral hypoglycemic

OHI ocular hypertension indicator
Oral Hygiene Index

OHIAA, OH-IAA hydroxyindoleacetic acid; also HIAA

OHI-S Oral Hygiene Index–Simplified

OHL oral hairy leukoplakia

ohm-cm ohm-centimeter

OHN Occupational Health Nurse

OHP hydroxyproline
orthogonal-hole test pattern
oxygen under high pressure

17-OHP 17-hydroxyprogesterone

OHRR open heart recovery room

OHS obesity hypoventilation syndrome
ocular hypoperfusion syndrome
open-heart surgery
ovarian hyperstimulation syndrome; also OHSS
Overcontrolled Hostility Scale

OHSS ovarian hyperstimulation syndrome; also OHS

OHT Occupational Health Technician
ocular hypertensive (glaucoma suspect)

OHU hydroxyurea; also OH-urea

OH-urea hydroxyurea; also OHU

OI objective improvement
obturator internus
occipito-iliacus
opportunistic infection
opsonic index
orgasmic impairment
Orientation Inventory (psychologic test)
ortho-iodohippurate; also OIH, OIHA
osteogenesis imperfecta
otitis interna
ouabain insensitive
oxygen income
oxygen intake

O-I outer-to-inner

OIC osteogenesis imperfecta congenita

OID optimal immunomodulating dose
organism identification (number)

OIF observed intrinsic frequency
oil immersion field

OIH ortho-iodohippurate; also OI, OIHA
ovulation-inducing hormone

OIHA ortho-iodohippurate; OI, OIH
ortho-iodohippuric acid

OIHP International Office of Public Hygiene [Fr. *Office Internationale d'Hygiene Publique*]

oint ointment

OIP organizing interstitial pneumonia

OIT Tien organic integrity test (psychiatry)

OJ, oj orange juice; also OrJ

OK, ok all right
approved
correct
optokinetic; also OPK

OKAN optokinetic after nystagmus

OKN optokinetic nystagmus

OKT Ollier-Klippel-Trenaunay (syndrome)
ornithine-ketoacid transaminase
Ortho-Kung T (cell)

OL left eye [L. *oculus laevus*]; also OS
other locations

Ol, ol oil [L. *oleum*]

OLA left occipito-anterior (fetal position)
[L. *occipitolaeva anterior*]

OLB olfactory bulb; also OB
open-liver biopsy

OLD obstructive lung disease

OLG oligodendrocyte; also ODC, OG

OLH ovine lactogenic hormone
ovine luteinizing hormone; also oLH

oLH ovine luteinizing hormone; also OLH

OLIB osmiophilic lamellar inclusion body

OLIDS open-loop insulin delivery system

OLMAT Otis-Lennon Mental Ability Test

ol oliv olive oil [L. *oleum olivae*]

OLP left occipitoposterior (fetal position) [L.
occipitolaeva posterior]

OLR otology, laryngology, and rhinology

ol res oleoresin

OLSIST Oral Language Sentence Imitation
Screening Test

OLT left occipitotransverse (fetal position) [L.
occipitolaeva transversa]
orthotopic liver transplantation; also Olt

Olt orthotopic liver transplantation; also OLT

OM obtuse marginal (coronary artery)
occipitomental
occupational medicine
oculomotor
Osborn-Mendel (rat)
osteomalacia
osteomyelitis; also osteo
osteopathic manipulation
otitis media
outer membrane
ovulation method (birth control)

om every morning [L. *omni mane*]; also
omn man

OMAC otitis media, acute, catarrhal

OMAD Oncovin, methotrexate, Adriamycin,
and dactinomycin

OMAS occupational maladjustment syndrome
otitis media, acute, suppurating

OMB Office of Management and Budget

OMC open mitral commissurotomy
osteo-meatal complex

OMCA otitis media, catarrhal, acute

OMCC otitis media, catarrhal, chronic; also
OMCCH

OMCCH otitis media, catarrhal, chronic;
also OMCC

OMChS otitis media, chronic, suppurating

OMD ocular muscle dystrophy
oculomandibulodyscephaly
organic mental disorder

OME Office of Medical Examiner
otitis media with effusion

3-OMG 3-*ortho*-methylglucose

om 1/4 h every quarter hour (every 15 minutes)
[L. *omni quadrante horae*]; also
om quad hor, omn quad hor

OMI old myocardial infarction

OMIM On-Line Mendelian Inheritance in Man

OML orbitomeatal line

OMM ophthalmomandibulomelic (dysplasia,
syndrome)
outer mitochondrial membrane

om mane vel noc every morning or night [L.
omni mane vel nocte]

OMN oculomotor nerve
oculomotor nucleus; also OCN

omn bid every two days [L. *omni biduo*]

omn bih every two hours [L. *omni bihora*]

omn hor every hour [L. *omni hora*]; also oh

omn 2 hor every second hour [L. *omni secunda
hora*]; also omn sec hor

omn man every morning [L. *omni mane*]; also
om

omn noct every night [L. *omni nocte*]; also
ON, on

omn quad hor every quarter hour (every 15
minutes) [L. *omni quadrante horae*];
also om 1/4 h, om quad hor

omn sec hor every second hour [L. *omni
secunda hora*]; also omn 2 hor

OMP olfactory marker protein
orotidylate

orotidylic acid
ortho-*N*-methylmorpholiniumpropylene
outer membrane protein

OMPA octamethyl pyrophosphoramide
otitis media, purulent, acute

OMPC otitis media, purulent, chronic;
also OMPCh
outer membrane protein complex

OMPCh otitis media, purulent, chronic;
also OMPC

om quad hor every quarter hour (every 15
minutes) [L. *omni quadrante horae*];
also om 1/4 h, omn quad hor

OMR operative mortality rate

OMS offshore medical school
organic mental syndrome
otomandibular syndrome

OM&S Osteopathic Medicine and Surgery

OMSA otitis media, suppurative, acute

OMSC otitis media, secretory, chronic; also
OMSCh
otitis media, suppurative, chronic;
also OMSCh

OMSCh otitis media, secretory, chronic;
also OMSC
otitis media, suppurative, chronic;
also OMSC

OMT, OM/T osteopathic manipulation
treatment

OMVC open mitral valve commissurotomy

OMVI operating motor vehicle while intoxicated

ON every night [L. *omni nocte*]; also omn
noct, on
occipitonuchal
office nurse
onlay
optic nerve
optic neuritis
optic neuropathy
oronasal
orthopedic nurse; also ORN
osteonecrosis
overnight

on every night [L. *omni nocte*]; also omn
noct, ON

ONC oncology; also onco, oncol
Oncology Nurse, Certified
Orthopedic Nursing Certificate
over-the-needle catheter

ONCG-A oncogenic virus battery–acute

onco oncology; also ONC, oncol

oncol oncology; also ONC, onco

ONCORNA oncogene ribonucleic acid

OND orbitonasal dislocation
other neurologic disease
other neurologic disorder

ONDS Oriental nocturnal death syndrome

ONH optic nerve head
optic nerve hypoplasia

ONP operating nursing procedure
ortho-nitrophenyl

ONPG *ortho*-nitro-phenyl-beta-galacto-
pyranoside
ortho-nitro-phenyl-beta-galactosidase;
also ONP-GAL
ortho-nitro-phenyl-beta-galactoside

ONP-GAL *ortho*-nitro-phenyl-beta-galacto-
sidase; also ONPG

ONA Oncology Nurses Association

ONTG oral nitroglycerin

ONTR orders not to resuscitate

OO oophorectomy
oral order(s)

O-O outer-to-outer

O&O off and on

o/o on account of

OOA outer optic anlage

OOB out of bed
out-of-body (experience)

OOBBRP out of bed with bathroom privileges

OOC onset of contractions
out of cast
out of control

OOD out of doors

OOH&NS ophthalmology, otorhinolaryngology, and head and neck surgery

OOL onset of labor

OOLR ophthalmology, otology, laryngology,
and rhinology

OOP out of pelvis
out of plaster (cast)
out on pass

OOR out of room

OOS out of stock; also OS

OOT out of town

OOW out of wedlock; also OW

OP oblique presentation
occipitoparietal
occipitoposterior

OP—cont'd
 occiput posterior
 old patient (previously seen)
 olfactory peduncle
 opening pressure
 operation; also op
 operational; also op
 operative; also op
 operative procedure
 operator; also O, op
 ophthalmology; also OPH, Oph, oph, Ophth, ophth
 opponens pollicis
 original package
 oropharynx
 orthostatic proteinuria
 oscillatory potential
 osmotic pressure
 osteoporosis
 other than psychotic
 outpatient; also O/P, OPT
 overproof
 ovine prolactin

O/P outpatient; also OP, OPT

O&P ova and parasites (stool exam)

Op opisthocranion

op operation; also OP
 operational; also OP
 operative; also OP
 operator; also O, OP
 opposite; also opp
 work [L. *opus*]

OPA oral pharyngeal airway
 outpatient anesthesia

OPAL Oncovin, prednisone, and L-asparaginase

OPB outpatient basis

OPC Outpatient Clinic

OPCA olivopontocerebellar atrophy; also OCA

op cit in the work cited [L. *opere citato*]

OPD obstetric prediabetes
 optical path difference
 original pack dispensing
 otopalatodigital (syndrome)
 Outpatient Department
 outpatient dispensary

o, p′-**DDD** 2,4′-dichlorodiphenyldichloroethane (mitotane)

OpDent operative dentistry

OPDG ocular plethysmodynamography

OPE outpatient evaluation

OPG ocular plethysmography

ocular pressure gradient
oculoplethysmograph
oculopneumoplethysmography; also OPPG
ophthalmoplethysmograph
oxypolygelatin (plasma volume extender)

opg opening; also O, o

OPG/CPA oculoplethysmography/carotid phonoangiography

OPH, Oph obliterative pulmonary hypotension
ophthalmia
ophthalmologist; also Ophth
ophthalmology; also OP, oph, Ophth, ophth
ophthalmoscope; also Ophth
ophthalmoscopy; also Ophth

oph ophthalmic
ophthalmologic
ophthalmology; also OP, OPH, Oph, Ophth, ophth

OphD Doctor of Ophthalmology

Ophth ophthalmologist; also OPH, Oph
ophthalmology; also OP, OPH, Oph, oph, ophth
ophthalmoscope; also OPH, Oph
ophthalmoscopy; also OPH, Oph

ophth ophthalmology; also OP, OPH, Oph, oph, Ophth

OPI oculoparalytic illusion
Omnibus Personality Inventory

OPK optokinetic; also OK, ok

OPL osmotic pressure of proteins in lymph
outer plexiform layer
ovine placental lactogen

OPLL ossification of posterior longitudinal ligament

OPM occult primary malignancy
ophthalmoplegic migraine

OPN ophthalmic nurse

OPP Oncovin, procarbazine, and prednisone
osmotic pressure of plasma
ovine pancreatic polypeptide
oxygen partial pressure

opp opposing
opposite; also op

OPPES oil-associated pneumoparalytic eosinophilic syndrome

OPPG oculopneumoplethysmography; also OPG

op reg operative region

oprg operating

OPRT orotate phosphoribosyltransferase

OPS operations
Outpatient Service
outpatient surgery

OPSA ovarian papillary serous cystadeno-
carcinoma

OpScan optical scanning

OPSI overwhelming postsplenectomy infection

OPSR Office of Professional Standards Review

OPSR-BQA Office of Professional Standards
Review–Bureau of Quality Assurance

OPT optimum; also opt
ortho-phthaladehyde
outpatient; also OP, O/P
outpatient treatment

Opt optometrist

opt best [L. *optimus*]
optical
optician
optics
optimal
optimum; also OPT
optional

OPT c̄ CA Ohio pediatric tent with compressed
air

OPT c̄ O₂ Ohio pediatric tent with oxygen

OPV oral attenuated poliovirus vaccine
oral poliovaccine
out-patient visit

OPW opiate withdrawal; also OPWL

OPWL opiate withdrawal; also OPW

OQSMAT Otis Quick Scoring Mental Abilities
Test

OR odds ratio
(o)estrogen receptor
oil-retention (enema)
open reduction
operating room
optic radiation
oral rehydration
organ recovery
orienting reflex
orienting response
orthopedic; also O, Orth, ortho
orthopedic research
own recognizance
oxidized-reduced

O-R, o/r oxidation-reduction

Or outflow rate

ORA occiput right anterior (fetal position)
opiate receptor antagonist

ORAN orthopedic resident admitting note

ORBC ox red blood cell

ORC order/results communication
ox red cell

ORCH orchiectomy

orch orchitis

ORD optical rotatory dispersion
oral radiation death

Ord orotidine; also O

ord orderly; also O
ordinate

OREF open reduction and external fixation
Orthopedic Research and Education
Foundation

OR en oil-retention enema

ORF open reading frame

OR&F open reduction and fixation

org organ
organic
organism

ORIF open reduction with internal fixation

orig origin
original

OrJ orange juice; also OJ, oj

ORL, orl otorhinolaryngology

ORN operating room nurse
ornithine; also Orn
orthopedic nurse; also ON

Orn ornithine; also ORN

ORO oil red O
orotate; also Oro
orotic acid; also OA, Oro

Oro orotate; also ORO
orotic acid; also OA, ORO

OROS oral osmotic

ORP occiput right posterior (fetal position)
oxidation-reduction potential

ORPM orthorhythmic pacemaker

ORS olfactory reference syndrome
oral rehydration salt
oral rehydration solution
oral surgeon
oral surgery; also OS
Orthopedic Research Society
orthopedic surgeon; also OS
orthopedic surgery; also OS

ORT objects relations techniques
operating room technician; also OR tech
oral rehydration therapy

OR tech operating room technician; also ORT

Orth orthopedic; also O, OR, ortho
orthopedics; also ortho
ORTHO American Orthopsychiatric
Association
ortho orthopedic; also O, OR, Orth
orthopedics; also Orth
orthot orthotonus
ORx oriented
OR x1 oriented to time
OR x2 oriented to time and place
OR x3 oriented to time, place, and person
OS left eye [L. *oculus sinister*]; also OL
in the left eye [L. *oculo sinistro*]
occipitosacral (fetal position)
occupational safety
opening snap (heart sound)
operating suite
oral surgery; also ORS
orthopedic surgeon; also ORS
orthopedic surgery; also ORS
Osgood-Schlatter (disease)
osteogenic sarcoma
osteoid surface
osteosarcoma
osteosclerosis
ouabain sensitive
out of stock; also OOS
overall survival
oxygen saturation; also O_2 sat, SaO_2, SO_2
Os osmium
os bone [L. *ossa*]
mouth [L. *os*]
OSA obstructive sleep apnea
Optical Society of America
OSAS obstructive sleep apnea syndrome
OSAT optimized sustained action technology
O_2 sat oxygen saturation; also OS, SaO_2, SO_2
OSBCL Ottawa School Behavior Check List
osc oscillate
OSCE objective structural clinical examination
OSCJ original squamocolumnar junction
OSD outside doctor
overside drainage
OSE ovarian surface epithelium
Ose glucose
OSF outer spiral fibers (of cochlea)
overgrowth-stimulating factor
OSFT outstretched fingertips
OSH Office on Smoking and Health

OSHA Occupational Safety and Health
Administration
OSIQ Offer Self-Image Questionnaire (for
Adolescents)
OSL Osgood-Schlatter lesion
OSM osmolarity
ovine submaxillary mucin
oxygen saturation meter
OsM osmolar; also osM
Osm osmole; also osmol
osM osmolar; also OsM
osm osmosis
osmotic
OSMF oral submucous fibrosis
Osm/kg osmoles per kilogram (osmolality)
Osm/L, Osm/l osmoles per liter (osmolarity)
osmol osmole; also Osm
OSM S osmolarity serum
OSM U osmolarity urine
OSN off-service note
OSRD Office of Scientific Research and
Development
OSS Object Sorting Scales (psychologic test)
osseous
over-shoulder strap
OS-SPT osmolarity urine spot (test)
OST object-sorting test
Ost osteotomy
Osteo osteopathologist; also osteopath
osteopathy
osteo osteoarthritis; also OA
osteomyelitis; also OM
osteopathology
osteocart osteocartilaginous
osteopath osteopathologist; also Osteo
OSUK Ophthalmological Society of the United
Kingdom
OT objective test
oblique talus
occiput transverse
occlusion time
occupational therapist; also OccTh, Occup Rx
occupational therapy; also OccTh, Occup Rx
ocular tension
Oestreicher-Turner (syndrome)
office treatment
old term (anatomy)
old terminology (anatomy)
old tuberculin (Koch's)

olfactory threshold
olfactory tubercle; also OTU
optic tract
orientation test
original tuberculin
orotracheal (tube)
orthopedic treatment
otolaryngology; also Ot, OTO, Oto, Otolar
otologist; also OTO, Oto, Otol
otology; also OTO, Oto, oto, Otol
oxytocin; also OX, OXT, OXY, oxy

O/T oral temperature

Ot otolaryngology; also OT, OTO, Oto, Otolar

OTA Office of Technology Assessment
open to air
Opinions Toward Adolescents (psychologic
  test)
ornithine transaminase
ortho-toluidine arsenite

OTC ornithine transcarbamylase (deficiency)
oval target cell
over-the-counter (nonprescription drug)
oxytetracycline

OTc heart-rate-corrected OT interval

OTCD over-the-counter drug (nonprescription)

OTC Rx over-the-counter prescription

OTD oral temperature device
organ tolerance dose
out the door

OTE optically transparent electrode

OTF oral transfer factor

OTH other; also O

OTI ovomucoid trypsin inhibitor

OTM orthotoluidine manganese (sulfate)

OTO, Oto otolaryngology; also OT, Ot, Otolar
otologist; also OT, Otol
otology; also OT, oto, Otol

oto otology; also OT, OTO, Oto, Otol

Otol otologist; also OT, OTO, Oto
otology; also OT, OTO, Oto, oto

Otolar otolaryngology; also OT, Ot, OTO, Oto

OTR Occupational Therapist, Registered
Ovarian Tumor Registry

OT/RT Occupational Therapy/Recreational
Therapy

OTS occipital temporal sulcus
orotracheal suction
ortho-toluenesulphonamide

OTSG Office of the Surgeon General

OTT, OT(T) orotracheal tube

OTU olfactory tubercle; also OT
operational taxonomic unit

OU both eyes (together) [L. *oculorum unitas*]
each eye [L. *oculus uterque*]
in each eye [L. *oculo utroque*]
Observation Unit
Oppenheim-Urbach (syndrome)

OULQ outer upper left quadrant

OURQ outer upper right quadrant

OV oculovestibular
office visit
Osler-Vaquez (disease)
osteoid volume
outflow volume; also O_v
ovalbumin; also OA, OVA
overventilation
ovulating
ovulation

O₂V oxygen ventilation equivalent

Ov ovary

O$_v$ outflow volume; also OV

ov egg [L. *ovum*]
ovarian

OVA ovalbumin; also OA, OV

OVAL ovalocyte

OVD occlusal vertical dimension

OvDF ovarian dysfunction

OVDQ Organizational Value Dimensions
Questionnaire

OVIS Ohio Vocational Interest Survey

OVIT Oral Verbal Intelligence Test

OVLT organum vasculosum of the lamina
terminalis

OVX ovariectomized

OW off work
once weekly
open wedge (osteotomy)
ordinary warfare
outer wall
out of wedlock; also OOW
oval window

O/W oil in water (emulsion)
oil to water (ratio)

o/w otherwise

OWA organics-in-water analyzer

OWNK out of wedlock and not keeping child

OWR ovarian wedge resection

OWS overwear syndrome

OWVI Ohio Work Values Inventory

OX optic chiasma; also OC
orthopedic examination; also OE
oxacillin
oxymel (honey, water, and vinegar); also ox
oxytocin; also OT, OXT, OXY, oxy

Ox oxygen; also O, O2, O_2, OXY, oxy

ox oxymel (honey, water, and vinegar); also OX

OXLAT oxalate

OXEA ox erythrocyte antibody

Oxi oximeter
oximetry

OXP oxypressin

OXPHOS oxidative phosphorylation

OXT oxytocin; also OT, OX, OXY, oxy

OXY, oxy oxygen; also O, O2, O_2, Ox
oxytocin; also OT, OX, OXT

OYE old yellow enzyme

oz ounce

oz ap ounce, apothecary

oz t ounce, troy

Φ phi, UPPER CASE, twenty-first letter of the Greek alphabet

φ phi, lower case, twenty-first letter of the Greek alphabet
ability continuum
file
magnetic flux
osmotic coefficient
phi coefficient (statistics)

φ phi, lower case, twenty-first letter of the Greek alphabet, variant
none

Π PI, UPPER CASE, sixteenth letter of the Greek alphabet
product of a sequence (math)

π pi, lower case, sixteenth letter of the Greek alphabet
3.1416 (3.1415926536), ratio of the circumference of a circle to its diameter
osmotic pressure

ϖ pi, lower case, sixteenth letter of the Greek alphabet, variant

Ψ PSI, UPPER CASE, twenty-third letter of the Greek alphabet
psychiatry; also P, PS, PSY, Psy, psychiat

ψ psi, lower case, twenty-third letter of the Greek alphabet
pseudo
pseudouridine
wave function

P after [L. *post*]; also p, p̄
by weight [L. *pondere*]; also p, Pond, pond
concentration by weight (after optical rotations); also p
father [L. *pater*]; also p
form perception (in General Aptitude Test Battery)
gas partial pressure
handful [L. *pugillus*]; also p
near [L. *proximum*]; also p
near point (of accommodation) [L. *punctum proximum*]; also p, PP, pp
P (blood group system)
page; also p, pg
pain
para (parity); also p
paraffin; also PAR, par
parent
parenteral; also parent
parietal electrode placement in electroencephalography

parity
parous
part; also p, pt
partial pressure (of a gas); also p, PP
passive; also pass
Pasteurella species; also *P, Past*
paternal
paternally contributing
patient; also PAT, PNT, Pnt, PT, Pt, pt
pelvis; also Pel
penicillin; also PC, Pc, PCN, pcn, Pen, pen, PN, PNC
per
percent; also pc, pct
percentile
perceptual speed
percussion; also percus, PERCUSS
perforation; also perf
peripheral; also p, peri
permeability
peta- (10^{15})
peyote
pharmacopeia; also PH, Ph, PHAR, phar, pharm
phenacetin
phenolphthalein
phenylalanine; also F, PA, PHA, PHE, Phe
phon (unit of loudness)
phosphate; also p, Ph, phos
phosphoric residue (nucleic acid terminology)
phosphorus; also PHP, phos
physiology; also PHY, PHYS, Phys, phys, Physiol, physiol
pico- (10^{-12}); also p (the preferred symbol)
pig
pilocarpine
pin
pink (indicator color)
pint; also O,Ō, oct, p, PT, pt
placebo; also PBO, PL, PLBO
plan
plasma; also Pl
Plasmodium species; also *P*
point; also pt
poise (unit of dynamic viscosity)
poison; also pois
poisoned; also pois
poisoning; also pois
polarity
polarization
pole
polymyxin

P—cont'd

  pons; also p

  poor

  popular response

  population; also Pop

  porcelain

  porcine

  porphyrin(s); also Porph

  position; also pos

  positive; also POS, pos

  posterior; also PO, post

  postpartum

  potency

  power

  precipitin

  prednisone; also PDN, PR, PRED, pred

  premolar; also PM

  presbyopia; also PR, Pr

  pressure; also p, PR, press

  primary; also Pr, prim

  primipara; (woman bearing first child); also I-para, primip, PRIMP

  primitive (hemoglobin)

  private (patient, room); also priv, PVT, pvt

  probability; also *P*, p, *p*, prob

  probable error; also p, PE

  product; also prod

  progesterone; also P_4, PROG

  prolactin; also PR, Pr, PRL, Prl

  proline (one-letter notation); also Pro

  properdin

  propionate

  protein; also PR, Pr, PRO, pro, Prot, prot

  Protestant

  Proteus species; also *P*

  proximal; also prox

  psoralen; also PSOR

  psychiatric; also PS, PSY, Psy, psychiat

  psychiatry; also Ψ, PS, PSY, Psy, psychiat

  psychosis

  pulmonary; also PUL, pul, PULM, pulm

  pulse

  punctum proximum

  pupil (of the eye); also p

  P wave (in electrocardiography)

  pyroplasty

  radiant flux

  radiant power

  significance probability (value)

  sound power

  weight [L. *pondus*]

P *Pasteurella* species; also P, *Past*

  Plasmodium species; also P

  probability; also P, p, *p*, prob

  Proteus species; also P

P/ partial upper denture

/P partial lower denture

~P high-energy phosphate bond

P_1 antigen in the P blood group system

  first parental generation

P-2 pulmonic second heart sound; also P_2

P_2 antigen in the P blood group system

  pulmonic second heart sound; also P-2

P_3 luminous flux

  proximal third (of bone); also P/3, proximal/3

P/3 proximal third (of bone); also P_3, proximal/3

P_4 progesterone; also P, PROG

^{32}P phosphorus 32, radioactive phosphorus: halflife, 14.3 days

P-50 oxygen half-saturation pressure of hemoglobin

P-55 hydroxypregnanedione

P_{700} pigment in chloroplasts bleached by light of wavelengths about 700 nm

P_{870} pigment in bacterial chromatophores bleached by light of wavelengths about 870 nm

p after [L. *post*]; also P, p̄

  antigen in the P blood group system

  atomic orbital with angular momentum quantum number 1

  by [L. *per*]

  by weight [L. *pondere*]; also P, Pond, pond

  concentration by weight (after optical rotations); also P

  father [L. *pater*]; also P

  freeze preservation

  frequency of the more common allele of a pair

  handful [L. *pugillus*]; also P

  momentum; also *p*

  near [L. *proximum*]; also P

  near point (of accommodation) [L. *punctum proximum*]; also P, PP, pp

  optic papilla

  page; also P, pg

  papilla; also pap

  para (parity); also P

  part; also P, pt

  partial pressure (of a gas); also P, PP

  peripheral; also P, peri

  phosphatej; also P, Ph, phos

  pico- (10^{-12}); also P (p is the preferred symbol)

  pint; also O, Ō, oct, P, PT, pt

  pons; also P

  pressure; also P, PR, press

probability; also P, *P*, *p*, prob
probable error; also P, PE
proton
pupil (of the eye); also P
sample proportion (in statistics)
short arm of chromosome
sound pressure

p   momentum; also p
    probability; also P, *P*, p, prob
    probability of success in independent trials
    pyranose

p-, *p*-   para- (chemical prefix for two symmetri-
    cal substitutions in benzene ring)

p̄   after [L. *post*]; also P, p
    mean pressure (of a gas)

PA   alveolar pressure
    panic attack
    pantothenic acid
    paralysis agitans
    paranoia
    parietal cell antibody; also PCA
    passive-aggressive
    paternal aunt
    pathology; also PATH, path
    pentemoic acid
    periarteritis
    peridural artery
    periodic acid
    periodontal abscess
    permeability area
    pernicious anemia
    peroxidatic activity
    phakic-aphakic
    phenol alcohol
    phenylalanine; also F, P, PHA, PHE, Phe
    phosphatidic acid
    phosphoarginine
    photoallergic
    photoallergy
    phthalic anhydride
    physical assistance
    Physician's Assistant
    Picture Arrangement (psychology)
    pineapple (test for butyric acid in stomach)
    pituitary-adrenal
    plasma aldosterone
    plasminogen activator
    platelet adhesiveness
    platelet aggregation
    platelet associated
    polyacrylamide; also PAA
    polyarteritis; also PAr
    polyarthritis

postaurale
posteroanterior; also P-A
prealbumin
predictive accuracy (probability)
pregnancy associated
presents again
primary aldosteronism
primary amenorrhea
primary anemia
prior to admission; also PTA
proactivator
proanthocyanidin
procainamide; also PCA
professional association
proinsulin antibody
prolonged action
prophylactic antibiotic
propionic acid
prostate antigen
proteolytic activity
prothrombin activity; also PTA
protrusio acetabuli
Pseudomonas aeruginosa
psychiatric aide
psychoanalysis; also PSAn, psychoan, PYA
psychogenic aspermia
pulmonary artery
pulmonary atresia
pulpoaxial
puromycin aminonucleoside; also PAN,
    PANS
pyrophosphate arthropathy
pyrrolizidine alkaloid
yearly [L. *per annum*]; also pa

P(*A*)   probability that event *A* occurs

P/A   percussion and auscultation; also P&A
    position and alignment; also P&A

P-A   posteroanterior; also PA

P&A   percussion and auscultation; also P/A
    position and alignment; also P/A
    present and active (reflex)

$P_2 > A_2$ pulmonic second heart sound greater
    than aortic second heart sound

$P_2 = A_2$ pulmonic second heart sound equal to
    aortic second heart sound

$P_2 < A_2$ pulmonic second heart sound less than
    aortic second heart sound

Pa   arterial pressure
    pascal (unit of pressure); also Pas
    protactinium
    pulmonary arterial (pressure)
    pulmonary artery (line)

pA picoampere

pA₂ affinity constant (binding drug to drug receptor)

pa after application [L. *post applicationem*]
  for the year [L. *pro anno*]
  yearly [L. *per annum*]; also PA

PAA partial agonal activity
  phenylacetic acid
  phosphoroacetic acid
  physical abilities analysis
  plasma angiotensinase activity
  polyacrylamide; also PA
  polyacrylic acid
  polyamino acid
  premarket approval application
  pyridineacetic acid

3-PAA 3-pyridineacetic acid

paa let it be applied to the affected area
  [L. *parti adfecta applicetur*]

P(A-aDO₂) alveolar-arterial oxygen tension
  difference; also P(A-a)O₂

P(A-a)O₂ alveolar-arterial oxygen tension
  difference; also P(A-aDO₂)

PAB *para*-aminobenzoic acid; also PABA
  polyacrylamide bead
  positive attention behavior
  premature atrial beat
  purple agar base (medium)

P(A\B) conditional probability that *A* occurs
  given that *B* has occured

PABA *para*-aminobenzoic acid; also PAB

PAC papular acrodermatitis of childhood
  para-aminoclonidine
  parent-adult-child (in transactional analysis)
  phenacetin, aspirin, and caffeine
  phenacetin, aspirin, and codeine
  plasma aldosterone concentration
  Platinol, Adriamycin, and cyclophosphamide
  political action committee
  preadmission certification
  premature atrial contraction
  premature auricular contraction
  Progress Assessment Chart of Social and
    Personal Development

PACC protein A immobilized in collodion
  charcoal

PACE Pacing and Clinical Electrophysiology
  performance and cost efficiency
  Personal Assessment for Continuing
    Education
  personalized aerobics for cardiovascular
    enhancement

promoting aphasics communicative effectiveness
  pulmonary angiotensin I converting enzyme

PACIA particle-counting immunoassay

PACO₂, PA_CO2 partial pressure of alveolar
  carbon dioxide

PaCO₂, Pa_CO2 partial pressure of arterial
  carbon dioxide

PACP pulmonary artery counterpulsation

PACS picture archiving and communications

PACT precordial acceleration tracing

PACVIS pathological cardiovascular ischemic
  states

PACU postanesthesia care unit

PAD per adjusted discharge
  percutaneous abscess drainage
  phenacetin, aspirin, and desoxyephedrine
  phonologic-acquisition device
  photon absorption densitometry
  pre-aid to the disabled
  preoperative autologous donation
  primary affective disorder
  psychoaffective disorder
  pulmonary artery diastolic; also PAd
  pulsatile assist device
  pulsed amperometric detection

PAd pulmonary artery diastolic; also PAD

PADDS photon-activated drug delivery system

PADP pulmonary artery diastolic pressure

PAE in equal parts [L. *partes aequales*]; also
    p ae, part aeq
  postanoxic encephalopathy
  postantibiotic effect
  progressive assistive exercise

p ae in equal parts [L. *partes aequales*]; also
    PAE, part aeq

paed paediatric; also PD, PED, ped, Peds, peds
  paediatrics; also PD, PED, ped, Peds, peds

PAEDP pulmonary artery end-diastolic
  pressure

PAF paroxysmal atrial fibrillation; also PAFIB
  paroxysmal auricular fibrillation
  phosphodiesterase-activating factor
  platelet-activating factor
  platelet-aggregating factor; also PAgF
  platelet aggregation factor
  pollen adherence factor
  premenstrual assessment form
  pseudoamniotic fluid
  pulmonary arteriovenous fistula; also PA-VF

PA&F percussion, auscultation, and fremitus

PAF-A platelet-activating factor of anaphylaxis

PAFD percutaneous abscess and fluid drainage
pulmonary artery filling defect

PAFG picric acid formaldehyde-glutaraldehyde

PAFI platelet-aggregation factor inhibitor

PAFIB paroxysmal atrial fibrillation; also PAF

PAFP pre-Achilles fat pad

PAG periaqueductal gray (matter)
phenylacetylglutamine
polyacrylamide gel
pregnancy-associated globulin

pAg protein A-gold (technique)

PAGE polyacrylamide gel electrophoresis

PAgF platelet-aggregating factor; also PAF

PAGG pentaacetylglucopyranosyl guanine

PAGIF polyacrylamide gel isoelectric focusing

PAGMK primary African green monkey kidney

PAH *para*-aminohippuric (acid); also PAHA
phenylalanine hydroxylase; also PH
polycyclic aromatic hydrocarbon
pulmonary artery hypertension
pulmonary artery hypotension

PAHA *para*-aminohippuric acid; also PAH

PAHO Pan American Health Organization

PAHVC pulmonary alveolar hypoxic vasoconstriction

PAI Pair Attraction Inventory
plasminogen activator inhibitor
platelet accumulation index

PAIDS pediatric acquired immunodeficiency syndrome

PAIgG platelet-associated immunoglobulin G

PAIR Personal Assessment of Intimacy in Relationships

PAIS Psychosocial Adjustment to Illness Scale

PAIVS pulmonary atresia with intact ventricular septum

PAJ paralysis agitans juvenilis

PAL pathology laboratory
phenylalanine ammonia lyase
posterior axillary line
product of activated lymphocyte
pulmonary air leak
pyogenic abscess of the liver

PAK *Pseudomonas aeruginosa* strain K

pal palate

PALA *N*-(phosphonacetyl)-L-aspartate

PA&Lat posteroanterior and lateral

PALN *para*-aortic lymph node

palp palpable
palpate
palpated
palpation
palpitation; also palpi

palpi palpitation; also palp

PALS Paired Associate Learning Subtest
pediatric advanced life support
periarterial lymphoid sheath
periarteriolar lymphocyte sheath
prison-acquired lymphoproliferative syndrome

PA-LS-ID pernicious anemia-like syndrome and immunoglobulin deficiency

PALST Picture Articulation and Language Screening Test

Palv alveolar pressure

PAM crystalline penicillin G in 2% aluminum monostearate
pancreatic acinar mass
penicillin aluminum monostearate
L-phenylalanine mustard (Melphalan); also Pam
postauricular myogenic
potential acuity meter
primary amebic meningoencephalitis; also PAME
pulmonary alveolar macrophage
pulmonary alveolar microlithiasis
pulmonary artery mean
pyridine aldoxime methiodide

Pam L-phenylalanine mustard (Melphalan); also PAM

PAMC pterygoarthromyodysplasia congenita

PAME primary amebic meningoencephalitis; also PAM

PAMIF Physical and Mental Impairment-of-Function (scale)

PAMP pulmonary artery mean pressure

PAN periarteritis nodosa; also PN
periodic alternating nystagmus
peroxyacetyl nitrate
peroxyacylnitrate
polyacrylonitrile
polyarteritis nodosa; also PN
positional alcohol nystagmus
puromycin aminonucleoside; also PA, PANS

pan pancreas
pancreatectomy
pancreatic

PAND primary adrenocortical nodular dysplasia

PANESS physical and neurologic examination for soft signs

PANS puromycin aminonucleoside; also PA, PAN

PAO peak acid output
peripheral airway obstruction
plasma amine oxidase
polyamine oxidase

PAO$_2$ partial pressure of oxygen in alveoli

PAO$_2$-PaO$_2$ alveolar-arterial difference in partial pressure of oxygen

PAo pulmonary artery occlusion (pressure)

Pao ascending aortic pressure

P$_{ao}$ airway opening pressure

PaO$_2$ partial pressure of arterial oxygen

PAOD peripheral arterial occlusive disease
peripheral arteriosclerotic occlusive disease

PAOI peak acid output insulin-induced

PAOP pulmonary artery occlusion pressure

PAOx phenylacetone oxime

PAP Papanicolaou (smear, stain, test); also Pap
papaverine
para-aminophenol
passive aggressive personality
Patient Assessment Program
peak airway pressure; also PAW
peroxidase antibody to peroxidase
peroxidase-antiperoxidase (technique)
Phytolacca americana protein
placental acid phosphatase
placental alkaline phosphatase; also PLAP
positive airway pressure
primary atypical pneumonia
prostatic acid phosphatase
pulmonary alveolar proteinosis
pulmonary artery pressure; also PPA, P$_{Pa}$
purified alternate pathway

Pap Papanicolaou (smear, stain, test); also PAP
papillary

pap papilla; also p

PAPF platelet adhesiveness plasma factor

Pap in canthus papilloma, inner canthus

PAPOVA, papova papilloma-polyoma-vacuolating agent (virus)

PAPP Pappenheimer's bodies
para-aminopropiophenone
pregnancy-associated plasma protein

PAPPC pregnancy-associated plasma protein C

PAPS adenosine 3'-phosphate 5'-phosphosulfate
phosphoadenosine diphosphosulfate
phosphoadenosine phosphosulfate
phosphoadenosylphosphosulfate

PA/PS pulmonary atresia/pulmonary stenosis

Paps papillomas

Pap sm Papanicolaou smear

PAPUFA physiologically active polyunsaturated fatty acid

Pa-Pv pulmonary arterial pressure–pulmonary venous pressure

PAPVC partial anomalous pulmonary venous connection

PAPVR partial anomalous pulmonary venous return

PAPW posterior aspect of the pharyngeal wall

PAQ Personal Attributes Questionnaire
Position Analysis Questionnaire (job analysis)

PAR pair [L. *par* (equal)]; also pr
paraffin; also P, par
parallel; also par
passive avoidance reaction
perennial allergic rhinitis
photosynthetically active radiation
physiologic aging rate
platelet aggregate ratio
positive attention received
postanesthesia recovery (room)
probable allergic rhinitis
problem-analysis report
Program for Alcohol Recovery
proximal alveolar region
pulmonary arteriolar resistance

PAr polyarteritis; also PA

Par paranoid

par paraffin; also P, PAR
parallel; also PAR
paralysis

Para number of pregnancies producing viable offspring [L. *parere* (to bring forth, to bear)]; also para
paraplegia; also para
paraplegic; also para
parous (having borne one or more viable offspring) [L. *parere* (to bring forth, to bear)]; also para
woman who has given birth [L. *parere* (to bring forth, to bear)]; also para

para number of pregnancies producing viable offspring [L. *parere* (to bring forth, to bear)]; also Para
paracentesis
paraparesis
paraplegia; also Para
paraplegic; also Para
parathyroid; also PT, PTH
parathyroidectomy; also PTX, PTx
parous (having borne one or more viable offspring) [L. *parere* (to bring forth, to bear)]; also Para
woman who has given birth [L. *parere* (to bring forth, to bear)]; also Para

I-para primipara (woman bearing first child) [L. *parere* (to bring forth, to bear)]; also P, primip, PRIMP

II-para secundipara (second pregnancy) [L. *parere* (to bring forth, to bear)]

III-para tertipara (third pregnancy) [L. *parere* (to bring forth, to bear)]

Para 0, para 0 nullipara (no child borne) [L. *parere* (to bring forth, to bear)]

Para I, para I unipara (having borne one child) [L. *parere* (to bring forth, to bear)]

Para II, para II bipara (having borne two children) [L. *parere* (to bring forth, to bear)]

Para III, para III tripara (having borne three children) [L. *parere* (to bring forth, to bear)]

Para IV, para IV quadripara (having borne four children) [L. *parere* (to bring forth, to bear)]

para C, para c paracervical; also PCX

par aff to the part affected [L. *pars affecta*]

para L paralumbar

parapsych parapsychology

parasit parasite
parasitic
parasitology

parasym parasympathetic (division of autonomic nervous system); also PS

para T parathoracic

PARD platelet aggregation as a risk of diabetes

parent parenteral; also P
parenterally

PARH plasminogen activator-releasing hormone

PARIS persantine/aspirin reinfarction study

PARNA peanut stunt virus-associated RNA

parox paroxysm
paroxysmal

PARR postanesthesia recovery room

PARS Personal Adjustment and Role Skills (scale)

PaRS pararectal space

part of a part [L. *partis*]
partly
parturition

part aeq in equal parts [L. *partes aequales*]; also PAE, p ae

part dolent painful parts [L. *partes dolentes*]

part vic in divided doses [L. *partitis vicibus*]

PARU postanesthetic recovery unit

parv small [L. *parvus*]

PAS *para*-aminosalicylic acid; also PASA
Parent Attitude Scale
patient appointments and scheduling
periodic acid-Schiff (method, reaction, stain, technique, test)
peripheral anterior synechia
persistent atrial standstill
personality assessment system
phosphatase acid serum
photoacoustic spectroscopy
Physician's Activity Study
pneumatic antiembolic stocking
postanesthesia score
posterior airway space
preadmission screening
pregnancy advisory service
premature atrial stimulus
premature auricular systole
Professional Activities Study
progressive accumulated stress
pseudoachievement syndrome
psychopathologic assessment scale
pulmonary arterial stenosis
pulmonary artery systolic

Pas pascal (unit of pressure); also Pa

Pa·s pascal-second

Pa x s pascals per second

PASA *para*-aminosalicylic acid; also PAS

PaSat saturation of oxygen in arterial blood

PASB Pan American Sanitary Bureau

PAS-C *para*-aminosalicylic acid crystallized (with ascorbic acid)

PASD after diastase digestion

P'ase alkaline phosphatase

Pas Ex passive exercise

PASG pneumatic antishock garment

PASH periodic acid-Schiff hematoxylin

PASI psoriasis area sensitivity index

PASM periodic acid-silver methenamine

PAS/MAP Professional Activities Study Medical Audit Program (medical records)

PASP pulmonary artery systolic pressure

pass here and there [L. *passim*]
passive; also P

PAST periodic acid-Schiff technique

Past *Pasteurella* species; also P, *P*

PASVR pulmonary anomalous superior venous return

PAT Pain Apperception Test
paroxysmal atrial tachycardia
paroxysmal auricular tachycardia
patella; also pat
patient; also P, PNT, Pnt, PT, Pt, pt
percentage of acceleration time
Photo Articulation Test (psychology)
physical abilities test
picric acid turbidity
platelet aggregation test
polyamine acetyltransferase
preadmission screening and assessment team
preadmission testing
Predictive Ability Test (psychology)
pregnancy at term
prism adaptation test
promoting activity test (Danz test)
propylaminotetraline
psychoacoustic testing
pulmonary artery trunk

pat patella; also PAT
patent
paternal origin

PATCO prednisone, Ara-C, thioguanine, cyclophosphamide, and Oncovin

PATE psychodynamic and therapeutic education
pulmonary artery thromboembolism
pulmonary artery thromboendarterectomy

PATH Partnership Approach to Health
pathologic; also path
pathologist; also path
pathology; also PA, path
pituitary adrenotropic hormone

path pathogen
pathogenesis
pathogenic
pathologic; also Path
pathologist; also Path
pathology; also PA, PATH

path fx pathologic fracture

PATLC Progressive Achievement Tests of Listening Comprehension

pat med patent medicine

PATS priority activity tracking system

PA-T-SP periodic acid-thiocarbohydrazide-silver proteinate

pat T patellar tenderness

PAT/TM patient's time

p aur behind the ear [L. *post aurem*]; also post aur

PAV partial atrioventricular
Pavulon (pancuronium bromide)
poikiloderma atrophicans vasculare
posterior arch vein

Pa Va Ex passive vascular exercise (a negative pressure)
passive venoarterial exercise (a negative pressure)

PAVe procarbazine, Alkeran, and Velban

PA-VF pulmonary arteriovenous fistula; also PAF

PAVM pulmonary arteriovenous malformation

PAVN paraventricular nucleus; also PVN

PAW peak airway pressure; also PAP
peripheral airways
pulmonary artery wedge

Paw mean airway pressure

Pawo pressure at airway opening

PAWP pulmonary arterial wedge pressure

PB British Pharmacopoeia [L. *Pharmacopoeia Britannica*]; also BP, PHB, PhB
pancreaticobiliary
paraffin bath
Paul-Bunnell (antibodies, test)
pentobarbital
perineal body
periodic breathing
peripheral blood
peroneus brevis
phenobarbital
phonetically balanced (word lists)
pinch biopsy
pinealoblastoma
piperonyl butoxide

polymyxin B; also PMB
posterior baffle
powder bed
powder board
power building
premature beat
pressure balanced
pressure breathing
protein binding
protein-bound
pudendal block
punch biopsy; also PBX

PB-7 pentagonal bipyramidal

PB% phonetically balanced percentage (of word lists)

P&B pain and burning
phenobarbital and belladonna

P$_B$ barometric pressure

Pb lead [L. *plumbum*]; also plumb
phenobarbital
presbyopia
probenecid

PBA percutaneous bladder aspiration
polyclonal B-cell activator
polyclonal B-cell activity
pressure breathing assister
prolactin-binding assay
prune belly anomaly
pulpobuccoaxial

P$_{BA}$ brachial arterial pressure

p-bars parallel bars

PBB polybrominated biphenyl(s)

PBBs polybrominated biphenyls

Pb-B lead level in blood

PBC packed blood cells
peripheral blood cell
point of basal convergence
prebed care
pregnancy and birth complications
primary biliary cirrhosis
progestin-binding complement

PBD percutaneous biliary drainage
postburn day

PBE partial breech extraction
tuberculin prepared from *Mycobacterium tuberculosis bovis* [Ger. *Perlsucht Bacillenemulsion*]

PBF peripheral blood flow
phosphate-buffered formalin
placental blood flow
pulmonary blood flow; also PF, Qp

PB-Fe protein-bound iron

PBG pedobarograph
Penassay broth plus glucose
porphobilinogen

PBGM Penassay broth plus glucose plus menadione

PBG-Q porphobilinogen-quantitative

PBG-S porphobilinogen synthase

PBI partial bony impaction
penile-brachial index
protein-bound iodine

PbI lead intoxication

PBK phosphorylase *b* kinase
pseudophakic bullous keratopathy

PBL peripheral blood leukocyte
peripheral blood lymphocyte

PBLI premature birth, live infant

PBLT peripheral blood lymphocyte transformation

PBM peripheral basement membrane
peripheral blood mononuclear (cell)
pharmacy benefit management

PBMC peripheral blood mononuclear cell; also PMNC

PBMV pulmonary blood mixing volume

PBN paralytic brachial neuritis
peripheral benign neoplasm
polymyxin B sulfate, bacitracin, and neomycin

PBNA partial body neutron activation (technique)

PBO penicillin in beeswax and oil
placebo; also P, PL, PLBO

PbO lead monoxide

PBP peak blood pressure
penicillin-binding protein
porphyrin biosynthetic pathway
progressive bulbar palsy
prostate-binding protein
pseudobulbar palsy
purified *Brucella* protein

PBPI penile-brachial pulse index

PBQ phenylbenzoquinone
Preschool Behavior Questionnaire

PBRT phonetically balanced rhyme test

PBS peripheral blood smear
phenobarbital sodium
phosphate-buffered saline
phosphate-buffered sodium

PBS —cont'd
polybrominated salicylanilide
primer-binding site
prune-belly syndrome
pulmonary branch stenosis

PBSC peripheral blood stem cells

PBSP prognostically bad signs during pregnancy

PBST phosphate-buffered saline/triton/EDTA

PBT Paul Bunnell test
phenacetin breath test
profile-based therapy

PBTI pancreatic basic trypsin inhibitor

PBT$_4$ protein-bound thyroxine

PBV percutaneous balloon valvuloplasty
Platinol, bleomycin, and vinblastine
predicted blood volume
pulmonary blood volume

PBW posterior bite wing

PBX punch biopsy; also PB

PBY post Baccalaureate year (postgraduate year)

PBZ phenoxybenzamine; also POB
phenylbutazone
pyribenzamine (tripelennamine)

PC avoirdupois weight [L. *pondus civile*]; also pc
packed cells
palmitoyl carnitine
paper chromatography
parent cell(s)
parent to child
particulate component
partition coefficient
patient's cells (cross-match)
pelvic cramp
penicillin; also P, Pc, PCN, pcn, Pen, pen, PN, PNC
pentose cycle
peritoneal cell
pharmacology
phosphate cycle
phosphatidylcholine (lecithin); also PtdCho
phosphocreatine; also PCR, PCr
phosphorylcholine
photoconductive
phrase construction
phycocyanin
Physician's Corporation
picryl chloride
picture completion
pill counter

piriform cortex
plasma concentration
plasma cortisol
plasmacytoma; also PCT
platelet concentrate
platelet count
Platinol and cyclophosphamide
pneumotaxic center; also PNC
polycentric
polyposis coli
poor condition
popliteal cyst
portacaval (shunt)
portal cirrhosis
postcoital; also PCT
posterior cervical
posterior chamber
posterior column
posterior commissure
posterior cortex
precordial
prepiriform cortex
present complaint
primary cleavage
primary closure
printed circuit
procollagen (ie, PC-I: type I procollagen)
producing cell
productive cough
professional corporation
proliferative capacity
prostatic carcinoma; also PCA
provisional cortex
proximal colon
pseudocyst; also Ps
pubococcygeus (muscle); also PCG
pulmonary capillary
pulmonic closure
Purkinje cell
pyloric canal
pyruvate carboxylase

P-C phlogistic corticoid

P&C prism and alternative cover-test (cross-over test, screen and cover test in ophthalmology)

Pc penicillin; also P, PC, PCN, pcn, Pen, pen, PN, PNC

pc after a meal [L. *post cibum*]
avoirdupois weight [L. *pondus civile*]; also PC
parsec
percent; also P, pct
picocurie; also pCi

pc1 platelet count pretransfusion

pc2 platelet count posttransfusion

PCA *para*-chloroamphetamine
parietal cell antibody; also PA
passive cutaneous anaphylaxis
patient care aide
patient care assistant
patient-controlled analgesia
perchloric acid
percutaneous carotid arteriogram
percutaneous coronary angioplasty
personal care attendant
phenylcarboxylic acid
photocontact allergic
porous-coated anatomic (prosthesis)
portacaval anastomosis
postconceptional age
posterior cerebral artery
posterior communicating artery; also
PCoA, PCom
posterior communication aneurysm
posterior cricoarytenoid
precoronary care area
President's Council on Aging
principal components analysis
procainamide; also PA
procoagulant activity
prostatic carcinoma; also PC
pyrrolidone carboxylic acid

PCAS Psychotherapy Competence Assessment
Schedule

PCAT Pharmacy College Admission Test

PCAVC persistent complete atrioventricular
canal

PCB pancuronium bromide
paracervical block
polychlorinated biphenyl(s)
portacaval bypass
prepared childbirth
procarbazine; also PCZ, PROC, Proc, Procarb

Pcb, PcB near point of convergence to the
intercentral baseline [L. *punctum
convergens basalis*]

PC-BMP phosphorycholine-binding myeloma
protein

PCC Pasteur Culture Collection
phenol, *m*-cresol, chloroform (interphase)
pheochromocytoma; also Pheo, pheo
phosphate carrier compound
plasma catecholamine concentration
Poison Control Center
precoronary care

premature chromosome condensation
prematurely condensed chromosome
primary care clinic
prothrombin-complex concentration

PCc periscopic concave

PCCC pediatric critical care center

PCCP percutaneous cord cyst puncture

PCCS parent-child communication schedule

PCCU post-coronary care unit

PCD papillary collecting duct
paroxysmal cerebral dysrhythmia
phosphate-citrate-dextrose
plasma cell dyscrasia
polycystic disease
posterior corneal deposits
postmortem cesarean delivery
primary ciliary dyskinesia
prolonged contractile duration
pulmonary clearance delay

PCDC plasma clot diffusion chamber
plasma clot diffusion culture

PCDD polychlorinated dibenzo-*p*-dioxins

PCDF polychlorinated dibenzofuran

PCDUS plasma cell dyscrasia of unknown
significance

PCE physical capacity evaluation
polymer-coated erythromycin
pseudocholinesterase; also PCHE; PsChE
pulmocutaneous exchange

PCEC purified chicken embryo culture
(rabies vaccine)

PCF peripheral circulatory failure
pharyngoconjunctival fever
posterior cranial fossa
prothrombin conversion factor

pcf pounds per cubic foot

PCFT platelet complement fixation test

PCG paracervical ganglion
phonocardiogram
Planning Career Goals (psychologic test)
pneumocardiogram
primate chorionic gonadotropin
pubococcygeus (muscle); also PC

PCGG percutaneous coagulation of gasserian
ganglion

PCH paroxysmal cold hemoglobinuria
polycyclic hydrocarbon(s)

PCHE pseudocholinesterase; also PCE, PsChE

PC&HS after meals and at bedtime [L. *post
cibum et hora somni*]

PCI pneumatosis cystoides intestinalis
posterior curve intermediate (cornea)
Premarital Communication Inventory
prophylactic cranial irradiation
prothrombin consumption index

pCi picocurie; also pc

PCIC Poison Control Information Center

PCILO perturbative configuration interaction using localized orbitals

PCIOL posterior chamber intraocular lens

PC-IRV pressure-controlled inverted ratio ventilation

PCIS Patient-Care Information System
post-cardiac injury syndrome

PCK polycystic kidney

PCKD polycystic kidney disease; also PKD

PCL pacing cycle length
persistent corpus luteum
plasma cell leukemia
posterior chamber lens
posterior cruciate ligament

P closure plastic closure

PCM primary cutaneous melanoma
protein-calorie malnutrition
protein carboxymethylase
pulse code modulation

PCMB, *p*-CMB *para*-chloromercuribenzoic acid

PCMC Primary Children's Medical Center

PCMBSA *para*-chloromercuribenzine sulfonic acid

PCMF perceptual cognitive motor function

PCMO Principal Clinical Medical Officer

PCMS *para*-chloromercuriphenylsulphonic acid

PCMX *para*-chloro-*m*-xylenol (chloroxylenol)

PCN penicillin; also P, PC, Pc, pcn, Pen, pen, PN, PNC
percutaneous nephrostomy
pregnenolone carbonitril
primary care network
primary care nursing

pcn penicillin; also P, PC, Pc, PCN, Pen, pen, PN, PNC

PCNA proliferating cell nuclear antigen

PCNB pentachloronitrobenzene

PCNL percutaneous nephrostolithotomy; also PNL

PCNV postchemotherapy nausea and vomiting

PCO patient complains of
photosynthetic carbon oxidation
polycystic ovary
predicted cardiac output
procytoxid

Pco, P_{CO} partial pressure of carbon monoxide

PCO_2, Pco_2, pCO_2, pco_2, p_{CO2}, pCO_2 partial pressure of carbon dioxide

PCoA posterior communicating artery; also PCA, PCom

PCOD polycystic ovarian disease

PCom posterior communicating artery; also PCA, PCoA

PCOS polycystic ovary syndrome; also POS

PCP *para*-chlorophenate
patient care plan
pentachlorophenol
peripheral coronary pressure
persistent cough and phlegm
1-(1-phenylcyclohexyl)piperidine (phencyclidine, angel dust)
pneumocystic pneumonia
Pneumocystis carinii pneumonia
primary care physician
prochlorperazine; also PCZ
procollagen peptide
pulmonary capillary pressure
pulse cytophotometry

PCPA *para*-chlorophenoxyacetic acid
para-chlorophenylalanine

PCPL pulmonary capillary protein leakage

pcpn precipitation; also pcpt, Ppt, ppt, pptn, precip

PCPQ Professional Corporation of Physicians of Quebec

PCPS phosphatidylcholine-phosphatidylserine

pcpt perception
precipitate; also Ppt, ppt, precip
precipitation; also pcpn, Ppt, ppt, pptn, precip

PCR pathologically confirmed complete remission
patient contact record
phosphocreatine; also PC, PCr
photosynthetic carbon reduction
plasma clearance rate
polymerase chain reaction (type of DNA testing)
probable causal relationship
protein catabolic rate

PCr phosphocreatine; also PC, PCR

PCS palliative care service

Patient Care System
patterns of care study
pharmacogenic confusional syndrome
piezoelectric crystal sensor
portable cervical spine
portacaval shunt
post-cardiac surgery
postcardiotomy syndrome
postcholecystectomy syndrome
postconcussion syndrome
precordial stethoscope
primary cancer site
primary cesarean section; also P c/s
Priority Counseling Survey
proportional counter spectrometer
proportional counter spectrometry
proximal coronary sinus
pseudotumor cerebri syndrome

Pcs, pcs preconscious

P c/s primary cesarean section; also PCS

PCSM percutaneous stone manipulation

PCT Patent Co-operation Treaty
Physiognomic Cue Test (psychology)
plasma clotting time
plasmacrit test (for syphilis)
plasmacytoma; also PC
platelet hematocrit
polychlorinated triphenyl
polychloroterphenyl
porcine calcitonin
porphyria cutanea tarda
portacaval transportation
portacaval transposition
positron computed tomography
postcoital; also PC
postcoital test
progestin challenge test
prothrombin consumption time
proximal convoluted tubule
pulmonary care team

pct percent; also P, pc

PCTA percutaneous coronary transluminal
angioplasty

PCU pain control unit
palliative care unit
patient care unit
primary care unit
progressive care unit
protective care unit
protein-calorie undernutrition
pulmonary care unit

p cut percutaneous; also PERC

PCV packed cell volume
parietal cell vagotomy
polychlorinated vinyl
polycythemia vera; also PV
postcapillary venule
procarbazine, CCNU (lomustine), vincristine

PCV-M polycythemia vera with myeloid
metaplasia

PCVP procarbazine, cyclophosphamide,
vinblastine, and prednisone

PCW pulmonary capillary wedge
purified cell walls

PCWP pulmonary capillary wedge pressure

PCX paracervical; also para C, para c

PCx periscopic convex

PCXR portable chest x-ray

PCZ procarbazine; also PCB, PROC, Proc,
Procarb
prochlorperazine; also PCP

PD by the day [L. *per diem*]; also pd
Doctor of Pharmacy [L. *Pharmaciae Doctor*];
also Phar D, Pharm D, PhD
interpupillary distance
Paget's disease
pancreatic duct
papilla diameter; also pd
paralyzing dose
Parkinsonian dementia
Parkinson's disease
paroxysmal discharge
pars distalis (pituitary)
patent ductus
patient day
patient demonstration
pediatric; also paed, PED, ped, Peds, peds
pediatrics; also paed, Pd, PED, ped, Peds,
peds
percutaneous drain
peritoneal dialysis
personality disorder
pharmacodynamics
phenyldichlorarsine
phosphate dehydrogenase; also PDH
photosensitivity dermatitis
Pick's disease
plasma defect
poorly differentiated
Porak-Durante (syndrome)
porphobilinogen deaminase
posterior division
postnasal drainage; also PND
postural drainage

PD—cont'd
  potential difference
  present disease
  pressor dose
  primary dendrite
  prism diopter; also pd
  problem drinker
  progression of disease
  protein degradation
  protein deprived
  protein diet
  provocation dose
  psychopathic deviate
  psychotic dementia
  psychotic depression
  pulmonary disease; also PN, PUD, PuD
  pulpodistal
  pulse duration
  pyloric dilator

P(D+) probability of having disease

P(D-) probability of not having disease

P/D packs per day (cigarettes); also p/d, PPD, ppd

PD$_{50}$ median paralyzing dose

Pd palladium
  pediatrics; also PD, PED, ped, Peds, peds

pd by the day [L. *per diem*]; also PD
  for the day [L. *pro die*]
  papilla diameter; also PD
  period
  prism diopter; also PD
  pupillary distance

p/d packs per day (cigarettes); also P/D, PPD, ppd

PDA parenteral drug abuser
  Parenteral Drug Association
  patent ductus arteriosus
  patient distress alarm
  pediatric allergy; also PdA
  posterior descending coronary artery
  predialyzed human albumin
  pulmonary disease anemia

PdA pediatric allergy; also PDA

PDAB *para*-dimethylaminobenzaldehyde

PDB Paget's disease of bone
  para-dichlorobenzene; also PDCB
  phosphorus-dissolving bacteria
  preventive dental health behavior
  Protein Data Bank

PDC pediatric cardiology; also PdC
  pentadecylcatechol
  physical dependence capacity

plasma digoxin concentration
  plasma disappearance curve
  postdecapitation convulsion
  preliminary diagnostic clinic
  private diagnostic clinic
  pyrindinol carbamate

PD&C postural drainage and clapping

PdC pediatric cardiology; also PDC

PDCB *para*-dichlorobenzene; also PDB

PDCD primary degenerative cerebral disease

PDD pervasive developmental disorder
  platinum diamminodichloride (cisplatin)
  primary degenerative dementia
  pyridoxine-deficient diet

PDDB phenododecinium bromide

PDDS Parasitic Disease Drug Service

PDE paroxysmal dyspnea on exertion
  phosphodiesterase; also PDIE
  progressive dialysis encephalopathy
  pulsed Doppler echocardiography

PdE pediatric endocrinology

PDF peritoneal dialysis fluid
  probability density function

PDFC premature dead female child

PDG Parkinsonism-dementia complex of Guam
  phosphate-dependent glutaminase
  phosphogluconate dehydrogenase;
    also PGD, PGDH
  pyruvate dehydrogenase; also PDH

PDGA pteroyldiglutamic acid

PDGF platelet-derived growth factor

PDGXT predischarge graded exercise test

PDH packaged disaster hospital
  past dental history
  phosphate dehydrogenase; also PD
  pyruvate dehydrogenase; also PDG

PDHC pyruvate dehydrogenase complex

PdHO pediatric hematology-oncology

PDI periodontal disease index
  plan-do integration
  protein disulfide isomerase
  Psychomotor Development Index

Pdi transdiaphragmatic pressure

PDIE phosphodiesterase; also PDE

P-diol pregnanediol

PDL periodontal ligament
  poorly differentiated lymphocyte
  population doubling level
  primary dysfunctional labor
  progressively diffused leukoencephalopathy

Pdl, pdl poundal (force of acceleration)
pudendal

pDL predicted diffusing capacity

PDLC poorly differentiated lung cancer

PDLD poorly differentiated lymphocytic
lymphoma–diffuse

PDLL poorly differentiated lymphocytic
lymphoma

PDLN poorly differentiated lymphocytic
lymphoma–nodular

PDLP predigested liquid protein

PDM polymyositis and dermatomyositis

PDMC premature dead male child

PDMEA phosphoryldimethylethanolamine

PDMS Patient Data Management Systems
pharmacokinetic drug-monitoring service
plasma desorption mass spectrometry

PDN prednisone; also P, PR, PRED, pred
private day nurse
private duty nurse

PdNEO pediatric neonatology

PdNEP pediatric nephrology

PDP pattern disruption point
piperidinopyrimidine
platelet-depleted plasma
primer-dependent deoxynucleic acid
polymerase
Product Development Protocol

PD&P postural drainage and percussion

PDPD prolonged-dwell peritoneal dialysis

PDPI primer-dependent deoxynucleic acid
polymerase index

PDQ parental development questionnaire
Prescreening Development Questionnaire
pretty damn quick
protocol data query

PDR pandevelopmental retardation
pediatric radiology; also PdR
peripheral diabetic retinopathy
Physician's Desk Reference
pleiotropic drug resistance
postdelivery room
primary drug resistance
proliferative diabetic retinopathy

PdR pediatric radiology; also PDR

pdr powder; also powd, pulv, pwd

PDRB Permanent Disability Rating Board

PDRc̄VH proliferative diabetic retinopathy
with vitreous hemorrhage

PDS pain-dysfunction syndrome

Paranoiddepressivitätsskala [Ger. (scale of
states paranoid depression)]
paroxysmal depolarizing shift
patient data system
pediatric surgery; also PdS, PS
peritoneal dialysis system
predialyzed human serum
primary dependence study

PdS pediatric surgery; also PDS, PS
psychiatric deviate, subtle

PDT phenyldimethyltriazine
photodynamic therapy
population doubling time

PDU pulsed Doppler ultrasonography

PDUF pulsed Doppler ultrasonic flowmeter

PDUR Predischarge Utilization Review

PDV peak diastolic velocity

PDW platelet distribution width

PDWHF platelet-derived wound healing factor

PE expiratory pressure; also P_E
pancreatic extract
paper electrophoresis
parallel elastic (component of muscle)
partial epilepsy
Pel-Ebstein (disease)
pelvic examination
penile erection
pericardial effusion
peritoneal exudate
phacoemulsification
pharyngoesophageal
phenylephrine
phosphatidylethanolamine; also PtdEtn
photographic effect
phycoerythrin
physical education; also PEd, P Ed, Phys Ed
physical evaluation
physical examination; also PEx, PX, Px, px
physical exercise
physiologic ecology
pigmented epithelium
plasma exchange
plating efficiency
Platinol and etoposide
pleural effusion
point of entry
polyethylene
polynuclear eosinophil
potential energy
powdered extract
pre-eclampsia
pre-excitation

PE—cont'd
present examination
pressure equalization
prior to exposure
probable error; also P, p
probe excision
protein electrophoresis; also PEP, Pro El
protein excretion
pulmonary edema
pulmonary embolism
pyramidal eminence
pyroelectric
pyrogenic exotoxin

P_E expiratory pressure; also PE

Pe Peclet number
perylene
pregnenolone; also Pg
pressure on expiration

pe for example [L. *per exemplum*]

PE2 secondary plating efficiency

PEA pelvic examination under anesthesia;
also PE↓A
phenylethyl alcohol
phenylethylamine
polysaccharide egg antigen

PE↓A pelvic examination under anesthesia;
also PEA

PEACH Preschool Evaluation and Assessment
for Children with Handicaps

PEAO phenylethylamine oxidase

PEAQ Personal Experience and Attitude
Questionnaire

PEARL pupils equal and react to light; also
PERL

PEARLA pupils equal and react to light and
accommodation

PEB Physical Evaluation Board
Platinol, etoposide, and bleomycin

PEBG phenethylbiguanide

PEC parallel elastic component
patient evaluation center
peduncle of cerebrum
peritoneal exudate cell
pulmonary ejection click
pyrogenic exotoxin C

PECHO, Pecho prostatic echogram

PECO₂ mixed expired carbon dioxide tension

PECT positron emission computed tomography

PED pediatric; also paed, PD, ped, Peds, peds
pediatrics; also paed, PD, Pd, ped, Peds, peds

peduncle (cerebral)
pharyngoesophageal diverticulum
pollution and environmental degradation
postentry day
postexertional dyspnea

PEd, P Ed physical education; also PE,
Phys Ed

ped pedangle
pedestrian
pediatric; also paed, PD, PED, Peds, peds
pediatrics; also paed, PD, Pd, PED,
Peds, peds

ped ed pedal edema

PEDG phenylethyldiguanide

PED/MVA pedestrian/motor vehicle accident
(pedestrian hit by motor vehicle)

PeDS Pediatric Drug Surveillance

Peds, peds pediatric; also paed, PD, PED, ped
pediatrics; also paed, PD, Pd, PED, ped

PEE parallel elastic element

PEEP peak end-expiratory pressure
positive end-expiratory pressure

PEER Pediatric Examination of Educational
Readiness

PEF peak expiratory flow
pharyngoepiglottic fold
Psychiatric Evaluation Form
pulmonary edema fluid

PEFR peak expiratory flow rate

PEFSR partial expiratory flow-static recoil
(curve)

PEFT peak expiratory flow time

PEFV partial expiratory flow volume

PEG Patient Evaluation Grid
percutaneous endoscopic gastrostomy
pneumoencephalogram
pneumoencephalography
polyethylene glycol

PEG-ELS polyethylene glycol and iso-osmolar
electrolyte solution

PEI phosphate excretion index
phosphorus excretion index
physical efficiency index
polyethyleneimine

PEIAS phenylephrine-activated isolated aortic
strip

PEJ percutaneous endoscopic jejunostomy

PEL peritoneal exudate lymphocyte
permissible exposure limit

Pel elastic recoil pressure of the lung

pelvic amputation
pelvis; also P

PELISA paper enzyme-linked immunosorbent assay

PEM peritoneal exudate macrophage
polyethylene matrix
precordial electrocardiographic mapping
prescription event monitoring
primary enrichment medium
probable error of measurement
production engineering measures
protein-energy malnutrition
pulmonary endothelial membrane

PEMA phenylethylmalonamide

PEMF pulsating electromagnetic field(s)

PEMS physical, emotional, mental, and safety

PEN parenteral and enteral nutrition

Pen penicillin; also P, PC, Pc, PCN, pcn, pen, PN, PNC

pen penetrating
penicillin; also P, PC, Pc, PCN, pcn, Pen, PN, PNC

PENG photoelectric nystagmography

PENS percutaneous epidural nerve stimulator

Pent, pent pentothal

PEO progressive external ophthalmoplegia

PEP peplomycin sulphate
peptidase; also Pep
performance evaluation procedure
phosphoenolpyruvate
polyestradiol phosphate
positive expiratory pressure
postencephalitic parkinsonism
pre-ejection period
protein electrophoresis; also PE, Pro El
Psychiatric Evaluation Profile

Pep peptidase; also PEP

PEPA peptidase A
protected environment units and prophylactic antibiotics

PEPAP 1-(2-phenethyl)-4-phenyl-4-acetoxy-piperidine

PEPC peptidase C
phosphoenol pyruvate carboxylase

PEPc corrected pre-ejection period

PEPCK phosphoenolpyruvate carboxykinase; also PEPK

PEPD peptidase D

PEPI pre-ejection period index

PEPK phosphoenolpyruvate carboxykinase; also PEPCK

PEP/LVET pre-ejection period/left ventricular ejection time

PEPP positive expiratory pressure plateau

PEPR precision encoder and pattern recognizer

PEPS peptidase S

PER peak ejection rate
pediatric emergency room
perineal; also per, peri
periodic evaluation record
postelectrophoresis relaxation
protein efficiency ratio
pudendal evoked response

per perineal; also PER, peri
periodic
periodicity
person
through, by [L. *per*]

per bid for a period of two days [L. *per bidum*]

PERC perceptual
percutaneous; also p cut
potential erythropoietin-responsive cell

perc disc percutaneous discectomy

percus percussion; also P, PERCUSS

PERCUSS percussion; also P, percus

PERD photoelectric registration device

perf perfect
perforation; also P

PERI peritoneal fluid; also PF, Peritf
Psychiatric Epidemiology Research Interview

peri perineal; also PER, per
peripheral; also P, p

periap periapical

perim perimeter

Peritf peritoneal fluid; also PERI, PF

Perio periodontics

PERK prospective evaluation of radial keratotomy

PERL pupils equal and react to light; also PEARL

PERLA pupils equal, react to light and accommodation

perm permanent
permutation

per op emet when the action of the emetic is over [L. *peracta operatione emetici*]

per os by mouth [L. per os]; also PO, po

perp perpendicular

Per pad, perpad perineal pad
PERR pattern evoked retinal response
PERRLA pupils equal, round, react to light and accommodation
PERS patient evaluation rating scale
pers personal
PERT program evaluation and review technique
pert pertussis (whooping cough)
PES photoelectron spectroscopy
postextrasystolic
pre-epiglottic space
pre-excitation syndrome
programmed electrical stimulation
programmed extrasystolic
pseudoexfoliation syndrome
PESP postextrasytolic potentiation
pe SPL peak equivalent sound pressure level
Pess pessary
PEST point estimation by sequential testing
PET parent effectiveness training
peak ejection time
pear-shaped extension tube
polyethylene terephthalates; also PETE
polyethylene tube
poor exercise tolerance
positron emission tomography
pre-eclamptic toxemia
pressure equalizing tube
progressive exercise test
Psychiatric Emergency Team
PETA pentaerythritol triacrylate
PETE polyethylene terephthalates; also PET
PETEG polyethylene terephthalate glycol
PETH pink-eyed, tan-hooded (rat)
PETLES peritoneal exudate T-lymphocyte-enriched system
PETN pentaerythritol tetranitrate
petr petroleum; also petrol
petrol petroleum; also petr
PETT pendular eye-tracking test
positron emission transaxial tomography
positron emission transverse tomography
PEU plasma equivalent unit
polyether urethane
PEV pulmonary extravascular fluid volume
PeV peripheral vein; also PV
pev, peV peak electron volt
PEVN periventricular nucleus

PEWV pulmonary extravascular water volume
PEx physical examination; also PE, PX, Px, px
PF parafascicular (nucleus)
parallel fiber
parotid fluid
partially follicular
patellofemoral (joint)
peak flow
pericardial fluid
peripheral field
peritoneal fluid; also PERI, Peritf
permeability factor
personality factor
phenol formaldehyde
L-phenylalanine mustard and 5-fluorouracil
physicians' forum
picture-frustration (study, test); also P-F
plantar flexion
plasma factor
plasma fibronectin
platelet factor
pleural fluid; also Pleur Fl, Plf
posterior fusion
power factor
precursor fluid
preservative free
proflavine
prostatic fluid
protection factor
pterygoid fossa
pulmonary blood flow; also PBF, Qp
pulmonary factor
pulmonary function
Purkinje fiber
purpura fulminans
push fluids
P-F picture-frustration (study, test); also PF
P/F pass/fail
PF$_{1-4}$ platelet factors 1 through 4
pF picofarad
PFA *para*-fluorophenylalanine
phosphonoformic acid
profunda femoris artery
PFAGH penalty, frustration, anxiety, guilt, hostility
PFAS performic acid-Schiff (reaction)
PFB properdin factor B
pseudofolliculitis barbae
PFC pelvic flexion contracture
perfluorocarbon
pericardial fluid culture
persistent fetal circulation
plaque-forming cell

pFc noncovalently bonded dimer of C-terminal immunoglobulin of Fc fragment

PFCPH persistent fetal circulation with pulmonary hypertension

PFD polyostotic fibrous dysplasia
primary flash distillate

PFEAAC posterior fossa extra-axial arachnoid cyst

PFFD proximal femur focal deficiency

PFFFP Pall-filtered fresh-frozen plasma

PFG peak-flow gauge
pulsed field gradient

PFH perifornical hypothalamus

PFI progression-free interval

PFIB perflouroisobutylene

PFJS patellofemoral joint syndrome

PFK phosphofructoaldolase
phosphofructokinase

PFKL phosphofructokinase, liver type

PFKM phosphofructokinase, muscle type

PFKP phosphofructokinase, platelet type

PFL Platinol, fluorouracil, and leucovorin calcium
profibrinolysin

PFM peak flow meter
porcelain fused to metal

PFN partially functional neutrophil

PFO patent foramen ovale

PFP pentafluoropropionyl
platelet-free plasma
pore-forming protein
preceding foreperiod

PFPC Pall-filtered packed cells

PFQ personality factor questionnaire

PFR parotid flow rate
peak filling rate
peak flow rate
pericardial friction rub

PFRC plasma-free red cell
predicted functional residual capacity

PFS penile flow study
primary fibromyalgia syndrome
protein-free supernatant
pulmonary function score

PFST positional feedback stimulation trainer

PFT pancreatic function test
parafascicular thalamotomy
posterior fossa tumor
prednisone, fluorouracil, and tamoxifen
pulmonary function test

PFT$_4$ proportion free thyroxin

PFTBE progressive form of tick-borne encephalitis

PFU plaque-forming unit(s); also pfu
pock-forming unit

pfu plaque-forming unit(s); also PFU

PFUO prolonged fever of unknown origin

PFV physiologic full value

PFW peak flow whistle

PFWB Pall-filtered whole blood

PG German Pharmacopeia [L. *Pharmacopoeia Germanica*]; also PhG
parapsoriasis guttata
paregoric
parotid gland
pentagastrin
pepsinogen
peptidoglycan
pergolide
phosphate glutamate
phosphatidyl-glycerol
phosphatidyl glycine
phosphogluconate
phosphoglycerate
pigment granule
pituitary gonadotropin
plasma gastrin
plasma glucose; also P$_G$
plasma triglyceride
polygalacturonate
postgraduate
postgraft
pregnanediol glucuronide
pregnant; also Pg, preg, pregn
propylene glycol
prostaglandin
proteoglycan
pyoderma gangrenosum

P$_G$ plasma glucose; also PG

3PG 3-phosphoglycerate

6PG 6-phosphogluconate

Pg gastric pressure
nasopharyngeal electrode placement in electroencephalography
petagram
pogonion; also Pog
pregnancy; also PR, preg, pregn
pregnant; also PG, preg, pregn
pregnenolone; also Pe

pg page; also P, p
picogram; also pgm

PGA phosphoglyceric acid
polyglandular autoimmune (syndrome)
polyglycolic acid
prostaglandin A
pteroylglutamic acid (folic acid)

PGA$_1$ prostaglandin A$_1$

PGA$_2$ prostaglandin A$_2$

PGA$_3$ prostaglandin A$_3$

PGAC phenylglycine acid chloride

PGAS persisting galactorrhea-amenorrhea syndrome

PGB prostaglandin B

PGB$_1$ prostaglandin B$_1$

PGB$_2$ prostaglandin B$_2$

PGC percentage of goblet cells
primordial germ cell
prostaglandin C
pure glycollide

PGC$_1$ prostaglandin C$_1$

PGC$_2$ prostaglandin C$_2$

PGC$_3$ prostaglandin C$_3$

PGD phosphogluconate dehydrogenase; also PDG, PGDH
phosphoglyceraldehyde dehydrogenase
prostaglandin D

PGD$_1$ prostaglandin D$_1$

PGD$_2$ prostaglandin D$_2$

PGDH phosphogluconate dehydrogenase; also PDG, PGD

PGDR plasma glucose disappearance rate

PGE platelet granule extract
posterior gastroenterostomy
primary generalized epilepsy
prostaglandin E

PGE$_1$ prostaglandin E$_1$

PGE$_2$ prostaglandin E$_2$

PGE$_3$ prostaglandin E$_3$

PGEM prostaglandin E metabolite

PGF paternal grandfather; also pgf
prostaglandin F

PGF$_1$ prostaglandin F$_1$

PGF$_{1\alpha}$ prostaglandin F$_1$ alpha

PGF$_2$ prostaglandin F$_2$

PGF$_{2\alpha}$ prostaglandin F$_2$ alpha

PGF$_3$ prostaglandin F$_3$

pgf paternal grandfather; also PGF

PGFM prostaglandin F and its metabolite

PGG polyclonal gamma globulin
prostaglandin G

PGG$_2$ prostaglandin G$_2$

PGH pituitary growth hormone
plasma growth hormone
porcine growth hormone
prostaglandin H

PGH$_2$ prostaglandin H$_2$

PGI pepsinogen I
phosphoglucose isomerase
potassium, glucose, and insulin
prostaglandin I

PGI$_2$ prostaglandin I$_2$ (prostacyclin)

PGK phosphoglycerate kinase
phosphoglycerokinase

PGL persistent generalized lymphadenopathy
phosphoglycolipid

PGlyM phosphoglyceromutase

PGM paternal grandmother; also pgm
phosphoglucomutase

pgm paternal grandmother; also PGM
picogram; also pg

PGMA polyglycerol methacrylate

PGN proliferative glomerulonephritis

PGO ponto-geniculo-occipital (spike)

PGP 3-phosphoglyceroyl phosphate
postgamma proteinuria
prepaid group practice; also PPGP

PGR progesterone receptor; also PgR
psychogalvanic response

PgR progesterone receptor; also PGR

P-GRN progranulocyte

PGS pineal gonadal syndrome
plant growth substance
prostaglandin synthetase
proteoglycan subunit

PGSR psychogalvanic skin resistance (test)
psychogalvanic skin response

PGT playgroup therapy

PGTR plasma glucose tolerance rate

PGTT prednisolone glucose tolerance test

PGU peripheral glucose uptake
postgonococcal urethritis

PGUT phosphogalactose uridyl transferase

PGV proximal gastric vagotomy

PGX prostaglandin X

PGY postgraduate year

PGYE peptone, glucose, and yeast extract (medium)

PH parathyroid hormone; also PTH
  partial hepatectomy
  partially hepatectomized
  passive hemagglutination; also PHA
  past history; also PHx, Px
  peliosis hepatitis
  perianal herpes
  persistent hepatitis
  personal history
  pharmacopeia; also P, Ph, PHAR, phar, pharm
  phenethicillin
  phenylalanine hydroxylase; also PAH
  pinhole
  polycythemia hypertonica
  poor health
  porphyria hepatica
  posterior hypothalamus
  post-history
  previous history
  primary hyperparathyroidism; also PHP, pHPT
  prolyl hydroxylase
  prostatic hypertrophy
  pseudohermaphroditism
  pubic hair
  public health
  pulmonary hypertension; also PHT
  punctate hemorrhage

Ph phalangeal amputation
  phalanx; also phal
  pharmacopeia; also P, PH, PHAR, phar, pharm
  phenanthrene
  phenyl
  phosphate; also P, p, phos

pH hydrogen ion concentration

Ph¹ Philadelphia chromosome

ph phase
  phial
  phote (unit of surface illumination)

PHA passive hemagglutination; also PH
  peripheral hyperalimentation
  phenylalanine; also F, P, PA, PHE, Phe
  phytohemagglutinin; also PHY, phy
  phytohemagglutinin activation
  phytohemagglutinin antigen
  pseudohypoaldosteronism
  pulse-height analyzer

pH$_A$ arterial blood hydrogen tension

pHa arterial pH

PHAL phytohemagglutinin-stimulated lymphocyte

phal phalanges
  phalanx; also Ph

PHAlb polymerized human albumin

PHA-M phytohemagglutinin M

PHA-m phytohemagglutinin-mucopolysaccharide (fraction)

PHA-P phytohemagglutinin-protein (fraction)

PHAR, phar pharmaceutical; also pharm
  pharmacopeia; also P, PH, Ph, pharm
  pharmacy; also PHARM, pharm
  pharynx; also Phx, phx

Phar B Bachelor of Pharmacy [L. *Pharmaciae Baccalaureus*]

Phar C Pharmaceutical Chemist; also PhC

Phar D Doctor of Pharmacy [L. *Pharmaciae Doctor*]; also PD, Pharm D, PhD

Phar G Graduate in Pharmacy; also PhG

Phar M Master of Pharmacy [L. *Pharmaciae Magister*]

PHARM pharmacy; also PHAR, phar, pharm

pharm pharmaceutical; also PHAR, phar
  pharmacopeia; also P, PH, Ph, PHAR, phar
  pharmacy; also PHAR, phar, PHARM

Pharm D Doctor of Pharmacy [L. *Pharmaciae Doctor*]; also PD, Phar D, PhD

PHB British Pharmacopoeia [L. *Pharmacopoeia Britannica*]; also BP, PB, PhB
  polyhydroxybutyrate
  preventive health behavior

PhB British Pharmacopoeia [L. *Pharmacopoeia Britannica*]; also BP, PB, PHB

PHBB propylhydroxybenzyl benzimidazole

PHC personal health cost
  posthospital care
  premolar aplasia, hyperhidrosis, and premature canities
  premolar hypodontia, hyperhidrosis, and canities prematura (Böök's syndrome)
  primary health care
  primary hepatic carcinoma
  primary hepatocellular carcinoma; also PHCC
  proliferative helper cell

PhC Pharmaceutical Chemist; also Phar C

PHCC primary hepatocellular carcinoma; also PHC

PHD photoelectron diffraction
  pulmonary heart disease

PhD Doctor of Pharmacy [L. *Pharmaciae Doctor*]; also PD, Phar D, Pharm D
Doctor of Philosophy [L. *Philosophiae Doctor*]

PHDD personal history of depressive disorders

PHDPE porous high-density polyethylene

PHE periodic health examination
phenylalanine; also F, P, PA, PHA, Phe
postheparin esterase
proliferative hemorrhagic enteropathy

Phe phenylalanine; also F, P, PA, PHA, PHE

PhEEM photoemission electron microscopy

PHF Potomac horse fever

Phen phenformin

Pheo, pheo pheochromocytoma; also PCC

PHF paired helical filaments
personal hygiene facility

PHFG primary human fetal glia (cells)

PhG German Pharmacopoeia [L. *Pharmacopoeia Germanica*); also PG
Graduate in Pharmacy; also Phar G

Phgly, phgly phenylglycine

PHH posthemorrhagic hydrocephalus

PHI passive hemagglutination inhibition
passive hemagglutination inhibitor
peptide histidine isoleucine
phosphohexoseisomerase
physiologic hyaluronidase inhibitor
prehospital index
Public Health Inspector

PhI International Pharmacopoeia [L. *Pharmacopoeia Internationalis*]; also PI

pH$_I$ isoelectric point; also PI, pIs

phial bottle [L. *phiala*]

PHIM posthypoxic intention myoclonus

PHIS post-head injury syndrome

PHK platelet phosphohexokinase
postmortem human kidney

PHKC postmortem human kidney cell

PHLA postheparin lipolytic activity

PHLS Public Health Laboratory Service (British)

PHM psyllium hydrophilic mucilloid
pulmonary hyaline membrane (syndrome)

PhM pharyngeal musculature

PHN passive Heymann nephritis
postherpetic neuralgia
public health nurse
public health nursing

PhNCS phenyl isothiocyanate; also PITC

PHO physician-hospital organization
public health official

PH$_2$O partial pressure of water vapor

phos phosphatase
phosphate; also P, p, Ph
phosphorus; also P, PHP

PHP passive hyperpolarizing potential
phosphorus; also P, phos
postheparin phospholipase
prehospital program
prepaid health plan
primary hyperparathyroidism; also PH, pHPT
pseudohypoparathyroidism; also PHPT

PHPA *para*-hydroxyphenylacetate; also PHPLA

PHPLA *para*-hydroxyphenylacetate; also PHPA

PHPP *para*-hydroxy-phenyl pyruvate oxidase; also p-HPPO

p-HPPO *para*-hydroxy-phenyl pyruvate oxidase; also PHPP

PHPPA *para*-hydroxyphenylpyruvic acid

PHPT pseudohypoparathyroidism; also PHP

pHPT primary hyperparathyroidism; also PH, PHP

PHPV persistent hyperplastic primary vitreous

PHR peak heart rate
photoreactivity

PHRT procarbazine, hydroxyurea, and radio-therapy (protocol)

PHS partial hospitalization program
patient-heated serum
phenylalanine hydroxylase stimulator
pooled human serum
posthypnotic suggestion
Public Health Service

PHSC pluripotent hemopoietic stem cell

pH-stat apparatus for maintaining pH of solution

PHT peroxide hemolysis test
phentolamine
phenytoin
portal hypertension; also PHTN
primary hyperthyroidism
pulmonary hypertension; also PH

PhTD Doctor of Physical Therapy

PHTN portal hypertension; also PHT

PHV persistent hypertrophic vitreous

PHx past history; also PH, Px

Phx, phx pharynx; also PHAR, phar
PHY pharyngitis
    physical; also Phys, phys
    physiology; also P, PHYS, Phys, phys,
        Physiol, physiol
    phytohemagglutinin; also PHA, phy
phy phytohemagglutinin; also PHA, PHY
PHYS physiology; also P, PHY, Phys, phys,
    Physiol, physiol
PhyS physiologic saline
Phys, phys physical; also PHY
    physician
    physiology; also P, PHY, PHYS, Physiol,
        physiol
phys dis physical disability
Phys Ed physical education; also PE, PEd,
    P Ed
physio physiologic
    physiotherapy; also PT
Physiol, physiol physiology; also P, PHY,
    PHYS, Phys, phys
Phys Med physical medicine; also PM
Phys Ther physical therapy; also PT
PI International Protocol [L. *Protocol*
    Internationalis]
    International Pharmacopoeia [L.
        Pharmacopoeia Internationalis]; also PhI
    isoelectric point; also pH_I, pIs
    pacing impulse
    package insert
    pancreatic insufficiency
    parainfluenza (virus)
    parallel importation
    pars intermedia
    paternity index
    patient's interest
    peptide inhibitor
    performance index
    performance intensity
    perinatal injury
    periodontal index
    peripheral iridectomy
    permanent incidence
    permeability index
    personal injury
    personality inventory
    phagocytic index
    phosphatidylinositol; also PtdIns
    physically impaired
    pineal body
    plaque index
    pneumatosis intestinalis

    poison ivy
    ponderal index
    postictal immobility
    postinfection
    post-injury
    postinoculation
    preinduction (examination)
    premature infant; also preemie
    prematurity index
    preparatory interval
    present illness
    pressure on inspiration
    primary infarction
    primary infection
    proactive inhibition
    proactive interference
    programmed instruction
    proinsulin
    prolactin inhibitor
    protamine insulin
    protease inhibitor; also Pi
    proximal intestine
    pulmonary incompetence
    pulmonary infarction
P_i inorganic phosphate; also Pi
Pi inorganic phosphate; also P_i
    pressure in inspiration
    protease inhibitor; also PI
pI pH value for isoelectric point
    platelet count increment; also pi
pi platelet count increment; also pI
PIA peripheral interface adapter
    phenylisopropyladenosine
    photoelectronic intravenous angiography
    plasma insulin activity
    porcine intestinal adenomatosis
    preinfarction angina
PIAT Peabody Individual Achievement Test
PIB psi-interactive biomolecules
PIC peripherally inserted catheter
    Personality Inventory for Children
    polymorphism information content
    postinflammatory corticoid
    postintercourse
PICA Porch Index of Communicative Ability
    posterior inferior cerebellar artery
    posterior inferior communicating artery
PICC peripherally inserted central catheter
PICD primary irritant contact dermatitis
PICU pediatric intensive care unit
    pulmonary intensive care unit

PID pain intensity difference (score)
pelvic inflammatory disease
photoionization detector
plasma iron disappearance
primary immunodeficiency disease
prolapsed intervertebral disk
proportional-integral-derivative
protruded intervertebral disk; also PIVD

PIDRA portable insulin dosage-regulating apparatus

PIDT plasma iron disappearance time

PIE postinfectious encephalomyelitis
preimplantation embryo
prosthetic infectious endocarditis
pulmonary infiltration with eosinophilia
pulmonary interstitial edema
pulmonary interstitial emphysema

PIEF isoelectric focusing in polyacrylamide

PIEP peripheral infarct epicardium

PIF peak inspiratory flow
pigment inspiratory factor
point of identical flow
premorbid inferiority feeling
proinsulin-free
prolactin-inhibiting factor
proliferation-inhibitory factor
prostatic interstitial fluid

PIFG poor intrauterine fetal growth

PIFR peak inspiratory flow rate

PIFT platelet immunofluorescence test

PIG pertussis immune globulin

Pig pigmentation

PIGI pregnancy-induced glucose intolerance

pigm pigment
pigmented

PIGPA pyruvate, inosine, glucose phosphate, adenine

PIH pregnancy-induced hypertension
prolactin-inhibiting hormone

PIHH postinfluenza-like hyposmia and hypogeusia

PII plasma inorganic iodine
primary irritation index

PIL patient information leaflet

Pil, pil pill
pills

PIIP portable insulin infusion pump

PIIS posterior inferior iliac spine

PIM penicillamine-induced myasthenia

PIMS programmable implantable medication system

PIN personal identification number

PINN proposed international nonproprietary name

PINS person in need of supervision

PINV postimperative negative variation

PIO progesterone in oil

PIO$_2$ inspired oxygen tension
intra-alveolar oxygen tension
partial pressure of inspiratory oxygen

PIP paralytic infantile paralysis
peak inflation pressure
peak inspiratory pressure
personal injury protection
phosphatidylinositol 4-phosphate
piperacillin
postinflammatory polyposis
postinfusion phlebitis
postinspiratory pressure
proximal interphalangeal (joint)
Psychotic Inpatient Profile

PIP$_2$ phosphatidylinositol 4,5-biphosphate

PIPA platelet ^{125}I-labeled staphylococcal protein A

PI-PB performance versus intensity function for phonetically balanced words

PIPIDA *N-para*-isopropylacetanilide-imino-diacetic acid (scan)

PIPJ proximal interphalangeal joint

pipsyl- *p*-iodophenyl sulfonyl-

PIQ Performance Intelligence Quotient

PIR piriform
postinhibition rebound
Protein Identification Resource

P-IRI plasma immunoreactive insulin

PIRS plasma immunoreactive secretion

PIS primary immunodeficiency syndrome
Provisional International Standard

pIs isoelectric point; also PI, pH$_I$

PISA phase-invariant signature algorithm

PISCES percutaneously inserted spinal cord electrical stimulation

PIT pacing-induced tachycardia
patellar inhibition test; also Pit
perceived illness threat
picture identification test
plasma iron turnover

Pit patellar inhibition test; also PIT

pit Pitocin
 pituitary
PITC phenyl isothiocyanate; also PhNCS
PIT (L) left partial inferior turbinectomy
PITP pseudoidiopathic thrombocytopenic
 purpura
PITR plasma iron turnover rate
PIT (R) right partial inferior turbinectomy
PITS parent-infant traumatic stress
PIU polymerase-inducing unit
PIV parainfluenza virus
 peripheral intravenous
PIVD protruded intervertebral disk; also PID
PIVH peripheral intravenous hyperalimentation
PIVKA protein-induced by vitamin K absence
 protein-induced by vitamin K antagonist
PIWT partially impacted wisdom teeth
PIXE particle-induced x-ray emission
 proton-induced x-ray emission; also PIXIE
pixel picture element
PIXIE proton-induced x-ray emission; also
 PIXE
PJ pancreatic juice
 Peutz-Jeghers (syndrome)
PJB premature junctional beat
PJC premature junctional contraction
PJP pancreatic juice protein
PJS peritoneojugular shunt
 Peutz-Jeghers syndrome
PJT paroxysmal junctional tachycardia
PJVT paroxysmal junctional-ventricular
 tachycardia
PK pack (cigarette)
 Parrot-Kauffman
 Paterson-Kelly (syndrome)
 penetrating keratoplasty; also PKP
 pericardial knock
 pharmacokinetic
 pig kidney
 Prausnitz-Küstner (reaction)
 protein kinase; also PKase
 psychokinesis
 psychokinetic
 pyruvate kinase
P$_K$ plasma potassium
P^k variant antigen in the P blood group system
pK ionization constant of acid
 negative logarithm of dissociation constant of
 an acid; also pK′

pK′ apparent value of pK
 negative logarithm of dissociation constant
 of an acid; also pK
pk peck
PKA prekallikrein activator
 prokininogenase
pKa measure of acid strength
pK$_a$ negative logarithm of acid ionization
 constant
pka International pressure units
PKAR protein kinase activation ratio
PKase protein kinase; also PK
PKB prone knee bend
PKC protein kinase C
PKD polycystic kidney disease; also PCKD
PKF phagocytosis and killing function
PKI potato kallikrein inhibitor
PKK plasma prekallikrein
 prekallikrein
PKN parkinsonism
PKP penetrating keratoplasty; also PK
PKR phased knee rehabilitation
PKT Prausnitz-Küstner test
PKU phenylketonuria
PKV killed poliomyelitis vaccine
pkV peak kilovoltage
PL palmaris longus
 pancreatic lipase
 perception of light
 peroneus longus
 phospholipase
 phospholipid; also PPL
 photoluminescence
 place; also pl
 placebo; also P, PBO, PLBO
 placental lactogen
 plantar
 plasmalemma
 plastic surgery; also PLS, PS, PSurg, P-Surg
 platelet(s); also pl, Plat, plats, PLT, Plt
 platelet lactogen
 plural; also pl
 polymer of lactic acid
 posterior lip (of acetabulum)
 preleukemia platelet
 premature labor
 problem list
 procaine and lactic acid
 product license
 psychosocial-labile

PL—cont'd
pulpolingual
pulpolinguoaxial; also PLA
Purkinje layer
transpulmonary pressure; also P_L, P_{TP}, P_{tp}

P_L pulmonary venous pressure; also PVP
transpulmonary pressure; also PL, P_{TP}, P_{tp}

PL/1 programming language 1

Pl petaliter
plasma; also P
Poiseuille (equation, law, space)

pL picoliter; also pl

pl picoliter; also pL
place; also PL
platelet(s); also PL, Plat, plats PLT, Plt
pleural; also PLEU
plural; also PL

PLA peroxidase-labeled antibodies (test)
phospholipase A
platelet antigen
polylactic acid
potentially lethal arrhythmia
pulpolabial; also PLa
pulpolinguoaxial; also PL

PLa pulpolabial; also PLA

Pla left atrial pressure

PLAP placental alkaline phosphatase; also PAP

Plat platelet(s); also PL, pl, plats, PLT, Plt

platinum/Vp-16 *cis*-diamminedichloro-
platinum (cisplatin) and VP-16-213
(etoposide)

PLAT-P plateau pressure

plats platelets; also PL, pl, Plat, PLT, Plt

PLAX parasternal long axis

PLB parietal lobe battery
phospholipase B
porous layer bead (in chromatography)

PLBO placebo; also P, PBO, PL

PLC personal locus of control
phospholipase C
primary liver cell
primed lymphocyte culture
proinsulin-like component
protein-lipid complex
pseudolymphocytic choriomeningitis

PLCC primary liver cell cancer

PLCL polyclonal gammopathy identified

PLCO postoperative low cardiac output

PL-CLP platelet clumps

PLD peripheral light detection
phospholipase D

platelet defect
posterior latissimus dorsi (muscle)
postlaser day
potentially lethal damage

PLDH plasma lactic dehydrogenase

PLDR potentially lethal damage repair

PLE panlobular emphysema
pleura
polymorphous light eruption; also PMLE
protein-losing enteropathy
pseudolupus erythematosus syndrome

PLED periodic lateralizing epileptiform
discharge

PLES parallel-line equal spacing

PLET polymyxin, lysozyme, EDTA, and
thallous acetate (in heart infusion agar)

PLEU pleural; also pl

Pleur Fl pleural fluid; also PF, Plf

PLEVA pityriasis lichenoides et varioliformis
acuta

PLF perilymphatic fistula
posterolateral fusion

Plf pleural fluid; also PF, Pleur Fl

PLFC premature living female child

PLG plasminogen

PLGV, P-LGV psittacosis–lymphogranuloma
venereum

PLH paroxysmal localized hyperhidrosis
placental lactogenic hormone

PLIF posterior lumbar interbody fusion
posterolateral interbody fusion

PLISSIT permission, limited information,
specific suggestions, intensive therapy

PLL peripheral light loss
poly-L-lysine
posterior longitudinal ligament
pressure length loop
prolymphocytic leukemia

PLM percentage of labeled mitoses
plasma level monitoring
polarized light microscopy

PLMC premature living male child

PLMT plasmacytoid lymphocyte

PLMV posterior-leaf mitral valve

PLN pelvic lymph node
peripheral lymph node
popliteal lymph node
posterior lip nerve

PLND pelvic lymph node dissection

PLO polycystic lipomembranous osteodysplasia

PLP paraformaldehyde-lysine-periodate
plasma leukapheresis
polystyrene latex particle(s)
proteolipid protein
pyridoxal phosphate; also PyrP

PLPD pseudoperiodic lateralized paroxysmal discharge

PLPI product license parallel importation

PLR product license of right
pronation-lateral rotation (fracture)
pupillary light reflex

PLS Papillon-Lefèvre syndrome
plastic surgery; also PL, PS, PSurg, P-Surg
preleukemic syndrome
Preschool Language Scale
primary lateral sclerosis
prostaglandin-like substance

pls please

PLSO posterior leafspring orthosis

PLT pancreatic lymphocytic infiltration
platelet(s); also PL, pl, Plat, plats, Plt
primed lymphocyte test
primed lymphocyte typing
psittacosis–lymphogranuloma venereum--trachoma (group)

Plt platelet(s); also PL, pl, Plat, plats, PLT

PLT EST platelet estimate

PLT-G giant platelet

plumb lead [L. *plumbum*]; also Pb

PLUT Plutchnik (geriatric rating scale)

PLV live poliomyelitis vaccine
panleukopenia virus
phenylalanine-lysine-vasopressin
posterior left ventricular

PLWS Prader-Labhart-Willi syndrome

plx plexus

PLYM prolymphocyte

PM after death [L. *post mortem*]
afternoon, evening [L. *post meridiem*]; also pm
pacemaker
papilla mammae
papillary muscle
papular mucinosis
paromomycin
partially muscular
partial meniscectomy
Pelizaeus-Merzbacher (disease)
perceptual motor

perinatal mortality; also PNM
peritoneal macrophage
petit mal (epilepsy)
photomultiplier (tube)
physical medicine; also Phys Med
plasma membrane
platelet membrane
platelet microsome
pneumomediastinum
poliomyelitis; also polio
polymorph
polymorphonuclear
polymyositis
poor metabolizer
porokeratosis of Mibelli
posterior mitral
postmenopausal
postmortem; also post
premamillary nucleus
premarketing (approval)
premolar; also P
presents mainly
presystolic murmur; also PSM
pretibial myxedema
preventive medicine; also PRM, PrM, PVMed
primary motivation
prostatic massage
protein methylesterase
pterygoid muscle
puberal macromastia
pulmonary macrophage
pulpomesial
purple membrane (protein)

P/M parent-metabolite ratio

Pm petameter
promethium

Pm² square petameter

Pm³ cubic petameter

pM picomolar

pm afternoon, evening [L. *post meridiem*]; also PM
picometer

pm² square picometer

pm³ cubic picometer

PMA papillary, marginal, attached (gingiva)
para-methoxyamphetamine
Pharmaceutical Manufacturers Association
phenylmercuric acetate; also PMAC
phorbol myristate acetate
phosphomolybdic acid
plasma membrane adenosinetriphosphatase
premenstrual asthma

PMA—cont'd
  Primary Mental Abilities (test)
  Prinzmetal's angina
  progressive muscular atrophy
  psychomotor agitation
  pyridylmercuric acetate

PMAC phenylmercuric acetate; also PMA

PMB papillomacular bundle
  para-hydroxymercuribenzoate
  polychrome methylene blue
  polymorphonuclear basophil(s)
  polymyxin B; also PB
  postmenopausal bleeding

PMC phenylmercuric chloride
  pleural mesothelial cell
  premature mitral closure
  pseudomembranous colitis

PMCP *para*-monochlorophenol

PMD perceptual motor development
  personal medical doctor
  posterior mandibular depth
  primary myocardial disease
  private medical doctor
  programmed multiple development (chromatography)
  progressive muscular dystrophy

PM/DM polymyositis/dermatomyositis

PMDS primary myelodysplastic syndrome

PME polymorphonuclear eosinophil(s)
  postmenopausal estrogen
  progressive myoclonus epilepsy

PMEA 9-(2-phosphonylmethoxyethyl)adenine

PMEC pseudomembranous enterocolitis

PMEDAP 9-(2-phosphonylmethoxyethyl)-2,6-diaminopurine

PMF Platinol, mitomycin C, and fluorouracil
  progressive massive fibrosis
  proton motive force; also pmf
  pterygomaxillary fossa

pmf proton motive force; also PMF

PMG *N*-phosphonomethylglycine

PMH past medical history; also PMHx
  posteromedial hypothalamus
  programmed medical history

PMHR predicted maximal heart rate

PMHx past medical history; also PMH

PMI past medical illness
  patient medical instructions
  patient medication instruction
  perioperative myocardial infarction
  phosphomannose isomerase
  plea of mental incompetence
  point of maximal impulse
  point of maximal intensity
  posterior myocardial infarction
  postmyocardial infarction
  present medical illness
  previous medical illness

PMIS postmyocardial infarction syndrome
  PSRO (Professional Standards Review Organization) Management Information System

PMK primary monkey kidney

PML polymorphonuclear leukocyte(s); also PMNL, POLY, poly
  posterior mitral leaflet
  progressive multifocal leukodystrophy
  progressive multifocal leukoencephalopathy
  pulmonary microlithiasis

pML posterior mitral valve leaflet; also PMVL, pMVL

PMLE polymorphous light eruption; also PLE

PMM pentamethylmelamine
  protoplast maintenance medium

PMMA polymethyl-methacrylate

PMMF pectoralis major myocutaneous flap

PMN polymorphonuclear; also POLY
  polymorphonuclear neutrophil(s); also M_7, PMNN
  polymorphonuclear neutrophilic (leukocyte)
  premanufacturing notification

PMNC percentage of multinucleated cells
  peripheral blood mononuclear cell; also PBMC
  pharmaceutical multinational company

PMNG polymorphonuclear granulocyte

PMNL polymorphonuclear leukocyte; also PML, POLY, poly

PMNN polymorphonuclear neutrophil(s); also M_7, PMN

PMNR periadenitis mucosa necrotica recurrens

PMO paramethadione
  perturbational molecular orbital
  postmenopausal osteoporosis
  Principal Medical Officer

pmol picomole

PMP pain management program
  past menstrual period
  patient management problem
  patient medication profile
  persistent mentoposterior (fetal position)
  previous menstrual period
  psychotropic medication plan

PMPO postmenopausal palpable ovary

PMQ phytylmenaquinone (vitamin K)

PMR patient medical record
perinatal morbidity rate
perinatal mortality rate
periodic medical review
physical medicine and rehabilitation; also PM&R
polymorphic reticulosis
polymyalgia rheumatica; also PR
prior medical record
proportionate morbidity ratio
proportionate mortality ratio
protein magnetic resonance
proton magnetic resonance
psychomotor retardation

PM&R physical medicine and rehabilitation; also PMR

PMRS physical medicine and rehabilitation service

PMS patient management system
phenazine methosulfate
postmarketing surveillance
postmenopausal stress
postmenopausal syndrome
postmitochondrial supernatant
pregnant mare's serum
premenstrual symptoms
premenstrual syndrome
pureed, mechanical, soft (diet)

PMSC pluripotent myeloid stem cell

PM-SCL polymyositis–scleroderma

PMSF phenylmethyl sulfonyl fluoride

PMSG pregnant mare's serum gonadotropin

PMT phenol-*o*-methyltransferase
photoelectric multiplier tube
photomultiplier tube
point of maximum tenderness
Porteus' maze test
premenstrual tension

PMTS premenstrual tension syndrome

PMTT pulmonary mean transit time

PMV paralyzed and mechanically ventilated
prolapse of mitral valve

PMVL, pMVL posterior mitral valve leaflet; also pML

PMW pacemaker wire(s)

PMZ pentamethylenetetrazol

PN nightmare [L. *pavor nocturnus*]
papillary necrosis
parenteral nutrition

Patte noire (test)
penicillin; also P, PC, Pc, PCN, pcn, Pen, pen, PNC
perceived noise
percussion note
percutaneous nephrostogram
periarteritis nodosa; also PAN
peripheral nerve
peripheral neuropathy; also PNP
peripheral node
phrenic nerve
plaque neutralization (test)
pneumonia; also Pn, pn, pneu, PNM
polyarteritis nodosa; also PAN
polynephritis
polyneuritis
pontine nucleus
poorly nourished
positional nystagmus
posterior nares
postnasal
postnatal
Practical Nurse
predicted normal
preemie nipple
primary nurse
progress note(s)
propoxyphene napsylate
psychiatry and neurology; also P&N
psychoneurotic
pulmonary disease; also PD, PUD, PuD
pyelonephritis
pyridine nucleotide
pyrrolnitrin

P/N positive to negative (ratio)

P&N psychiatry and neurology; also PN

P$_{N2}$ partial pressure of nitrogen

Pn, pn pneumonia; also PN, pneu, PNM

PNA Parisiensia Nomina Anatomica (Anatomical Names, Paris)
peanut agglutinin
pediatric nurse associate
pentosenucleic acid

PNA, P$_{Na}$ plasma sodium [L. *natrium* (sodium)]

PNAB percutaneous needle aspiration biopsy

PNAH polynuclear aromatic hydrocarbon

PNAS prudent no added salt (diet)

PNAvQ positive-negative ambivalent quotient

PNB percutaneous needle biopsy
polymyxin, neomycin, bacitracin
premature newborn
premature nodal beat

PNBT *para*-nitroblue tetrazolium

PNC penicillin; also P, PC, Pc, PCN, pcn, Pen, pen, PN
peripheral nerve conduction
peripheral nucleated cell
pneumotaxic center; also PC
postnecrotic cirrhosis
premature nodal contraction
prenatal care
purine nucleotide cycle

PND paroxysmal nocturnal dyspnea
pelvic node dissection
postnasal drainage; also PD
postnasal drip
postneonatal death
pregnancy, not delivered
pronatriodilatin

pnd pound; also L, lb, lib

PNdb perceived noise decibel

PNDO partial neglect of differential orbital

PNE plasma norepinephrine

PNET peripheral neuroectodermal tumor
permeative neuroectodermal tumor

PNET-MB permeative neuroectodermal tumor–medulloblastoma

pneu pneumonia; also PN, Pn, pn, PNM

PNF prenatal fluoride
proprioceptive neuromuscular facilitation (reaction)
proprioceptive neuromuscular fasciculation

PNG penicillin G
pneumogram

PNH paroxysmal nocturnal hemoglobinuria
polynuclear hydrocarbons

PNI peripheral nerve injury
postnatal infection
prognostic nutrition index
pseudoneointimal
psychoneuroimmunology

PNID Peer Nomination Inventory for Depression

PNK polynucleotide kinase

PNL percutaneous nephrostolithotomy; also PCNL
peripheral nerve lesion
polymorphonuclear neutrophilic leukocyte

PNLA percutaneous needle lung aspiration

PNM perinatal mortality; also PM
peripheral nerve myelin
pneumonia; also PN, Pn, pn, pneu
postneonatal mortality

PNMG persistent neonatal myasthenia gravis

PNMT phenylethanolamine-*N*-methyltransferase

PNO Principal Nursing Officer

PNP *para*-nitrophenol; also P-NP
peak negative pressure
Pediatric Nurse Practitioner
peripheral neuropathy; also PN
platelet neutralization procedure
polyneuropathy
progressive nuclear palsy
psychogenic nocturnal polydipsia
purine nucleoside phosphorylase
purine nucleotide phosphorylase

P-NP *para*-nitrophenol; also PNP

PNPB positive-negative pressure breathing

PNPG *para*-nitrophenyl-β-galactoside

p-NPGB *para*-nitrophenyl-*p*′guanidobenzoate

PNPP, pNPP, $_p$NPP *para*-nitrophenyl-phosphate

PNPR positive-negative pressure respiration

PNPS, P-NPS *para*-nitrophenylsulfate

PNRS premature nursery

PNS parasympathetic nervous system; also PSNS
partial nonprogressive stroke
peripheral nerve stimulator
peripheral nervous system
polynucleotide sequence
posterior nasal spine

PNT partial nodular transformation
percutaneous nephrostomy tube
patient; also P, PAT, Pnt, PT, Pt, pt

Pnt patient; also P, PAT, PNT, PT, Pt, pt

p-NTV *para*-nitrotetrazolium violet

PNU protein nitrogen unit

PNV prenatal vitamins

PNVX pneumococcus vaccine; also PV

Pnx pneumonectomy
pneumothorax; also PT, PTX, Px, px

PNZ posterior necrotic zone

PO by mouth, orally [L. *per os*]; also per os, po
parapineal organ
parietal operculum
parieto-occipital
perceptual organization
period of onset
perioperative
phone order; also P/O
physician only
portal

posterior; also P, post
postoperative; also P-O, POP, POp, postop, post-op
predominating organism

P-O postoperative; also PO, POP, POp, postop, post-op

P/O oxidative phosphorylation ratio
phone order; also PO
protein to osmolar (ratio)

P&O parasites and ova

PO₂, Po₂, P_{O2}, pO₂ partial pressure of oxygen

PO₄ phosphate

Po polonium
porion
position response

po by mouth, orally [L. *per os*]; also per os, PO

POA pancreatic oncofetal antigen
phalangeal osteoarthritis
point of application
preoptic area
primary optic atrophy

POAG primary open-angle glaucoma

POA-HA preoptic anterior hypothalamic area

POB penicillin, oil, beeswax
phenoxybenzamine; also PBZ
place of birth
prevention of blindness

POBE Profile of Out-of-Body Experience(s)

POC particulate organic carbon
postoperative care
potential operated channel
procarbazine, Oncovin, and CCNU (lomustine)
products of conception

Po/C ocular pressure

POCA 2-(5-[4-chlorophenyl] pentyl)oxirane-2-carboxylate

POCC procarbazine, Oncovin, CCNU (lomustine), and Cytoxan

Pocill, pocill small cup [L. *pocillum*]

Pocul, pocul cup [L. *poculum*]

POCY postoperative chronologic year

POD pacing on demand
peroxidase; also PX
place of death
podiatry; also Pod
polycystic ovary disease
postoperative day
postovulatory day

Pod podiatry; also POD

Pod D Doctor of Podiatry

PODx preoperative diagnosis

POE port of entry
position of ease
postoperative endophthalmitis
proof of eligibility

POEMS polyneuropathy, organomegaly, endocrinopathy, monoclonal gammopathy (M protein), skin changes (syndrome)

POET pulse oximeter/end tidal (carbon dioxide)

POEx postoperative exercise

POF position of function
primary ovarian failure
pyruvate oxidation factor

PofE portal of entry

POG Pediatric Oncology Group
polymyositis ossificans generalisata
products of gestation

Pog pogonion; also Pg

pOH hydroxyl ion concentration

POHI physically or otherwise health-impaired

POHS presumed ocular histoplasmosis syndrome

POI Personal Orientation Inventory

POIK, poik poikilocyte
poikilocytosis

pois poison; also P
poisoned; also P
poisoning; also P

POL premature onset of labor

pol polish
polishing

polio poliomyelitis; also PM

POLY polymorphonuclear; also PMN
polymorphonuclear leukocyte; also PML, PMNL, poly

poly polymorphonuclear leukocyte; also PML, PMNL, POLY

poly-A, poly(A) polyadenylate
polyadenylic acid

poly-C, poly(C) polycytidylic acid

POLY-CHR polychromatophilia

poly-G, poly(G) polyguanylic acid

poly-I, poly(I) polyinosinic acid

poly-IC copolymer of poly-I and poly-C; also poly-I:C

poly-I:C copolymer of poly-I and poly-C; also poly-IC

% POLYS percent of polymorphonuclear leukocytes

polys polymorphonuclear leukocytes

polys(segs) polymorphonuclear segmented neutrophils

poly-T, poly(T) polythymidylic acid

poly-U, poly(U) polyuridylic acid

POM pain on motion
polyoximethylene
prescription only medicine

POMC propiomelanocortin

POMP prednisone, Oncovin, methotrexate, and Purinethol (6-mercaptopurine)
principal outer material protein

POMR problem-oriented medical record; also POR

POMS Profile of Mood States

PON paraxonase
particulate organic nitrogen

Pond, pond by weight [L. *pondere*]; also P, p

PONI postoperative narcotic infusion

POOH postoperative open-heart (surgery)

POOR poor clot

POP diphosphate group; also PP
pain on palpation
paroxypropione
persistent occipitoposterior (fetal position)
pituitary opioid peptide
plasma oncotic pressure
plasma osmotic pressure
plaster of paris; also PP
polymyositis ossificans progressiva
popliteal; also Pop, pop, poplit
postoperative; also PO, P-O, POp, postop, post-op

POp postoperative; also PO, P-O, POP, postop, post-op

Pop popliteal; also POP, pop, poplit
population; also P

pop popliteal; also POP, Pop, poplit

poplit popliteal; also POP, Pop, pop

POPOP 1,4-bis(5-phenoxazol-2-yl) benzene 2,2'-(phenylene)-bis(5-phenyloxazole)

POR physician of record
postocclusive oscillatory response
problem-oriented medical record; also POMR

PORH postocclusive reactive hyperemia

PORP partial ossicular replacement prosthesis

Porph porphyrin(s); also P

PORT perioperative respiratory therapy
postoperative respiratory therapy

port portable

POS paraosteal osteosarcoma
polycystic ovary syndrome; also PCOS
positive; also P, pos
psycho-organic syndrome

pos position; also P
positive; also P, POS

POSC problem-oriented system of charting

POSM patient-operated selector mechanism

Pos pr, pos pr positive pressure

POSS percutaneous on-surface stimulation
proximal over-shoulder strap

poss possible

post posterior; also P, PO
postmortem; also PM

post aur behind the ear [L. *post aurem*]; also p aur

postgangl postganglionic

postop, post-op postoperative; also PO, P-O, POP, POp

post prand after meals [L. *post prandia*]; also PP, pp, p̄p̄, PPD

POSTS positive occipital sharp transients of sleep

post sag D posterior sagittal diameter; also PSD

post sing sed liq after every loose stool [L. *post singulas sedes liquidas*]

POT periostitis ossificans toxica
postoperative treatment
potion[L. *potio* (a draft, a large dose of medicine to be taken at once)]; also pot
purulent otitis media

pot a drink [L. *potus*]
potash
potassa
potassium; also K, potass
potential; also poten
potion [L. *potio* (a draft, large dose of medicine to be taken at once)]; also POT

potass potassium; also K, pot

PotAGT, pot AGT potential abnormality of glucose tolerance

poten potential; also pot

POU placenta, ovaries, and uterus

PoV portal vein; also PV

POVT puerperal ovarian vein thrombophlebitis

POW Powassan's (encephalitis, virus)
prisoner of war

powd powder; also pdr, pulv, pwd

PP diphosphate group; also POP
near point (of accommodation) [L. *punctum proximum*]; also P, p, pp
pacesetter potential; also PSP
pancreatic polypeptide
paradoxical pulse
parietal pleura
partial pressure (of a gas); also P, p
pathology point
pedal pulse
pellagra preventive
pentose pathway
perfusion pressure
peripheral pulse
peritoneal pseudomyxoma
permanent partial
persisting proteinuria
Peyer's patch
phosphorylase phosphatase
pink puffer(s) (emphysema)
pinpoint
pinprick
placental protein
plane polarization
planned parenthood
plasma pepsinogen
plasmapheresis
plasma protein
plaster of paris; also POP
polypeptide
polystyrene agglutination plate
poor person
population planning
porcine pancreatic
posterior papillary
posterior pituitary
postpartum; also pp
postprandial [L. *post prandia* (after meals)];
also pp, p̄p̄, PPD, post prand
preferred provider
presenting part
private practice
private patient; also pp
prothrombin-proconvertin; also PTP
protoporphyria
protoporphyrin; also PROTO
proximal phalanx
pseudomyxoma peritonei
pterygoid process
pulse pressure
pulsus paradoxus
purulent pericarditis

push pills
pyrophosphate; also PYP, Pyro

P&P pins and plaster
policy and procedure
prothrombin and proconvertin (test)

PP$_i$ inorganic pyrophosphate

P-5′-P pyridoxal-5′-phosphate

PP5 placental protein 5

pp near point (of accommodation) [L. *punctum proximum*]; also P, p, PP
pages
polyphosphate
postpartum; also PP
postpill (amenorrhea)
postprandial [L. *post prandia* (after meals)];
also PP, p̄p̄, PPD, post prand
private patient; also PP

p̄p̄ postprandial (after meals) [L. *post prandia* (after meals)]; also PP, pp, PPD, post prand

PPA after shaking or shake well [L. *phiala prius agitata* (the vessel first having been shaken)]; also ppa
palpation, percussion, and auscultation;
also PP&A, pp&a
pepsin A
phenylpropanolamine
phenylpyruvic acid
Pittsburgh pneumonia agent
polyphosphoric acid
postpartum amenorrhea
postpill amenorrhea
pure pulmonary atresia

PP&A, pp&a palpation, percussion, and auscultation; also PPA

P$_{PA}$, P$_{Pa}$ pulmonary artery pressure; also PAP

ppa after shaking or shake well [L. *phiala prius agitata* (the vessel first having been shaken)]; also PPA

PPAS peripheral pulmonary artery stenosis
postpolio atrophy syndrome

PPB parts per billion; also ppb
platelet-poor blood
positive pressure breathing

ppb parts per billion; also PPB

PPBE postpartum breast engorgement
proteose-peptone beef extract

PPBS postprandial blood sugar

PPC pentose phosphate cycle
plasma prothrombin conversion
plaster of paris cast
platinum-palladium colloid

PPC—cont'd
pneumopericardium
pooled platelet concentrate
progressive patient care
proximal palmar crease

PPCA plasma prothrombin conversion
accelerator
proserum prothrombin conversion accelerator

PPCE postproline cleaving enzyme

PPCF peripartum cardiac failure
plasmin prothrombin conversion factor

PPCH piperazinylmethyl cyclohexanone

PPCM postpartum cardiomyopathy

PPD packs per day (cigarettes); also P/D,
p/d, ppd
paraphenylenediamine
percussion and postural drainage; also P&PD
permanent partial disability
phenyldiphenyloxadiazole
posterior polymorphous dystrophy
postpartum day
postprandial [L. *post prandia* (after meals)];
also PP, pp, p̄ p̄, post prand
primary physical dependence
progressive perceptive deafness
Seibert's purified protein derivative (tuberculin)

P&PD percussion and postural drainage;
also PPD

ppd packs per day (cigarettes); also P/D,
p/d, PPD
prepared (for procedure); also Ppt, ppt,
prepd, prepped

PPD-B purified protein derivative, Battey

PPDR preproliferative diabetic retinopathy

PPD-S purified protein derivative, standard

PPE partial plasma exchange
permeability pulmonary edema
polyphosphoric ester
porcine pancreatic elastase
programmed physical examination

PPF pellagra preventive factor
phagocytosis-promoting factor
plasma protein fraction

PPFA Planned Parenthood Federation of
America

PPG photoplethysmography
polymorphonuclear cells per glomerulus
polyurethane-polyvinyl graphite
postprandial glucose
pretragal parotid gland

ppg picopicogram

PPGA postpill galactorrhea/amenorrhea

PPGF polypeptide growth factor

PPGI psychophysiologic gastrointestinal
(reaction)

PPGP prepaid group practice; also PGP

ppGpp guanosine 3′,5′-diphosphate

PPH persistent pulmonary hypertension
postpartum hemorrhage
primary pulmonary hypertension
protocollagen proline hydroxylase

pphm parts per hundred million

PPHN persistent pulmonary hypertension
of the newborn

PPHP pseudopseudohypoparathyroidism

ppht parts per hundred thousand

PPHx previous psychiatric history

PPI partial permanent impairment
patient package insert
plan-position-indication
potato protease inhibitor
preceding preparatory interval
preproinsulin
present pain intensity
purified porcine insulin

PPi, PP$_i$ inorganic pyrophosphate; also IPP

PPID peak pain intensity difference (score)

PPIM postperinatal infant mortality

PPK palmoplantar keratosis
partial penetrating keratoplasty

PPL pars plana lensectomy
penicilloyl-polylysine
phospholipid; also PL
protein polysaccharide

Ppl intrapleural pressure

PPLF postperfusion low flow

PPLO pleuropneumonia-like organism(s)

PPM parts per million; also ppm
permanent pacemaker
phosphopentomutase
pigmented pupillary membrane
posterior papillary muscle

ppm parts per million; also PPM
pulses per minute

PPMA postpoliomyelitis muscular atrophy
progressive postmyelitis muscular atrophy

PPMD posterior polymorphous dystrophy of
cornea

PPMM postpolycythemia myeloid metaplasia

PPMS psychophysiologic musculoskeletal (reaction)

PPN partial parenteral nutrition
pedunculopontine nucleus
pyramidopallidonigral

PPNA peak phrenic nerve activity

PPNAD primary pigmented nodular adreno-cortical disease

PPNG penicillinase-producing *Neisseria gonorrhoeae*

PPO 2,5-diphenyloxazole (scintillator)
peak pepsin output
platelet peroxidase
pleuropneumonia organism
preferred provider organization

PPP palatopharyngoplasty
palmoplantar pustulosis
Pariser-Parr-Pople (method in quantum chemistry)
passage, power, and passenger (progress of labor)
pedal pulse present
pentose phosphate pathway
peripheral pulse palpable
Pickford projective pictures
plasma protamine precipitating
platelet-poor plasma
polyphoretic phosphate
porcine pancreatic polypeptide
postpartum psychosis
protamine paracoagulation phenomenon
purified placental protein
pustulosis palmaris et plantaris

PPPBL peripheral pulses palpable both legs

PPPG postprandial plasma glucose

PPPH purified placental protein, human

PPPI primary private practice income

PPPPP pain, pallor, pulse loss, paresthesia, and paralysis

PPPPPP pain, pallor, pulse loss, paresthesia, paralysis, and prostration

PPR patient-physician relationship
patient progress record
photopalpebral reflex
poor partial response
Price precipitation reaction

PPr paraprosthetic

PPRC Physician Payment Review Commission

PPRF paramedian pontine reticular formation
postpartum renal failure

PPRibp 5-phospho-α-D-ribosyl pyrophosphate; also PPRP

PPROM prolonged premature rupture of membranes

PPRP 5-phospho-α-D-ribosyl pyrophosphate; also PPRibp

PPRWP poor precordial R-wave progression

PPS pepsin
pepsin A
peripheral pulmonary stenosis
Personal Preference Scale
phosphoribosylpyrophosphate synthetase
polyvalent pneumococcal polysaccharide
postpartum sterilization
postperfusion syndrome
postpericardiotomy syndrome
postpolio syndrome
postpump syndrome
primary acquired preleukemic syndrome
primary physician services
prospective payment system
prospective pricing system
protein plasma substitute

PPSB prothrombin, proconvertin, Stuart factor, antihemophilic B factor

PPSH pseudovaginal perineoscrotal hypospadias

PPT parietal pleural tissue
partial prothrombin time
peak-to-peak threshold
plant protease test
potassium phosphotungstate
preprotachykinin
pulmonary platelet trapping

Ppt, ppt precipitate; also pcpt, precip
precipitation; also pcpn, pcpt, pptn, precip
prepared (for procedure) [L. *praeparatus*]; also ppd, prepd, prepped

pptd precipitated; also precip

pptg precipitating

PPTL postpartum tubal ligation

pptn precipitation; also pcpn, pcpt, Ppt, ppt, precip

PPTT postpartum painless thyroiditis with transient thyrotoxicosis

PPU perforated peptic ulcer

PPV porcine parvovirus
positive predictive value
positive-pressure ventilation
progressive pneumonia virus

PPVT Peabody Picture Vocabulary Test

PPVT-R Peabody Picture Vocabulary Test, Revised

Ppw pulmonary wedge pressure; also PWP

PPZ perphenazine

PPZSO perphenazine sulfoxide

PQ paraquat
permeability quotient
plastoquinone
pronator quadratus
pyrimethamine-quinine

PQ-9 plastoquinone-9

PQD protocol data query

PQNS protein, quantity not sufficient

PQQ pyrroloquinolinequinone (coenzyme)

PR by way of rectum [L. *per rectum*]; also pr, p rec, pro rect
far point (of accommodation) [L. *punctum remotum*]; also pr
Panama red (variety of marijuana)
parallax and refraction
pars recta
partial reinforcement; also PRF
partial remission
partial response
pathology report
patient relations
peer review
pelvic rock
percentile rank
peripheral resistance
peripheral rheumatism
phenol red
photoreaction
photoreactivating
photoreactivation
physical rehabilitation
physician reviewer
pityriasis rosea
polymyalgia rheumatica; also PMR
posterior root
postural reflex
potency ratio
potential relation
prednisone; also P, PDN, PRED, pred
preference record (test)
pregnancy; also Pg, preg, pregn
pregnancy rate
premature; also Pr, prem
presbyopia; also P, Pr
pressoreceptor
pressure; also P, p, press
prevention; also prev
Preyer's reflex

proctologist; also Pr
proctology; also Proct
production rate
professional relations
profile
progesterone receptor
progressive relaxation
progressive resistance
prolactin; also P, Pr, PRL, Prl
prolonged remission
propicillin
propranolol; also PROP
prosthion
protein; also P, Pr, PRO, pro, Prot, prot
psychotherapy responder
public relations
Puerto Rican
pulmonary regurgitation
pulmonary rehabilitation
pulse rate
pulse repetition
pyramidal response

P-R time between P wave and beginning of QRS complex in electrocardiography

P/R productivity to respiration (ratio)

P&R pelvic and rectal (examination)
pulse and respiration

Pr praseodymium
premature; also PR, prem
presbyopia; also P, PR
primary; also P, prim
prism
proctologist; also PR
production rate (of steroid hormones)
prolactin; also P, PR, PRL, Prl
propyl (normal)
protein; also P, PR, PRO, pro, Prot, prot

pr by way of rectum [L. *per rectum*]; also PR, p rec, pro rect
far point (of accommodation) [L. *punctum remotum*]; also PR
pair; also PAR

PRA panel reactive antibodies
percent reactive antibody (cytotoxic screen)
phonation, respiration, articulation-resonance
phosphoribosylamine
plasma renin activity
progesterone receptor assay

PRACT practolol

prac practice; also pract
practioner; also pract

pract practice; also prac
practitioner; also prac

PrA-HPA protein A hemolytic plaque assay

prand dinner [L. *prandium*]

PRAS prereduced anaerobically sterilized (media)

PRAT platelet radioactive antiglobulin test

p rat aetat in proportion to age [L. *pro ratione aetatis*]

PRB Population Reference Bureau
Prosthetics Research Board

PRBC packed red blood cells; also PRC

PRBV placental residual blood volume

PRC packed red blood cells; also PRBC
peer review committee
phase response curve
plasma renin concentration
prime responder cell

PRCA pure red cell agenesis
pure red cell aplasia

PRCN porcine respiratory coronavirus

PRD partial reaction of degeneration
phosphate restricted diet
polycystic renal disease
postradiation dysplasia

PRE passive resistance exercise
photoreacting enzyme
physical reconditioning exercise
pigmented retina epithelial (cell)
progressive resistive exercise

pre preliminary; also prelim

pre-AIDS pre-acquired immune deficiency syndrome

p rec by way of rectum [L. *per rectum*]; also PR, pr, pro rect

precip precipitate; also pcpt, Ppt, ppt
precipitated; also pptd
precipitation; also pcpn, pcpt, Ppt, ppt, pptn

PRED prednisone; also P, PDN, PR, pred

pred predicted
prednisone; also P, PDN, PR, PRED

PREE partial reinforcement extinction effect

preemie premature infant; also PI

prefd preferred

PREG pregnelone

preg pregnancy; also Pg, PR, pregn
pregnant; also PG, Pg, pregn

pregn pregnancy; also Pg, PR, preg
pregnant; also PG, Pg, preg

prelim preliminary; also pre

prem premature; also PR, Pr
prematurity

preop, pre-op preoperative

prep preparation; also prepn
preparatory
prepare (for procedure)
preposition

prepd prepared (for procedure); also ppd, Ppt, ppt, prepped

prepped prepared (for procedure); also ppd, Ppt, ppt, prepd

prepn preparation; also prep

PRERLA pupils round, equal, react to light and accommodation

PREs progressive resistive exercises (ophthalmology)

pres president

preserv preservation
preserve

press pressure; also P, p, PR

prev prevention; also PR
preventive
previous

PrevAGT, prev AGT previous abnormality of glucose tolerance

PREVMEDU preventive medicine unit

PRF partial reinforcement; also PR
patient report form
pontine reticular formation
progressive renal failure
prolactin-releasing factor
pyrogen-releasing factor

pRF polyclonal rheumatoid factor

PRFA plasma-recognition-factor activity

PRFM premature rupture of fetal membranes; also PROM
prolonged rupture of fetal membranes; also PROM

PRFN percutaneous radiofrequency

PRFR pressure-retaining flow-relieving

PRFRT partially relaxed Fourier transform

PRG phleborheogram
phleborheography
purge

PRGI percutaneous retrogasserian glycerol injection

PRH past relevant history
preretinal hemorrhage
prolactin-releasing hormone

PRHBF peak reactive hyperemia blood flow

PRI Pain Rating Index
personal resource inventory
phosphate reabsorption index
phosphoribose isomerase
plexus rectales inferiores

PRIAS Packard's radioimmunoassay system

PRIH prolactin release-inhibiting hormone

prim primary; also P, Pr

PRIME Prematriculation Program in Medical Education

primip primipara (woman bearing first child); also I-para, P, PRIMP

prim luc early in the morning [L. *prima luce* (at first light)]

prim m first thing in the morning [L. *primo mane*]

PRIMP primipara (woman bearing first child); also I-para, P, primip

primus the first [L. *primus*]

PRIND prolonged reversible ischemic neurologic deficit

PRISM Pediatric Risk of Mortality Score

PRIST paper radioimmunosorbent technique
paper radioimmunosorbent test

prius before, former [L. *prius*]

priv private (patient, room); also P, PVT, pvt

PRK primary rabbit kidney

PRL, Prl prolactin; also P, PR, Pr

PRLA pupils react to light and accommodation

PRM phosphoribomutase
photoreceptor membrane
premature rupture of membranes
preventive medicine; also PM, PrM, PVMed
Primary Reference Material
primidone

PrM preventive medicine; also PM, PRM, PVMed

PRM-SDX pyrimethamine sulfadoxine; also PRM-SOX

PRM-SOX pyrimethamine sulfadoxine; also PRM-SDX

PRN as the occasion arises, as necessary [L. *pro re nata*]; also prn
polyradiculoneuropathy

prn as the occasion arises, as necessary [L. *pro re nata*]; also PRN

PRNT plaque reduction neutralization test

PRO peer review organization
professional review organization

projection
prolapse
pronation; also pron
pronator; also pron
protein; also P, PR, Pr, pro, Prot, prot

Pro proline; also P
prophylactic; also prop, proph, prophy
prophylaxis; also prop
prothrombin

pro protein; also P, PR, Pr, PRO, Prot, prot

prob probability; also P, *P*, p, *p*
probable
problem

PROC, Proc procarbazine; also PCB, PCZ, Procarb

proc procedure
proceedings
process

Proc AACR Proceedings of the American Association for Cancer Research

Procarb procarbazine; also PCB, PCZ, PROC, Proc

Proc ASCO Proceedings of the American Society of Clinical Oncology

Proct proctology; also PR

procto proctoscopy

prod product; also P
production

pro dos for a dose [L. *pro dose*]

Pro El protein electrophoresis; also PE, PEP

prof professor
professorship

PROG progesterone; also P, P_4
prognathism
program
progressive

prog prognosis; also progn, Px, px

progn prognosis; also prog, Px, px

progr progress

prolong prolongation
prolonged

PROM passive range of motion
premature rupture of fetal membranes; also PRFM
programmable read-only memory
prolonged rupture of fetal membranes; also PRFM

ProMACE prednisone, methotrexate, Adriamycin, cyclophosphamide, etoposide, and leucovorin calcium

ProMACE-CytaBOM ProMACE + cytarabine, bleomycin, and Oncovin

ProMACE-MOPP ProMACE + mechlorethamine, Oncovin, procarbazine, and prednisone

PROMIN programmable multiple ion monitor

PROMIS Problem-oriented Medical Information System

Promy promyelocyte

pron pronation; also PRO
pronator; also PRO

PROP propranolol; also PR

prop prophylactic; also Pro, proph, prophy
prophylaxis; also Pro

ProPAC, ProPac Prospective Payment Assessment Commission

proph prophylactic; also Pro, prop, prophy

prophy prophylactic; also Pro, prop, proph

PROPLA prophospholipase A

pro rat aet according to age [L. *pro ratione aetatis*]

pro rect by rectum [L. *pro recto*]; also PR, pr, p rec

PROSO protamine sulfate; also PS

pros prostate; also prostat
prostatic; also prostat

prostat prostate; also pros
prostatic; also pros

prosth prothesis
prosthetic

Prot, prot protein; also P, PR, Pr, PRO, pro

pro time, pro-time, proTime, protime prothrombin time; also PT

PROTO protoporphyrin; also PP

pro-UK prourokinase

pro us ext for external use [L. *pro usu externo*]

prov provisional (diagnosis)

PROVIMI proteins, vitamins, and minerals; also PVM

prox proximal; also P

proximal/3 proximal third (of bone); also P_3, P/3

prox luc the day before [L. *proxima luce*]

PRP panretinal photocoagulation
penicillinase-resistant penicillin
phosphosylribitol phosphate
physiologic rest position
pityriasis rubra pilaris
platelet-rich plasma
polymer of ribose phosphate
polyribophosphate
polyribosyl ribitol phosphate
postreplication repair
postural rest position
pressure rate product
problem reporting program
progressive rubella panencephalitis
proliferative retinopathy photocoagulation
proline-rich protein
Psychotic Reaction Profile
pulse repetition frequency

PRPP 5′-phosphoribosyl-1-pyrophosphate

PRR proton relaxation rate

PRRE pupils round, regular, and equal

PR-RSV Prague Rous sarcoma virus

PRS parents' rating scale
Personality Rating Scale
plasma renin substrate
positive rolandic spike
pupil rating scale

PRSA plasma renin substrate activity

PRSIS Prospective Rate Setting Information System

PRSM peripheral smear; also PS

PRSP penicillinase-resistant synthetic penicillin

PRT *Penicillium roqueforti* toxin
pharmaceutical research and testing
phosphoribosyltransferase; also PRTase
photoradiation therapy
postoperative respiratory treatment

PRTA proximal renal tubular acidosis

PRTase phosphoribosyltransferase; also PRT

PRTH-C prothrombin time control; also PT-C, PT-CT

PRU peripheral resistance unit

PRV polycythemia rubra vera
pseudorabies virus

PRVEP pattern reversal visual evoked potential(s)

PRVR peak-to-resting velocity ratio

PrVS prevesicle space

PRW polymerized ragweed

PRWP poor R-wave progression (electrocardiogram)

PRZ prazepam

PRZF pyrazofurin

PS Paget-Schroetter (syndrome)
Paltauf-Sternberg (disease)
paired stimulation
paradoxical sleep
paralaryngeal space
paranoid schizophrenia
paraseptal
parasternal
parasympathetic (division of autonomic nervous system); also parasym
partial shoulder
pathologic stage
patient's serum (crossmatch)
pediatric surgery; also PDS, PdS
Pellegrini-Stieda (disease)
performance status
performing scale (IQ)
periodic syndrome
peripheral smear; also PRSM
permeability surface
phosphate saline (buffer)
phosphatidyl serine
photosynthesis
phrenic nerve stimulation
physical status
pigeon serum
plastic surgery; also PL, PLS, PSurg, P-surg
point of symmetry
polysaccharide
polystyrene; also PS1
population sample
Porter-Silber (chromogen); also P-S
postanesthesia shivering
postmaturity syndrome
pregnancy serum
prescription; also Ps, Rx
pressure support
prestimulus
principal sulcus
programmed symbols
prostatic secretion
protamine sulfate; also PROSO
protective services
protein synthesis
Pseudomonas species, also Ps, *Ps*
psychiatric; also P, PSY, Psy, psychiat
psychiatry; also *Ψ*, P, PSY, Psy, psychiat
pulmonary stenosis
pulse sequence
pyloric stenosis

P-S pancreozymin-secretin
Porter-Silber (chromogen); also PS
pyramid surface

P/S polisher-stimulator
polyunsaturated to saturated (fatty acid ratio)

P&S pain and suffering
paracentesis and suction
permanent and stationary
pharmacy and supply

PS1 polystyrene; also PS

Ps prescription; also PS, Rx
pseudocyst; also PC
Pseudomonas species; also PS, *Ps*

Ps *Pseudomonas* species, also PS, Ps

ps per second
picosecond; also psec

PSA paired sample advised (acute & convalescent)
picryl sulfonic acid
polyethylene sulfonic acid
product selection allowed
progressive spinal ataxia
prolonged sleep apnea
prostate specific antigen
public service announcement

PsA psoriatic arthritis

Psa systemic blood pressure; also SBP

PSAGN poststreptococcal acute glomerulonephritis

PSAn psychoanalysis; also PA, psychoan, PYA
psychoanalytic

PSAP prostate specific acid phosphatase
pulmonary surfactant apoprotein

PSAX parasternal short axis

PSB protected specimen brush

PSBO partial small-bowel obstruction

PSC partial subligamentous calcification
patient services coordination
physiologic squamocolumnar
pluripotential stem cell
Porter-Silber chromogen
posterior semicircular canal
posterior subcapsular cataract; also PSCC
primary sclerosing cholangitis
pulse-synchronized contractions

PSCC posterior subcapsular cataract; also PSC

PSCE presurgical coagulation evaluation

PsChE pseudocholinesterase; also PCE, PCHE

Psci pressure at slow component intercept

PSCM pokeweed-activated spleen-conditioned medium

PSCP posterior subscapular cataractous plaque

PSCT peripheral stem cell transplant

P/score pressure score

PSD particle size distribution
peptone-starch-dextrose
periodic synchronous discharge
phosphate supplemental diet
photon-stimulated desorption
posterior sagittal diameter; also post sag D
poststenotic dilation
postsynaptic density

PSDES primary symptomatic diffuse
esophageal spasm

PSE paradoxical systolic expansion
partial splenic embolization
penicillin-sensitive enzyme
point of subjective equality
portal systemic encephalopathy
postshunt encephalopathy
proximal stimulating electrode
purified spleen extract

PSEC poststress ethanol consumption

psec picosecond; also ps

PSF peak scatter factor
point spread function
posterior spinal fusion
prostacyclin production-stimulating factor
pseudosarcomatous fasciitis

psf pounds per square foot

PSG peak systolic gradient
phosphate, saline, glucose
polysomnogram
presystolic gallop

PSGN poststreptococcal glomerulonephritis

PSH past surgical history
postspinal headache (anesthetic)

PsHD pseudoheart disease

PSI personal security index
physiologic stability index
posterior sagittal index
posterior-superior iliac (spine)
pounds per square inch; also lb/in^2, psi
Problem Solving Information
prostaglandin synthetic inhibitor
psychologic screening inventory
psychosomatic inventory

psi pounds per square inch; also lb/in^2, PSI

psia pounds per square inch absolute

PSIFT platelet suspension immunofluorescence test

psig pounds per square inch gauge

PSIL preferred frequency speech interference
level

PSIS posterior-superior iliac spine

PSL parasternal line
percent stroke length
potassium, sodium chloride, and sodium
lactate (solution)

PSLI physalemin-like immunoreactivity

PSLT Picture-Story Language Test

PSM presystolic murmur; also PM

PSMA progressive spinal muscular atrophy
proximal spinal muscular atrophy

PSMed psychosomatic medicine; also
PsychosMed

PSMF protein-sparing modified fast

PSMRD postsurgical minimum residual
disease

PSMT psychiatric services management team

PSNS parasympathetic nervous system;
also PNS

PSO physostigmine salicylate ophthalmic
proximal subungual onychomycosis

Psol partly soluble

PSOR psoralen; also P

P/sore pressure sore

PSP pacesetter potential; also PP
pancreatic spasmolytic peptide
paralytic shellfish poisoning
parathyroid secretory protein
periodic short pulse
phenolsulfonphthalein (phenol red)
positive spike pattern
posterior spinal sclerosis
postsynaptic potential; also psp
professional simulated patient
progressive supranuclear palsy
pseudopregnancy

psp posterior subscapular plague
postsynaptic potential; also PSP

PSPF prostacyclin synthesis-stimulating
plasma factor

PSQ Parent Symptom Questionnaire
patient satisfaction questionnaire

PSR extrahepatic portal-systemic resistance
pain sensitivity range
problem status report
proliferative sickle retinopathy
pulmonary stretch receptor

PSRBOW premature spontaneous rupture of
bag of waters

PSRC Plastic Surgery Research Council

PSRO Professional Standards Review Organization

PSS painful shoulder syndrome
physiologic saline solution
progressive systemic scleroderma
progressive systemic sclerosis
psoriasis severity scale
Psychiatry Status Schedule

PST pancreatic suppression test
paroxysmal supraventricular tachycardia; also PSVT
Pascal-Suttle Test (psychiatry)
penicillin, streptomycin, and tetracycline
perceptual span time
peristimulus time
phenolsulfotransferase
phonemic segmentation test
platelet survival time
poststenotic
poststimulus time
prefrontal sonic treatment
protein-sparing therapy
proximal straight tubule

PSTH poststimulus time histogram

PSTI pancreatic secretory trypsin inhibitor

PSTP pentasodium triphosphate

PSTV potato spindle tuber viroid

PSU photosynthetic unit
postsurgical unit
primary sampling unit
primary site undetermined

PSurg, P-Surg plastic surgery; also PL, PLS, PS

PSV papillitis stenosans Vateri
pressure supported ventilation
psychological, social, and vocational (adjustment factors)

PSVER pattern-shift visual-evoked response

PSVT paroxysmal supraventricular tachycardia; also PST

PSW past sleepwalker
primary surgical ward
Psychiatric Social Worker

PSY, Psy psychiatric; also P, PS, psychiat
psychiatry; also Ψ, P, PS, psychiat
psychology; also Psych, psych, psychol

Psych, psych psychologic; also psychol
psychology; also PSY, Psy, psychol

psychiat psychiatric; also P, PS, PSY, Psy
psychiatry; also Ψ, P, PS, PSY, Psy

psychoan psychoanalysis; also PA, PSAn, PYA
psychoanalytical

psychol psychologic; also Psych, psych
psychology; also PSY, Psy, Psych, psych

psychopath psychopathologic; also psy-path
psychopathology; also psy-path

PsychosMed psychosomatic medicine; also PSMed

psychother psychotherapeutic
psychotherapy

psy-path psychopathologic; also psychopath
psychopathology; also psychopath

PT parathormone; also PTH
parathyroid; also para, PTH
paroxysmal tachycardia
patient; also P, PAT, PNT, Pnt, Pt, pt
pericardial tamponade
permanent and total; also P&T
pharmacy and therapeutics; also P&T
phenytoin
phonation time
photophobia
phototoxicity
physical therapist
physical therapy; also Phys Ther
physical training
physiotherapy; also physio
pine tar
pint; also O,Ō,oct, P, p, pt
planium temporale
plasma thromboplastin
pneumothorax; also Pnx, PTX, Px, px
polyvalent tolerance
posterior tibial (artery pulse)
posttransplantation
preterm
pronator teres
propylthiouracil; also PTU
prothrombin time; also pro time, pro-time, proTime, protime
protriptyline; also PTL
pulmonary thrombosis
pulmonary toilet
pulmonary trunk
pulmonary tuberculosis; also PTB
pure tone (audiometry)
pyramidal tract
temporal plane

P&T paracentesis and tubing (of ears)
peak and trough
permanent and total; also PT
pharmacy and therapeutics; also PT

Pt let it be continued [L. *perstetur*]; also pt
patient; also P, PAT, PNT, Pnt, PT, pt
platinum
psychasthenia

pt let it be continued [L. *perstetur*]; also Pt
part; also P, p
patient; also P, PAT, PNT, Pnt, PT, Pt
pint; also O, , oct, P, p, PT
point; also P

PTA parathyroid adenoma
percutaneous transluminal angioplasty
persistent trigeminal artery
persistent truncus arteriosus
phosphotungstic acid
physical therapy assistant
plasma thromboplastin antecedent (coagulation factor XI)
platelet thromboplastin antecedent
post-traumatic amnesia
post-traumatic arthritis
pretreatment anxiety
prior to admission; also PA
prior to arrival
prothrombin activity; also PA
pure tone acuity
pure tone average; also PT(A)

PT(A) pure tone average; also PTA

PTAF policy target adjustment factor

P-TAG target-attaching globulin precursor

PTAH phosphotungstic acid hematoxylin

PTAP purified diphtheria toxoid precipitated by aluminum phosphate

PTB patellar tendon-bearing (cast prosthesis)
prior to birth
pulmonary tuberculosis; also PT

PTBA percutaneous transluminal balloon angioplasty

PTBD percutaneous transhepatic biliary drainage; also PTHBD

PTBD-EF percutaneous transhepatic biliary drainage–enteric feeding

PTBE pyretic tick-borne encephalitis

PTBP *para*-tertiary butylphenol

PTBS post-traumatic brain syndrome

PTC patient to call
percutaneous transhepatic cholangiogram
percutaneous transhepatic cholangiography; also PTHC
phase transfer catalyst
phenylthiocarbamide
phenylthiocarbamoyl

pheochromocytoma, thyroid carcinoma (syndrome)
plasma thromboplastin component (coagulation factor IX)
premature tricuspid closure
prior to conception
prothrombin complex
pseudotumor cerebri

PT-C prothrombin time control; also PRTH-C, PT-CT

PTCA percutaneous transluminal coronary angioplasty

PTCL peripheral T-cell lymphoma

PtcCO₂ partial pressure of transcutaneous carbon dioxide

PTCP pseudothrombocytopenia

PTC peptide phenylthiocarbamoyl peptide

PTCR percutaneous transluminal coronary recanalization

PT-CT prothrombin time control; also PRTH-C, PT-C

PTCV Plowright tissue culture vaccine

PTD percutaneous transluminal dilation
period to discharge
permanent and total disability
prior to delivery
prior to discharge

Ptd phosphatidyl

PtdCho phosphatidylcholine (lecithin); also PC

PtdEtn phosphatidylethanolamine; also PE

PtdIns phosphatidylinositol; also PI

PTDP permanent transvenous demand pacemaker

PtdSer phosphatidylserine

PTE parathyroid extract
post-traumatic endophthalmitis
pretibial edema
proximal tibial epiphysis
pulmonary thromboembolism

PTED pulmonary thromboembolic disease

PteGlu pteroylglutamic (acid)

pter end of short arm of chromosome

PTF patient treatment file
plasma thromboplastin factor (coagulation factor VIII)

PTFA prothrombin time fixing agent

PTFE polytetrafluoroethylene

PTG parathyroid gland

PTGA pteroyltriglutamic acid

PTH parathormone; also PT
parathyroid; also para, PT
parathyroid hormone; also PH
phenylthiohydantoin
plasma thromboplastin (component)
post-transfusion hepatitis
prior to hospitalization

PTh primary thrombocythemia

PTHBD percutaneous transhepatic biliary drain
percutaneous transhepatic biliary drainage;
also PTBD

PTHC percutaneous transhepatic cholangiography; also PTC

PTHS parathyroid hormone secretion (rate)

PTI pancreatic trypsin inhibitor
persistent tolerant infection
Pictorial Test of Intelligence
pressure time index

PTJV percutaneous transtracheal jet ventilation

PTK protein tyrosine kinase

PTL perinatal telencephalic leukoencephalopathy
pharyngotracheal lumen
posterior tricuspid valve leaflet; also pTL
preterm labor
protriptyline; also PT
Sodium Pentothal

pTL posterior tricuspid valve leaflet; also PTL

PTLC precipitation thin-layer chromatography
preparative thin-layer chromatography

PTM posterior trabecular meshwork
post-transfusion mononucleosis
post-traumatic meningitis
pressure time per minute
preterm milk

Ptm pterygomaxillary (fissure)
transmural pressure (airway, blood vessel)

PTMA phenyltrimethylammonium

PTMDF pupils, tension, media, disc, fundus

PTN pain transmission neuron

pTNM postsurgical: tumor, nodes, metastases
(postsurgical staging of cancer)

PTO Klemperer's tuberculin [Ger. *Perlsucht Tuberculin Original*]
percutaneous transhepatic obliteration
personal time off
please turn over

PTP percutaneous transhepatic portography
posterior tibial pulse
post-tetanic potentiation

post-transfusion purpura
prior to program
prothrombin-proconvertin; also PP
proximal tubular pressure

P_{TP} transpulmonary pressure; also PL, P_L, Ptp

Ptp transpulmonary pressure; also PL, P^L, P_{TP}

PTPI post-traumatic pulmonary insufficiency

PTPM post-traumatic progressive myelopathy

PTPN peripheral vein total parenteral nutrition

PTR patella tendon reflex
patient termination record
patient to return
peripheral total resistance
prothrombin time ratio
psychotic trigger reaction
tuberculin prepared from *Mycobacterium tuberculosis bovis* (in the same manner of Koch's new tuberculin) [Ger. *Perlsucht Tuberculin Rest*]

PTr porcine trypsin

PTRA percutaneous transluminal renal angioplasty

PTRIA polystyrene-tube radioimmunoassay

PTS painful tonic seizure
para-toluenesulfonic acid
patella tendon socket
patella tendon suspension
patients; also Pts, pts
permanent threshold shift
phosphotransferase system
post-thrombotic syndrome
prior to surgery

Pts, pts patients; also PTS

PTSD post-traumatic stress disorder

PTSM pyruvaldehyde-bis-(*N*-4-methylthiosemicarbazone)-

PTT partial thromboplastin time
particle transport time
patellar tendon transfer
platelet transfusion therapy
portable transcription terminator
posterior tibial transfer
pulmonary transit time
pulse transmission time

PTT-CT partial thromboplastin time control

PTTH prothoracicotropic hormone

PTU pain treatment unit
propylthiouracil; also PT

PTV posterior tibial vein

PTWTKG patient's weight in kilograms

PTX parathyroidectomy; also para, PTx
pelvic traction
pertussis toxin
phototoxic reaction
picrotoxinin
pneumothorax; also Pnx, PT, Px, px

PTx parathyroidectomy; also para, PTX

PTXA parathyroidectomy and autotrans-
plantation

PTZ pentamethylenetetrazole
pentylenetetrazol
phenothiazine

PU by way of urethra [L. *per urethra*]
passed urine
paternal uncle
pelvic-ureteric
pepsin unit
peptic ulcer
posterior urethra
precursor uptake
pregnancy urine

Pu plutonium
purple (indicator color); also Pur
putrescine; also PUT

pub public; also publ

publ public; also pub

PUBS percutaneous umbilical cord blood
sampling

PUC pediatric urine collector

PUD peptic ulcer disease
pulmonary disease; also PD, PN, PuD

PuD pulmonary disease; also PD, PN, PUD

PUE pyrexia of unknown etiology

PUFA polyunsaturated fatty acid

PUH pregnancy urine hormone

PUL pubourethral ligament

PUL, pul pulmonary; also P, PULM, pulm

PULM, pulm gruel [L. *pulmentum*]
pulmonary; also P, PUL, pul
pulmonic

PULSES general physical, upper extremities,
lower extremities, sensory, excretory, social
support (physical profile)

pulv powder [L. *pulvis*]; also pdr, powd, pwd

pulv gros coarse powder [L. *pulvis grossus*]

pulv subtil smooth powder [L. *pulvis subtilis*]

pulv tenu very fine powder [L. *pulvis tenuis*]

PUM peanut lectin-binding urinary mucins

PUMC Peking Union Medical College

PUN plasma urea nitrogen

PUNL percutaneous ultrasonic
nephrolithotripsy

PUO pyrexia of uncertain origin
pyrexia of undetermined origin
pyrexia of unknown origin

PUP percutaneous ultrasonic pyelolithotomy

PU-PC polyunsaturated phosphatidylcholine

PUPPP pruritic urticarial papules and plaques
of pregnancy

PUR polyurethane

Pur purine
purple (indicator color); also Pu

purg cathartic, purgative [L. *purgativus*]

PUT putamen
putrescine; also Pu

PUVA psoralen plus ultraviolet light of A
wavelength (therapy)
pulsed ultraviolet actinotherapy

PUVD pulsed ultrasonic blood velocity
detector

PUW pick-up walker

PV by way of vagina [L. *per vaginam*]; also pv
pancreatic vein
papilloma virus
paraventricular
pemphigus vulgaris
peripheral vascular
peripheral vein; also PeV
peripheral venous
peripheral vessel(s)
phonation volume
photovoltaic
pinocytotic vesicle
pityriasis versicolor
plasma viscosity
plasma volume
Plummer-Vinson (syndrome)
pneumococcus vaccine; also PNVX
polio vaccine
polycythemia vera; also PCV
polyoma virus
polyvinyl
popliteal vein
portal vein; also PoV
postvasectomy
postvoiding
predictive value
pressure-volume
Proteus vulgaris
pulmonary vein
pure vegetarian

P-V Panton-Valentine (leukocidin)
pressure volume (curve)

P/V pressure to volume (ratio)

P&V peak and valley
percuss and vibrate
pyloroplasty and vagotomy

Pv venous pressure; also VP

pv by way of vagina [L. *per vaginam*]; also PV

PVA partial villous atrophy
polyvinyl alcohol (fixative)
Prinzmetal's variant angina

PVAc polyvinyl acetate

PVAS postvasectomy specimen

PVB Platinol, vinblastine, and bleomycin
premature ventricular beat

PVBS possible vertebral-basilar system

PVC persistent vaginal cornification
polyvinyl chloride
postvoiding cystogram
predicted vital capacity
premature ventricular complex
premature ventricular contraction
primary visual cortex
pulmonary venous capillary
pulmonary venous congestion

PVCM paradoxical vocal cord motion

PVCO$_2$, Pv$_{CO2}$ partial pressure of carbon
dioxide in mixed venous blood

PVD patient very disturbed
peripheral vascular disease
portal vein dilation
posterior vitreous detachment
postural vertical dimension
postvagotomy diarrhea
premature ventricular depolarization
pulmonary vascular disease

PVDF polyvinylidenefluoride

PVE perivenous encephalomyelitis
periventricular echogenicity
premature ventricular extrasystole
prosthetic valve endocarditis

PVED periventricular echo density

PVEP pattern visual-evoked potential

PVF peripheral visual field
portal venous flow
primary ventricular fibrillation

PVFS postviral fatigue syndrome

PVH papilloma virus hominis
periventricular hemorrhage
pulmonary vascular hypertension

PVI peripheral vascular insufficiency
periventricular inhibitor

PVK penicillin V potassium [L. *kalium* (potassium)]; also PVP

PVL periventricular leukomalacia

P-VL Panton-Valentine leukocidin

PVM pneumonia virus of mice
proteins, vitamins, and minerals; also
PROVIMI

PVMed preventive medicine; also PM, PRM,
PrM

PVN paraventricular nucleus; also PAVN
predictive value of a negative test

PVNPS post-Viet Nam psychiatric syndrome

PVNS pigmented villonodular synovitis; also
PVS

PVO peripheral vascular occlusion
pulmonary venous obstruction
pulmonary venous occlusion
pyogenic vertebral osteomyelitis

PVO$_2$, Pv$_{O2}$ partial pressure of oxygen in
mixed venous blood

PVOD peripheral vascular occlusive disease
pulmonary vascular obstructive disease
pulmonary veno-occlusive disease

PVP penicillin V potassium; also PVK
peripheral vein plasma
peripheral venous pressure
polyvinyl-pyrrolidone (povidone)
portal venous pressure
predictive value of a positive test
pulmonary venous pressure; also P$_L$

PVP-I polyvinylpyrrolidone-iodine (povidone-
iodine)

PVR peripheral vascular resistance
postvoiding residual
proliferative vitreoretinopathy
pulmonary vascular resistance
pulmonary venous redistribution
pulse-volume recording

PVRA peripheral vein renin activity

PVRI peripheral vascular resistance index

PVRV purified vero-cell rabies vaccine

PVS paravesicle space
percussion, vibration, and suction
peritoneovenous shunt
periventricular nuclear stratum
persistent vegetative state
pigmented villonodular synovitis; also PVNS
Plummer-Vinson syndrome

poliovirus sensitivity
polyvinyl sponge
premature ventricular systole
programmed ventricular stimulation
pulmonary vein stenosis
pulmonic valve stenosis

PVT paroxysmal ventricular tachycardia
physical volume test
portal vein thrombosis
pressure, volume, temperature
private (patient, room); also P, priv, pvt

pvt private (patient, room); also P, priv, PVT

PVW posterior vaginal wall

PW pacing wire
Parkes-Weber (syndrome)
patient waiting
peristaltic wave
plantar wart
posterior wall (of heart)
Prader-Willi (syndrome); also P-W
pulmonary wedge (pressure)
pulsed wave
puncture wound

P-W Prader-Willi (syndrome); also PW

P&W pressures and waves

Pw progesterone withdrawal

PWA person with acquired immunodeficiency
syndrome (person with AIDS)

PWB partial weight-bearing
psychologic well-being

PWBC peripheral white blood cell(s)

PWBRT prophylactic whole-brain radiation
therapy

PWC peak work capacity
Pfeiffer-Weber-Christian (syndrome)
physical work capacity

PWD precipitated withdrawal diarrhea
pulsed-wave Doppler

pwd powder; also pdr, powd, pulv

PWE posterior wall excursion

PWI posterior wall infarct

PWLV posterior wall of left ventricle

PWM pokeweed mitogen

PWP pulmonary wedge pressure; also Ppw

PWR pressurized water reactor

PWS port wine stain
Prader-Willi syndrome
pulse-wave speed

pwt pennyweight

PWV peak weight velocity

polistes wasp venom
posterior wall velocity
pulse wave velocity

PX pancreatectomized
peroxidase; also POD
physical examination; also PE, PEx, Px, px

Px past history; also PH, PHx
physical examination; also PE, PEx, PX, px
pneumothorax; also Pnx, PT, PTX, px
prognosis; also prog, progn, px

px physical examination; also PE, PEx, PX, Px
pneumothorax; also Pnx, PT, PTX, Px
prognosis; also prog, progn, Px

PXE pseudoxanthoma elasticum

Pxl pyridoxal

PXM projection x-ray microscopy

Pxm pyridoxamine

PY, P/Y pack-year (cigarettes)
person-year

Py phosphopyridoxal
polyoma (virus)
pyrene
pyridine; also Pyr

PYA psychoanalysis; also PA, PSAn, psychoan

PYC proteose-yeast Castione (medium)

PyC pyogenic culture

PYE peptone yeast extract

PYG peptone-yeast-glucose (broth)

PYGM peptone-yeast-glucose-maltose (broth)

PYLL potential years of life lost

PYM psychosomatic

PYP pyrophosphate; also PP, Pyro

PYR person-year rad

Pyr pyridine; also Py
pyrimidine
pyruvate

Pyro pyrophosphate; also PP, PYP

PyrP pyridoxal phosphate; also PLP

PYS parietal yolk sac (cells)
pyriform sinus

PZ pancreozymin
peripheral zone
prazosin
pregnancy zone
proliferative zone

Pz electrode placement in electroencephalography
parietal midline (zero)
4-phenylazobenzyloxycarbonyl

pz   pieze (unit of pressure)

PZA   pyrazinamide

PzB   parenzyme, buccal

PZ-CCK   pancreozymin-cholecystokinin

PZD   piperazinedione

PZE   piezoelectric

PZI   protamine zinc insulin

PZP   pregnancy zone protein

Q

Q cardiac output; also CO, QT
clerical perception (General Aptitude Test Battery)
coenzyme Q (ubiquinone); also CoQ, q
coulomb; also C
each, every [L. *quisque*]; also q, qq
1,4-glucan branching enzyme
glutamine (one-letter notation); also GLN, Gln, GLU, Glu, Glx
perfusion (flow)
quantitative; also qt, quant
quantity; also Q, q, q, qt, qty, quant
quantity of electric charge
quantity of heat
quart; also q, qt
quarter; also q, qr
quartile
Query (fever)
question; also quest
quinacrine (fluorescent method)
quinidine
quinone
quotient; also quot
Q wave (electrocardiographic wave)
radiant energy
reaction energy
reactive power
volume of blood flow

Q electric charge; also q, q
heat
quantity; also Q, q, q, qt, qty, quant
reaction quotient

$\dot{Q}$ rate of blood flow

Q°, q° every hour around the clock [L. *quaque* (every)]; also Q1°

Q1° every hour around the clock [L. *quaque* (every)]; also Q°, q°

Q2° every two hours around the clock [L. *quaque* (every)]

Q-6, Q$_6$ ubiquinone-6; also q
ubiquinone-Q$_6$

Q$_9$ ubichromenol-9

Q$_{10}$ temperature coefficient (increase in rate of a process produced by raising the temperature 10°C)
ubiquinone-10
ubiquinone (50)
ubiquinone-Q$_{10}$

q each, every [L. *quisque*]l also Q, qq

electric charge; also Q, q
four [L. *quattuor*]; also Quat, quat
frequency of rarer allele of a gene pair
quantity; also Q, Q, q, qt, qty, quant
quart; also Q, qt
quarter; also Q, qr
quintal
the long arm of a chromosome
volume; also V, vol

q coenzyme Q (ubiquinone); also CoQ, Q
electric charge; also Q, q
probability of an alternative event
quantity; also Q, Q, q, qt, qty, quant

q 28 days every 28 days [L. *quisque* (every)]

QA quality assessment
quality assurance
quinaldic acid
quisqualic acid

QAC quaternary ammonium compound

qad every other day [L. *quaque altera die*]; also qod

qah every other hour [L. *quaque altera hora*]; also qoh

QALE quality-adjusted life expectancy

QALY quality-adjusted life years

QAM every morning [L. *quaque ante meridiem*]; also Qam, qAM, qam, qm
quality assurance monitor

Qam, qAM, qam every morning [L. *quaque ante meridiem*]; also QAM, qm

qan every other night [L. *quaque altera nocte*]; also qon

Q angle Quatrefages' angle (parietal angle)

QAP quality assurance program
quinine, Atabrine (quinacrine hydrochloride), and pamaquine

QAR quality assurance reagent
quantitative autoradiographic

QA/RM quality assurance/risk management

QAS quality assurance standards

QAT quality assurance technical (material)

QAUR quality assurance and utilization review

QB Quantitative Electrophysiological Battery
whole blood; also WB, W Bld

Q$_B$ blood flow; also BF
total body clearance; also TBC

QBC quality buffy coat

QBCA quantitative buffy-coat analysis

QBV whole blood volume

QC quality control
quick catheter
quinine and colchicine

Qc pulmonary capillary blood flow (perfusion)

QCA quantitative coronary angiography

QCD quantum chromodynamics

QCIM Quarterly Cumulative *Index Medicus*

Qco$_2$, Q$_{CO2}$ microliters of carbon dioxide (at standard temperature and pressure, dry) given off per milligram of dry weight of tissue per hour

Q$_{CSF}$ rate of bulk flow of cerebrospinal fluid from cerebrospinal space by arachnoid villi uptake

QCT quantitative computerized tomography

qd every day [L. *quaque die*]; also qqd

qds four times a day [L. *quater die sumendum*]

QED quantum electrodynamics
that which is to be demonstrated [L. *quod erat demonstrandum*]; also qed

qed that which is to be demonstrated [L. *quod erat demonstrandum*]; also QED

QEE quadriceps extension exercise

QEF quail embryo fibroblast

Q fever Query fever (Queensland fever); also QF, QuF

QET Quality Extinction Test

QEW quick early warning

QF quality factor (relative biologic effectiveness)
Query fever (Queensland fever); also Q fever, QuF
quick freeze

Q fract quick fraction

Q-H$_2$ ubiquinol

qh every hour [L. *quaque hora*]; also qq hor

q2h every two hours [L. *quaque* (every)]

q3h every three hours [L. *quaque* (every)]

q4h every four hours [L. *quaque* (every)]; also qqh

QHS Qinghaosu (artemisinin)

qhs every night [L. *quaque hora somni* (every hour of sleep)]; also qn

qid four times daily [L. *quater in die*]

QIg quantitative immunoglobulin

QJ quadriceps jerk

QJM *Quarterly Journal of Medicine*

ql as much as desired [L. *quantum libet*]; also qp

QLS Quality of Life Scale

qlty quality; also qual

QM Quénu-Muret (sign)
quinacrine mustard

qm every morning [L. *quaque mane*]; also QAM, Qam, qAM, qam

QMI Q-wave myocardial infarction

q month every month [L. *quaque* (every)]

QMT quantitative muscle testing

QMWS quasi-morphine withdrawal syndrome

qn every night [L. *quaque nocte*]; also qhs

QNB quinuclidinyl benzilate

QNOD normalized absorbance of the chromosome long arm

QNS quantity not sufficient; also qns
Queen's Nursing Sister (of Queen's Institute of District Nursing)

qns quantity not sufficient; also QNS

Qo oxygen consumption; also QO$_2$, Qo$_2$, Q$_{O2}$, qO$_2$

QO$_2$, Qo$_2$, Q$_{O2}$, qO$_2$ oxygen consumption; also Qo
oxygen quotient
oxygen utilization

QOC Quality of Contact

qod every other day [L. *quaque* (every)]; also qad

qoh every other hour [L. *quaque* (every)]; also qah

qon every other night [L. *quaque* (every)]; also qan

QP quadrant pain
Qualified Psychiatrist
quanti-Pirquet (reaction)

Qp pulmonary blood flow; also PBF, PF

qp as much as desired [L. *quantum placeat*]; also ql

QPC quadrigeminal plate cistern
quality of patient care

Qpc pulmonary capillary blood flow

QPEEG quantitative pharmacoelectroencephalography

Qpm, qPM, qpm each evening [L. *quaque post meridiem*]

QP/QS ratio of pulmonary to systemic circulation

Qp/Qs left-to-right shunt ratio (electro-cardiography)

QPVT Quick Picture Vocabulary Test

qq also [L. *quoque*]
each, every [L. *quisque*]; also Q, q

qqd every day [L. *quaque die*]; also qd

qqh every four hours [L. *quaque quattuor hora*]; also q4h

qq hor every hour [L. *quaque hora*]; also qh

qqv which see (plural) [L. *quae vide, quod vide*]

QR quadriradial
quality review
quantity is correct [L. *quantitas recta*]; also qr
Quick Recovery (defibrillator)
quieting reflex
quieting response
quiet room
quinaldine red

qr quantity is correct [L. *quantitas recta*]; also QR
quarter; also Q, q

QRB Quality Review Bulletin

Q-RB electrocardiographic time-wave interval

QRN quasiresonant nucleus

QRS Q wave, R wave, and S wave (electro-cardiographic wave complex or interval)

QRS-ST electrocardiographic junction between QRS complex and ST segment

QRS-T electrocardiographic angle between QRS and T vectors

QRZ wheal reaction time [Ger. *Quaddel Reaktion Zeit*]

QS quantity sufficient
quiet sleep

QS2, QS$_2$ total electromechanical systole

Qs systemic blood flow

qs as much as may suffice [L. *quantum sufficiat*]
sufficient quantity [L. *quantum satis*]; also q sat

qs ad sufficient quantity to make [L. *quantum sufficiat ad*]
to a sufficient quantity [L. *quantum satis ad*]

QSAR quantitative structure–activity relationship

q sat sufficient quantity [L. *quantum satis*]; also qs

QSC quasi-static compliance

QS$_2$I shortened electrochemical systole

Qsp physiologic shunt flow

QSPR quantitative structure–pharmacokinetic relationship

QSPV quasistatic pressure volume

Qs/Qt intrapulmonary shunt fraction
right-to-left shunt ratio

Qsrel relative shunt flow

QSS quantitative sacroiliac scintigraphy

Q's sign Quant's sign

Q-S test Queckenstedt-Stookey test

q suff as much as suffices [L. *quantum sufficit*]

QT blood volume (quantity) per unit time
cardiac output; also CO, Q
qualification test
Queckenstedt's test
Quick's Test (psychology, pregnancy, pro-thrombin); also Q-T

Q-T electrocardiographic interval from the beginning of QRS complex to end of T wave
Quick's Test (psychology, pregnancy, pro-thrombin); also QT

Qt quiet; also qt

qt quantitative; also Q, quant
quantity; also Q, *Q*, q, *q*, qty, quant
quart; also Q, q
quiet; also Qt

QTC quantitative tip culture

QT$_c$ QT interval corrected for heart rate

qter end of long arm of chromosome

qty quantity; also Q, *Q*, q, *q*, qt, quant

Quad quadriplegia; also quad
quadriplegic; also quad

quad quadrant
quadriceps (muscle)
quadrilateral
quadriplegia; also Quad
quadriplegic; also Quad

quad ex quadriceps exercise

quadrupl four times as much [L. *quadrupli-cato*]

qual qualitative
quality; also qlty

qual anal qualitative analysis

quant quantitative; also Q, qt
quantity; also Q, *Q*, q, *q*, qt, qty

quar quarantine

quart fourth [L. *quartus*]
  quadrantectomy, axillary dissection, and radiotherapy
  quarterly

Quat, quat four [L. *quattuor*]; also q

QUATS, quats quaternary ammonium compounds

quer querulous

QUEST quality, utilization, effectiveness, statistically tabulated

quest question; also Q
  questionable

QuF Query fever (Queensland fever); also QF, Q fever

QUICHA quantitative inhalation challenge apparatus

quinq five [L. *quinque*]

quint fifth [L. *quintus*]

quor of which [L. *quorum*]

quot as often as necessary [L. *quoties*]; also quot op sit, quot o s
  daily [L. *quotidie*]; also quotid
  quotient; also Q

quotid daily [L. *quotidie*]; also quot

quot op sit as often as necessary [L. *quoties opus sit*]; also quot, quot o s

quot o s as often as necessary [L. *quoties opus sit*]; also quot, quot op sit

qv as much as you desire [L. *quantum vis*]
  which see (literature citation) [L. *quod vide, quae vide*]

QW quality of working (life)

qwk once a week [L. *quisque* (each, every)]

q 4 wk every 4 weeks [L. *quisque* (each, every)]

QWL quality of working life

R

P RHO, UPPER CASE, seventeenth letter of the Greek alphabet

ρ rho, lower case, seventeenth letter of the Greek alphabet
  correlation coefficient
  electrical resistivity
  electric charge density
  mass density
  population correlation coefficient
  reactivity

ϱ rho, lower case, seventeenth letter of the Greek alphabet, variant

R arginine (one-letter notation); also ARG, Arg
  Behnken's unit (of roentgen-ray exposure)
  Broadbent registration point
  drug-resistant plasmid
  electrical resistance (ohm): also *R*, RES
  electrocardiographic wave in QRS complex
  far point (of vision) [L. *remotum*]; also r
  gas constant (8.315 joules); also *R*
  general symbol for the remainder of a chemical formula
  metabolic respiratory quotient
  organic radical
  race
  racemic; also r, *r-*, rac
  rad
  radical; also RAD, rad
  radioactive; also RA
  radioactive material; also RAM
  radiology; also RAD, Rad, Radiol
  radius; also r, Ra, rad
  radius, complete (congenital absence of limb)
  ramus
  range
  Rankine (temperature scale)
  rare
  rate
  ratio
  rationale
  raw
  reaction; also RXN
  reading
  Réaumur (temperature scale)
  recessive
  rectal; also (R), rect, rtl
  rectified average
  rectum; also RECT, rect
  rectus (muscle); also rect
  red (indicator color); also rub
  reference; also ref

regimen
registered; also Reg
registered trademard; also RTM, ℝ
regression coefficient
regular; also reg
regulator (gene)
rejection (factor)
relapse
relaxation
release (factor)
remission; also Rm
remote point of convergence
repressor
resazurin
resident; also RES, res
residuum
resistance (determinant) (plasmid)
resistance (factor)
resistance unit (in cardiovascular system); also RU
resistant
respiration; also Resp, resp
respiratory; also Resp, resp
respiratory exchange ratio; also R_E, RER
response; also resp, Rs
rest (cell cycle)
resting
restricted
reticulocyte; also RET, RETIC, retic
reverse; also REV, rev
review; also REV, rev
rhythm
rib
ribose; also r, Rib
Rickettsia species; also *R*
right; also (R), ℝ, RT, Rt, rt
Rinne (hearing test)
roentgen; also r, ROE, roent
rough (bacterial colony)
routine; also rout, RTN
rub
side chain in amino acid formula
stimulus [Ger. *Reiz* (stimulus)]; also S, ST
take [L. *recipe*]; also Rx
total response; also TR

R electrical resistance (ohm); also R, RES
  gas constant (8.315 joules); also R
  Rickettsia species; also R

ℝ real number

+R Rinne's test positive

-R Rinne's test negative

R✓ receipt done

(R) rectal; also R, rect, rtl
right; also R, Ⓡ, RT, Rt, rt

Ⓡ right; also R (R), RT, Rt, rt

Ⓡ registered trademark; also R, RTM

°R degree Rankine
degree Réaumur

R#1 good risk (for anesthesia)

R#2 fairly good risk (for anesthesia)

R#3 poor risk (for anesthesia)

R#4 very poor risk (for anesthesia)

r angle of refraction
applied shear stress
drug resistance; also *r*
far point (of vision) [L. *remotum*]; also R
racemic; also R, *r*-, rac
radius; also R, Ra, rad
radius, incomplete (congenital absence of limb)
reproductive potential
ribose; also R, Rib
ring chromosome
roentgen (former symbol; now "R"); also R, ROE, roent
round
sample correlation coefficient; also *r*

r distance radius
drug resistance; also r
sample correlation coefficient; also r

r- racemic; also R, r, rac

r², r² coefficient of determination

RA radioactive; also R
radionuclide angiography; also RNA, RNG
radium; also Ra, Rad
ragocyte (cell)
ragweed antigen
rales
Raynaud (phenomenon)
reading age; also RdA
reciprocal asymmetrical
refractory anemia
refractory ascites
regular army
remittance advice
renal artery
renin activity
renin-angiotensin
repeat action (drugs)
residual air
retinoic acid
rheumatic arthritis
rheumatoid agglutinin

rheumatoid arthritis; also RhA
rifampicin
right angle
right angulation
right aortic
right arm
right atrial
right atrium
right auricle
Rokitansky-Aschoff (sinuses)
room air

R$_A$ airway resistance; also AR, RAW, R(AW), R$_{AW}$

Ra radial; also rad
radium; also RA, Rad
radius; also R, r, rad
Rayleigh number

rA riboandenylate

RAA Regression-associated antigen
renin-angiotensin-aldosterone (system)
right atrial abnormality

RAAGG rheumatoid arthritis agglutination
rheumatoid arthritis agglutinin

RAAS renin-angiotensin-aldosterone system

RAB rice, applesauce, and banana (diet)
remote afterload brachy (therapy)

Rab rabbit

RABA rabbit anti-bladder antibody

RABBI Rapid Access Blood Bank Information

RABCa rabbit anti-bladder cancer

RABG room air blood gas

RAbody right atrium body

RABP retinoic acid-binding protein

RAC radial artery catheter
right atrial contraction

rac racemate
racemic; also R, r, *r*-

RACCO right anterior caudocranial oblique

RA cell rheumatoid arthritis cell

RACT recalcified wholeblood activated clotting time

RAD radiation absorbed dose; also rad
radical; also R, rad
radiology; also R, Rad, Radiol
reactive airway disease
right anterior descending (coronary artery); also RADCA
right atrial diameter
right axis deviation
roentgen administered dose

Rad radiologist; also Radiol
radiology; also R, RAD, Radiol
radiotherapist
radiotherapy; also RADIO, Rad Ther, RT, Rx
radium; also RA, Ra

rad radial; also Ra
radian
radiation absorbed dose; also RAD
radical; also R, RAD
radiculitis
radius; also R, r, Ra
root [L. *radix*]

RADA right acromiodorso-anterior (fetal position)

RADCA right anterior descending coronary artery; also RAD

rad imp radium implant

RADIO radiotherapy; also Rad, Rad Ther, RT, Rx

Radiol radiologist; also R, Rad
radiology; also RAD, Rad

RAD ISO VENO BILAT radioactive isotopic venogram, bilateral

RADISH rheumatoid arthritis diffuse idiopathic skeletal hyperostosis

RadLV radiation leukemia virus

RADP right acromiodorso-posterior (fetal position)

RADS reactive airway disease syndrome
retrospective assessment of drug safety

rad/s radians per second

Rad Ther radiotherapy; also Rad, RADIO, RT, Rx

RADTS rabbit anti-dog-thymus serum

Rad Ul radius-ulna

RADWASTE radioactive waste

RAE right atrial enlargement

RaE rabbit erythrocyte

RAEB refractory anemia, erythroblastic
refractory anemia with excess blasts

RAEB-T refractory anemia with excess of blasts in transformation

RAEM refractory anemia with excess myeloblasts

RAF rheumatoid arthritis factor

Ra-F radium-F

RAG ragweed; also RW
ragweed pollen antigen
room air gas

Ragg rheumatoid agglutinator

RAH radioactive Hippuran (test)
regressing atypical histiocytosis
right anterior hemiblock; also RAHB
right atrial hypertrophy

RAHB right anterior hemiblock; also RAH

RAHO rabbit antibody to human ovary

RAHTG rabbit anti-human-thymocyte globulin

RAI radioactive iodine
rapid attentional integration
resting ankle index
right atrial involvement

RAID radioimmunodetection; also RID

RAIT radioimmunotherapy

RAIU radioactive iodine uptake; also RIU

RAL resorcylic acid lactone

RALS rabbit antiserum to rat lymphocytes
reflection-absorption infrared spectroscopy

RALT Riley Articulation and Language Test
routine admission laboratory tests

RAM nucleus raphe magnus
rabbit anti-mouse
radioactive material; also R
random-access memory
random alternating movements
rapid alternating movements
research aviation medicine
right anterior measurement

RAMC Royal Army Medical Corps

RAMI Risk-adjusted Mortality Index

RAMP radioactive antigen microprecipitin
rapid absorbent matrix pad
right atrial mean pressure

RAMT rabbit anti-mouse thymocyte

RAN resident's admission notes

RANA rheumatoid arthritis nuclear antigen

RAND random (sample, specimen)

RANT right anterior

RAO right anterior oblique
right anterior occipital

RaONC radiation oncology

RAP recurrent abdominal pain
regression-associated protein
renal artery pressure
rheumatoid arthritis precipitin
right atrial pressure

RAPD relative afferent pupillary defect

RAPE right atrial pressure elevation

RAPM refractory anemia with partial myeloblastosis

RAPO rabbit antibody to pig ovary

RAPS Rapid Acute Physiology Score

RAQ right anterior quadrant

RAR rat insulin receptor
relative adherence ratio
retinoic acid receptor
right arm, reclining (blood pressure, pulse measurement)
right arm, recumbent (blood pressure, pulse measurement)

RARLS rabbit anti-rat-lymphocyte serum

RARTS rabbit anti-rat-thymocyte serum

RAS recurrent aphthous stomatitis
reflex-activating stimulus
renal artery stenosis
renin-angiotensin system
reticular activating system
rheumatoid arthritis serum (factor)
right arm, sitting (blood pressure, pulse measurement)

ras scrapings, filings [L. *rasurae*]

RASP rapidly alternating speech
rheumatoid arthritis specific protein

RASS rheumatoid arthritis and Sjögren syndrome

RAST radioallergosorbent test

RASV recovered avian sarcoma virus

RAT rat aortic tissue
repeat action tablet
rheumatoid arthritis test
right anterior thigh
right atrial (pressure)

RATA radioimmunologic assay antithyroid antibody

RATG rabbit anti-thymocyte globulin

RATHAS rat thymus antiserum

RATS rabbit anti-thymocyte serum

RATx radiation therapy; also RT, RTx, RXT

RAU radioactive uptake; also RU

RAUC raw area under curve

RAV Rous-associated virus

RAW, R(AW), R$_{AW}$ airway resistance; also R$_A$

RAZ razoxane

RB rating board
rebreathing
Renaut's body
respiratory bronchiole
respiratory burst

reticulate body
retinoblastoma
retrobulbar
right breast
right bundle
right buttock
Roth-Bernhardt (disease)
round body

R&B right and below

Rb rubidium

RBA relative binding affinity
rescue breathing apparatus
right basil artery
right brachial artery
rose bengal antigen

RBAF rheumatoid biologically active factor

RBAP repetitive bursts of action potential

RBB retrobulbar block
right breast biopsy
right bundle-branch

RBBB right bundle-branch block

RBBsB right bundle-branch system block

RBBX right breast biopsy examination

RBC red blood cell
red blood cell count

RBC-ADA red blood cell adenosine deaminase

RBCD right border cardiac dullness

RBC FO red blood cell fallout

RBC frag red blood cell fragility

RBC/hpf red blood cells per high power field

RBC IT red blood cell iron turnover

RBCM red blood cell mass

RBC/P red blood cells to plasma (ratio)

RBC s/f red blood cells spun filtration

RBCV red blood cell volume

RBD right border dullness (percussion of heart)

RBE relative biological effectiveness

RBF regional blood flow
renal blood flow
riboflavin; also RF
rice bran factor

RBG random blood glucose

Rb Imp rubber base impression

RBL rat basophilic leukemia (cells)
Reid's baseline

RBM Raji cell-binding material
regional bone mass

RBME regenerating bone marrow extract

RBN retrobulbar neuritis

RBOW rupture of bag of waters

RBP resting blood pressure
retinol-binding protein
riboflavin-binding protein

RBR radiation bowel reaction

RBRVS resource-based relative value scale

RBS random blood sugar
ribosome-binding site
Rutherford backscattering (method)

RbSA rabbit serum albumin; also RSA

RBTC round-bottom tissue culture (tubes)

RBU Raji cell-binding unit

Rbu ribulose

RBV right brachial vein

RB-V right bundle ventricular

RBW relative body weight

Rby ribitol

RBZ rubidazone (zorubicin)

RC radiocarpal
Raymond-Céstan (syndrome)
reaction center
receptor-chemoeffector (complex)
recrystallized
red cell
red cell cast; also RCC
Red Cross
referred care
reflection coefficient
regenerated cellulose
resistance and capacitance
respiration cease
respiratory care
respiratory center
response, conditioned; also Rc
rest cure
retention catheter; also ret cath
retrograde cystogram
rib cage
right ear, cold stimulus
Roman Catholic
root canal
rotator cuff
Roussy-Cornil (syndrome)
routine cholecystectomy

R/C reclining chair

Rc receptor; also REC
response, conditioned; also RC

RCA radionuclide cerebral angiogram
Raji cell assay
red cell adherence
red cell agglutination
relative chemotactic activity
renal cell carcinoma; also RCC
Ricinus communis agglutinin
right carotid artery
right coronary artery

RCBF regional cerebral blood flow

RCBV regional cerebral blood volume

RCC radiographic coronary calcification
radiologic control center
rape crisis center
ratio of cost to charges
receptor-chemoeffector complex
red cell cast; also RC
red cell concentrate
red cell count
renal cell carcinoma; also RCA
right common carotid
right coronary cusp

Rcc radiochemical

RCCA right common carotid artery

RCCT randomized controlled clinical trial
results of clinical controlled trial

RCD relative area of cardiac dullness
Ringer, citrate, dextrose (buffer)

RCDR relative corrected death rate

RCE reasonable compensation equivalent

RCF recombinant cloning factor
red cell filterability
red cell folate
Reiter complement fixation
relative centrifugal field
relative centrifugal force
ristocetin cofactor; also RCoF

RCFS reticulocyte cell-free system

RCG radioelectrocardiography; also RECG

RCH rectocolic hemorrhage

RCHF right-sided congestive heart failure

RCI rate change induced
respiratory control index

RCIA red cell immune adherence

RCIT red cell iron turnover

RCITR red cell iron turnover rate

RCL range of comfortable loudness
renal clearance

RCLAAR red cell-linked antigen-antiglobulin
reaction

RCM radiocontrast material
radiographic contrast medium
red cell mass
reinforced clostridial medium

RCM—cont'd
 replacement culture medium
 retinal capillary microaneurysm
 rheumatoid cervical myelopathy
 right costal margin
 Roux's conditioned medium
 Royal College of Midwives

RCMI red cell morphology index

rCMRO₂ regional cerebral metabolic rate
 for oxygen

RCN right caudate nucleus
 Royal College of Nursing

RCO aliphatic acyl radical

RCoF ristocetin cofactor; also RCF

RCOG Royal College of Obstetricians and
 Gynaecologists (England)

RCP random chemistry profile
 reciprocity (test)
 retrocorneal pigmentation
 riboflavin carrier protein
 Royal College of Physicians (England)

rcp reciprocal (translocation)

RCPE, RCP(E) Royal College of Physicians
 (Edinburgh); also RCP(Edin)

RCP(Edin) Royal College of Physicians
 (Edinburgh); also RCPE, RCP(E)

RCPH red cell peroxide hemolysis

RCP(I) Royal College of Physicians (Ireland)

RCPM raven colored progressive matrix

RCPs Respiratory Care Practioners

RCPSC Royal College of Physicians and
 Surgeons of Canada

RCQG right caudal quarter ganglion

RCR relative consumption rate
 respiratory control ratio

RCRA Resource Conservation and Recovery
 Act

RCRS Rehabilitation Client Rating Scale

RCS rabbit aorta-contracting substance
 red cell suspension
 repeat cesarean section; also R/CS
 reticulum cell sarcoma; also RSA
 right coronary sinus
 Royal College of Surgeons (England)

R/CS repeat cesarean section; also RCS

RCS(E) Royal College of Surgeons
 (Edinburgh); also RCS(Edin)

RCS(Edin) Royal College of Surgeons
 (Edinburgh); also RCS(E)

RCSI, RCS(I) Royal College of Surgeons
 (Ireland)

RCT randomized clinical trial
 red colloidal test
 retrograde conduction time
 root canal therapy
 Rorschach content test

RC TNTC red cells too numerous to count

RCU red cell utilization
 respiratory care unit

RCV red cell volume

RCVS Royal College of Veterinary Surgeons

RD radial deviation
 rate difference
 Raynaud's disease
 reaction of degeneration
 reaction of denervation
 reflex decay
 Registered Dietician
 Reiter's disease
 renal disease
 Rénon-Delille (syndrome)
 resistance determinant
 respiratory disease
 respiratory distress
 retinal detachment
 Reye's disease
 rheumatoid disease
 right deltoid
 right dorsoanterior
 Riley-Day (syndrome)
 rubber dam
 ruptured disk

R&D research and development

Rd reading; also rd
 rutherford (unit of radioactivity); also rd

rd reading; also Rd
 rutherford (unit of radioactivity); also Rd

RDA recommended daily allowance
 recommended dietary allowance
 Registered Dental Assistant
 right dorso-anterior (fetal position)
 rubidium dihydrogen arsenate

RdA reading age; also RA

RDB randomized double-blind (trial)
 research and development board

RDC research diagnostic criteria

RDDA recommended daily dietary allowance

RDDP ribonucleic acid-dependent deoxynucleic acid polymerase
 ribonucleic acid-directed deoxynucleic acid
 polymerase

RDE receptor-destroying enzyme

RDEB recessive dystrophic epidermolysis bullosa

RDES remote data entry system

RDFC recurring digital fibroma of childhood

RDFS ratio of decayed and filled surfaces (teeth)

RDFT ratio of decayed and filled teeth

RDG Research Discussion Group
right dorsogluteal

RDH Registered Dental Hygienist

RDHBF regional distribution of hepatic blood flow

RDI recommended daily intake
recommended dietary intake
rupture-delivery interval

RDIH right direct inguinal hernia

RDLBBB rate-dependent left bundle-branch block

RDLS Reynell Development Language Scales (psychologic test)

RDM readmission; also Rdm, RE, readm
rod disk membrane

Rdm readmission; also RDM, RE, readm

RDMS Registered Diagnostic Medical Sonographer

rDNA recombinant deoxyribonucleic acid
ribosomal deoxyribonucleic acid

RDOD retinal detachment, right eye [L. *oculus dexter* (right eye)]

RDOS retinal detachment, left eye [L. *oculus sinister* (left eye)]

RDP radiopharmaceutical drug product
right dorsoposterior (fetal position)

RDPase ribonucleic acid-dependent deoxy-ribonucleic acid polymerase

RDPE reticular degeneration of pigment epithelium

RDQ respiratory disease questionnaire

RdQ reading quotient; also RQ

RDRC radioactive drug research committee

RDRV rhesus diploid cell strain rabies vaccine

RDS research diagnostic (criteria)
respiratory distress syndrome
reticuloendothelial depressing substance

RDT regular hemodialysis treatment
retinal damage threshold
routine dialysis therapy

RDTD referral, diagnosis, treatment, and discharge

RDVT recurrent deep vein thrombosis

RDW red blood cell distribution width (index)

RE racemic epinephrine
radium emanation
random error
readmission; also RDM, Rdm, readm
recording electrode
rectal examination
reflux esophagitis
regarding, concerning, in reference to; also re, reg
regional enteritis
regular education
renal and electrolyte
renal excretion
resting energy
reticuloendothelial
retinol equivalent
right ear
right eye
ring enhancement
rostral end

R$_E$ respiratory exchange ratio; also R, RER

R&E research and education
rest and exercise
round and equal

R↑E right upper extremity; also RUE, RUX

R↓E right lower extremity; also RLE, RLX

RE✓ recheck

Re rhenium

R$_e$ Reynold's number

re regarding, concerning, in reference to; also RE, reg

REA radiation emergency area
radioenzymatic assay
renal anastomosis
right ear advantage

REACH Reassurance to Each (assistance to family of mentally ill)

readm readmission; also RDM, Rdm, RE

REAS reasonably expected as safe

REAT radiologic emergency assistance team

REB roentgen-equivalent biologic

R-EBD-HS recessive epidermolysis bullosa dystrophica–Hallopeau-Siemens (syndrome)

REC radioelectrocomplexing
rear end collision
receptor; also Rc

REC—cont'd
recommend
record; also rec
recovery
recreation; also rec
recur
right external carotid

rec fresh [L. *recens*]; also recen
reactive
recent
recombinant (chromosome)
recommendation
record; also REC
recreation; also REC
recurrence; also recur
recurrent; also recur

RECA right external carotid artery

recd, rec'd received

RE CEL reticulum cell(s); also RETUL

RECG radioelectrocardiography; also RCG

recip recipient
reciprocal

recen fresh [L. *recens*]; also rec

recon smallest unit of DNA capable of recombination ["rec" (recombination) + Ger. *on* (quantum)]

recond reconditioned
reconditioning

reconstr reconstruction

recryst recrystallization

RECT rectum; also R, rect

rect rectal; also R, (R), rtl
rectification
rectified
rectum; also R, RECT
rectus (muscle); also R

recur recurrence; also rec
recurrent; also rec

RED radiation experience data
rapid erythrocyte degeneration

Re-D re-evaluation deadline

red reduce
reducing
reduction; also redn

redig in pulv let it be reduced to powder [L. *redigatur in pulverem*]

red in pulv reduced to powder [L. *reductus in pulverem*]

redn reduction; also red

redox reduction-oxidation

REE rapid extinction effect
rare earth element
resting energy expenditure

re-ed re-education

REEDS retention of tears, ectrodactyly, ectodermal dysplasia, and strange hair, skin, and teeth (syndrome)

REEG radioelectorencephalography

R-EEG resting electroencephalogram

REELS Receptive-Expressive Emergent Language Scale

REEP right end-expiratory pressure
role exchange/education-practice

ReEND reproductive endocrinology

REF ejection fraction at rest
rat embryo fibroblast
referred
refused
renal erythropoietic factor

ref reference; also R
reflex; also Refl

Ref Doc referring doctor

REFI regional ejection fraction image

ref ind refractive index; also RI

Refl reflect
reflection
reflex; also ref

REFMS Recreation and Education for Multiple Sclerosis (Victims)

Ref Phys referring physician

REFRAD released from active duty

REG Radiation Exposure Guide
radioencephalogram
radioencephalography
rheoencephalography

Reg registered; also R

reg regarding; also RE, re
region
regular; also R
regulation

regen regenerate
regeneration

reg rhy regular rhythm

reg R&R regular rate and rhythm

reg umb umbilical region [L. *regio umbilici*]

regurg regurgitation

REH renin essential hypertension

REHAB, rehab rehabilitated
rehabilitation

REL rate of energy loss

recommended exposure limit
relative; also rel
religion
resting expiratory level

rel related
relation
relative; also REL

RELE resistive exercises, lower extremities

reliq remainder [L. *reliquus*]

REM radiation-equivalent-man
rapid eye movement (sleep)
recent event memory
reticular erythematous mucinosis
return electrode monitor
roentgen-equivalent-man; also rem

Rem removal; also rem

rem removal; also Rem
roentgen-equivalent-man; also REM

REMA repetitive excess mixed anhydride
(method)

REMAB radiation-equivalent-manikin absorption

REMCAL radiation-equivalent-manikin
calibration

REMP roentgen-equivalent-man period

REMPI resonant enhanced multiphoton
ionization

REMS rapid eye movement sleep

REN renal; also ren, RN

ren renal; also REN, RN
renew [L. *renovetur* (let it be renewed]

ren ∠ renal angle

ren sem renew only once [L. *renovetur semel*
(let it be renewed once)]

REO respiratory enteric orphan (virus)

REP repair (surgical)
repeat; also rept, rpt
report; also rep, rept, rpt
rest-exercise program
retrograde pyelogram; also Retro Pyelo, RGP,
RP, RPG
roentgen-equivalent-physical; also rep

rep replication
report; also REP, rept, rpt
roentgen-equivalent-physical; also REP
to be repeated [L. *repetatur* (let it be
repeated)]; also repet

rep B&S repetitive bending and stooping

REPC reticuloendothelial phagocytic capacity

repet to be repeated [L. *repetatur* (let it be
repeated)]; also rep

repol repolarization

REPS reactive extensor postural synergy
repetitions

rept repeat; also REP, rpt
report; also REP, rep, rpt

req requested
required

REQF wrong test requested–floor error

RER renal excretion rate
respiratory exchange ratio; also R, R_E
rough endoplasmic reticulum

RES electrical resistance (ohm); also R, R
resection
resident; also R, res
respiratory emergency syndrome
reticuloendothelial system

Res research; also res

res research; also Res
reserve
residence
resident; also R, RES
residue

RESA ring-infected erythrocyte surface antigen

RESC, resc resuscitation; also resus

resist ex resistive exercise

Resp respective; also resp
respectively; also resp
respiration; also R, resp
respiratory; also R, resp

resp respective; also Resp
respectively; also Resp
respiration; also R, Resp
respiratory; also R, Resp
respiratory rate; also RR
response; also R, Rs
responsible

RESP-A respiratory battery, acute

REST Raynaud's phenomenon, esophageal
motor dysfunction, sclerodactyly, and
telangiectasia (syndrome)
regressive electric shock therapy
restoration
reticulospinal tract

resus resuscitation; also RESC, resc

RET rational-emotive therapy
retention
reticulocyte; also R, RETIC, retic
retina
retired; also ret, Rtd

RET—cont'd
return; also rtn
right esotropia

ret rad equivalent therapeutic
retired; also RET, Rtd

RETC rat embryo tissue culture

ret cath retention catheter; also RC

RETIC, retic reticulocyte; also R, RET

Retro Pyelo retrograde pyelogram; also REP,
RGP, RP, RPG

RETUL reticulum cell(s); also RE CEL

REUE resistive exercises, upper extremities

REV reticuloendotheliosis virus
reversal
reverse; also R, rev
review; also R, rev
revolution; also rev

rev reverse; also R, REV
review; also R, REV
revolution; also REV

REVL to be reviewed by laboratory
(pathologist)

rev/min revolutions per minute; also
RPM, rpm

Rev of Sym review of symptoms; also
ROS, RS

Rev of Sys review of systems; also ROS, RS

re-x re-examination

RF radial fiber (of cochlea)
radiofrequency; also rf
rate of flow (symbol denoting movement of a
substance in paper chromatography relative
to the solvent front); also R_F, R_f, R_f
ratio of cortical blood flows (outer cortex to
inner cortex)
receptive field (of visual cortex)
receptor floor
recognition factor
reflecting (platelet)
regurgitant fraction
Reitland-Franklin (unit)
relative flow
relative fluorescence
releasing factor
renal failure
replicative form
resistance factor
resorcinol formaldehyde
respiratory failure
respiratory frequency; also Rf
retardation factor (chromatography); also
Rf, R-F

reticular formation
retroflexed
retroperitoneal fibromatosis
rheumatic fever
rheumatoid factor
riboflavin; also RBF
Riga-Fede (syndrome)
right foot
risk factor
root canal filling
rosette formation
Rundles-Falls (syndrome)

R&F radiographic and fluoroscopic

R-F retardation factor (chromatography);
also RF, Rf

R_F, R_f, R_f rate of flow (symbol denoting movement of a substance in paper chromatogra-
phy relative to the solvent front); also RF

Rf respiratory frequency; also RF
retardation factor (chromatography); also
RF, R-F
rutherfordium

rf radiofrequency; also RF

RFA right femoral artery
right forearm
right fronto-anterior (fetal position)

RFB retained foreign body
rheumatoid factor binding

RFC retrograde femoral catheter
right frontal craniotomy
rosette-forming cell

RFE relative fluorescence efficiency

RFFIT rapid fluorescent focus inhibition test

RFI recurrence-free interval
renal failure index

RFL Reiter-Fiessinger-Leroy syndrome
right frontolateral (fetal position)

RFLA rheumatoid-factor-like activity

RFLC resistant Friend leukemia cell

RFLP restriction fragment length polymor-
phism (type of DNA testing)

RFLS rheumatoid-factor-like substance

RFM, Rfm rifampin; also RIF, RMP

RFN Registered Fever Nurse

RFOL results to follow

RFP request for payment
request for proposal
right frontoposterior (fetal position)

RFPS (Glasgow) Royal Faculty of Physicians
and Surgeons of Glasgow

RFR rapid filling rate
  refraction

RFS rapid frozen section
  relapse-free survival
  renal function study

RFT right fibrous trigone
  right frontotransverse (fetal position)
  rod-and-frame test
  routine fever therapy

RFTB riboflavin tetrabutyrate

RFTSW right foot switch

RFV right femoral vein

RFW rapid filling wave (cardiology)

RG retrograde
  right gluteal
  right gluteus

R/G red/green

Rg Rodgers antibodies

RGA retrograde to the atria

RGAS retained gastric antrum syndrome

RGBMT renal glomerular basement membrane
  thickness

RGC radio-gas chromatography
  reaction-gas chromatography
  remnant gastric cancer
  retinal ganglion cell
  right giant cell

RGD range-gated Doppler

RGE relative gas expansion
  respiratory gas equation

RGH rat growth hormone

RGM Rietti-Greppi-Micheli (syndrome)
  right gluteus maximus

RGMT reciprocal geometric mean titer

RGN Registered General Nurse (Scotland)

RGO reciprocating gait orthosis

RGP retrograde pyelogram; also REP,
  Retro Pyelo, RP, RPG
  rural general practitioner

RGR relative growth rate

RGT reversed gastric tube

RH radial hemolysis
  radiant heat
  radiologic health
  reactive hyperemia
  recurrent herpes
  reduced haloperidol
  regional heparinization
  regulatory hormone

relative humidity
  releasing hormone
  rest home
  retinal hemorrhage
  Richner-Hanhart (syndrome)
  right hand
  right hemisphere
  right hyperphoria
  room humidifier

Rh Rhesus (blood factor)
  rheumatoid; also rheu, rheum
  rheumatology; also RHU
  rhinion (craniometric point)
  rhodium
  rhonchus [Gr. *rhonchos* (a snoring sound)]

106Rh rhodium 106, radioactive rhodium;
  halflife, 30 seconds

Rh+ Rhesus positive

Rh- Rhesus negative

rh rales [Fr. râle (rattle)]
  rheumatic; also rheu, rheum

r/h roentgens per hour; also r/hr

RHA right hepatic artery

RhA rheumatoid arthritis; also RA

RHB raise head of bed
  right heart bypass

RHBF reactive hyperemia blood flow

RHBV right heart blood volume

RHC resin hemoperfusion column
  respiration has ceased
  right heart catheterization
  right hypochondrium

RHD radial head dislocation
  radiologic health data
  relative hepatic dullness
  renal hypertensive disease
  rheumatic heart disease; also rheu ht dis
  round heart disease

RhD Rhesus (hemolytic) disease

RHE respiratory heat exchange

RHEED reflection high-energy electron diffraction

rheo rheostat

rheu rheumatic; also rh, rheum
  rheumatism; also rheum
  rheumatoid; also Rh, rheum

rheu ht dis rheumatic heart disease; also RHD

rheum rheumatic; also rh, rheu
  rheumatism; also rheu
  rheumatoid; also Rh, rheu

RHF restricted Hartree-Fock
right heart failure

RHG radial hemolysis in gel
relative hemoglobin
right-hand grip

RHH right homonymous hemianopsia

Rhi rhinology; also Rhin

RhIG Rhesus immune globulin

Rhin rhinologist
rhinology; also Rhi

rhin rhinitis

rhino rhinoplasty

Rhiz *Rhizobium* species

RHL recurrent herpes labialis
right hemisphere lesion
right hepatic lobe

RHLN right hilar lymph node

rhm roentgens per hour at 1 meter

rHm EPO recombinant human erythropoietin;
also r-HuEPO

RhMK, RhMk Rhesus monkey kidney; also
RhMkK, RMK

RhMkK Rhesus monkey kidney; also RhMK,
RhMk, RMK

RHMV right heart mixing volume

RHN Rockwell hardness number

Rh neg Rhesus factor negative

Rh$_{null}$ Rhesus factor null (all Rh factors are
lacking)

RHO right heel off

rhom rhomboid (muscle)

RHP *Rhodospirillum* heme protein
right hemiparesis
right hemiplegia

RHPA reverse hemolytic plaque assay

Rh pos Rhesus factor positive

RHR renal hypertensive rat
resting heart rate

r/hr roentgens per hour; also r/h

RHS right-hand side
right heel strike
rough hard sphere

RHT renal homotransplantation
right hypertropia

RHU Registered Health Underwriter
rheumatology; also Rh

r-HuEPO recombinant human erythropoietin;
also rHm EPO

RHW radiant heat warmer

RI input resistor
radiation intensity
radioimmunology
radioisotope
recession index
recombinant inbred (strain)
refractive index; also ref ind
regenerative index
regional ileitis
regular insulin
relative intensity
release inhibiting
release inhibition
remission induced
remission induction
renal insufficiency
replicative intermediate
respiratory illness
respiratory index
reticulocyte index
retroactive inhibition
retroactive interference
ribosome
right iliac (crest)
right injured
right involved
rooming in
rosette inhibition

R/I rule in

RIA radioimmune assay
radioimmunoassay
reversible ischemic attack
right iliac artery

RIA-DA radioimmunoassay double antibody
(test)

RIAST Reitan Indiana Aphasic Screening Test

RIAT radioimmune antiglobulin test

Rib ribose; also R, r

RIBS Rutherford ion backscattering

RIC radioimmunoconjugate
renomedullary interstitial cell
right iliac crest
right internal capsule
right internal carotid
Royal Institute of Chemistry

RICA reverse immune cytoadhesion
right internal carotid artery

RICE rest, ice, compression, elevation

RICM right intercostal margin

RICS right intercostal space; also RIS

RICU respiratory intensive care unit

RID radial immunodiffusion
radioimmunodetection; also RAID
radioimmunodiffusion
remission-inducing drug
remove intoxicated driver
right ventricular internal diameter
ruptured intervertebral disk; also RIVD

RIDCSF radial immunodiffusion cerebrospinal
fluid

RIE rocket immunoelectrophoresis; also RIEP

RIEP rocket immunoelectrophoresis; also RIE

RIF release-inhibiting factor
rifampin; also RFM, Rfm, RMP
right iliac fossa
right index finger
rigid internal fixation
rosette inhibitory factor

RIFA radioiodinated fatty acid

RIFC rat intrinsic factor concentrate

RIG rabies immune globulin

RIGH rabies immune globulin, human

RIH right inguinal hernia

RIHSA radioactive iodinated human serum
albumin

RIJ right internal jugular (catheter, vein)

RIL recombinant interleukin

RILT rabbit ileal loop test

RIM radioisotope medicine
recurrent induced malaria
relative-intensity measure

RIMA right internal mammary anastomosis
right internal mammary artery

RIMR Rockefeller Institute for Medical
Research

RIMS resonance ionization mass spectrometry

RIN rat insulinoma

RIND resolving incomplete neurologic deficit
resolving ischemic neurologic deficit
reversible ischemic neurologic deficit

RINN recommended international nonproprietary name

RIO right inferior oblique (muscle)

RIOJ recurrent intrahepatic obstructive
jaundice

RIP radioimmunoprecipitation (test)
radioimmunoprecipitin (test)
rapid infusion pump
reflex-inhibiting pattern
respiratory inductance plethysmography

RIPA radioimmunoprecipitation assay

RIPH Royal Institute of Public Health (now:
RIPHH, Royal Institute of Public Health
and Hygiene)

RIPHH Royal Institute of Public Health and
Hygiene

RIR right iliac region
right inferior rectus

RIRB radioiodinated rose bengal (dye)

RIS rapid immunofluorescence staining
resonance ionization spectroscopy

RISA radioactive iodinated serum albumin
radioimmunosorbent assay

RIST radioimmunosorbent test

RIT radioiodinated triolein
Rorschach Inkblot Test; also Ror
rosette inhibition titer

RITC rhodamine isothiocyanate
rhodamine isothiocyanate conjugated

RIU radioactive iodine uptake; also RAIU

RIV ramus interventricularis
right innominate vein

RIVC radionuclide imaging of inferior vena cava
right inferior vena cava

RIVD ruptured intervertebral disk; also RID

RIVS ruptured interventricular septum

RJ radial jerk (reflex)

RJI radionuclide joint imaging

RK rabbit kidney
radial keratotomy
rhodopsin kinase
right kidney; also RKID

RKG radioelectrocardiogram

RKH Rokitansky-Küster-Hauser (syndrome)

RKID right kidney; also RK
right kidney (urine sample)

RKS renal kidney stone
retrograde kidney study

RKV rabbit kidney vacuolating (virus)

RKW renal potassium wasting (L. *kalium*
(potassium)]

RKY roentgen kymography

RL coarse rales [Fr. *râle* (rattle)]
radiation laboratory
reduction level
resistive load
reticular lamina
right lateral; also R LAT, R Lat, RT LAT,
rt lat
right leg
right lower
right lung

RL—cont'd
Ringer's lactate (solution); also RLS
Roussy-Lévy (syndrome)

R L right to left; also R-L, R/L, R➡L

R-L right to left; also R L, R/L, R➡L

R/L right to left; also R L, R-L, R➡L

R➡L right to left; also R L, R-L, R/L

R$_L$ pulmonary resistance; also R$_p$

RL$_3$ numerous coarse rales

Rl medium rales

Rl$_2$ moderate number of medium rales

rl fine rales

rl$_1$ few fine rales

RLA radiographic lung area

R LAT, R Lat right lateral; also RL, RT LAT, rt lat

RLB remontant-leukocytes Beljansky

RLBCD right lower border cardiac dullness

RLC Rapaport-Luebering cycle
reaction liquid chromatography
rectus and longus capitis
residual lung capacity
rhodopsin-lipid complex

RLD related living donor
resistive load detection
right lateral decubitus (position)
round vesicles, large profile and dark mitochondria (synaptic terminals)
ruptured lumbar disk

RLE Recent Life Events
right lower extremity; also RLX, R⬇E

RLF retained lung fluid
retrolental fibroplasia
right lateral femoral (site of injection)
right lateral flexion

RLL radiolucent line
right liver lobe
right lower limb
right lower lobe (of lung)

RLM rat liver mitochondria

RLMD rat liver mitochondria (and submitochondrial particles derived by) digitonin (treatment)

RLN recurrent laryngeal nerve
regional lymph node

RLNC regional lymph node cell

RLND regional lymph node dissection
retroperitoneal lymph node dissection; also RPLND

RLO residual lymphocyte output

RLP radiation leukemia protection
ribosome-like particle
round vesicles, large profile and pale mitochondria (synaptic terminals)

RLQ right lower quadrant (of abdomen)

RLR right lateral rectus (eye muscle)
right lumbar region

RLS person with stammers, having difficulty in enunciating R, L, and S
rat lung strip
restless leg syndrome
Ringer's lactate solution; also RL

RLSB right lower scapular border
right lower sternal border

rl-sh right-left shunt

RLT right lateral thigh

RLTCS repeat low transverse cesarean section

RLV Rauscher's leukemia virus

RLWD routine laboratory work done

RLX right lower extremity; also RLE, R⬇E

RM radical mastectomy
random migration
range of movement; also ROM
red marrow
reference material
regional myocardial
rehabilitation medicine
repetition maximum
resistive movement
respiratory metabolism
respiratory movement
right median
risk management
room; also rm
Rosenthal-Melkersson (syndrome)
Rothmann-Makai (syndrome)
ruptured membranes

R&M routine and microscopic (urinalysis)

Rm relative mobility
remission; also R

rm room; also RM

RMA Registered Medical Assistant
relative medullary area (of kidney)
right mento-anterior (fetal position)

RMB right main-stem bronchus

RMBF regional myocardial blood flow

RMC right middle cerebral (artery)

RMCA right main coronary artery
right middle cerebral artery

RMCAT right middle cerebral artery thrombosis

RMCL right midclavicular line

RMCP rat mast cell protease

RMCT rat mast cell technique

RMD rapid movement disorder
ratio of midsagittal diameters
retromanubrial dullness
right manubrial dullness

RME rapid maxillary expansion
resting metabolic expenditure
right mediolateral episiotomy; also RMLE

RMEE right middle ear exploration

RMF right middle finger

RMI Reading Miscue Inventory

RMK Rhesus monkey kidney; also RhMK, RhMk, RhMkK

RML radiation myeloid leukemia
right mediolateral
right mentolateral (fetal position)
right middle lobe (of lung)

RMLB right middle lobe bronchus

RMLE right mediolateral episiotomy; also RME

RMLS right middle lobe syndrome

RMLV Rauscher's murine leukemia virus; also RMuLV

RMM rapid micromedia method

RMN Registered Mental Nurse (England and Wales)

RMO Regional Medical Office (British)
Resident Medical Officer

RMP rapidly miscible pool
resting membrane potential
rifampin; also RFM, Rfm, RIF
right mentoposterior (fetal position)

RMR resting metabolic rate
right medial rectus (eye muscle)

RMS rectal morphine sulfate (suppository)
repetitive motion syndrome
respiratory muscle strength
rheumatic mitral stenosis
rhodomyosarcoma
root-mean-square; also rms
Ruvalcaba-Myrhe-Smith (syndrome)

rms root-mean-square; also RMS

RMSD root-mean-square deviation

RMSE root-mean-square error

RMSF Rocky Mountain spotted fever

RMT Registered Music Therapist

relative medullary thickness
retromolar trigone
right mentotransverse (fetal position)

RMUI relief medication unit index

RMuLV Rauscher's murine leukemia virus; also RMLV

RMV respiratory minute volume

RN radionuclide
red nucleus
reflex nephropathy
Registered Nurse
renal; also REN, ren
reticular nucleus

Rn radon

RNA radionuclide angiography; also RA, RNG
Registered Nurse Anesthetist
ribonucleic acid
rough, noncapsulated, avirulent (bacterial culture)

RNAA radiochemical neutron activation analysis

RNAase ribonuclease; also RNase

RNase ribonuclease; also RNAase

RNC Registered Nurse Clinician

RND radical neck dissection
reactive neurotic depression

RNEF resting radionuclide ejection fraction; also RREF

RNG radionuclide angiography; also RA, RNA

RNICU regional neonatal intensive care unit

RNL renal laboratory profile

RNMS Registered Nurse for the Mentally Subnormal

RNMT Registered Nuclear Medicine Technologist

RNP Registered Nurse Practitioner
ribonucleoprotein

RNR ribonucleotide reductase

RNS reference normal serum

RNSC radionuclide superior cavography

RNT radioassayable neurotensin

Rnt roentgenology; also roent

RNTC rat nephroma tissue culture

RNV radionuclide venography
radionuclide ventriculography; also RNVG, RVG

RNVG radionuclide ventriculogram; also RVG
radionuclide ventriculography; also RNV, RVG

RO reality orientation
relative odds
reverse osmosis
Ritter-Oleson (technique)
routine order
rule out; also R/O

R/O rule out; also RO

R₀ resting radium

ROA right occipito-anterior (fetal position)

ROAC repeated oral doses of activated charcoal

ROAD reversible obstructive airway disease

ROATS rabbit ovarian antitumor serum

rob Robertsonian (translocation)

ROC receiver operating characteristic(s)
receptor-operated channel
relative operating characteristic(s)
resident on call
residual organic carbon

roc reciprocal ohm centimeter

ROD renal osteodystrophy

RODAC replicate organism detection and counting

ROE return on equity
roentgen; also R, r, roent

roent roentgen; also; R, r, ROE
roentgenology; also Rnt

ROH rat ovarian hyperemia (test)

ROI region of interest

ROIDS hemorrhoids

ROIH right oblique inguinal hernia

ROL right occipitolateral (fetal position)

ROM range of motion
range of movement; also RM
reaction oxygen metabolite
read-only memory
right otitis media
rupture of membranes

Rom Romberg's (sign); also Romb

rom reciprocal ohm meter

Romb Romberg's (sign); also Rom

ROM C P range of motion complete and pain-free

ROMI rule out myocardial infarction

ROMSA right otitis media, suppurative, acute

ROMSC right otitis media, suppurative, chronic

ROM WNL range of motion within normal limits

ROP retinopathy of prematurity
right occipitoposterior (fetal position)

Ror Rorschach (Inkblot Test); also RIT

ROS rat osteosarcoma
review of symptoms; also RS, Rev of Sym
review of systems; also RS, Rev of Sys
rod outer segment(s)

RoS rostral sulcus

ROSC restoration of spontaneous circulation

ROSE reconstruction by optimized series expansion

ROSS review of subjective symptoms
review other subjective symptoms

ROT real oxygen transport
remedial occupational therapy
right occipitotransverse (fetal position)
rotating; also Rot, rot
rotation; also Rot, rot
rotator
rule of thumb

Rot, rot rotate
rotating; also ROT
rotation; also ROT

rot ny rotatory nystagmus

ROU recurrent oral ulcer

rout routine; also R, RTN

ROW rat ovarian weight
Rendu-Osler-Weber (disease, syndrome)

RP (certificate in) radiologic physics
radial pulse
radiographic planimetry
radiopharmaceutical
rapid processing (film)
Raynaud's phenomenon
reaction product
reactive protein
readiness potential
rectal prolapse
re-entrant pathway
refractory period
regulatory protein
relapsing polychondritis; also RPC
relative potency
respiratory rate:pulse rate (index)
resting potential
resting pressure
rest pain
retinitis pigmentosa
retinitis proliferans; also R Pr
retractor penis

retrograde pyelogram; also REP, Retro Pyelo, RGP, RPG
retroperitoneal
reversed phase (chromatography)
rheumatoid polyarthritis
ribose phosphate
roentgenographic pelvimetry

R-5-P ribose-5-phosphate

R$_P$ pulmonary resistance; also R$_L$

RPA radial photon absorptiometry
random phase approximation
resultant physiologic acceleration
12-retinolphorbol-13-acetate
reverse passive anaphylaxis
right pulmonary artery

RPAW right pulmonary artery withdrawal

rPBF regional pulmonary blood flow

RPC relapsing polychondritis; also RP
relative proliferative capacity

RPCF Reiter protein complement fixation (test)

RPCFT Reiter protein complement fixation test

RPCGN rapidly progressive crescenting glomerulonephritis

RPCH rural primary care hospital

RPCU retropubic cytourethropexy

RPD removable partial denture

RPE rate of perceived exertion
recurrent pulmonary emboli
retinal pigment epithelium

RPF relaxed pelvic floor
renal plasma flow
retroperitoneal fibrosis

RPF^a arterial renal plasma flow

RPF^v venous renal plasma flow

RPG radiation protection guide
retrograde pyelogram; also REP, Retro Pyelo, RGP, RP
rheoplethysmography

RPGG retroplacental gamma globulin

RPGN rapidly progressive glomerulonephritis
right pedal giant neuron

RPH retroperitoneal hemorrhage
reverse passive hemagglutination; also RPHA

RPh, R Ph Registered Pharmacist

RPHA reverse passive hemagglutination; also RPH

RPHAMFCA reverse passive hemagglutination by miniature fast centrifugal analysis (test)

RP-HPLC reversed phase high-performance liquid chromatography

RPI reticulocyte production index

R2PI resonant two-photon ionization

RPICA right posterior internal carotid artery

RPICCE round pupil intracapsular cataract extraction

RPIPP reversed phase ion-pair partition

RPL retroperitoneal lymphadenectomy; also RPLAD

RPLAD retroperitoneal lymphadenectomy; also RPL

RPLC reversed-phase liquid chromatography

RPLD repair of potentially lethal damage

RPLND retroperitoneal lymph node dissection; also RLND

RPM, rpm radical pair mechanism
rapid processing mode
revolutions per minute; also rev/min

RPMD rheumatic pain modulation disorder

RPMI Roswell Park Memorial Institute (medium)

RPN renal papillary necrosis
resident's progress note(s)

RPO right posterior oblique (radiologic view)

RPP heart rate–systolic blood pressure product
reductive pentose phosphate (cycle)
retropubic prostatectomy

RPPC regional pediatric pulmonary center

RPPI role perception picture inventory

RPPR red cell precursor production rate

RPR rapid plasma reagin (test)
Reiter protein reagin

R Pr retinitis proliferans; also RP

RPRC rapid plasma reagin card (test)

RPRCF rapid plasma reagin complement fixation

RPRCT rapid plasma reagin card test

RPS renal pressor substance
revolutions per second; also rps

rps revolutions per second; also RPS

RPT rapid pull-through
refractory period of transmission
Registered Physical Therapist

rpt repeat; also REP, rept
 report; also REP, rep, rept

RPTA renal percutaneous transluminal angioplasty

Rptd ruptured; also rupt

RPU retropubic urethropexy

RPV right portal vein
 right pulmonary vein(s)
 Rinderpest virus

RPVP right posterior ventricular pre-excitation

RQ reading quotient; also RdQ
 recovery quotient
 respiratory quotient

RR radial rate
 radiation reaction
 radiation response
 rapid radiometric
 rate ratio
 rate-responsive (pacemaker code)
 reading retarded
 recovery room
 red reflex
 regular rate
 regular respiration
 relative response
 relative risk
 renin release
 respiratory rate; also resp
 respiratory reserve
 response rate
 retinal reflex
 rheumatoid rosette
 right rotation
 risk ratio
 Riva-Rocci (sphygmomanometer); also RRS
 road rash
 ruthenium red

R/R rales/rhonchi

R&R rate and rhythm
 recent and remote
 recession and resection
 rest and recuperation

Rr rami

RRA radioreceptor activity
 radioreceptor assay
 Registered Record Administrator
 right renal artery

RRAM rapid rhythmic alternating movements

RRBC rabbit red blood cell

RRC residency review committee
 risk reduction component
 routine respiratory care

RRCT no(m) regular rate, clear tones, no
 murmurs

RRE radiation-related eosinophilia
 regressive resistive exercise
 round, regular, and equal (pupils); also RR&E

RR&E round, regular, and equal (pupils); also
 RRE

RREF resting radionuclide ejection fraction;
 also RNEF

RRF residual renal function

RR-HPO rapid recompression–high-pressure
 oxygen

RRI reflex relaxation index
 relative response index

RRL Registered Record Librarian

RRm right radical mastectomy

rRNA ribosomal ribonucleic acid

RRND right radical neck dissection

RROM resistive range of motion

RRP relative refractory period

RRQG right rostral quarter ganglion

RRR regular rhythm and rate
 renin-release rate
 risk rescue rating

RRRN round, regular, react normally (pupils)

RRS retrorectal space
 Richards-Rundle syndrome
 Riva-Rocci sphygmomanometer

RRSW Rosin-Rammler-Sperling-Weibull
 (equation for microcapsules)

RRT randomized response technique
 Registered Respiratory Therapist
 relative rate test
 relative retention time
 resazurin reduction time

RRU respiratory resistance unit

RRV Rhesus monkey rotavirus
 right renal vein

RS random sample
 rapid smoking
 rating schedule
 Rauwolfia serpentina
 Raynaud's syndrome
 reading of standard
 recipient's serum
 rectal sinus
 rectosigmoid
 Reed-Sternberg (cell)
 reinforcing stimulus
 Reiter's syndrome
 relative survival

remnant stomach
renal specialist
Repression-Sensitization (scale)
reproductive success
resolved sarcoidosis
resorcinol-sulfur
respiratory syncytial (virus); also Rs
respiratory system
response to stimulus (ratio)
reticulated siderocyte; also R-S
review of symptoms; also Rev of Sym, ROS
review of systems; also Rev of Sys, ROS
Reye's syndrome
rhinal sulcus
rhythm strip
right sacrum
right septum
right side
right stellate (ganglion)
right subclavian
Riley-Schwachmann (syndrome)
Ringer's solution
Ritchie's sedimentation
Robert's syndrome

R-S reticulated siderocyte; also RS
rough-smooth (variation)

R/S rest stress
rupture spontaneous

R&S restraint and seclusion

Rs respiratory syncytial (virus); also RS
respond
response; also R, resp
total systemic resistance

R$_s$ resolution

R/s roentgens per second

r$_s$, r_s Spearman's rank correlation coefficient

RSA rabbit serum albumin; also RbSA
rat serum albumin
regular spiking activity
relative specific activity
relative standard accuracy
respiratory sinus arrhythmia
reticulum cell sarcoma; also RCS
right sacro-anterior (fetal position)
right subclavian artery
roentgen stereophotogrammetric analysis

Rsa total systemic arterial resistance

RSB Regimental Stretcher Bearer
reticulocyte standard buffer
right sternal border

RSBT rhythmic sensory bombardment therapy

RSC rat spleen cell
rested-state contraction

reversible sickle cell
right side colon (cancer)

RSCA, RScA right scapulo-anterior (fetal position)

RSCN Registered Sick Children's Nurse

RSCP, RScP right scapuloposterior (fetal position)

rscu-PA recombinant, single-chain, urokinase-type plasminogen activator

RSD Ratoon stunting disease
reflex sympathetic dystrophy
relative sagittal depth
relative standard deviation
round vesicles, small profile and dark mitochondria (synaptic terminals)

RSDS reflex sympathetic dystrophy syndrome

RSDV respiratory sialodacryoadenitis virus

RSE rat synaptic ending
reference standard endotoxin
reverse sutured eye
right sternal edge

RSEP right somatosensory evoked potential

RSES Rosenberg Self-Esteem Scale

RSF raw soybean flour

RSG Reitan Strength of Grip

RSI repetition strain injury

R-SICU respiratory-surgical intensive care unit

RSIVP rapid-sequence intravenous pyelogram
rapid-sequence intravenous pyelography

RSL right sacrolateral (fetal position)

R SL right short-leg (brace)

RSLD repair of sublethal damage

RSM risk-screening model
Royal Society of Medicine

RSMR relative standardized mortality ratio

RSN right substantia nigra

RSNA Radiological Society of North America

RSO Resident Surgical Officer
right salpingo-oophorectomy
right superior oblique (muscle)

RSP recirculating single pass
removable silicone plug
rhinoseptoplasty
right sacroposterior (fetal position)

RSPK recurrent spontaneous psychokinesis

RSR regular sinus rhythm
relative survival rate
response-stimulus ratio
right superior rectus (muscle)

RSS rat stomach strip
  rectosigmoidoscope
  Russian spring-summer (encephalitis)

RSSE Russian spring-summer encephalitis

RSSR relatively slow sinus rate

RST radiosensitivity test
  rapid surfactant test
  reagin screen test
  right sacrotransverse (fetal position)
  rubrospinal tract

RSTL relaxed skin tension lines

RSTMH Royal Society of Tropical Medicine
  and Hygiene

RSTs Rodney Smith tubes

RSV respiratory syncytial virus
  right subclavian vein
  Rous sarcoma virus

RSVC right superior vena cava

RSVCEF Rous's sarcoma virus-transformed
  chick embryo fibroblast

RSVM Ram seminal vesicle microsomal
  (preparation)

RSW right-sided weakness

RT rabbit trachea
  radiation therapy; also RATx, RTx, RXT
  Radiologic Technologist
  radiologic technology
  radiotelemetry
  radiotherapy; also Rad, RADIO, Rad Ther,
   Rx
  radium therapy
  random transfusion
  raphe transection
  reaction time
  reading task
  reading test
  reading time
  receptor transforming
  reciprocating tachycardia
  recreational therapy
  rectal temperature; also R/T
  red tetrazolium
  reduction time
  Registered Technician
  Registered Technologist
  relaxation time
  renal transplant
  repetition time
  Reporter's Test
  reptilase time
  resistance transfer
  respiratory technology

  Respiratory Therapist
  Respiratory Therapy
  respiratory tract
  rest tremor
  retransformation
  re-transformed (cell-lines)
  right; also R, (R), $\circledR$, Rt, rt
  right thigh
  right triceps
  room temperature
  Rubinstein-Taybi (syndrome)
  running total

R/T rectal temperature; also RT
  related to; also R/t

R$_T$ total pulmonary resistance

RT$_3$ reverse triiodothyronine; also rT$_3$
  serum resin triiodothyronine (uptake)

rT$_3$ reverse triiodothyronine; also RT$_3$

RT$_4$ resin thyroxin

Rt, rt right; also R, $\circledR$, (R), RT

R/t related to; also R/T

rT ribothymidine

RTA renal tubular acidosis
  renal tubular antigen
  road traffic accident

RT(ARRT) Registered Technologist (certified
  by American Registry of Radiologic
  Technologists)

RTC (a)round the clock
  randomized trial, controlled
  renal tubular cell
  research and training center
  residential treatment center
  return to clinic

RTCS Roske-De Toni-Caffey-Smith (disease)

RTD resubmission turnaround document
  routine test dilution

Rtd retarded
  retired; also RET, ret

RTE rabbit thymus extract

RTECS Registry of Toxic Effects of Chemical
  Substances

RTER return to emergency room

RTF replication and transfer
  residential treatment facility
  resistance transfer factor
  respiratory tract fluid
  return to flow

RT + 5-Fu radiation therapy and 5-fluorouracil

RTI respiratory tract infection

RtH right-handed

Rti tissue resistance

RTKP radiothermokeratoplasty

RTL reactive to light (pupils)

rtl rectal; also R, (R), rect

RT LAT, rt lat right lateral; also RL, R LAT, R Lat

RTLC reaction thin-layer chromatography

RTM registered trademark; also R, ®
routine medical care

R$_{tmf}$ total matrix formation rate

RTMN retreatment (staging of cancer)

rTMP ribothymidylic acid

RTN renal tubular necrosis
routine; also R, rout

RT(N) Registered Technologist in Nuclear Medicine

rtn return; also RET

RT(N)(ARRT) Registered Technologist in Nuclear Medicine (certified by American Registry of Radiologic Technologists)

RTO return to office
right toe off

RTOG Radiation Therapy Oncology Group

RTP renal transplant patient
reverse transcriptase-producing (agent)

RTPA, rt PA, rt-PA recombinant tissue-type plasminogen activator

RTPS radiation therapy planning system

RTR Recreational Therapist, Registered
red blood cell turnover rate
retention time ratio
return to room

RT(R)(ARRT) Registered Technologist in Radiography (certified by American Registry of Radiologic Technologists)

RTRR return to recovery room

RTS real-time scan
relative tumor size
return to sender
right toe strike

rTSAB rodent thyroid-stimulating antibody

rt scap bord right scapular border

RT(T)(ARRT) Radiologic Technologist in Radiation Therapy (certified by American Registry of Radiologic Technologists)

r$_{tt}$ obtained coefficient
reliability coefficient

RTU ready to use

real-time ultrasonography; also RTUS
relative time unit

RT$_3$U resin triiodothyronine uptake

RT$_3$UR resin triiodothyronine uptake ratio

rTU ribosomal ribonucleic acid transcription unit

RTUS real-time ultrasonography; also RTU

RTV room temperature vulcanization

RTW return to work; also R/W

RTWD return to work determination

RTx radiation therapy; also RATx, RT, RXT

RU radioactive uptake; also RAU
radioulnar
rat unit
reading of unknown
rectourethral
recurrent ulcer
residual urine
resin uptake
resistance unit (in cardiovascular system);
also R
retrograde urethrogram
retrograde urogram
retroverted uterus
right uninjured
right uninvolved
right upper
rodent ulcer
roentgen unit
routine urinalysis

RU-1 human embryonic lung fibroblast

Ru ruthenium

RUA routine urine analysis

rub red [L. *ruber*]; also R

RUBIDIC rubidazone/dacarbazine (DIC)

RuBP ribulose bisphosphate

RUD rational use of drugs

RUE right upper extremity; also RUX, R↑ E

RUG resource utilization group
retrograde urethrogram

RUL right upper (eye)lid
right upper lateral
right upper limb
right upper lobe (of lung)
right upper lung

RUM right upper medial

RUO right ureteral orifice

RUOQ right upper outer quadrant

RUP right upper pole

rupt ruptured; also Rptd

RUQ right upper quadrant

RUR resin-uptake ratio

RURTI recurrent upper respiratory tract infection

RUS radioulnar synostosis
recurrent ulcerative stomatitis

RUSB right upper sternal border

RUSS recurrent ulcerative scarifying stomatitis

RUV residual urine volume

RUX right upper extremity; also RUE, R↑E

RV random variable
rat virus
Rauscher's virus
recreational vehicle
rectal vault
rectovaginal
reinforcement value
relative viscosity
renal venous
reovirus
reserve volume
residual volume
respiratory volume
retinal vasculitis
retrovaginal
retroversion
retrovirus
return visit
rheumatoid vasculitis
rhinovirus
right ventricle
right ventricular
rubella vaccine
rubella virus
Russell viper

R$_V$ radius of view

RVA rabies vaccine, adsorbed
re-entrant ventricular arrhythmia
right ventricular activation
right ventricular apical
right vertebral artery

RVAD right ventricular assist device

RVAW right ventricular anterior wall

RVB red venous blood

RVC radioactivity of vegetative cells
respond to verbal command

RVD relative vertebral density
relative volume decrease
right ventricular dimension
right vertebral density

RVDO right ventricular diastolic overload

RVDV right ventricular diastolic volume

RVE right ventricular enlargement

RVECP right ventricular endocardial potential

RVEDD right ventricular end-diastolic diameter

RVEDP right ventricular end-diastolic pressure

RVEDV right ventricular end-diastolic volume

RVEF right ventricular ejection fraction
right ventricular end-flow

RVESVI right ventricular end-systolic volume index

RVET right ventricular ejection time

RVF Rift Valley fever
right ventricular failure
right visual field

RVFP right ventricular filling pressure

RVG radionuclide ventriculogram; also RNVG
radionuclide ventriculography; also RNV, RNVG
relative value guide
right ventrogluteal
right visceral ganglion

RVH renovascular hypertension
right ventricular hypertrophy

RVHD rheumatic valvular heart disease

RVI relative value index
right ventricle infarction

RVID right ventricular internal dimension

RVIDd right ventricular internal dimension diastole

RVIDP right ventricular initial diastolic pressure

RVIT right ventricular inflow tract (view)

RVL right vastus lateralis (muscle)

RVLG right ventrolateral gluteal (injection site)

RVO relaxed vaginal outlet
retinal vein occlusion
right ventricular outflow
right ventricular overactivity

RVOT right ventricular outflow tract

RVP rat ventral prostate
red veterinary petrolatum
renovascular pressure
resting venous pressure
right ventricular pressure

RVPFR right ventricular peak filling rate

RVPRA renal vein plasma renin activity

RVR rapid ventricular response
reduced vascular response
reduced vestibular response
renal vascular resistance
renal vein renin
repetitive ventricular response (test)
resistance to venous return

RVRA renal vein renin activity
renal venous renin assay

RV/RA renal vein/renal activity (ratio)

RVRC renal vein renin concentration

RV/RF retroverted/retroflexed

RVS relative value scale
relative value schedule
relative value study
reported visual sensation
retrovaginal space
Rokeach Value Survey (psychologic test)

RVSO right ventricular stroke output

RVSW right ventricular stroke work

RVSWI right ventricular stroke work index

RVT renal vein thrombosis
Russell's viper venom time; also RVVT

RVTE recurring venous thromboembolism

RV/TLC residual volume to total lung capacity (ratio)

RVU relative value unit

RVV rubella vaccine virus
Russell's viper venom

RVVL rubella virus vaccine live

RVVT Russell's viper venom time; also RVT

RVWD right ventricular wall device

RW radiologic warfare
ragweed; also RAG
respiratory work

right ear, warm stimulus
Romano-Ward (syndrome)
Rothmund-Werner (disease)
round window

R-W Rideal-Walker (coefficient)

R/W return to work; also RTW

RWAGE ragweed antigen E

RWIS restraint and water immersion stress

RWM regional wall motion

RWP ragweed pollen
R-wave progression (electrocardiography)

RWS ragweed sensitivity

RWT R-wave threshold (electrocardiography)

Rx drug
medication
pharmacy
prescribe
prescription; also PS, Ps
prescription drug
radiotherapy; also Rad, RADIO, Rad ther, RT
take [L. *recipe*]; also R
therapy
treatment

r(X) right X (chromosome)

Rxd treated

Rx'd US, diath, trx treated with ultrasound, diathermy, traction

RXLI recessive X-linked ichthyosis

RXN reaction; also R

Rx Phys treating physician

RXT radiation therapy; also RATx, RT, RTx
right exotropia

R-Y Roux-en-Y (anastomosis)

Σ SIGMA, UPPER CASE, eighteenth letter of the Greek alphabet
foaminess
sigmoid
sigmoidoscopy; also sig
sum
summation of all quantities following the symbol
syphilis; also SY, syph

σ sigma, lower case, eighteenth letter of the Greek alphabet
conductivity; also cond
cross-section
millisecond (0.001 seconds); also msec, ms
population standard deviation
Stefan-Boltzmann constant
stress
surface tension; also ST
type of molecular bond
wave number

σ^2 population variance

σ_{diff} standard error of difference between scores

σ_{est} standard error of the estimate; also SEE

σ_{meas} standard error of measurement

Σ SIGMA, UPPER CASE, eighteenth letter of the Greek alphabet, terminal

ς sigma, lower case, eighteenth letter of the Greek alphabet, terminal

ϲ sigma, eighteenth letter of the Greek alphabet, variant

S apparent power
area; also A, a
entropy (in thermodynamics); also *S*
exposure time (radiology)
half [L. *semis*]; also HF, hf, s, sem, semi, ss, s̄s̄, s̈s̈
label [L. *signa* (mark, write on)]; also s, Sig, sig
left [L. *sinister*]; also s
length of path; also s
mean dose per unit cumulated activity
midpoint of sella turcica (point)
relative storage capacity
response to white space
sacral
saline; also SA, Sa, SAL, sal
same
saturated; also SAT, Sat, sat, satd, sat'd, std
saturation (of hemoglobin)

schizophrenia; also SC, SCHIZ, schiz
screen-containing cassette
scruple; also s, SC, scr
second (1/60 minute); also s, sec
section; also s, SEC, sec, sect
sedimentation coefficient
sella (turcica)
semilente (insulin)
senile
senility
sensation; also s, sens
sensitivity; also sen, sens
sensory; also sens
septum; also sept
sequential (analysis)
series; also s, ser
serine (one-letter notation); also Ser
serum
sick
siderocyte; also SIDER
Siemen's (unit)
sign [L. *signa* (mark, write on)]; also /S/, /s/, s
signature (prescription); also /S/, /s/, Sig
signed [L. *signa* (mark, write on)]; also /S/, /s/, s, Sig
silicate
single (marital status)
singular; also sing
sinus
sister; also SIS
small; also SM, Sm, sm
smooth (bacterial colony)
soft
soil
solid
soluble; also Sol, sol
solute; also solu
son
sone (unit of loudness)
space; also sp
spasm
spatial aptitude (in General Aptitude Test Battery)
specific activity; also SA
spherical; also Sph, sph
spherical lens; also Sph, sph
spleen; also SP, sp
sporadic
standard; also *S,* std
standard normal deviation
steady state; also s, SS, ss

stem (cell)
stimulus; also R, ST
storage
streptomycin; also SM, STM, strep
subject
subjective (findings)
substrate
suckling; also s
suction; also SUX, SZ
sulcus
sulfur
sum of arithmetic series
supervision; also sup
supravergence
surface
surgery; also SURG, surg, Sx, S_x, sx
suture
Svedberg unit of sedimentation coefficient
   (10^{-13} sec)
swine; also Sw
Swiss (mouse)
symmetrical; also s, sym, *sym*
sympathetic; also sympath
synthesis (phase in cell cycle)
systole; also syst
without [L. *sine*, Fr. *sans*]; also s, s̄,WO, w/o,
write [L. *signa* (mark or write on)]; also s,
   Sig, sig

Ŝ symbol for spatial vector (in electro-
   cardiology)

S denoting attachment to sulfur
entropy (in thermodynamics); also S
Salmonella species
Schistosoma species
Spirillum species; also Sp
standard; also S, std
Staphylococcus species; also Staph, staph
Streptococcus species; also Str, strep
Streptomyces species

/S/ sign; also S, /s/, s
signature; also S, /s/, Sig
signed; also S, /s/, s, Sig

S1 - S5 first through fifth sacral nerves or
   vertebrae

S_1, S_2, S_3, S_4 suicide risk classification

S_1 first heart sound
first sacral nerve or vertebra

S_2 second heart sound
second sacral nerve or vertebra

S_{2P} pulmonic valve closure component of
   the second heart sound

S_3 third heart sound

third sacral nerve or vertebra
ventricular gallop sound

S_4 atrial gallop
fourth heart sound
fourth sacral nerve or vertebra

S_5 fifth sacral nerve or vertebra

s atomic orbital with angular momentum quantum number zero
distance
half [L. *semis*]; also HF, hf, S, sem, semi, ss,
   s̄s̄, s̄ s̄
label [L. *signa* (mark or write on)]; also S,
   Sig, sig
left [L. *sinister*]; also S
length of path; also S
sample standard deviation; also s
sample variance; also s^2
satellite (chromosome)
scruple; also S, SC, scr
second (1/60 minute); also S, sec
section; also S, SEC, sec, sect
sensation; also S, sens
series; also S, ser
sign [L. *signa* (mark or write on)]; also S,
   /S/, /s/
signed [L. *signa* (mark, write on)]; also S,
   /S/, /s/, Sig
steady state; also S, SS, ss
suckling; also S
without [L. *sine*, Fr. *sans*]; also S, s̄ , sin,
   WO, w/o
write [L. *signa* (mark or write on)]; also S,
   Sig, sig

s sample standard deviation; also s
symmetrical; also S, sym, *sym*

s̄ without [L. *sine*, Fr. *sans*]; also S, s, sin,
   WO, w/o
without spectacles

s^{-1} reciprocal second

s^2 sample variance; also s

/s/ sign; also S, /S/, s
signature; also S, /S/, Sig
signed; also S, /S/, s, Sig

SA by skill [L. *secundum artem* (according to
   art)]; also sa, sec a
salicylamide; also SAM
salicylic acid; also S-A
saline; also S, Sa, SAL, sal
salt added
sarcoma; also sarc
second antibody
secondary amenorrhea

SA—cont'd
secondary anemia
secondary arrest
self-agglutinating
self-analysis
semen analysis
sensitizing antibody
serum albumin; also SAB
serum aldolase
short acting
sialic acid; also Sia
sialoadenectomy
siblings raised apart
simian adenovirus
sinoatrial; also S-A
sinus arrest
sinus arrhythmia
skeletal age
sleep apnea
slightly active
social acquiescence
soluble in alkaline (medium)
Spanish-American
spatial average
specific activity; also S
spectrum analysis
sperm abnormality
spermagglutinin
spiking activity
splenic artery
standard accuracy
Staphylococcus aureus
stimulus artifact
Stokes-Adams (disease)
suicide alert
suicide attempt
surface antigen
surface area; also S-A
surgeon's assistant
surgical assistant
sustained action; also S-A
sympathetic activity
systemic artery
systemic aspergillosis

S-A salicylic acid; also SA
sinoatrial; also SA
sinoauricular
surface area; also SA
sustained action; also SA

S/A same as
sugar and acetone; also S&A

S&A sickness and accident (insurance)
sugar and acetone; also S/A

Sa most anterior point of anterior contour of
the sella turcica (point)
saline; also S, SA, SAL, sal
samarium; also Sm

sa by skill [L. *secundum artem* (according to
art)]; also SA, sec a

sA statampere

SA-8 square antiprismatic

SAA same as above
serum amyloid-A
severe aplastic anemia
Stokes-Adams attack

SAAABB Subcommittee on Accreditation of
the American Association of Blood Banks

SAARD slow-acting antirheumatic drug

SAAST self-administered alcohol screening
test

SAB serum albumin; also SA
significant asymptomatic bacteriuria
sinoatrial block; also S-AB
Society of American Bacteriologists
spontaneous abortion; also spont Ab
subarachnoid bleed
subarachnoid block

S-AB sinoatrial block; also SAB

SABHI Sabouraud dextrose and brain heart
infusion (agar)

SABP spontaneous acute bacterial peritonitis

SABRS social adjustment behavior rating scale

SAC saccharin
screening and acute care
short-arm cast
splenic adherent cell
subarea advisory council
substance abuse counselor

SACC short-arm cylinder cast

sacc cogwheel respiration [Fr. *saccade* (jerk)]

SACD subacute combined degeneration; also
SCD

SACE serum angiotensin-converting enzyme
(activity)

SACH single axis, cushion heel (foot)
small animal care hospital
solid ankle, cushion heel (orthopedic appliance)

SACHT serum anti-chymotrypsin

sac-il sacroiliac; also SI

SACS secondary anticoagulation system

SACSF subarachnoid cerebrospinal fluid

SACT sinoatrial conduction time

SAD seasonal affective disorder
Self-Assessment Depression (scale)
separation anxiety disorder
sinoaortic denervated (rat)
small airway dysfunction
social avoidance and distress
source-to-axis distance
subacute dialysis
sugar, acetone, diacetic acid (test)
suppressor-activating determinant

SADBE squaric acid dibutylester

SADD Standardized Assessment of Depressive Disorders
Students Against Drunk Driving

SADL simulated activities of daily living

SADQ Self-Administered Dependency Questionnaire

SADR suspected adverse drug reaction

SADS Schedule for Affective Disorders and Schizophrenia
Shipman Anxiety Depression Scale

SADS-C Schedule for Affective Disorders and Schizophrenia - Change

SADS-L Schedule for Affective Disorders and Schizophrenia - Lifetime (version)

SADT Stetson Auditory Discrimination Test

SAE short above-elbow (cast)
specific action exercise
subcortical atherosclerotic encephalopathy
supported arm exercise

SAEB sinoatrial entrance block

SAECG signal-averaged electrocardiogram

SAEP *Salmonella abortus equi* pyrogen

SAF self-articulating femoral (hip prosthesis)
serum accelerator factor
simultaneous auditory feedback
Spanish-American female

SAFA soluble antigen fluorescent antibody (test)

SAFE simulated aircraft fire and emergency

SAG Swiss-type agammaglobulinemia

sag sagittal

Sag D sagittal diameter

SAGM sodium chloride, adenine, glucose, mannitol

SAH *S*-adenosyl-L-homocysteine
subarachnoid hemorrhage
systemic arterial hypertension

SAHS sleep apnea–hypersomnolence syndrome

SAI Self-Analysis Inventory

Sexual Arousability Inventory
Social Adequacy Index
Sodium Amytal interview
systemic active immunotherapy
without other qualification [L. *sine altera indicatione*]

SAICAR succinoaminoimidazole carboxamide ribonucleotide

SAID sexually acquired immunodeficiency (syndrome)

SAIDS simian acquired immunodeficiency syndrome

SAKK Swiss Group for Clinical Cancer Research

SAL according to the rules of the art [L. *secundum artis leges*]; also sal
salbutamol
salicylate; also Sal, sal
saline; also S, SA, Sa, sal
sensorineural acuity level
specified antilymphocytic
suction-assisted lipectomy

SAL 12 sequential analysis of twelve chemistry constituents

Sal salicylate; also SAL, sal
salicylic; also sal
Salmonella species

sal according to the rules of the art [L. *secundum artis leges*]; also SAL
salicylate; also SAL, Sal
salicylic; also Sal
saline; also S, SA, Sa, SAL
saliva
salt

SAM *S*-adenosyl-L-methionine
salicylamide; also SA
scanning acoustic microscope
scanning Auger microscopy
self-administered medication
sex arousal mechanism
Spanish-American male
sulfated acid mucopolysaccharide
surface-active material
synthetic, adhesive, moisture (vapor permeable)
systolic anterior motion (of mitral valve)

SAMA Student American Medical Association (now: AMSA, American Medical Student Association)

SAMD *S*-adenosyl-L-methionine decarboxylase; also SAM-DC

SAM-DC *S*-adenosyl-L-methionine decarboxylase; also SAMD

SAMF single antibody millipore filtration

SAMI socially acceptable monitoring instrument

SAMO Senior Administrative Medical Officer

S-AMY serum amylase

SAN side-arm nebulizer
sinoatrial node
sinoauricular node
slept all night
solitary autonomous nodule

SANA sinoatrial node artery

Sanat sanatorium

SANC short-arm navicular cast

SANDR sinoatrial nodal re-entry

sang sanguinous

sanit sanitarium
sanitary
sanitation

SANS Scale for the Assessment of Negative
Symptoms

SAO small airway obstruction
splanchnic artery occlusion

SaO$_2$, S$_{AO2}$ oxygen percent saturation (arterial); also OS, O$_2$ sat, SO$_2$

SAP sensory action potential
serum acid phosphatase
serum alkaline phosphatase
serum amyloid P (component)
situs ambiguus with polysplenia
Staphylococcus aureus protease
systemic arterial pressure

sap saponification; also sapon
saponify

SAPD self-administration of psychotropic drug

SAPH saphenous

SAPMS short-arm posterior-molded splint

sapon saponification; also sap

SAPP sodium acid pyrophosphate

SAPS short-arm plaster splint
Simplified Acute Physiology Score

SAQ short-arc quadriceps (test)

SAQC statistical analysis and quality control

SAR seasonal allergic rhinitis
sexual attitude reassessment
sexual attitude restructuring
structure-activity relationship

Sar sulfarsphenamine

SARA sexually acquired reactive arthritis
system for anesthetic and respiratory
administration

sarc sarcoma; also SA

SART sinoatrial recovery time

SAS salicylazosulfapyridine; also SASP
saline, agent, and saline
self-rating anxiety scale
short-arm splint
Sklar Aphasia Scale
sleep apnea syndrome
small animal surgery
small aorta syndrome
social adjustment scale
sodium amylosulfate
space-adaptation syndrome
Statistical Analysis System
sterile aqueous solution
sterile aqueous suspension
subaortic stenosis; also SS
subarachnoid space
sulfasalazine; also SAZ, ss
supravalvular aortic stenosis; also SVAS
surface-active substance

SASDRA sample acquisition system for
dissolution rate analysis

SASH saline, agent, saline, and heparin

SASP salazosulfapyridine
salicylazosulfapyridine; also SAS

SAT satellite
saturated; also S, Sat, sat, satd, sat'd, std
saturation; also Sat, sat, satn
Scholastic Aptitude Test
School Ability Test
School Attitude Test
Senior Apperception Technique
serum antitrypsin
Shapes Analysis Test
single-agent chemotherapy
slide agglutination test
specific antithymocytic
speech awareness threshold
spermatogenic activity test
spontaneous activity test
spontaneous autoimmune thyroiditis
Stanford Achievement Test
structural atypia
subacute thyroiditis
symptomless autoimmune thyroiditis
systematized assertive therapy
systemic assertive therapy

Sat saturated; also S, SAT, sat, satd, sat'd, std
saturation; also SAT, sat, satn

sat satisfactory
saturated; also S, SAT, Sat, satd, sat'd, std
saturation; also SAT, Sat, satn
without thymonucleic acid [L. *sine acido
thymonucleinico*]

SATA spatial average/temporal average

SATB Special Aptitude Test Battery

sat cond satisfactory condition

satd, sat'd saturated; also S, SAT, Sat, sat, std

SATL surgical Achilles tendon lengthening

SATM sodium aurothiomalate

satn saturation; also SAT, Sat, sat

SATP spatial average temporal peak

sat sol saturated solution; also sat soln, SS

sat soln saturated solution; also sat soln, SS

SAU statistical analysis unit

SAV sequential atrioventricular (pacing)
streptavidin
supra-annular valve

SAVD spontaneous assisted vaginal delivery

SAZ sulfasalazine; also SAS, SS

SB safety belt
sandbag
Schwartz-Bartter (syndrome)
scleral buckle
Sengstaken-Blakemore (tube); also S-B
serum bilirubin
shortness of breath; also SOB
sick bay (Navy)
sideroblast
Silvestroni-Bianco (syndrome)
single blind
single-breath
sinus bradycardia
small bowel
sodium balance
soybean
spina bifida
spontaneous blastogenesis
spontaneously breathing
stand-by; also ST BY
Stanford-Binet (Intelligence Scale); also S-B
stereotyped behavior
sternal border
stillbirth
stillborn; also STB, Stb, stillb
suction biopsy
surface binding (protein)

SB- not wearing seat belt

+SB wearing seat belt

S-B Sengstaken-Blakemore (tube); also SB
Stanford-Binet (Intelligence Scale); also SB

S/B seen by
side bending

Sb antimony [L. *stibium*]
strabismus; also strab

sb stilb (unit of luminous intensity)

SBA serum bactericidal activity
serum bile acid
soybean agglutinin
spina bifida aperta
stand-by assistance
summary basis for approval

SBB simultaneous binaural bithermal
small-bowel biopsy
stimulation-bound behavior

SBC serum bactericidal concentration
standard bicarbonate
strict bed confinement
sunburn cell

SBD straight bag drainage
suggested brain dysfunction

S-BD seizure-brain damage

SBDCo single-breath diffusing capacity for
carbon monoxide

SbDH sorbitol dehydrogenase; also SDH

SBE breast self-examination
short below-elbow (cast)
shortness of breath on exertion; also SOBE,
SOBOE
subacute bacterial endocarditis

SBEP somatosensory brainstem-evoked
potential(s)

S/β sickle-cell beta

SBF serologic-blocking factor
serum blocking factor
specific blocking factor
splanchnic blood flow
splenic blood flow

SBFT small bowel follow-through; also
SMBFT

SBG selenite brilliant green
stand-by guard

SBGM self blood-glucose monitoring

SBH sea-blue histiocyte
State Board of Health

SBI serious bacterial infection
soybean trypsin inhibitor; also SBTI, STI
systemic bacterial infection

SBIS Stanford-Binet Intelligence Scale

SBJ skin, bones, joints

SBL serum bactericidal level
soybean lecithin

SBMPL simultaneous binaural midplace localization

SBMV southern bean mosaic virus

SBN single-breath nitrogen (test); also SBN_2, SB_{N2}

SBN_2, SB_{N2} single-breath nitrogen (test); also SBN

SBNT single-breath nitrogen test

SBNW single-breath nitrogen washout

SBO small bowel obstruction
spina bifida occulta

SBOD scleral buckle, right eye [L. *oculus dexter* (right eye)]

SBOM soybean oil meal

SBOS scleral buckle, left eye [L. *oculus sinister* (left eye)]

SBP school breakfast program
scleral buckling procedure
serotonin-binding protein
spontaneous bacterial peritonitis
steroid-binding plasma (protein)
sulfobromophthalein
systemic blood pressure; also Psa
systolic blood pressure; also SYS BP

SBPC sulfobenzylpenicillin

SBQC small-based quad cane

SBR spleen to body weight ratio
stillbirth rate
stimulus-bound repetitive
strict bed rest
styrene-butadiene rubber

SBS shaken baby syndrome
short bowel syndrome
side-by-side (structure)
side to back to side
small bowel series
social breakdown syndrome
staff burn-out scale
straight back syndrome

SBSM self blood-sugar monitoring

SBSRT Spreen-Benton Sentence Repetition Test

SBSS Seligmann buffered salt solution

SBT serum bactericidal test
serum bacteriocial titer
single-breath test
sulbactam

SBTI soybean trypsin inhibitor; also SBI, STI

SBTPE State Boards Test Pool Examination

SBTT small bowel transit time

SBW spectral bandwidth

SC sacrococcygeal
Sanetis-Cacchione (syndrome)
Sanitary Corps
schedule change
schizophrenia; also S, SCHIZ, schiz
Schüller-Christian (disease)
Schwann cell
Scianna (blood group)
sciatic (nerve)
science; also Sc, Sci, sci
scruple; also S, s, scr
secondary cleavage
secretory coil
secretory component
self-care
self-control
semicircular
semiclosed
semilunar valve closure
serum complement
serum creatinine; also SCr
service-connected
sex chromatin
Sézary cell
shallow compartment
short circuit
sick call
sickle cell; also S-C
silicone coated
single chemical
skin conduction
slow component
Smeloff-Cutter (prosthesis, valve)
Snellen's chart
sodium citrate
soluble complex
special care
specific characteristic
spinal cord; also sp cd
spleen cell; also SPC
squamous carcinoma
statistical control
stellate cell
stepped care
sternoclavicular
stimulus, conditioned
stratum corneum
streptococcus
stroke count

subcellular

subclavian

subcorneal

subcortical

subcostal (view)

subcutaneous; also sc, SQ, Sq, subcu, subcut, subq, sub-q

succinylcholine; also SCH, SUCC, SUX

sugar coated

sulfur colloid

sulfur containing

superior colliculus

superior constrictor (muscles of pharynx)

superior cornu

supportive care

suppressor cell

surface colony

surgical cone

systemic candidiasis

systolic click

without correction (without glasses) [L. *sine correctione*]; also s̄ gl

S-C sickle cell; also SC

S&C sclerae and conjunctivae

singly and consensually

Sc scandium

scapula

science; also SC, Sci, sci

scientific; also Sci, sci

sC statcoulomb

sc one may know [L. *scilicet* (certainly, evidently, of course)]

scant

sclera

subcutaneous; also SC, SQ, Sq, subcu, subcut, subq, sub-q

SCA School and College Ability (tests)

self-care agency

severe congenital anomaly

sickle cell anemia; also SSA

single-channel analyzer

sperm-coating antigen

spleen colony assay

steroidal-cell antibody

subclavian artery

subcutaneous abdominal (block)

superior cerebellar artery

suppressor cell activity

SCa, S$_{Ca}$ serum calcium

SCAB streptozotocin, CCNU, Adriamycin, bleomycin sulfate

SCAb autoantibody to stratum corneum

SCABG single coronary artery bypass graft

SCAG sandoz clinical assessment–geriatric (rating)

single coronary artery graft

SCAN suspected child abuse and neglect

systolic coronary artery narrowing

SCAS semicontinuous activated sludge

SCAT sheep cell agglutination test

sheep cell agglutination titer

sickle cell anemia test

scat box [L. *scatula*]

scat orig original package [L. *scatula originalis*]

SCB sedative cabinet bath

stratum corneum basic

strictly confined to bed

SCBA self-contained breathing apparatus

SCBC small cell bronchogenic carcinoma

SCBE single-contrast barium enema

SCBF spinal cord blood flow

SCBG symmetrical calcification of basal cerebral ganglia

SCBH systemic cutaneous basophil hypersensitivity

SCBP stratum corneum basic protein

SCBU special care baby unit

ScBU screening bacteriuria

SCC sequential combination chemotherapy

Services for Crippled Children

short circuit current

short course chemotherapy

sickle cell crisis

small cell carcinoma

small cleaved cell

squamous carcinoma of cervix

squamous cell cancer

squamous cell carcinoma; also SCCA, SqCCA, sq cell ca

SCCA semiclosed circle absorber system

squamous cell carcinoma; also SCC, SqCCA, sq cell ca

SCCB small cell carcinoma of bronchus

SCCH sternocostoclavicular hyperostosis

SCCHN squamous cell carcinoma of head and neck

SCCL small cell carcinoma of the lung

SCCM Sertoli cell culture medium

SCD sequential compression device

service-connected disability

SCD—cont'd
sickle cell disease; also SSD
spinal cord disease
spinocerebellar degeneration
subacute combined degeneration; also SACD
sudden cardiac death
sudden coronary death
sulfur-carbon drug
systemic carnitine deficiency

ScD Doctor of Science

ScDA right scapulo-anterior (fetal position)
[L. *scapulodextra anterior*]

ScDP right scapuloposterior (fetal position)
[L. *scapulodextra posterior*]

SCE saturated calomel electrode
secretory carcinoma of the endometrium
sister chromatid exchange
subcutaneous emphysema

SCEP sandwich counterelectrophoresis
somatosensory cortical-evoked potential

SCER sister chromatid exchange rate

SCF supercritical fluid

SCFA short-chain fatty acid

SCFE slipped capital femoral epiphysis

SCFI specific clotting factor and inhibitor

SCG serum chemistry graft
serum chemogram
sodium cromoglycate
superior cervical ganglion

SCH Schirmer's (test)
sole community hospital
succinylcholine; also SC, SUCC, SUX
suprachiasmatic

SCh succinylcholine chloride

SChE serum cholinesterase

sched schedule

SCHISTO schistocyte (schizocyte); also SCHIZ

SCHIZ schistocyte (schizocyte); also
SCHISTO
schizophrenia; also S, SC, schiz

schiz schizophrenia; also S, SC, SCHIZ

SCHL subcapsular hematoma of liver

SCHLP supracricoid hemilaryngopharyn-
gectomy

SCI Science Citation Index
short crus of incus
spinal cord injury
structured clinical interview

Sci, sci science; also SC, Sc
scientific; also Sc

SCIBTA stem cell indicated by transplantation
assay

SCID severe combined immunodeficiency
disease

SCII Strong-Campbell Interest Inventory

SCIPP sacrococcygeal to inferior pubic point

SCIS severe combined immunodeficiency
syndrome

SCIU spinal cord injury unit

SCIV subcutaneous intravenous

SCJ squamocolumnar junction
sternoclavicular joint

SCK serum creatine kinase

SCL scleroderma; also SD
serum copper level
sinus cycle length
skin conductance level
soft contact lens
spinocervicolemniscal
symptom checklist
syndrome checklist

Scl, scl sclerosis
sclerotic

ScLA left scapulo-anterior (fetal position)
[L. *scapulolaeve anterior*]

SCLAX subcostal long axis

SCLC small cell lung cancer

SCLE subcutaneous lupus erythematosus

ScLP left scapuloposterior (fetal position)
[L. *scapulolaeva posterior*]

SCM Schwann cell membrane
sensation, circulation, and motion
Society of Computer Medicine
soluble cytotoxic medium
spleen cell-conditioned medium
spondylitic caudal myelopathy
State Certified Midwife
steatocystoma multiplex
sternocleidomastoid
streptococcal cell membrane
structure of the cytoplasmic matrix
surface-connecting membrane

S colony smooth colony

ScM scalene muscle

SCMC S-carboxymethylcysteine
sodium carboxymethyl-cellulose
spontaneous cell-mediated cytotoxicity

SCMD senile choroidal macular
degeneration

SCMO Senior Clerical Medical Officer

SCMS sodium colistin methanesulfonate

SCN serum thiocyanate
  sodium thiocyanate
  special care nursery
  suprachiasmatic nucleus
  thiocyanate

SC$_{Na}$ sieving coefficient for sodium

SCNS subcutaneous nerve stimulation

SCO somatic crossing-over
  subcommissural organ

SCOP, scop scopolamine

SCP single-celled protein
  sodium cellulose phosphate
  soluble cytoplasmic protein
  Standardized Care Plan
  submucous cleft palate
  superior cerebellar peduncle

scp spherical candle power

SCPK, S-CPK serum creatine phosphokinase

SCPN serum carboxypeptidase N

SCPNT Southern California Postrotary
  Nystagmus Test

SCR silicon-controlled rectifier
  skin conductance response
  special care room
  spondylitic caudal radiculopathy

SCr serum creatinine; also SC

scr scruple; also S, s, SC

SCRAM speech-controlled respirometer for
  ambulation measurement

SCRAP Simple-Complex Reaction-Time
  Apparatus

SCRS Short Clinical Rating Scale

SCS Saethre-Chotzen syndrome
  silicon-controlled switch
  Society of Clinical Surgery
  surface connecting system

SCSAX subcostal short axis

SCSP supracondylar suprapatellar

SCT salmon calcitonin
  Sentence Completion Test
  sex chromatin test
  sickle cell trait
  sperm cytotoxic
  spinal computed tomography
  spinocervicothalamic
  staphylococcal clumping test
  sugar-coated tablet

SCTAT sex cord tumor with anular tubules

SCU self-care unit
  special care unit

SCUBA self-contained underwater breathing
  apparatus

SCUD septicemic cutaneous ulcerative disease

SCUF slow continuous ultrafiltration

SCUM secondary carcinoma of the upper
  mediastinum

scu-PA single chain urokinase-type plasminogen activator

SCUT schizophrenia, chronic undifferentiated
  type

SCV sensory conduction velocity
  smooth, capsulated, virulent (bacteria)
  squamous-cell carcinoma of vulva
  subclavian vein; also SV
  subcutaneous vaginal (block)

SCV-CPR simultaneous compression ventilation–cardiopulmonary resuscitation

SD sagittal depth (of cornea)
  Sandhoff's disease
  scleroderma; also SCL
  secretion droplet
  senile dementia
  septal defect
  serologically defined
  serologically detectable
  serologically determined
  serum defect
  severely disabled
  shoulder disarticulation
  shoulder dislocation
  Shy-Drager (syndrome)
  skin destruction
  skin dose
  socialized delinquency
  somadendritic
  spontaneous delivery
  sporadic depression
  Sprague-Dawley (rat)
  spreading depression
  stable disease
  standard deviation
  standard diet
  statistical documentation
  Stensen's duct
  sterile dressing
  Still's disease
  stimulus drive; also Sd
  stone disintegration
  straight drainage
  streptodornase

SD—cont'd
streptozocin and doxorubicin
succinate dehydrogenase; also SDG, SDH
sudden death
sulfadiazine
superoxide dismutase; also SOD
surgical drain
systolic discharge

S-D sickle cell–hemoglobin D
strength-duration (curve)

S/D sharp/dull
systolic to diastolic (ratio)

S&D stomach and duodenum

Sd stimulus drive; also SD

S^d stimulus, discriminative

SDA right sacro-anterior (fetal position) [L. *sacrodextra anterior*]
Sabouraud dextrose agar
salt-dependent agglutinin
Seventh-Day Adventist
sialodacryoadenitis (virus)
specific dynamic action
steroid-dependent asthmatic
succinic dehydrogenase activity
superficial distal axillary (node)

SDAT senile dementia, Alzheimer type

SDB sleep-disordered breathing

SDBP seated diastolic blood pressure
standing diastolic blood pressure
supine diastolic blood pressure

SDC sensitivity depth compensation (ramp)
serum digoxin concentration
size/date consistency
sodium deoxycholate
succinyldicholine
sulfodeoxycholate

SD&C suction, dilation, and curettage

SDCL symptom distress checklist

SDD selective digestive tract decontamination
sporadic depressive disease
sterile dry dressing

SDDS 2-sulfamoyl-4,4′-diaminodiphenyl-sulphone

SDE specific dynamic effect

SDEEG stereotactic depth electroencephalo-gram

SDES symptomatic diffuse esophageal spasm

SDF slow death factor
stream dilution factor
stress distribution factor

SDFP single-donor frozen plasma

SDG short distance group
succinate dehydrogenase; also SD, SDH
sucrose density gradient

SDGC sucrose density gradient centrifugation

SDGU sucrose density gradient ultracentri-fugation

SDH serine dehydrase
sorbitol dehydrogenase; also SbDH
spinal dorsal horn
subdural hematoma
subjacent dorsal horn
succinate dehydrogenase; also SD, SDG

SDHD sudden death heart disease

SDI size/date inconsistency
standard deviation interval (index)
Surtees Difficulties Index

SDIHD sudden death ischemic heart disease

SDL self-directed learning
serum digoxin level
serum drug level
speech discrimination loss

SDLRS self-directed-learning readiness scale

sdly sidelying

SDM sensory detection method
single, divorced, married
standard deviation of the mean
sulfadimidine

SDMS Society of Diagnostic Medical Sonographers

SDMT Symbol Digit Modalities Test

SDN sexually dimorphic nucleus

SDNA single-strand deoxyribonucleic acid

SDO sudden-dosage onset

SDP right sacroposterior (fetal position) [L. *sacrodextra posterior*]
single-donor platelets
stomach, duodenum, and pancreas

SDPH sodium diphenylhydantoin

SDR spontaneously diabetic rat
surgical dressing room

SDRS social dysfunction rating scale

SDRT Stanford Diagnostic Reading Test

SDS same day surgery
school dental service
Self-Rating Depression Scale
sensory deprivation syndrome
sexual differentiation scale
Shy-Drager syndrome
simple descriptive scale

single dose suppression
sodium dodecyl sulfate
specific diagnosis service
speech discrimination score
standard deviation score
sudden death syndrome
sulfadiazine silver
sustained depolarizing shift

Sds, sds sounds

SD-SK streptodornase-streptokinase

SDS/PAGE sodium dodecyl sulfate/polyacrylamide gel electrophoresis; also SDS-PGE

SDS-PGE sodium dodecyl sulfate/polyacrylamide gel electrophoresis; also SDS/PAGE

SDT right sacrotransverse (fetal position) [L. *sacrodextra transversa*]
sensory decision theory
single-donor transfusion
speech detection threshold

SDU short double upright
Standard Deviation Unit
step-down unit

SDW separated, divorced, widowed

SE saline enema
sanitary engineering
Seeing Eye
self-explanatory
sheep erythrocyte
side effect(s)
smoke exposure
smoke extract
soft exudate
solid extract
sphenoethmoidal (suture)
spherical equivalent
spin-echo
spongiform encephalopathy
Spurway-Eddowes (syndrome)
squamous epithelium
standard error
starch equivalent
Starr-Edwards (pacemaker, prosthesis, valve); also S-E
status epilepticus
sterol ester
subendocardial
subendothelial
supernormal excitability
sustained engraftment
systematic error

S-E Starr-Edwards (pacemaker, prosthesis, valve); also SE

S&E safety and efficiency

Se selenium

SEA screening experiment analysis
sheep erythrocyte agglutination
shock-elicited aggression
soluble egg antigen
Southeast Asia
spontaneous electrical activity
staphylococcal enterotoxin A

SEAR Southeast Asia refugee

SEAT sheep erythrocyte agglutination test

SEB Scale for Emotional Blunting
staphylococcal enterotoxin B

SEBA staphylococcal enterotoxin B antiserum

seb derm seborrheic dermatitis

seb ker seborrheic keratosis; also SK

SEBL self-emptying blind loop

SEBM Society of Experimental Biology and Medicine

SEC according to [L. *secundum*]
secondary; also sec, *sec*
secretin
secretion
section; also S, s, sec, sect
series elastic component (of muscles)
Singapore epidemic conjunctivitis
size exclusion chromatography
soft elastic capsule
squamous epithelial cell
strong exchange capacity (resin)

Sec Seconal

sec second (1/60 minute); also S, s
secondary; also SEC, *sec*
secretary
section; also S, s, SEC, sect

sec secondary; also SEC, sec

sec a by skill [L. *secundum artem* (according to art)]; also SA, sa

SECG stress electrocardiography

SECPR standard external cardiopulmonary resuscitation

SECSY spin-echo correlated spectroscopy

sect section; also S, s, SEC, sec

SED sedimentation; also sed
sedimentation (rate)
side effects of drugs
skin erythema dose
spondyloepiphyseal dysplasia
standard error of difference
staphylococcal enterotoxin D

SED—cont'd
strain energy density
suberythemal dose
surgical emergency department

Sed stool [L. *sedes*]; also sed

sed sedate
sedative
sedimentation; also SED
stool [L. *sedes*]; also Sed

SEDD Szondi's Experimental Diagnostics of
Drives

sed rate sedimentation rate; also sed rt, SR

sed rt sedimentation rate; also sed rate, SR

SEE scopolamine-Eukodal-Ephetonin
series elastic element
standard error of the estimate; also σ_{est}

SEEP small end-expiratory pressure

SEER Surveillance, Epidemiology, and End
Results (Program)

SEF somatically evoked field
staphylococcal enterotoxin F

SEG segment; also segm
soft elastic gelatin (capsule)
sonoencephalogram
Southeastern Cancer Study Group

seg segmented neutrophil (segmented leukocyte)

segm segment; also SEG
segmented

SEGS, segs segmented neutrophils (polymorphonuclear leukocytes)

SEH subependymal hemorrhage

SEI Self-Esteem Inventory
subepithelial corneal infiltrate
Suretee's Events Index

SELFVD sterile elective low forceps vaginal
delivery

SEM scanning electron microscope
scanning electron microscopy
secondary enrichment medium
semen; also sem
serum methylguanidine
smoke exposure machine
standard error of the mean
systolic ejection murmur
verbal sample evaluation method

sem half [L. *semis*]; also HF, hf, S, s, semi, ss,
s̄ s̄, s̈ s̈
semen; also SEM
seminal

SEMDJL spondyloepimetaphyseal dysplasia
with joint laxity

semel in d once a day [L. *semel in die*]; also
sem in d, sid

Semf seminal fluid; also SF

SEMI subendocardial myocardial infarction
subendocardial myocardial injury

semi half [L. *semis*]; also HF, hf, S, s, sem, ss,
s̄ s̄, s̈ s̈

semid half a drachm [L. *semidrachma*]

semih half an hour [L. *semihora*]

sem in d once a day [L. *semel in die*]; also
semel in d, sid

SEN State Enrolled Nurse

sen sensitive
sensitivity; also S, sens

SENA sympathetic efferent nerve activity

sens sensation ; also S, s
sensitivity; also S, sen
sensorium
sensory; also S

SEO surgical emergency officer

SEOG Southeastern Oncology Group

SEP sensory evoked potential
separate
serum electrophoresis
somatosensory evoked potential; also SSEP
sperm entry point
spinal evoked potential
surface epithelium
systolic ejection period

sep separated

separ separately
separation; also sepn

sepn separation; also separ

SEPS selenium-containing protein saccharide

sept septum; also S
seven [L. *septem*]

septo septoplasty

SEQ side-effects questionnaire
simultaneous equation
that which follows [L. *sequela*]; also seq

Seq sequential

seq sequel
sequelae
sequence
sequestrum
that which follows [L. *sequela*]; also SEQ

seq dev ex sequential development exercises

seq luce the following day [L. *sequenti luce*]

SER scanning equalization radiography
sebum excretion rate
sensory evoked response
service; also serv
smooth endoplasmic reticulum; also sER
somatosensory evoked response; also SSER
supination external rotation (type of fracture)
systolic ejection rate

Ser serine; also S

sER smooth endoplasmic reticulum; also SER

ser serial
series; also S, s

SERHOLD National Biomedical Serials Holding Database

SERI Spondee Error Index

ser ind serum index

SERLINE Serials on Line

sero serologic; also serol
serology; also serol

serol serologic; also sero
serology; also sero

ser sect serial sections

SERS surface-enhanced Raman spectroscopy

SERT sustained ethanol release tube

serv keep, preserve [L. *serva*]
service; also SER

SERVHEL Service and Health (Records)

SES socioeconomic status
spatial emotional stimuli
subendothelial space

SESAP Surgical Education and Self-Assessment Program

sesquih an hour and a half [L. *sesquihora*]

sesquiunc an ounce and a half [L. *sesquiuncia*]; also sesunc

Sess sessile

sesunc an ounce and a half [L. *sesuncia*]; also sesquiunc

SET skin endpoint titration
systolic ejection time

sev sever
several
severe; also SV
severed

SEWHO shoulder-elbow-wrist-hand orthosis

SEXAF surface extended x-ray absorption fine (structure)

SeXO serum xanthine oxidase

s expr without expressing, without pressing [L. *sine expressione*]

SF Sabin-Feldman (dye test)
safety factor
salt free
saturated fat
scarlet fever
Schilder-Foix (disease)
seizure frequency
seminal fluid; also Semf
serosal fluid
serum factor
serum ferritin
serum fibrinogen
sham feeding
shell fragment
shrapnel fragment
shunt flow
sickle cell–hemoglobin F
simian foam-virus
skin fibroblast
skin fluorescence
slow function
slow initial function
snack food
sodium azide, fecal (medium)
soft feces
spinal fluid; also sp fl
spontaneous fibrillation
spontaneous fission (radioactive isotopes)
spontaneous fluctuation
spontaneous fracture
stable factor
sterile female
Still-Felty (syndrome)
Streptococcus faecalis
stress formula
sugar free
sulfation factor (of blood serum)
superior facet
suppressor factor
suprasternal fossa
survival fraction
surviving factor
Svedberg flotation (unit)
symptom free
synovial fluid; also Synf, Syn Fl, syn fl

Sf Svedberg flotation unit; also S_f

S&F shave and fulguration

SF% shortening fraction percentage

s&f soft and flat

S_f Svedberg flotation unit; also Sf
negative sedimentation Svedberg unit

SFA saturated fatty acid
　seminal fluid assay
　serum folic acid
　stimulated fibrinolytic activity
　superficial femoral angioplasty
　superficial femoral artery

SFB Sanfilippo syndrome, type B
　surgical foreign body

SFBL self-filling blind loop

SFC serum fungicidal
　soluble fibrin-fibrinogen complex
　spinal fluid count; also sfc
　superficial fluid chromatography

sfc spinal fluid count; also SFC

SFD sheep factor delta
　short foot drape
　skin-film distance
　small for dates (gestational age)
　soy-free diet
　spectral frequency distribution

SFEMG single-fiber electromyography

SFF speaking fundamental frequency

SFFA serum-free fatty acid

SFFF sedimentation field flow fractionation

SFFV spleen focus-forming virus
　spleen focus Friend virus

SFFV-F spleen focus-forming virus in Friend
　virus complex

SFG spotted fever group

SFH schizophrenia family history
　serum-free hemoglobin
　stroma-free hemoglobin; also SFHb

SFHb stroma-free hemoglobin; also SFH

SFI Sexual Functioning Index
　Social Function Index

SFL synovial fluid lymphocyte

SFLE Stress From Life Experience

SFM serum-free medium
　soluble fibrin monomer

SFMC soluble fibrin monomer complex

SFN sensitivity or negative force

SFO subfornical organ

SFP screen filtration pressure
　simultaneous foveal perception
　spinal fluid pressure
　stopped flow pressure

SFPT standard fixation preference test

SFR screen-filtration resistance
　stroke with full recovery

SFS serial focus seizures
　serum fungistatic
　skin and fascia stapler
　split function study

SFT sensory feedback therapy
　serum-free thyroxin
　skinfold thickness

SFTR sagittal, frontal, transverse, rotation

SFV Semliki Forest virus
　shipping fever virus
　Shope's fibroma virus
　squirrel fibroma virus
　superficial femoral vein

SFW sexual function of women
　shell fragment wound
　shrapnel fragment wound
　slow filling wave

SG Sachs-Georgi (reaction, test); also S-G
　salivary gland
　secretory granule
　serous granule
　serum globulin
　serum glucose
　sign(s)
　skin graft
　soluble gelatin
　specific gravity; also SPG, SpG, SpGr, sp gr
　Strandberg-Groenblad (syndrome)
　substantia gelatinosa (of Rolando)
　Surgeon General
　Swan-Ganz (catheter); also S-G

S-G Sachs-Georgi (reaction, test); also SG
　Swan-Ganz (catheter); also SG

SGA small for gestational age
　Student Government Association

SGAW, SG$_{AW}$ specific airway conductance

SGC spermicide-germicide compound
　Swan-Ganz catheter

SG-C serum gentamicin concentration

SGc specific conductance

SGD straight gravity drainage

SGE secondary generalized epilepsy
　significant glandular enlargement

SGF sarcoma growth factor
　silica gel filtered
　skeletal growth factor

SGFR single nephron glomerular filtration rate;
　also SNGFR

SGGT serum gamma-glutamyltransferase

SGH stable-type glycated hemoglobin
　subgaleal hematoma

s̄ gl without glasses (without correction) [L. *sine* (without)]

SGL salivary gland lymphocyte

SGO Surgeon General's Office
surgery, gynecology, and obstetrics

SGOT serum glutamic oxaloacetic transaminase (aspartate aminotransferase)

SGP serine glycerophosphatide
sialoglycoprotein
Society of General Physiologists
soluble glycoprotein

SGPT serum glutamic pyruvic transaminase (alanine aminotransferase)

SGR Sachs-Georgi reaction
Shwartzman's generalized reaction
submandibular gland renin
substantia gelatinosa Rolando

SGS second generation sulfonylurea
subglottic stenosis

S-Gt Sachs-Georgi test

SGTT standard glucose tolerance test

SGTX surugatoxin

SGV salivary gland virus
selective gastric vagotomy
small granular vesicle

SH Salter-Harris (fracture)
Schönlein-Henoch (purpura)
serum hepatitis
service hours
sex hormone
sexual harassment
sham operated
shared haplotypes
Sherman (rat)
short; also Sh, sh
shoulder; also Sh, sh, SHLD
shower
sick in hospital
sinus histiocytosis
social history; also SHx
somatotropic hormone; also STH
spontaneously hypertensive (rat)
State Hospital
Student Health
sulfhydryl
surgical history
symptomatic hypoglycemia
systemic hyperthermia

S/H sample and hold
suicidal/homicidal ideation

S&H speech and hearing

Sh sheep
short; also SH, sh
shoulder; also SH, sh, SHLD
shoulder amputation

sh short; also SH, Sh
shoulder; also SH, Sh, SHLD

SHA ship his ass (out of here)
soluble HLA antigen
staphylococcal hemagglutinating antibody
super-heated aerosol

SHAA serum hepatitis-associated antigen

SHAA-Ab serum hepatitis-associated antigen antibody

SHAM salicylhydroxamic acid

SHARP School Health Additional Referral Program
small histidine-alanine-rich protein

SHAV superior hemiazygos vein

SHB sequential hemibody (irradiation)
subacute hepatitis with bridging
sulfhemoglobin; also S Hb, S-Hb, SULFHB

S Hb sickle hemoglobin
sulfhemoglobin; also SHB, S-Hb, SULFHB

S-Hb sulfhemoglobin; also SHB, S Hb, SULFHB

SHBD serum hydroxybutyric dehydrogenase

SHBG sex hormone-binding globulin

SHCO sulfated hydrogenated caster oil

SHDI supraoptical hypophysial diabetes insipidus

SHE super-heavy element
Syrian hamster embryo

SHEA sheep erythrocyte antibody
sheep erythrocyte antigen

SHEENT skin, head, eyes, ears, nose, and throat

SHF simian hemorrhagic fever

shf super-high frequency

SHG Sauerbruch-Hermannsdorfer-Gerson (diet)
synthetic human gastrin

SHHP semihorizontal heart position

Shk shikimic acid

SHL sensorineural hearing loss; also SNHL
supraglottic horizontal laryngectomy

SHLD shoulder; also SH, Sh, sh

SHML sinus histiocytosis with massive lymphadenopathy

SHMO Senior Hospital Medical Officer

SHMT serine hydroxymethyltransferase

SHN spontaneous hemorrhagic necrosis
subacute hepatic necrosis

SHO secondary hypertrophic osteoarthropathy
Senior House Officer
Student Health Organization

SHORT, S-H-O-R-T short stature, hyperexten-
sibility of joints or hernia (or both), ocular
depression, Rieger's anomaly, teething
delayed

SHP Schönlein-Henoch purpura
secondary hyperparathyroidism; also sHPT
state health plan
surgical hypoparathyroidism

SHPDA State Health Planning and
Development Agency

sHPT secondary hyperparathyroidism; also SHP

SHR spontaneously hypertensive rat

SHRC shortened, held, resisted, contracted

SHS Sayre's head sling
sheep hemolysate supernatant
Shipley-Hartford Scale
student health service
super-high speed

SHSP spontaneously hypertensive stroke-prone
(rat)

SHSS Stanford Hypnotic Susceptibility Scale

SHT simple hypocalcemic tetany
subcutaneous histamine test

SHUR System for Hospital Uniform Reporting

SHV simian herpesvirus

SHx social history; also SH

SI International System of Units [Fr. *Système
Internationale d' Unités*]
sacroiliac; also sac-il
saline infusion
saline injection
saturation index
self-inflicted
sensitive index
serious illness
seriously ill
serum insulin
serum iron
service index
severity index
sex inventory
Singh Index
single injection
small intestine
social introversion

soluble insulin
special intervention
spirochetosis icterohaemorrhagica
stimulation index
streptozotocin induced
stress incontinence
strict isolation
stroke index
suicidal ideation
sulfated insulin
suppression index
systolic index

S/I sucrose to isomaltose (ratio)

S&I suction and irrigation

Si most anterior point on lower contour of
sella turcica (point)
silicon
venous sinus

SIA serum inhibitory activity
stimulation-induced analgesia
stress-induced analgesia
stress-induced anesthesia
subacute infectious arthritis
synalbumin-insulin antagonism
syncytia induction assay

Sia sialic acid; also SA

SIADH syndrome of inappropriate antidiuretic
hormone (secretion)

SIB self-injurious behavior

sib sibling

sibs siblings; also SS

SIC dry [L. *siccus*]; also sic
serum inhibitory concentration
serum insulin concentration

sic dry [L. *siccus*]; also SIC

SICD Sequenced Inventory of Communication
Development
serum isocitric dehydrogenase

SICRI substance immunologically cross-
reactive with insulin

SICSVA sequential impaction cascade sieve
volumetric air (sampler)

SICT selective intracoronary thrombolysis

SICU spinal intensive care unit
surgical intensive care unit

SID Society for Investigative Dermatology
sucrase-isomaltase deficiency
sudden inexplicable death
sudden infant death
suggested indication of diagnosis
systemic inflammatory disease

sid once a day [L. *semel in die*]; also
semel in d, sem in d

SIDER siderocyte; also S

SIDS sudden infant death syndrome

SIE stroke in evolution

SIECUS Sex Information and Educational
Council of the United States

SIF serum inhibitory factor
small, intensely fluorescent (ganglia)

Sif segment inferior

SIFT selected ion flow tube

SIG silver-intensified gold (staining)
sigmoidoscope
special interest group

SIg serum immune globulin
surface immunoglobulin; also sIg

Sig label [L. *signa* (mark, write on)]; also
S, s, sig
signature; also S, /S/, /s/
signed; also S, /S/, /s/, s
write [L. *signa* (mark, write on)]; also
S, s, sig

sIg surface immunoglobulin; also SIg

sig label [L. *signa* (mark, write on)]; also
S, s, Sig
sigmoidoscopy; also Σ
signal
significant
write [L. *signa* (mark, write on)]; also
S, s, Sig

SIgA surface immunoglobulin A

S-IgA secretory immunoglobulin A

sig n pro label with proper name [L. *signa
nomine proprio*]

SIH stimulation-induced hypalgesia

SIhPTH serum immunoreactive human
parathyroid hormone

SIJ sacroiliac joint; also SI jt

SI jt sacroiliac joint; also SIJ

SIL seriously ill list
speech interference level

SILD Sequenced Inventory of Language
Development

SILFVD sterile indicated low forceps vaginal
delivery

SILS Shipley Institute of Living Scale

SIM selective ion monitoring
Similac
Society for Industrial Microbiology

specific ion monitoring
sucrose-isomaltose
sulfide, indole, motility (medium)

Simkin simulation kinetics (analysis)

simp simple

SIMS secondary ion mass spectroscopy

simul at once, at the same time [L. *simul* (at
once, together)]
simultaneously

SIMV synchronized intermittent mandatory
ventilation

sin six times a night [L. *sex in nocte*]
without [L. *sine*]; also S, s, s̄, WO, w/o

sing of each [L. *singulorum*]
singular; also S

sing aur every morning [L. *singulis auroris*]

sing hor quad every quarter hour [L. *singulis
horae quadrantibus*]

si non val if it is not enough [L. *si non valeat*]

si op sit if it is necessary [L. *si opus sit*]; also
s op s, s op sit, SOS, sos

SIP segment inertial properties
Sickness Impact Profile
slow-inhibitory potential
surface inductive plethysmography

SIPSP slow-inhibitory postsynaptic potential

SIPTH serum immunoreactive parathyroid
hormone

SIQ sick in quarters (military)

SIR single isomorphous replacement
specific immune release
standardized incidence ratio

SIREF specific immune-response-enhancing
factor

SIRF severely impaired renal function

SIRS soluble immune response suppressor

SIS sisomicin
sister; also S
social information system
spontaneous interictal spike
sterile injectable solution
sterile injectable suspension

SISI short increment sensitivity index

SISS serum inhibitor of streptolysin S

SISV, SiSV simian sarcoma virus; also SSV

SIT serum inhibiting titer
Slosson Intelligence Test
sperm immobilization test

SIT BAL sitting balance

SIT-F Sperm Immobilization Test - Fjabrant

SIT-I Sperm Immobilization Test - Isojima

SIT TOL sitting tolerance

SIV simian immunodeficiency virus
Sprague-Dawley-Ivanovas (rat)

si vir perm if strength will permit [L. *si vires permitant*]

SIVP slow intravenous push

SIW self-inflicted wound

SIWIP self-induced water intoxication and psychosis

SJ, S-J Stevens-Johnson (syndrome)

SJR Shinowara-Jones-Reinhart (unit)

SJS Stevens-Johnson syndrome;
Swyer-James syndrome

SjS Sjögren's syndrome; also SS

SK seborrheic keratosis; also seb ker
senile keratosis
serum potassium
skin; also Sk, SKI
Sloan-Kettering (Institute) (used with numbers to designate various experimental compounds used in treating cancer)
solar keratosis
spontaneous killer (cell)
streptokinase; also STK
striae keratopathy
substance K
swine kidney

Sk skin; also SK, SKI

sk skeletal; also skel
skimmed

SKA supracondylar knee-ankle (orthosis);
also SKAO

SKAB skeletal antibody

SKAO supracondylar knee-ankle orthosis;
also SKA

SKAT Sex Knowledge and Attitude Test

skel skeletal; also sk
skeleton

SKI skin; also SK, Sk
Sloan-Kettering Institute

SKL serum-killing level

SKSD, SK-SD, SK/SD streptokinase–streptodornase

sk tr skeletal traction

SKW Sturge-Kalischer-Weber (syndrome)

SL according to law [L. *secundum legem*];
also sl
according to rule [L. *secundum legem*];
also sl
salt loser
sarcolemma
satellite-like
sclerosing leukoencephalopathy
sensation level (of hearing)
sensory latency
serious list
short-leg (cast)
Sibley-Lehninger (unit)
signal level
Sinding-Larsen (syndrome)
Sjögren-Larsson (syndrome)
slight; also Sl, sl
slit lamp (examination); also S/L
small leukocyte
small lymphocyte
soda lime
sodium lactate
solidified liquid
sound level
Stein-Leventhal (syndrome)
streptolysin
Strümpell-Lorrain (disease)
sublingual; also sL, sl, subl, subling

S/L slit lamp (examination); also SL
sucrase to lactase (ratio); also S:L

S:L sucrase to lactase (ratio); also S/L

Sl slight; also SL, sl
Steel (mouse)

sL sublingual; also SL, sl, subl, subling

sl according to law [L. *secundum legem*];
also SL
according to rule [L. *secundum legem*];
also SL
slice
slight; also SL, Sl
slow
slyke (unit of buffer value)
sublingual; also SL, sL, subl, subling

SLA left sacro-anterior (fetal position)
[L. *sacrolaeva anterior*]
single-cell liquid cytotoxic assay
slide latex agglutination
surfactant-like activity
swine lymphocyte antigens

SLAM scanning laser acoustic microscope

SLAP serum leucine aminopeptidase

SLB short-leg brace

SLC short-leg cast
Sociopolitical Locus of Control
sodium lithium countertransport

SLCC short-leg cylinder cast
sulfated lithocholic conjugate

SLCG sulfolithocholylglycine

SLD serum lactate dehydrogenase; also SLDH

SLDH serum lactate dehydrogenase; also SLD

SLE slit-lamp examination
St. Louis encephalitis; also STLE
systemic lupus erythematosus

SLEP short latent-evoked potential

SLEV St. Louis encephalitis virus

SLFIA substrate-labeled fluorescent
immunoassay
substrate-linked fluorescent immunoassay

SLFVD sterile low forceps vaginal delivery

SLGXT symptom-limited graded exercise test

SLHR sex-linked hypophosphatemic rickets

SLI secretin-like immunoreactivity
selective lymphoid irradiation
somatostatin-like immunoreactivity; also
SLIR
speech and language impaired
splenic localization index

SLIP Singer-Loomis Inventory of Personality

SLIR somatostatin-like immunoreactivity;
also SLI

SLK superior limbic keratoconjunctivitis;
also SLKC

SLKC superior limbic keratoconjunctivitis;
also SLK

SLM sound level meter

SLMC spontaneous lymphocyte-mediated
cytotoxicity

SLMFD sterile low midforceps vaginal delivery

SLMP since last menstrual period

SLN sublentiform nucleus
superior laryngeal nerve

SLNTG sublingual nitroglycerin

SLNWBC short-leg non-weight-bearing cast

SLNWC short-leg non-walking cast

SLO streptolysin O

SLP left sacroposterior (fetal position)
[L. *sacrolaeva posterior*]
segmental limb systolic pressure
sex-limited protein

short luteal phase
speech-language pathologist
subluxation of patella

SLPP serum lipophosphoprotein

SLPMS short-leg posterior-molded splint

SLR Shwartzman's local reaction
single lens reflex
straight-leg raising
Streptococcus lactis-resistant

SLRT straight-leg raising tenderness
straight-leg raising test

SLS segment long-spacing (collagen fibers)
short-leg splint
single limb support
Sjögren-Larsson syndrome
Stein-Leventhal syndrome

SLSG S-locus specific glycoprotein

SLSQ Speech and Language Screening
Questionnaire

SLT left sacrotransverse (fetal position)
[L. *sacrolaeva transversa*]
Shiga-like toxin
sodium levothyroxine
swing light test

SlTr silent treatment

SLUD salivation, lacrimation, urination,
defecation

S-L-V solid-liquid-vapor

SLWC short-leg walking cast

SLZ serum lysozyme

SM sadomasochism
Scheuthauer-Marie (syndrome)
self-monitoring
semimembranous
Sexual Myths (Scale)
Shigella mutant
shine mold (medium)
simple mastectomy
skim milk
small; also S, Sm, sm
smoker
smooth muscle
somatomedin
space medicine
sphingomyelin; also SPH, Sph
splenic macrophage
sports medicine
stapedius muscle
staphylococcus medium
streptomycin; also S, STM, strep

SM—cont'd
  Strümpell-Marie (disease)
  submandibular; also submand
  submucosal
  submucous
  substituted metabolite
  substitute for morphine
  suckling mouse; also sM
  sucrose medium
  suction method
  sulfamerazine
  superior mesenteric
  supramammillary (nucleus)
  sustained medication
  symptom(s); also Sm, sym, symp,
    sympt, Sx, S_x, sx
  synaptic membrane
  synovial membrane
  systolic mean (pressure)
  systolic motion
  systolic murmur

S/M sadism/masochism

SM service mark

Sm samarium; also Sa
  small; also S, SM, sm
  Smith (antigen)
  symptom(s); also SM, sym, symp, sympt, Sx,
    S_x, sx

sM suckling mouse; also SM

sm small; also S, SM, Sm

SMA schedule of maximal allowance
  Sequential Multichannel Autoanalyzer
  Sequential Multiple Analysis
  Sequential Multiple Analyzer
  serial multiple analysis
  serum muramidase activity
  simultaneous multichannel autoanalyzer
  smooth muscle antibody
  smooth muscle autoantibody
  spectral map analysis
  spinal muscular atrophy
  spontaneous motor activity
  standard method agar
  superior mesenteric artery
  supplementary motor area

SM-A somatomedin A

SMA-6 Sequential Multiple Analysis (six different tests)

SMA 6/60 Sequential Multiple Analysis (six tests in sixty minutes)

SMA-12 Sequential Multiple Analysis (twelve different tests)

SMA 12/60 Sequential Multiple Analysis (twelve tests in sixty minutes)

SMA-20 Sequential Multiple Analysis (twenty different tests)

SMA-60 Sequential Multiple Analysis (sixty different tests)

SMABF superior mesenteric artery blood flow; also SMAF

SMABV superior mesenteric artery blood velocity

SMAC Sequential Multiple Analyzer plus Computer

SMAE superior mesenteric artery embolus

SMAF smooth muscle activating factor
  specific macrophage arming factor
  superior mesenteric artery blood flow; also SMABF

SMAL serum methyl alcohol level

sm an small animal

SMAO superior mesenteric artery occlusion

SMART simultaneous multiple-angle reconstruction technique

SMAS submucosal aponeurotic system (flap)
  superior mesenteric artery syndrome

SMAST Short Michigan Alcoholism Screening Test

SMAT School Motivation Analysis Test

SMB selected mucosal biopsy
  standard mineral base

sMB suckling mouse brain

SMBFT small bowel follow-through; also SBFT

SMBG self-monitored blood glucose

SMBP serum myelin basic protein

SMBV suckling mouse brain vaccine

SMC selenomethylnorcholesterol
  single mixing coil
  smooth muscle cell
  special monthly compensation
  special mouth care
  succinlymonocholine

SM-C, Sm-C somatomedin C

SMCA smooth muscle contracting agent
  suckling mouse cataract agent

SMCD senile macular chorioretinal degeneration

SM-C/IGF somatomedin C/insulin-like growth factor

SMD senile macular degeneration

sternocleidomastoid diameter
submanubrial dullness

SMDA starch methylenedianiline

SME stalk median eminence

SMEDI stillbirth, mummification, embryonic death, infertility (syndrome)

SMEM supplemented Eagle minimal essential medium

SMEPP subminiature end-plate potential

SMF streptozotocin, mitomycin C, fluorouracil

SMFP state medical facilities plan

SMFVD sterile midforceps vaginal delivery

SMG submandibular gland

SMH state mental hospital
strongyloidiasis with massive hyperinfection

SMI Senior Medical Investigator
sensory motor integration
severely mentally impaired
silent myocardial ischemia
stress myocardial image
Style of Mind Inventory
supplementary medical insurance
sustained maximal inspiration

SmIg surface membrane immunoglobulin

SMILE sustained maximal inspiratory lung exercises

SML single major locus

SMMD specimen mass measurement device

SMN second malignant neoplasm

SMNB submaximal neuromuscular block

SMO Medical Officer of Schools
Senior Medical Officer (Navy)
serum monoamine oxidase
slip made out

SMOH Senior Medical Officer of Health

SMON subacute myelo-optical neuropathy

SMOS Society of Military Orthopaedic Surgeons

SMP self-management program
slow-moving protease
special monthly pension
standard medical practice
standard medical procedure
submitochondrial particle

SMR Senior Medical Resident
sensorimotor rhythm
severe mental retardation
skeletal muscle relaxant
somnolent metabolic rate
standard metabolic rate

standard morbidity ratio
standard mortality ratio
stroke with minimal residuum
submucosal resection

SMRR submucosal resection and rhinoplasty

SMRV squirrel monkey retrovirus

SMS Scheuthauer-Marie-Sainton (syndrome)
senior medical student
somatostatin; also SS, SST
State Medical Society
stiff-man syndrome
supplemental minimal sodium

SMSA standard metropolitan statistical area

SMSV San Miguel sea-lion virus

SMT Sertoli cell mesenchyme tumor
Snider Match Test
spindle microtubule
spontaneous mammary tumor

SMuLV Scripps murine leukemia virus

SMV slow-moving vehicle
small volume
spontaneous minute volume
submental vertex (view)
submentovertical
superior mesenteric vein

SMVT sustained monomorphic ventricular tachycardia

SMX sulfamethoxazole; also SMZ

SMZ sulfamethazine
sulfamethoxazole; also SMX

SN according to nature [L. *secundum naturam*]; also sn
school of nursing
sciatic notch
sclerema neonatorum
scrub nurse
second nucleotide
sensorineural
sensory neuron
seronegative
serum neutralization
serum neutralizing
single nephron
sinus node
spinal needle
spontaneous nystagmus
staff nurse
Standard Nomenclature
streptonigrin
Student Nurse
subnormal

SN—cont'd
　substantia nigra
　supernatant
　supernormal
　suprasternal notch; also SSN

SN 7618 chloroquine

SN 13,272 primaquine

SN 13,276 pentaquine

S-N sella to nasion (cephalometrics)

S/N sample to negative control (ratio)
　signal to noise (ratio)
　speech to noise (ratio)

Sn subnasale
　tin [L. *stannum*]

sn according to nature [L. *secundum naturam*]; also SN

SNA specimen not available
　superior nasal artery
　systems network architecture

S-N-A sella-nasion-subspinale point A (in cephalometrics)

SNa serum sodium (concentration)

SNAFU situation normal, all fouled up
　situation normal, all fucked up

SNagg serum normal agglutinator

SNAI Standard Nomenclature of Athletic Injuries

SNAP sensory nerve action potential

SNAT suspected non-accidental trauma

SNB scalene node biopsy
　Silverman needle biopsy
　spinal nucleus of the bulbocavernosus

S-N-B sella-nasion-supramentale point B (in cephalometrics)

SNC central nervous system [L. *sistema nervosum centrale*]; also CNS
　skilled nursing care
　spontaneous neonatal chylothorax

SNCL sinus node cycle length

SNCV sensory nerve conduction velocity

SND single needle device
　sinus node dysfunction
　striatonigral degeneration

SNDO Standard Nomenclature of Diseases and Operations; also SNODO

SNDS supplementary new drug submission

SNE sinus node electrogram
　spatial nonemotional (stimuli)
　subacute necrotizing encephalomyelopathy

SNEF skilled nursing extended care facility

SNF sinus node formation
　skilled nursing facility

SNFH schizophrenia non-family history

SNGBF single nephron glomerular blood flow

SNGFR single nephron glomerular filtration rate; also SGFR

SNGPF single nephron glomerular plasma flow

SNHL sensorineural hearing loss; also SHL

SNIVT Society of Non-Invasive Vascular Technology (now: SVT, Society of Vascular Technology)

SNK Student-Newman-Keuls (procedure)

SNM Society of Nuclear Medicine
　sulfanilamide

SNM-TS Society of Nuclear Medicine - Technologists Section (also: TSSNM, Technologists Section of the Society of Nuclear Medicine)

SNOBOL String-Oriented Symbolic Language

SNODO Standard Nomenclature of Diseases and Operations; also SNDO

SNOMED Standardized Nomenclature of Medicine

SNOOP Systematic Nursing Observation of Psychopathology

SNOP Systematized Nomenclature of Pathology

SNP School Nurse Practitioner
　sinus node potential
　sodium nitroprusside

SNQ superior nasal quadrant

SNR signal-to-noise ratio

snRNA small nuclear ribonucleic acid

snRNP small nuclear ribonucleoprotein

SNRT sinus node recovery time; also SRT

SNRTd sinus node recovery time, direct (measuring)

SNS Society of Neurological Surgeons
　sterile normal saline
　sympathetic nervous system

SNSA seronegative spondyloarthropathy

SNT sinuses, nose, throat

SNV spleen necrosis virus
　superior nasal vein

SO salpingo-oophorectomy; also S-O, S&O
　salpingo-oophoritis
　Schlatter-Osgood (disease)

second opinion
sex offender
shoulder orthosis
significant other; also S/O
slow oxidative (muscle fiber)
spheno-occipital (synchondrosis)
sphincter of Oddi
standing orders
stitches out
suboccipital
superior oblique (muscle)
supraoptic (nucleus)
supraorbital
sutures out

S/O significant other; also SO

S-O salpingo-oophorectomy; also SO, S&O

S&O salpingo-oophorectomy; also SO, S-O

SO$_2$ oxygen saturation; also OS, O$_2$ sat,
SaO$_2$, S$_{AO2}$

So socialization; also SOC

SOA serum opsonic activity
spinal opioid analgesia
supraorbital artery
swelling of ankles

SOAA signed out against medical advice;
also SOAMA

SOAM stitches out in morning
sutures out in morning

SOAMA signed out against medical advice;
also SOAA

SOA-MCA superficial occipital artery to
middle cerebral artery

SOAP subjective data, objective data, assessment, and plan (problem-oriented record)

SOAPIE subjective data, objective data, assessment, plan, implementation, and evaluation
(problem-oriented record)

SOAPS suction, oxygen, apparatus, pharmaceuticals, saline (anesthesia equipment)

SOB see order blank
see order book
shortness of breath; also SB
side of bed
suboccipitobregmatic

SOBE shortness of breath on exertion;
also SBE, SOBOE

SOBOE shortness of breath on exertion;
also SBE, SOBE

SOC sequential-type oral contraceptive
socialization; also So
standard of care

state of consciousness; also SoC
syphilitic osteochondritis

S&OC signed and on chart

SoC state of consciousness; also SOC

soc social
society

SOCD Separation of Circle-Diamond

SocSec Social Security; also SS

soc serv social services; also SS

S-OCT serum ornithine carbamoyltransferase

SOD sinovenous occlusive disease
spike occurrence density
superoxide dismutase; also SD
surgical officer of the day

sod sodium; also Na, natr

SODAS spheroidal oral drug absorption system

sod bicarb sodium bicarbonate

SODIS soluble ophthalmic drug insert

SOFS spontaneous osteoporotic fracture of
sacrum

SOFT Sorting of Figures Test

SOG suggestive of good

SOH sympathetic orthostatic hypotension

SOHN supraoptic hypothalamic nucleus

SOL solution; also Sol, sol, soln
space-occupying lesion

Sol, sol soluble; also S
solution; also SOL, soln

SOLER squarely face person, open posture,
lean toward person, eye contact, relaxed

solidif solidification
solidifies

soln solution; also SOL, Sol, sol

SOLST Stephens Oral Language Screening
Test

solu solute; also S

solv dissolve [L. *solve*]
solvent

soly solubility

SOM scanning optical microscope
secretory otitis media
sensitivity of method
serous otitis media
somatotropin
somnolent
sulformethoxine

somat somatic

SOMI sternal-occipital-mandibular immobilization

SON supraoptic nucleus

SONH supraopticoneurohypophysial

SONK spontaneous osteonecrosis of knee

sono sonogram
sonography

SONP soft organs not palpable
solid organs not palpable

SOP standard operating procedure

SOPA syndrome of primary aldosteronism

SOPM stitches out in afternoon
sutures out in afternoon

SOPP splanchnic occluded portal pressure

s op s if it is necessary [L. *si opus sit*]; also
si op sit, s op sit, SOS, sos

s op sit if it is necessary [L. *si opus sit*]; also
si op sit, s op s, SOS, sos

SOQ Suicide Opinion Questionnaire

SOR sign own release
stimulus-organism response

SOr supraorbitale

Sorb, sorb sorbitol

SOREMP sleep-onset rapid eye movement
period

SOS if it is necessary [L. *si opus sit*]; also
si op sit, s op s, s op sit, sos
self-obtained smear
stimulation of senses
supplemental oxygen system

sos if it is necessary [L. *si opus sit*]; also
si op sit, s op s, s op sit, SOS

SOT something other than
stream of thought
systemic oxygen transport

SOTT synthetic medium old tuberculin
trichloroacetic acid precipitated

SP sacral promontory
sacrum posterior
sacrum to pubis
salivary progesterone
Schick-positive
schizotypal personality
secretory piece
semiprivate; also S/P
senile plaque
septal pore
septum pellucidum
sequential pulse
serine proteinase

seropositive
serum protection
serum protein; also S/P
shunt pressure
shunt procedure
silent period
sinus pause
skin potential
sleep deprivation
sleep deprived
small protein
soft palate
solid phase
spatial peak
speech; also Sp
speech pathology
spike potential
spinal; also S/P, sp, spin
spine; also Sp, sp, spin
spiramycin
spirometry
spleen; also S, sp
spouse
square planar (complex)
stand and pivot; also S/P
standard of performance
standard practice
standard procedure
staphylococcal protease
status post; also S/P, s/p
steady potential
stool preservative
subliminal perception
substance P
subtilopeptidase
suicide precautions; also S/P
sulfapyridine
summating potential
suprapatellar pouch
suprapubic; also S/P
suprapubic puncture
symphysis pubis
synthase phosphatase
systolic pressure; also S/P

SP-4 square planar

SP-5 square pyramidal

S/P semiprivate; also SP
serum protein; also SP
spinal; also SP, sp, spin
stand and pivot; also SP
status post; also SP, s/p
suicide precautions; also SP
suprapubic; also SP
systolic pressure; also SP

2-S P transport medium used for mycoplasma isolation

Sp most posterior point on posterior contour of sella turcica
sacropubic
species (singular); also sp
speech; also SP
spine; also SP, sp, spin
Spirillum species; also S
summation potential

sP senile parkinsonism

sp space; also S
species (singular); also Sp
specific; also spec
sperm
spinal; also SP, S/P, spin
spine; also SP, Sp, spin
spirit, alcohol [L. *spiritus*]; also spir, Spt
spleen; also S, SP

s/p status post; also SP, S/P

SPA salt-poor albumin
schizophrenia with premorbid asociality
serum prothrombin activity
sheep pulmonary adenomatosis
single photon absorptiometry
sperm penetration assay
spinal progressive amyotrophy
spondyloarthropathy
spontaneous platelet aggregation
staphylococcal protein A
stimulation-produced analgesia
suprapatellar amputation
suprapubic aspiration

SpAb specifically purified antibody

SPAC sectionally processed, antibody coated

SPAD stenosing peripheral arterial disease
subcutaneous peritoneal administration device

SPAG small particle aerosol generator

SPAI steroid protein activity index

SPAM scanning photoacoustic microscopy

SPAMM spatial modulation of magnetization

span spansule

SPAR sensitivity prediction by acoustic reflex

SPAT slow paroxysmal atrial tachycardia

SPBI serum protein-bound iodine

S-PBIgG serum-platelet bindable immuno-globulin G

SPBT suprapubic bladder tap

SPC salicylamide, phenacetin, and caffeine
saturated phosphatidylcholine concentration

Schick-positive compound
serum phenylalanine concentration
sickle-shaped particle cell
single palmar crease
single photoelectron counting
single proton counting
small pyramidal cell
spike-processed contraction
spleen cell; also SC
standard plate count
synthesizing protein complex

SPCA serum prothrombin conversion accelerator (factor VII)

sp cd spinal cord; also SC

SPD salmon-poisoning disease
silicon photodiode
sociopathic personality disorder
specific paroxysmal discharge
spectral power distribution
spermidine; also Spd
standard peak dilution
subcorneal pustular dermatosis

Spd spermidine; also SPD

SPDC striopallidodentate calcinosis

SPDT single-pole, double-throw (switch)

SPE septic pulmonary edema
serum protein electrophoresis; also SPEP
streptococcal pyrogenic exotoxin
subjective paranormal experience
sucrose polyester

SPEC specimen; also spec

Spec specialist
specialty

spec special
specific; also sp
specimen; also SPEC
spectroscopy

Spec Ed special education

SPECT single photon emission computed tomography

SPEG serum protein electrophoretogram

SPEM smooth pursuit eye movement

SPEP serum protein electrophoresis; also SPE

SPET single photon emission tomography

SPF skin protection factor
specific pathogen free
spectrofluorometry
spectrophotofluorometer
split products of fibrin
standard perfusion fluid
streptococcal proliferative factor

SPF—cont'd
  Stuart-Prower factor
  sun protection factor
  suntan photoprotection factor

sp fl spinal fluid; also SF

SPFT Sixteen Personality Factors Test

SPG *Schizophyllum* polyglucosan
  serine phosphoglyceride
  specific gravity, also SG, SpG, SpGr, sp gr
  sphenopalatine ganglion
  sucrose-phosphate-glutamate
  symmetrical peripheral gangrene

SpG specific gravity; also SG, SPG, SpGr,
  sp gr

spg sponge

SpGr, sp gr specific gravity; also SG, SPG,
  SpG

SPH secondary pulmonary hemosiderosis
  severely and profoundly handicapped
  spherocyte(s); also SPHE, SPHER
  sphingomyelin; also SM, Sph

Sph sphenoidale
  spherical; also S, sph
  spherical lens; also S, sph
  spherocytosis
  sphingomyelin; also SM, SPH
  sphingosine

sph spherical; also S, Sph
  spherical lens; also S, Sph
  spheroid

SPHE Society of Public Health Educators
  spherocyte(s); also SPH, SPHER

SPHER spherocyte(s); also SPH, SPHE

sp ht specific heat

SPI selective protein index
  serum precipitable iodine
  Shipley Personal Inventory
  somatotyping ponderal index
  speech processor interface
  subclinical papilloma virus infection

SPIA solid-phase immunoabsorbent assay
  solid-phase immunoassay

SPID summed pain intensity difference

SPIF solid-phase immunoassay fluorescence
  spontaneous peak inspiratory force

SPIH superimposed pregnancy-induced hypertension

spin spinal; also SP, S/P, sp
  spine; also SP, Sp, sp

sp indet species indeterminate [L. *species
  indeterminata*]

sp inquir species of doubtful status [L. *species
  inquirendae*]

spir spiral
  spirit, alcohol [L. *spiritus*]; also sp, Spt

spiss dried [L. *spissus*]
  inspissated, thickened by evaporation [L.
  spissatus]

SPK serum pyruvate kinase
  spinnbarkheit
  superficial punctate keratitis

spkr speaker

SPL skin potential level
  sound pressure level
  splanchnic
  spontaneous lesion
  staphylococcal phage lysate

SPLATT split anterior tibial tendon (transfer)

SPLI substance P-like immunoreactivity

SPLV serum parvovirus-like virus

SPM self-phase modulation
  shocks per minute
  significance probability mapping
  spectinomycin; also SPT
  spermine
  subhuman primate model
  suspended particulate matter
  syllables per minute
  synaptic plasma membrane
  synaptosomal plasma membrane

SpM spiriformis medialis (nucleus)

spm gene that leads to suppression and mutation of mutants that are unstable

SPMA spinal progressive muscular atrophy

SPMB strong partial maternal behavior

SPMI status postmyocardial infarction

SPMR standardized proportionate mortality

SPN solitary pulmonary nodule
  student practical nurse
  supplementary parenteral nutrition
  sympathetic preganglionic neuron

sp n new species [L. *species novum*]

SPO status post-operative

SPOD spouse's perception of disease

spon spontaneous; also spont

spont spontaneous; also spon

spont Ab spontaneous abortion; also SAB

SPOOL simultaneous peripheral operation
  on-line

SPORO sporotrichosis

SPP Sexuality Preference Profile
skin perfusion pressure
suprapubic prostatectomy

Spp, spp species (plural)
subspecies; also SPPP, Ssp, ssp, subsp

SPPP subspecies; also Spp, spp, Ssp, ssp, subsp

SPPS solid phase peptide synthesis
stable plasma protein solution

SPPT superprecipitation (response)

SPR scan projection radiography
serial probe recognition (task)
skin potential reflex
solid phase radioimmunoassay; also SPRIA
solid phase receptacle

SPRIA solid phase radioimmunoassay; also SPR

SPRINT Special Psychiatric Rapid Intervention Team

SPROM spontaneous premature rupture of membranes

SPRT sequential probability ratio test

SPS shoulder pain and stiffness
simple partial seizure
slow-progressive schizophrenia
sodium polyanetholesulfonate
sodium polyethylene sulfonate
sodium polystyrene sulfonate
sound production sample (test)
special Pap smear
status postsurgery
stimulated protein synthesis
sulfite-polymyxin-sulfadiazine (agar)
Symonds Picture-Story (Test)
systemic progressive sclerosis

SpS sphenoid sinus

spSHT stroke-prone spontaneous hypertensive

SPSS Statistical Package for the Social Sciences

SPST single-pole, single-throw (switch)
Symonds Picture-Story Test

SPT skin prick test
slow pull-through
sound production tasks
spectinomycin; also SPM
spinal tap; also Sp tap
Spondee Picture Test
standing pivotal transfer
Supervisory Practices Test
Symbolic Play Test

Spt spirit, alcohol [L. *spiritus*]; also sp, spir

SPTA spacial peak temporal average

Sp tap spinal tap; also SPT

SPTI systolic pressure time index

SPTP spatial peak temporal peak

SPTS subjective post-traumatic syndrome

SPTURP status post-transurethral resection of prostate

SPTx static pelvic traction

SPU short procedure unit

SPUT sputum

SPV Shope's papilloma virus
slow-phase velocity
sulfophosphovanillin

SPVR systemic peripheral vascular resistance

SPZ secretin pancreozymin
sulfinpyrazone

SQ social quotient
squalene
square; also sq
status quo
subcutaneous; also SC, sc, Sq, subcu, subcut, subq, sub-q
survey question
symptom questionnaire

Sq squamous; also sq
subcutaneous; also SC, sc, SQ, subcu, subcut, subq, sub-q

sq squamous; also Sq
square; also SQ

SQC semi-quantitative culture

SqCCA squamous cell carcinoma; also SCC, SCCA, sq cell ca

sq cell ca squamous cell carcinoma; also SCC, SCCA, SqCCA

sq cm square centimeter; also cm^2

sq m square meter; also m^2

sq mm square millimeter; also mm^2

sqq, *sqq* and following [L. *sequentia*]

SQUID superconducting quantum-interference device

SR sarcoplasmic reticulum
saturation-recovery
scanning radiometer
Schmidt-Ruppin (strain)
screen
secretion rate
sedimentation rate; also sed rate, sed rt
see report
seizure resistant

SR—cont'd
self-recording
senior
sensitivity response
sensitization response (cell)
sentence repetition
service record
sex ratio
short hair (guinea pig)
side rails
sigma reaction
silicone rubber
simple reaction
sinus rhythm
skin resistance
slow release
smooth-rough (bacterial colony); also S-R
soluble repository
specific release
specific resistance
specific response
stage of resistance
stimulation ratio
stimulus response
stomach rumble
Stransky-Regala (syndrome)
stress relaxation
stretch reflex
sulfonamide-resistant
superior rectus
supply room
sustained release
systemic reaction
systemic resistance
systems review

S-R smooth-rough (bacterial colony); also SR

S&R seclusion and restraint(s)

Sr strontium

85Sr strontium 85, radioactive strontium; halflife, 64 days

sr steradian (unit of three-dimensional measure)

SRA segmented renal artery
spleen repopulating activity

SRAI social role adjustment instrument

SRAM static random access memory

SRAN surgical resident's admission note

SR$_{AW}$ specific airway resistance

SRBC sheep red blood cells; also SRC
sickle red blood cell

SRBOW spontaneous rupture of bag of waters

SRC sedimented red cells
sheep red blood cells; also SRBC

SRCA specific red cell adherence
subrenal capsule assay

SRCBC serum reserve cholesterol binding capacity

SRD service-related disability
sodium-restricted diet
specific reading disability

SRDD sorbent regenerated dialysate delivery

SRDT single radial diffusion test

SRE Schedule of Recent Experiences

SRF severe renal failure
skin reactive factor
slow-reacting factor
somatotropin-releasing factor
split renal function
subretinal fluid

SRF-A slow-reacting factor of anaphylaxis; also SRFOA

SRFC sheep red cell rosette-forming cell

SRFOA slow-reacting factor of anaphylaxis; also SRF-A

SRFS split renal function study

SRH signs of recent hemorrhage
single radial hemolysis
somatotropin-releasing hormone
spontaneously responding hyperthyroidism
stigmata of recent hemorrhage

SRI severe renal insufficiency

SRID single radial immunodiffusion

SRIF somatotropin-release inhibiting factor (somatostatin)

SRM Standard Reference Material
superior rectus muscle

SMRD stress-related mucosal damage

SRN State Registered Nurse (England and Wales)
Student Registered Nurse
subretinal neovascularization; also SRNV

sRNA soluble ribonucleic acid (now known as transfer RNA)

SR/NE sinus rhythm, no ectopy

SRNG sustained release nitroglycerin

SRNP soluble ribonuclear protein

SRNS steroid-responsive nephrotic syndrome

SRNV subretinal neovascularization; also SRN

SRNVM senile retinal neovascular membrane
subretinal neovascular membrane

SRO single room occupancy

SROM spontaneous rupture of membranes

SRP short rib–polydactyly (syndrome)
signal recognition particle
signal recognition protein
simple response paradigm
stapes replacement prosthesis
State Registered Physiotherapist

SRPS short rib–polydactyly syndrome

SRR slow rotation room
stabilized relative response
standardized rate ratio
steroid-resistant rejection
stimulus response ratio
surgical recovery room

SRRS Social Readjustment Rating Scale

SR-RSV Schmidt-Ruppin strain Rous
sarcoma virus

SRS schizophrenic residual state
septal rage syndrome
sex reassignment surgery
Silver-Russell syndrome
slow-reacting substance
Social and Rehabilitation Service
Symptom Rating Scale

SRSA, SRS-A slow-reacting substance of
anaphylaxis

SRT sedimentation rate test
sick role tendency
simple reaction time
sinus node recovery time; also SNRT
speech reception test
speech reception threshold
spontaneously resolving thyrotoxicosis
Stroke Rehabilitation Technician
sustained release theophylline
Symptom Rating Test

SRU side rails up
solitary rectal ulcer
structural repeating unit

SRUS solitary rectal ulcer syndrome

SRV Schmidt-Ruppin virus
superior radicular vein

SRVT sustained re-entrant ventricular
tachyarrhythmia

SRW short ragweed (test)

SRY sex-determining region Y

SS sacrosciatic
saline soak
saline solution
saliva sample

saliva substitute
Salmonella-Shigella (agar)
salt substitute
Sanarelli-Shwartzman (phenomenon)
saturated solution; also sat sol, sat soln
schizophrenia spectrum
Schizophrenia Subscale
seizure sensitive
serum sickness
Sézary's syndrome
Shigella sonnei
siblings; also sibs
sickle cell (anemia)
side-to-side
signs and symptoms; also S/S, s/s, S&S,
S/SX, S&Sx
Simmonds-Sheehan (syndrome)
single-stranded (DNA); also ss
Sjögren's syndrome; also SjS
sliding scale
slip sent
slow-wave sleep; also SWS
soapsuds; also ss
Social Security; also SocSec
social services; also soc serv
somatostatin; also SMS, SST
sparingly soluble
special service
Spillinger-Stock (disease, syndrome)
stable sarcoidosis
staccato syndrome
Stainer-Scholte (medium)
standard score
statistically significant
steady state; also S, s, ss
sterile solution
steroid sensitivity
steroid sulfurylation
Stickler syndrome
Strachan-Scott (syndrome)
subaortic stenosis; also SAS
subscapularis
subsegmental
subsequent sibling
substernal
suction socket
sulfasalazine; also SAS, SAZ
sum of squares
supersaturated
support and stimulation; also S&S
susceptible
Sweet's syndrome
symmetrical strength
systemic sclerosis; also SSc

S/S, s/s signs and symptoms; also SS, S&S, S/SX, S&Sx

S&S shower and shampoo
signs and symptoms; also SS, S/S, s/s, S/SX, S&Sx
support and stimulation; also SS

Ss serum soluble (antigen)
subjects

ss half [L. *semis*]; also HF, hf, S, s, sem, semi, s̄
s̄, s̈ s̄
single-stranded (DNA); also SS
soapsuds; also SS
steady state; also S, s, SS
subspinale

s̄s̄, half [L. *semis*]; also HF, hf, S, s, sem, semi, ss, s̈ s̄

s̈ s̄ half [L. *semis*]; also HF, hf, S, s, sem, semi, ss, s̄ s̄

SSA sagittal split advancement
salicylsalicylic acid (salsalate)
Salmonella-Shigella agar
sickle cell anemia; also SCA
Sjögren's syndrome antigen A
skin-sensitizing antibody
skin sympathetic activity
Smith surface antigen
Social Security Administration
special somatic afferent
sperm-specific antigen
sperm-specific antiserum
subsegmental airway
subsegmental atelectasis
sulfosalicylic acid

SS-A Sjögren's syndrome A (antibody)

SSAO semicarbazide-sensitive amine oxidase

SSAV simian sarcoma-associated virus

SSB short spike burst
stereospecific binding

SS-B Sjögren's syndrome B (antibody)

SSBG sex steroid-binding globulin

SSBR see separate bacteriology report

SSC somatosensory cortex
standard saline citrate
Stein Sentence Completion (test)
superior semicircular canal
syngeneic spleen cell

SSc systemic sclerosis; also SS

SSCA sensitized sheep cell agglutination
single shoulder contrast arthrography
spontaneous suppressor cell activity

SSCCS slow spinal cord compression syndrome

SSCF sleep stage change frequency

SSCP substernal chest pain

SSCPE standard saline, citrate, phosphate, EDTA

SSCr stainless steel crown

SSCVD sterile spontaneous controlled vaginal delivery

SSD shock-induced suppression of drinking
sickle cell disease; also SCD
silver sulfadiazine
single saturating dose
Social Security Disability
source to skin distance
source to surface distance
speech-sound discrimination
succinate semialdehyde dehydrogenase
sudden sniffing death
sum of square deviations
syndrome of sudden death

SSDI Social Security disability income

SSDMAE dimethylaminoethanol succinyl-succinate

SS-DNA, ssDNA single-stranded deoxyribonucleic acid

SSE saline solution enema
skin self-examination
soapsuds enema
steady-state exercise
systemic side effects

SSEA stage-specific embryonic antigen

SSEP somatosensory evoked potential; also SEP

SSER somatosensory evoked response; also SER

SSF soluble suppressor factor
subscapular skinfold (thickness)
supplementary sensory feedback

SSFI social stress and functionability inventory

SSG sublingual salivary gland

SSH snowshoe hare (virus)

SSHb homozygous for sickle cell hemoglobin

SSHL severe sensorineural hearing loss

SSI segmental sequential irradiation
small-scale integration
Social Security income
stuttering severity instrument
subshock insulin
subunit-subunit interface
Supplemental Security Income
synthetic sentence identification
System Sign Inventory

SSIAM Structured and Scaled Interview to Assess Maladjustment

SSIDS sibling of sudden infant death syndrome (victim)

SSIE Smithsonian Science Information Exchange

SSII Safran Student's Interest Inventory

SSIT subscapularis, supraspinatus, infraspinatus, teres minor (muscles)

SSKI saturated solution of potassium iodide

SSL skin surface lipid
synthetic sentence list

SSM subsynaptic membrane
superficial spreading malignant melanoma

SSN severely subnormal
Social Security number
suprasternal notch; also SN

SSNS steroid-sensitive nephrotic syndrome

SSO Spanish-speaking only
special sense organs

SSOP Second Surgical Opinion Program

SSP Sanarelli-Shwartzman phenomenon
single-stranded polypeptide
small spherical particle
subacute sclerosing panencephalitis; also SSPE
supersensitivity perception

Ssp, ssp subspecies; also Spp, spp, SPPP, subsp

SSPE subacute sclerosing panencephalitis; also SSP

SSPG steady-state plasma glucose

SSPI steady-state plasma insulin

SSPL saturation sound pressure level

SSPP subsynaptic plate perforation

SSPS side-to-side portacaval shunt

SS-PSE Schizophrenic Subscale of Present State Examination

SSPU surgical short procedure unit

SSR somatosensory response
steady-state rest
surgical supply room

SSRA Sjögren's syndrome–RA (rheumatoid arthritis)

ssRNA single-stranded RNA

SSS layer upon layer [L. *stratum super stratum*]; also sss
scalded skin syndrome
sensation-seeking scale
sick sinus syndrome
specific soluble substance

Stanford Sleepiness Scale
sterile saline soak
strong soap solution
structured sensory stimulation
systemic sicca syndrome

sss layer upon layer [L. *stratum super stratum*]; also SSS

SSSB sagittal split setback

SS-SC Sjögren's syndrome–Sicca complex

SSSS staphylococcal scalded skin syndrome

SSST superior sagittal sinus thrombosis

SSSV superior sagittal sinus velocity

SST sagittal sinus thrombosis
sodium sulfite titration
somatosensory thalamus
somatostatin; also SMS, SS

s str in the strict sense [L. *sensu stricto*]

SSU self-service unit
sterile supply unit

SSV Schoolman-Schwartz virus
sheep seminal vesicle
simian sarcoma virus; also SISV, SiSV
Stock-Spielmeyer-Vogt (syndrome)
under a poison label [L. *sub signo veneni*]; also ssv

ssv under a poison label [L. *sub signo veneni*]; also SSV

SSW staggered spondaic word (test)

SSX sulfisoxazole

S/SX signs and symptoms; also SS, S/S, s/s, S&S, S&Sx

S&Sx signs and symptoms; also SS, S/S, s/s, S&S, S/SX

ST electrocardiographic wave segment
esotropia
esotropic
heat-stable enterotoxin
sacrum transverse
Salmonella typhi
scala tympani
sclerotherapy
sedimentation time
semitendinosus
septal thickness
serum transferrin
shock therapy
siblings raised together
similarly tested
sinus tachycardia
sinus tympani
skin temperature

ST—cont'd
  skin test
  skin thickness
  slight trace
  slow twitch (muscle fiber)
  smokeless tobacco
  sore throat
  Spanlang-Tappeiner (syndrome)
  speech therapist
  speech therapy
  sphincter tone
  split thickness

  standardized test
  starting time
  sternothyroid
  Stewart-Treves (syndrome)
  stimulus; also R, S
  stomach; also St, st, stom
  store; also STO
  straight; also St, st
  stress test
  stretcher
  striatum; also Str
  sublingual tablet
  subtalar
  subtotal
  sulfathiazole
  surface tension; also σ
  surgical therapy
  survival time
  systolic time

S-T sickle cell thalassemia; also STh, S-Thal

St, st let it stand [L. *stet*]; also stet
  let them stand [L. *stent*]
  stage of (disease)
  stere (measure of capacity)
  stoke (unit of kinematic viscosity)
  stomach; also ST, stom
  stomion (median point of oral slit when lips
    are closed)
  stone (unit)
  straight; also ST
  stroke
  subtype

ST37 hexylresorcinol

STA second trimester abortion
  serum thrombotic accelerator
  serum tobramycin assay
  superficial temporal artery
  superior temporal artery

Sta staphylion
  station

stab stabilization
  stab neutrophil [Ger. *stabkernige* (staff
    nuclear)]

STACL Screening Test for Auditory
  Comprehension of Language

St AE standard above-elbow (cast)

STAG slow target-attaching globulin
  split thickness autogenous graft

S-TAG slow-binding target-attaching globulin

STAI State Trait Anxiety Inventory

STAI-I State Trait Anxiety Index–I

STA-MCA superficial temporal artery to
  middle cerebral artery

StanPsych standard psychiatric (nomenclature)

Staph, staph *Staphylococcus* species; also *S*

STAT at once [L. *statim*]; also stat
  Suprathreshold Adaptation Test

stat at once [L. *statim*]; also STAT
  radium emanation unit (a German unit for
    measuring the amount of radium emana-
    tion, equivalent to 0.364 microcurie)

STB, Stb stillborn; also SB, stillb

STBAL standing balance

ST BY stand-by; also SB

STC serum theophylline concentration
  sexually transmitted condition
  soft-tissue calcification
  stimulate to cry
  Stroke Treatment Center
  subtotal colectomy
  sugar tongue cast

STD sexually transmitted disease
  skin test done
  skin test dose
  skin to tumor distance
  sodium tetradecyl (sulfate)
  standard density (reference)
  standard test dose

std saturated; also S, SAT, Sat, sat, satd, sat'd
  standard; also S, *S*
  standardized

STDH skin test for delayed-type hypersensitivity

STDT standard tone-decay test

STD TF standard tube feeding; also STF

STEAM stimulated-echo acquisition mode
  streptonigrin, thioguanine, Endoxan, actino-
    mycin, mitomycin C

STEL short-term exposure limit

STEM scanning transmission electron microscope

sten stenosed
stenosis

STEP sequential tests of educational progress

STEPS sequential treatment employing pharmacologic support

stereo stereogram
stereophonic

STESS subject's treatment-emergent symptom scale; also STRESS

STET submaximal treadmill exercise test

stet let it stand [L. *stet*]; also St, st

STETH stethoscope

STF serum thymus factor
slow twitch fiber
small third-trimester fetus
specialized treatment facility
special tube feeding
standard tube feeding; also STD TF
sudden transient freezing

ST FeSv Synder-Thielen feline sarcoma virus

STG short-term goal
split-thickness graft
stomatogastric ganglion

STGC syncytiotrophoblastic giant cell

STH soft-tissue hemorrhage
somatotropic hormone (somatotropin); also SH
subtotal hysterectomy
supplemental thyroid hormone

STh sickle cell thalassemia; also S-T, S-Thal

S-Thal sickle cell thalassemia; also S-T, STh

STHB said to have been

STHRF somatotropin hormone-releasing factor

STI scientific and technical information
serum trypsin inhibitor
soft tissue injury
soybean trypsin inhibitor; also SBI, SBTI
systolic time interval

STIC serum trypsin inhibition capacity
solid-state transducer intracompartment

stillat drop by drop [L. *stillatim*]

stillb stillborn; also SB, STB, Stb

stim stimulation; also stimn, stm, stmn

stimn stimulation; also stim, stm, stmn

STIP (basophilic) stippling

STJ subtalar joint

STK streptokinase; also SK

STL serum theophylline level
status thymicolymphaticus
swelling, tenderness, limited (motion)

STLE St. Louis encephalitis; also SLE

STLI subtotal lymphoid irradiation

STLOM swelling, tenderness, limitation of motion

STLV simian T-cell lymphotropic virus

STM scanning tunneling microscope
short-term memory
spore tip mucilage
streptomycin; also S, SM, strep

stm stimulation; also stim, stimn, stmn

stmn stimulation; also stim, stimn, stm

StMPM syncytiotrophoblast microvillar plasma membrane

STN subthalamic nucleus; also SubN
supratrochlear nucleus

STNR symmetrical tonic neck reflex

STNS sham transcutaneous nerve stimulation

STNV satellite tobacco necrosis virus

STO Slater-type orbital
store; also ST

stom stomach; also ST, St, st

STORCH syphilis, toxoplasmosis, rubella, cytomegalovirus, and herpesvirus

STP scientifically treated petroleum
serenity, tranquility, peace (user's term for 2,5-dimethoxy-4-methylamphetamine)
Sibling Training Program
sodium thiopental
standard temperature and pressure
standard temperature and pulse

STPD standard temperature and pressure, dry (0° C, 760 mm Hg)

STPI State-Trait Personality Inventory

STPP sodium tripolyphosphate

STPS specific thalamic projection system

STQ superior temporal quadrant

STR soft tissue rheumatism
special treatment room

str *Streptococcus* species; also *S*, strep
striatum; also ST

strab strabismus; also Sb

strep *Streptococcus* species; also *S*, Str
streptomycin; also S, SM, STM

STRESS subject's treatment-emergent symptom scale; also STESS

STRT skin temperature recovery time

struct structural
structure; also STX

STS sequence-tagged site
serologic test for syphilis
sexual tubal sterilization
short-term storage
Society of Thoracic Surgeons
sodium tetradecyl sulfate
sodium thiosulfate
soft tissue swelling
standard test for syphilis
steroid sulphatase
sugar-tong splint

STSG split thickness skin graft

STSS staphylococcal toxic shock syndrome

STT sensitization test
serial thrombin time
skin temperature test
standard triple therapy

STTOL standing tolerance

STU shock trauma unit
skin test unit

STV short-term variability
soft tissue view
superior temporal vein

STVA subtotal villous atrophy; also SVA

STVS short-term visual storage

STX saxitoxin
structure; also struct

STYCAR Screening Tests for Young Children
and Retardates

STZ streptozocin; also stz, SZ, Sz, SZN
streptozyme

stz streptozocin; also STZ, SZ, Sz, SZN

sU salicyluric (acid)
Senear-Usher (syndrome)
sensation unit
sensory urgency
solar urticaria
Somogyi unit
sorbent unit
spectrophotometric unit
stress ulcer
strontium unit
subunit
sulfonamide; also Su, sulfa
sulfonylurea
supine

S&U supine and upright

Su sulfonamide; also SU, sulfa

su let him take [L. *sumat*]; also sum

SUA serum uric acid
single umbilical artery
single unit activity

SUB Skene, urethral and Bartholin (glands)

subac subacute

subconj subconjunctival

subcu subcutaneous; also SC, sc, SQ, Sq,
subcut, subq, sub-q

subcut subcutaneous; also SC, sc, SQ, Sq,
subcu, subq, sub-q

sub fin coct toward the end of boiling [L. *sub
finem coctionis*]

subl sublimes
sublingual; also SL, sL, sl, subling

subling sublingual; also SL, sL, sl, subl

submand submandibular, ; also SM

subN subthalamic nucleus; also STN

subq, sub-q subcutaneous; also SC, sc, SQ,
Sq, subcu, subcut

subsp subspecies; also Spp, spp, SPPP, Ssp, ssp

substc substance concentration

substd substandard

substfr substance fraction

suc juice [L. *succus*]

SUCC succinylcholine; also SC, SCH, SUX

Succ succinate
succinic

SUD skin unit dose
sudden unexpected death
sudden unexplained death

SUDS single-unit delivery system
Subjective Unit of Distress Scale
sudden unexplained death syndrome

SUF sequential ultrafiltration

Suff sufficient

SUHT subject's height (in inches)

SUI stress urinary incontinence
suicide

SUID sudden unexpected infant death
sudden unexplained infant death

sulf sulfate

sulfa sulfonamide; also SU, Su

SULFHB sulfhemoglobin; also SHB, S Hb,
S-Hb

SULF-PRIM sulfamethoxazole and trimethoprim

sum let him take [L. *sumat*]; also su
summation
to be taken [L. *sumendum*]

SUMIT streptokinase-urokinase myocardial
infarction trial

sum tal let him take one like this [L. *sumat
talem*]

SUN serum urea nitrogen
Standard Units and Nomenclature

SUO syncope of unknown origin

SUP superficial; also sup
superior; also sup
supination; also supin
supinator (muscle); also sup
symptomatic uterine prolapse

sup above [L. *supra*]
superficial; also SUP
superior; also SUP
supervision; also S
supervisor
supinator (muscle); also SUP

supin supination; also SUP

supp support
suppository; also suppos

suppl supplement
supplementary

suppos suppository; also supp

SUPT-P pressure support

SURG, surg surgeon
surgery; also S, Sx, S$_x$, sx
surgical

SURS solitary ulcer of rectum syndrome

SUS solitary ulcer syndrome
stained urinary sediment
suppressor sensitive

susp suspended
suspension

SUTI symptomatic urinary tract infection

SUUD sudden unexpected, unexplained death

SUV small unilamellar vesicle

SUX succinylcholine; also SC, SCH, SUCC
suction; also S, SZ

SV saphenous vein
sarcoma virus
satellite virus
selective vagotomy
semilunar valve
seminal vesicle
Sendai virus
severe; also sev
sigmoid volvulus
simian virus
single ventricle
single vessel
sinus venosus
snake venom
spatial velocity
Spielmeyer-Vogt (disease)
spirit of wine (alcoholic spirit) [L. *spiritus
vini*]; also sv
splenic vein
spoken voice
spontaneous ventilation
stroke volume
subclavian vein; also SCV
subventricular
supravital

S/V surface to volume (ratio)

SV40 simian vacuolating virus 40

Sv sievert (unit); also sv

sv sievert (unit); also Sv
single vibration
spirit of wine (alcoholic spirit) [L. *spiritus
vini*]; also SV

SVA selective vagotomy with antrectomy
selective visceral angiography
sequential ventriculoatrial (pacing)
spatial voltage at maximal anterior (force)
special visceral afferent
subtotal villous atrophy; also STVA
supraventricular activity

SVAS subvalvular aortic stenosis
supravalvular aortic stenosis; also SAS

SVB saphenous vein bypass
supraventricular beats

SVBG saphenous vein bypass graft

SVC segmental venous capacitance
slow vital capacity
Spiroplasmavirus citri
subclavian vein catheterization
superior vena cava
suprahepatic vena cava

SVCG spatial vectorcardiogram

SVCO superior vena cava obstruction

SVCP Special Virus Cancer Program

SVC-PA superior vena cava–pulmonary artery
(shunt)

SVCR segmented venous capacitance ratio

SVC-RPA superior vena cava–right pulmonary artery (shunt)

SVCS superior vena cava syndrome

SVD single vessel disease
singular value decomposition
small vessel disease
spontaneous vaginal delivery
spontaneous vertex delivery
swine vesicular disease

SVE slow volume encephalography
soluble viral extract
special visceral efferent
sterile vaginal examination
Streptococcus viridans endocarditis
supraventricular ectopy

SVG saphenous vein graft

SVI stroke volume index
systemic vascular index
systolic velocity integral (Doppler)

SVL severe visual loss
superficial vastus lateralis

SVM seminal vesicle microsome
spatial voltage at maximal (posterior force)
standard Volvox medium
syncytiovascular membrane

SVN small volume nebulizer

SvO$_2$, S$_{VO2}$ venous oxygen saturation

SVOM sequential volitional oral movement

SVP selective vagotomy with pyloroplasty
small volume parenteral (infusion)
spatial voltage at maximal posterior (force)
spontaneous venous pulse
standing venous pressure
static volume pressure
superficial vascular plexus

SVPB supraventricular premature beat

SVPC supraventricular premature contraction

SVR rectified spirit of wine (distilled) [L. *spiritus vini rectificatus*]; also svr
sequential vascular response
supraventricular rhythm
systemic vascular resistance

svr rectified spirit of wine (distilled) [L. *spiritus vini rectificatus*]; also SVR

SVRI systemic vascular resistance index

SVS slit ventricle syndrome
Society for Vascular Surgery

SVSe supravaginal septum

SVT sinoventricular tachyarrhythmia
sinoventricular tachycardia
Society of Vascular Technology
subclavian vein thrombosis
supraventricular tachyarrhythmia
supraventricular tachycardia
thin spirit of wine (diluted, proof spirit)
[L. *spiritus vini tenuis*]; also svt

svt thin spirit of wine (diluted, proof spirit)
[L. *spiritus vini tenuis*]; also SVT

SW Schwartz-Watson (test)
seawater
seriously wounded
short wave
slow-wave
Social Worker
spherule wall
spike wave
spiral wound
stab wound
sterile water
stroke work
Sturge-Weber (syndrome)
Swiss Webster (mouse)

Sw swine; also S

sw switch

SWAG scientific wise-ass guess

SWAMP swine-associated mucoprotein

SWC submaximal working capacity

SWD short-wave diathermy

SWFI sterile water for injection; also SWI

SWG standard wire gauge

SWI skin and wound isolation
sterile water for injection; also SWFI
stroke work index
surgical wound infection

SWIM sperm-washing insemination method

SWM segmental wall motion

SWO superficial white onychomycosis

SWOG Southwest Oncology Group

SWP small whirlpool

SWR serum Wassermann reaction

SWS slow-wave sleep; also SS
spike-wave stupor
steroid wasting syndrome
Sturge-Weber syndrome

SWT sine-wave threshold
Speech Weber Test
stab wound of throat

SWU septic work-up

SX sulfamethoxypyridazine

Sx, S$_x$, sx signs
    surgery; also S, SURG, surg
    symptom(s); also SM, Sm, sym, symp, sympt

SXR skull x-ray

SXT sulfamethoxazole/trimethoprim

SY syphilis; also syph, Σ
    syphilitic; also syph

SYA subacute yellow atrophy (of the liver)

SYC small, yellow, constipated (stool)

sym symmetrical; also S, *s*, *sym*
    symptom(s); also SM, Sm, Sx, S$_x$, sx, symp, sympt

sym symmetrical; also S, *s*, sym

symb symbol
    symbolic

symp symptom(s); also SM, Sm, Sx, S$_x$, sx, sym, sympt

sympath sympathetic; also S

symph symphysis

sympt symptom(s); also SM, Sm, Sx, S$_x$, sx, sym, symp

syn syndrome; also synd
    synonym
    synovial

sync synchronous

synd syndrome; also syn

Synf synovial fluid; also SF, Syn Fl, syn fl

Syn Fl, syn fl synovial fluid; also SF, Synf

synth synthetic

syph syphilis; also SY, Σ
    syphilitic; also SY

SYR Syrian (hamster)

Syr syrup; also syr

syr syringe
    syrup; also Syr

SYS stretching-yawning syndrome

sys system; also syst
    systemic; also syst

SYS BP systolic blood pressure; also SBP

syst system; also sys
    systemic; also sys
    systole; also S
    systolic

SZ schizophrenic; also Sz
    seizure; also Sz
    Skevas-Zerfus (disease)
    streptozocin; also STZ, stz, Sz, SZN
    streptozotocin
    suction; also S, SUX
    sulfamethizole

Sz schizophrenic; also SZ
    seizure; also SZ
    skin impedance
    streptozocin; also STZ, stz, SZ, SZN

SZD streptozocin diabetes

SZN streptozocin; also STZ, stz, SZ, Sz

T

T TAU, UPPER CASE, nineteenth letter of the Greek alphabet

τ tau, lower case, nineteenth letter of the Greek alphabet
life (lifetime of radioisotope); also T, t
mean life
relaxation time
shear stress
spectral transmittance
torque; also T
transmission coefficient

τ ½ halflife (of radioactive isotopes); also T½, t½, t½

Θ THETA, UPPER CASE, eighth letter of the Greek alphabet
thermodynamic termperature

θ theta, lower case, eighth letter of the Greek alphabet
angular coordinate variable
customary temperature
latent trait (statistics)
temperature interval

ϑ theta, lower case, eighth letter of the Greek alphabet, variant

T absolute temperature (Kelvin); also T
electrocardiographic wave corresponding to repolarization of the ventricles
interocular tension; also TEN
life (lifetime of radioiostopes); also t, τ
obtained under test conditions
period (time)
ribosylthymine
ribothymidine (thymidine); also Thd
tablespoon; also TBS, tbs, tbsp
tamoxifen; also TAM, TMX
tanycyte (ependymal cell)
T-bandage
T-bar
telomere or terminal banding
temperature; also T°, t, TEMP, temp, TPR
temporal electrode placement in electro-encephalography
temporary; also TEMP, temp
tender
tension
tera- (10^{12})
terminal (congenital absence of limb)
tertiary; also t, ter, tert, *tert*
Tesla
testes both down

testicle
testosterone; also testos
tetra
tetracycline; also TC, Tc, TCN, TCNE, TE, TETCYC
T-fiber
theophylline; also TH, TL
thoracic; also Th, th, thor
thoracoabdominal (stapler)
thorax; also TH, Th, th, thor
threatened (animal)
threonine (one-letter notation); also Thr
thrombus; also throm, thromb
thymidine (thymine-2-desoxyriboside); also TdR
thymine; also Thy
thymus; also thy
thymus (cell); also thy
thymus derived (lymphocyte)
thyroid; also thr
tidal gas
tidal volume (subscript)
tight
time; also *t*
timolol
tincture; also tinc, tinct, TR, Tr, tr
tissue
tocopherol
tone
tonometer reading
topical; also top
torque; also τ
total
toxicity; also Tox, tox
trace; also TR, Tr, tr
training (group)
transition elements
transition (point); also TP
transmittance; also *T*
transverse; also trans
tray
triangulation
triggered
tritium; also t
tuberculin; also TB
tuberculosis; also TB, Tb, tb, TBC, Tbc, tbc, tuberc
tuberculous; also TB, Tb, tb, TBC, Tbc, tbc, tuberc
tuberculum
tuberosity

tumor; also TM
turnkey system
type; also Ty

T absolute temperature (Kelvin); also T
Taenia species
transmittance; also T
Treponema species
Trichomonas species
Trichophyton species
Trypanosoma species

T° temperature; also T, *t*, TEMP, temp, TPR

T- decreased intraocular tension

T+ increased intraocular tension

T^1/$_2$ halflife (of radioactive isotopes); also $\tau^1/_2$, t^1/$_2$, $t^1/_2$
halftime (of radioactive isotopes); also t^1/$_2$, $t^1/_2$
mitral pressure half-time (Doppler)
terminal halflife (of isotopes)

T$_1$ monoiodotyrosine
tricuspid first heart sound

T1 spin-lattice or longitudinal relaxation time (MRI scan)

T1 thru T12 first to twelfth thoracic nerves
first to twelfth thoracic vertebrae

T+1, T+2, T+3 first, second, and third stages of increased intraocular tension

T-1, T-2, T-3 first, second, and third stages of decreased intraocular tension

T$_2$ diiodothyronine
tricuspid second heart sound

T2 spin-spin or transverse relaxation time (MRI scan)

T$_3$ triiodothyronine; also TIT, TITh, TRIT

T3 Tylenol with codeine (30 mg)

T$_4$ levothyroxine
tetrahedral
tetraiodothyronine (thyroxine)

T-7 free thyroxine factor

2,4,5-T 2,4,5-trichlorophenoxy acetic acid

T-1824 Evans blue (dye)

%T percent transmittance

t duration
life (lifetime of radioisotopes);also T, τ
student test variable; also *t*
teaspoon; also ts, tsp
temperature (Celsius, Fahrenheit)
temporal; also TEMP, temp
telephoned
terminal; also term, TRML, Trml
tertiary; also T, ter, tert, *tert*

test of significance
three times [L. *ter*]; also ter
ton
tonne
translocation
Treponema
Trichophyton
tritium; also T
Trypanosoma

t^1/$_2$ halflife (of radioactive isotopes); also $\tau^1/_2$, T^1/$_2$, $t^1/_2$
halftime (of radioactive isotopes); also T^1/$_2$, $t^1/_2$
reaction halftime
time taken for half of initial concentration of deoxyribonucleic acid to renature

t student test variable; also t
student's *t* statistic
temperature; also T, T°, TEMP, temp, TPR
time; also T

t^1/$_2$ halflife (of radioactive isotopes); also $\tau^1/_2$, T^1/$_2$, $t^1/_2$
halftime (of radioactive isotopes); also T^1/$_2$, $t^1/_2$

tγ shear rate

TA alkaline tuberculin
tactile afferent
Takayasu's arteritis
tarsal amputation
tarsus
technical assistance
teichoic acid
temperature, axillary; also T(A)
temporal arteritis
temporal average
tendon of Achilles
tension, arterial
tension by applanation; also Ta, TAP
terminal antrum
test age
therapeutic abortion; also TAB, TAb
thermophilic Actinomyces
thymocytotoxic autoantibody
thyroglobulin autoprecipitation
thyroglobulin autoprecipitin
thyroid antibody
thyroid autoantibody
tibialis anterior
titratable acid
total alkaloids
toxic adenoma
toxin-antitoxin; also T-A, TAT
tracheal aspirate

TA—cont'd
  traffic accident; also T/A
  transactional analysis
  transaldolase; also TRA
  transantral
  transplantation antigen
  trapped air
  treatment assignment
  triamcinolone acetonide; also TAA
  tricholomic acid
  tricuspid annuloplasty
  tricuspid atresia; also TCA
  trophoblast antigen
  true anomaly
  truncus arteriosus
  tryptamine
  tryptophan-acid (reaction)
  tryptose agar
  tube agglutination
  tumor antigen
  tumor associated

T-A toxin-antitoxin; also TA, TAT

T/A time and amount
  traffic accident; also TA

T&A tonsillectomy and adenoidectomy
  tonsils and adenoids

T(A) temperature, axillary; also TA

TA₄ tetraiodothyroacetic acid: also TETRAC

Ta T-amplifier
  tantalum
  tension by applanation; also TA, TAP
  tonometry applanation

TAA thoracic aortic aneurysm
  total ankle arthroplasty
  transverse aortic arch
  triamcinolone acetonide; also TA
  tumor-associated antigen

TAAF thromblastic activity of amniotic fluid

TAANA The American Association of Nurse Attorneys

TAB tablet; also tab
  therapeutic abortion; also TA, TAb
  triple antibiotic
  typhoid, paratyphoid A, and paratyphoid B (vaccine)

TAb therapeutic abortion; also TA, TAB

tab tablet; also TAB

TABC total aerobic bacteria count
  typhoid, paratyphoid A, paratyphoid B, and paratyphoid C (vaccine)

tabs tablets

TABT typhoid, paratyphoid A, paratyphoid B, and tetanus (vaccine)

TABTD typhoid, paratyphoid A, paratyphoid B, tetanus toxoid, and diphtheria toxoid (vaccine)

TAC terminal antrum contraction
  tetracaine, Adrenalin, and cocaine
  thyroid-adrenocortical (syndrome)
  time-activity curve
  total abdominal colectomy
  total aganglionosis coli
  Toxicant Analysis Center
  triamcinolone acetonide cream

TACE teichoic acid crude extract
  trianisylchloroethylene

tach tachycardia; also tachy

tachy tachycardia; also tach

TACL Test for Auditory Comprehension of Language

TAD thioguanine, Ara-C, and daunorubicin
  thoracic asphyxiant dystrophy
  total administered dose
  transient acantholytic dermatosis
  transverse abdominal diameter
  tricyclic antidepressant drug

TADAC therapeutic abortion, dilation, aspiration, and curettage

TAE transcatheter arterial embolization

TAF albumose-free tuberculin [Ger. *Tuberculin Albumose frei*]
  tissue angiogenesis factor (British abbreviation)
  toxoid-antitoxin floccules
  trypsin-aldehyde-fuchsin
  tumor angiogenesis factor; also TAGF

TAG target-attaching globulin
  thymine, adenine, guanine
  triacylglycerol; also TG

TAGF tumor angiogenesis factor; also TAF

TAGH triiodothyronine, amino acids, glucagon, heparin

TAH total abdominal hysterectomy
  total artificial heart
  transabdominal hysterectomy

TAHBSO total abdominal hysterectomy and bilateral salpingo-oophorectomy

TAI tissue antagonist of interferon

TAL tendo Achilles lengthening
  thick ascending limb (of Henle's loop)
  thymic alymphoplasia
  total arm length

tal of such, such a one [L. *talis*]

tal dos such doses [L. *talis dosis*]

talc talcum

TALH thick ascending limb of Henle's loop

TALL, T-ALL T-cell acute lymphoblastic leukemia

TALTFR tendo Achilles lengthening and toe flexor release

TAM tamoxifen; also T, TMX
teenage mother
thermoacidurans agar modified
total active motion
toxoid-antitoxoid mixture
transient abnormal myelopoiesis

TAME toluenesulfonylarginine methyl ester
toluene-sulfo-trypsin arginine methyl ester

TAMe toxoid-antitoxoid mixture esterase

TAMI thrombolysis in acute myocardial infarction

TAMIS Telemetric Automated Microbial Identification System

TAML, t-AML therapy-related acute myeloid leukemia

TAN tonically autoactive neuron
total adenine nucleotide
total ammonia nitrogen

tan tandem translocation
tangent

TANI total axial lymph node irradiation

TAO thromboangiitis obliterans
triacetyloleandomycin
turning against object

TAP tension by applanation; also TA, Ta
tonometry by applanation
2,5,6-triamino-4(1-*H*)-pyrimidinone

TAPS training and placement service
trial assessment procedure scale

TAPVC total anomalous pulmonary venous connection

TAPVD total anomalous pulmonary venous drainage

TAPVR total anomalous pulmonary venous return

TAQW transient abnormal Q wave

TAR thrombocytopenia with absent radii (syndrome)
tissue-to-air ratio
total abortion rate
total ankle replacement
Treatment Authorization Request

TARA total articular replacement arthroplasty
tumor-associated rejection antigen

TAS test for ascendance-submission
tetanus antitoxin serum
Therapeutic Activities Specialist
turning against self
typical absence seizure

TASA tumor-associated surface antigen

T'ase, Tase tryptophan synthetase

TAT Tell a Tale (psychiatry)
tetanus antitoxin
Thematic Apperception Test
Thematic Aptitude Test
thromboplastin activation test
till all taken
total antitryptic (activity)
toxin-antitoxin; also TA, T-A
transaxial tomogram
transverse axial tomography
tray agglutination test
tryptone-azolectin-tween (broth)
tumor activity test
turnaround time
tyrosine aminotransferase

TATA transanal abdominal transanal proctosigmoidectomy and coloanal anastomosis
tumor-associated transplantation antigen

TATBA triamcinolone acetonide *tert*-butyl acetate

TATR tyrosine aminotransferase regulator

TATST tetanus antitoxin skin test

TAV trapped air volume

TB Tapes for the Blind
Taussig-Bing (syndrome)
terminal bronchiole
thromboxane B
thymol blue
toluidine blue
total base
total bilirubin; also TBIL, T Bili, T bili
total body
tracheal bronchiolar (region)
tracheobronchitis
trapezoid body
trigonal bipyramid (complexes)
tub bath
tubercle bacillus; also Tb, tb, TBA
tuberculin; also T
tuberculosis; also T, Tb, tb, TBC, Tbc, tbc, tuberc
tuberculous; also T, Tb, tb, TBC, Tbc, tbc, tuberc
tumor-bearing

TB-5 trigonal bipyramidal

T-B Thomas-Binetti (test)

Tb Tbilisi (phage)
terbium
tubercle bacillus; also TB, tb, TBA
tuberculosis; also T, TB, tb, TBC, Tbc, tbc, tuberc
tuberculous; also T, TB, tb, TBC, Tbc, tbc, tuberc

T$_b$ body temperature

tb biologic halflife(time)
tubercle bacillus; also TB, Tb, TBA
tuberculosis; also T, TB, Tb, TBC, Tbc, tbc, tuberc
tuberculous; also T, TB, Tb, TBC, Tbc, tbc, tuberc

TBA tertiary butylacetate
testosterone-binding affinity
thiobarbituric acid
thyroxine-binding albumin
to be absorbed
to be added
to be administered
to be admitted
total bile acid
total-body surface area; also TBSA
traditional birth attendant
trypsin-binding activity
tubercle bacillus; also TB, Tb, tb
tumor-bearing animal

TBAB tryptose blood agar base

T banding telomere banding (of chromosomes)
terminal banding (of chromosomes)

TBB transbronchial biopsy

TBB 1-698 tibione

TBBC total vitamin B$_{12}$ binding capacity

TBBM total-body bone mineral

TBC thyroxine-binding coagulin
total body calcium
total body clearance; also Q$_B$
total body counting
tubercidin
tuberculosis; also T, TB, Tb, tb, Tbc, tbc, tuberc
tuberculous; also T, TB, Tb, tb, Tbc, tbc, tuberc

Tbc, tbc tuberculosis; also T, TB, Tb, tb, TBC, tuberc
tuberculous; also T, TB, Tb, tb, TBC, tuberc

TBD total body density

TBE tick-borne encephalitis
tuberculin bacillen emulsion; also TBN

TBES total-body exchangeable sodium

TBF total body fat
tuberculin bouillon filtrate

TBFB tracheobronchial foreign body

TBG testosterone-binding globulin
thermobarogravimetry
thyroxine-binding globulin
tracheobronchogram
tris-buffered Grey's solution

TBG cap T$_4$-binding capacity (of thyroxine-binding globulin assays)

TBGE thyroxine-binding globulin, estimated

TBGI thyroid-binding globulin index
thyroxine-binding globulin index

TBGP total blood granulocyte pool

TBH total-body hematocrit

TBHT total-body hyperthermia

TBI thyroid-binding index
thyroxine-binding index
tooth-brushing instruction
total body involved
total body irradiation; also TBX
traumatic brain injury

TBII TSH-binding inhibitory immunoglobulin

TBIL total bilirubin; also TB, T Bili, T bili

T Bili, T bili total bilirubin; also TB, TBIL

TBK total-body potassium [L. *kalium* (potassium)]

TBLB transbronchial lung biopsy

TBLC term birth, living child

TBLF term birth, living female

TBLI term birth, living infant

TBLM term birth, living male

TBLN tracheobronchial lymph node

TBM thyroxine-binding meningitis
total body mass
tracheobronchomalacia
tuberculous meningitis
tubular basement membrane

TBN total-body nitrogen
tuberculin bacillen emulsion; also TBE

TBNA total-body neutron activation
total-body sodium
transbronchial needle aspiration
treated but not admitted

TBNAA total-body neutron activation analysis

t-BOC, *t*-BOC *N*-tertiary butoxycarbonyl; also BOC, Boc

TBP testosterone-binding protein

thiobisdichlorophenol (bithionol)
thyroxine-binding protein
total-body photograph
total bypass
tributyl phosphate
tuberculous peritonitis

TBPA thyroxine-binding prealbumin

TBPT total-body protein turnover

TBR total bed rest
tumor-bearing rabbit

TB-RD, TB-Rd tuberculosis-respiratory disease

TBRS Timed Behavioral Rating Sheet

TBS tablespoon; also T, tbs, tbsp
The Bethesda System (cytopathology)
total-body solids
total-body solute
total body surface
total burn side
tracheal bronchial submucosa
tracheobronchoscopy
tribromsalan (tribromosalicylanilide)
triethanolamine-buffered saline
tris-buffered saline

tbs tablespoon; also T, TBS, tbsp

TBSA total body surface area; also TBA
total burn surface area

tbsp tablespoon; also T, TBS, tbs

TBSV tomato bushy shunt virus

TBT, TbT tolbutamide test
tracheobronchial toilet
tracheobronchial tree

TBTNR Toronto Biculture Test of Nonverbal Reasoning

TBTT tuberculin tine test

t bu tert-butyl (1,1-dimethylethyl)

TBUT tear break-up time

TBV total blood volume
transluminal balloon valvuloplasty

TBV$_P$ total blood volume predicted (from body surface)

TBW total body washout
total body water; also TBWA, TW
total body weight

TBWA total body water; also TBW, TW

TBX thromboxane; also Thx, TX
total body irradiation; also TBI

TBZ tetrabenazine
thiabendazole

TC target cell

taurocholate
taurocholic (acid)
telephone call; also T/C
temperature compensation
teratocarcinoma
tertiary cleavage
tetracycline; also T, Tc, TCN, TCNE, TE, TETCYC
therapeutic category
therapeutic community
therapeutic concentrate
thermal conductivity; also λ
thioquanine and cytarabine
thoracic cage
throat culture; also TH-CULT
thyrocalcitonin; also TCA, TCT
tissue culture
to contain (pipette)
total calcium
total capacity
total cholesterol; also TOTAL-C
total colonoscopy
total correction
transcobalamin; also Tc
transcutaneous; also tc
transplant center
transverse colon
trauma center
Treacher Collins (syndrome)
treatment completed
true conjugate
tuberculin, contagious
tuberculosis, contagious
tubocurarine
tumor cell
type and cross-match; also T&C, T&M, T&X, TXM

T/C telephone call; also TC
to consider

T&C test and cross-match
turn and cough
type and cross-match; also TC, T&M, T&X, TXM

TC I transcobalamin I

TC II transcobalamin II

TC$_{50}$ median toxic concentration

T$_4$(C) serum thyroxine measured by column chromatography

Tc core temperature
T-cell cytolytic
T-cell cytotoxic
technetium
temporal complex

Tc—cont'd
tetracycline; also T, TC, TCN, TCNE, TE,
TETCYC
transcobalamin; also TC

T_c generation time of cell cycle

tc transcutaneous; also TC
translational control

^{99m}Tc technetium 99_m, radioactive technetium;
halflife, 6.0 hours

TCA taurocholic acid
terminal cancer
terminal carcinoma
tetracyclic antidepressant: also TTA
thioguanine and cytarabine
thyrocalcitonin; also TC, TCT
tissue culture assay
total cholic acid
total circulating albumin
total circulatory arrest
transluminal coronary angioplasty
tricalcium aluminate
tricarboxylic acid
trichloroacetic acid
trichloroacetate
tricuspid atresia; also TA
tricyclic amine
tricyclic antidepressant; also TCAD

TCABG triple coronary artery bypass graft;
also TCAG

TCAD tricyclic antidepressant; also TCA

TCAG triple coronary artery bypass graft; also
TCABG

TCAP trimethylcetylammonium pen-
tachlorophenate

TCB beta strep throat culture
tetrachlorobiphenyl
to call back
total cardiopulmonary bypass
transcatheter biopsy
tumor cell burden

TCBS thiosulfate-citrate-bile salts-sucrose
(agar)

TCC thromboplastic cell component
toroidal coil chromatography
transitional cell carcinoma
trichlorocarbanilide
triclocarban; also Tcc

Tcc triclocarban; also TCC

TCCA transitional cell cancer-associated
(virus)

TCCAV transitional cell cancer-associated
virus

TCCB transitional cell carcinoma of the bladder

TCCL T-cell chronic lymphocytic (leukemia)

TC CO_2 transcutaneous carbon dioxide
(monitor)

TCD thermal conductivity detector; also TC
detector
tissue culture dose
transcranial Doppler
transverse cardiac diameter

TCD$_{50}$ 50% long-term tumor control dose
median tissue culture dose

TCDB, TC&DB turn, cough, and deep breathe

TCDC taurochenodeoxycholate

TCDD tetrachlorodibenzodioxin (dioxin)

TC detector thermal conductivity detector;
also TCD

TcDISIDA technetium diisopropyliminodiacetic acid (scan)

TCE T-cell enriched
tetrachlorodiphenylethane; also TDE
trichloroethanol
trichloroethylene

T-cell thymus-derived cell

TCES time-controlled explosion system (galen-
ics)
transcutaneous cranial electrical stimulation

TCESOM trichloroethylene-extracted soybean-
oil meal

TCET transcerebral electrotherapy

TCF tissue-coding factor; also TSF
total coronary flow
Treacher-Collins-Franceschetti (syndrome)

TCFU tumor colony-forming unit

TCG time compensation gain

TCGF thymus cell growth factor

TCH tanned cell hemagglutination
total circulating hemoglobin
turn, cough, and hyperventilate

TChE total cholinesterase

TcHIDA technetium hepatoiminodiacetic acid
(scan)

TCI T-cell immunity
to come in (to hospital)
total cerebral ischemia
Totman's Change Index
transient cerebral ischemia
tricuspid insufficiency; also TI

TCi teracurie

TCID tissue culture infective dose
tissue culture inoculated dose

TCID$_{50}$ median tissue culture infective dose

TcIDA technetium iminodiacetic acid

TCIE transient cerebral ischemic episode

TCIPA tumor-cell-induced platelet aggregation

TCL thermochemiluminescence
total capacity of the lung
triazine chlorguanide

T-CLL T-cell chronic lymphatic leukemia

TCLo toxic concentration low

TCM tissue culture medium
traditional Chinese medicine
transcutaneous monitor

TCMA transcortical motor aphasia

TCMH tumor-direct cell-mediated hypersensitivity

TCMI T-cell-mediated immunity

TCMP thematic content modification program

TCMZ trichloromethiazide

TCN tetracycline; also T, TC, Tc, TCNE, TE, TETCYC

TCNE tetracycline; also T, TC, Tc, TCN, TE, TETCYC

TCNS transcutaneous nerve stimulation; also TNS

TCO total contact orthosis

TCOM transcutaneous oximetry
transcutaneous oxygen monitor; also TOM

TCP teacher-child-parent
therapeutic class profile
therapeutic continuous penicillin
total circulating protein
tranylcypromine
tricalcium phosphate
trichlorophenol
tricresyl phosphate

TCPA tetrachlorophthalic anhydride

T$_4$CPB T$_4$ by competitive protein binding

TCPCO$_2$, TcPCO$_2$, tcPCO$_2$ transcutaneous partial pressure of carbon dioxide

TCPE trichlorophenoxyethanol

TCPO$_2$, TcPO$_2$, tcPO$_2$ transcutaneous partial pressure of oxygen

TCR T-cell antigen receptor
T-cell reactivity
T-cell rosette
thalamocortical relay
total cytoplasmic ribosome

tcRNA translational control ribonucleic acid

TCRP total cellular receptor pool

TCS T-cell supernatant
total cellular score
total coronary score

Tcs T-cell-mediating contact sensitivity

TCSA tetrachlorosalicylanilide

TCT thrombin clotting time
thyrocalcitonin; also TC, TCA

TCTFE 1,1,2-trichloro-1,2,2-trifluoroethane

TCu copper T

TCV thoracic cage volume
three-concept view
turnip crinkle virus

TCVA thromboembolic cerebral vascular accident

TD Takayasu's disease
tardive dyskinesia; also TDK
T-cell dependent
temporary disability
teratoma differentiated
terminal device
tetanus and diphtheria toxoid (pediatric use)
tetrodotoxin; also TTX
therapeutic dietitian
therapy discontinued
thermal dilution
thoracic duct
three times daily [L. *ter die*]; also td
threshold dose
threshold of detectability
threshold of discomfort
thymus-dependent
tibial dyschondroplasia
timed diathermocoagulation
timed disintegration
tocopherol deficient
to deliver (pipette)
tolerance dose
tone decay
torsion dystonia
total disability
total dose
totally disabled
toxic dose
tracheal diameter
tracking dye
transdermal
transverse diameter; also trans D
traveler's diarrhea
treatment discontinued
tuberoinfundibular dopaminergic
tumoral dose
typhoid dysentery

T_D time required to double the number of cells in a given population

T₄D, T₄(D) serum thyroxine measured by displacement analysis

TD₅₀ median toxic dose

Td tetanus-diphtheria toxoid (adult type)

td three times daily [L. *ter die*]; also TD

TDA therapeutic drug assay
thyroid-stimulating-hormone displacing antibody
thyrotropin-displacing activity
tryptophan deaminase agar
TSH-displacing antibody

TDAK tumor-derived activated killer

TDB Toxicology Data Bank

TDC taurodeoxycholate
taurodeoxycholic (acid)
total dietary calories

TDD telecommunication device for the deaf
tetradecadiene
thoracic duct drainage
total digitalizing dose

tdd three times a day [L. *ter de die*]; also TID, tid

TDDA tetradecadienyl acetate

TDE tetrachlorodiphenylethane; also TCE
time-delayed exponential
total daily energy (requirement)
total digestible energy
triethylene glycol diglycidyl ether

TDEC test declined (no longer offered)

TDF testis-determining factor
Thinking Disturbance Factor
thoracic duct fistula
thoracic duct flow
time-dose fractionation (factor)
tissue-damaging factor; also TF
tumor dose fractionation

TDGA tetradecyglycidate

TDH threonine dehydrogenase
total decreased histamine
toxic dose, high

TDI temperature difference integrator
toluene 2,4-diisocyanate
total dose infusion

TDK tardive dyskinesia; also TD

TDL thoracic duct lymph
thoracic duct lymphocyte
thymus-dependent lymphocyte; also TL, T-L
toxic dose, low

TDM tartaric dimalonate
therapeutic drug monitoring
trehalose dimycolate

TDN total digestible nutrients
transdermal nitroglycerin; also TDNTG

tDNA transfer deoxyribonucleic acid

TDNTG transdermal nitroglycerin; also TDN

TDO thichodento-osseous (syndrome)

TDP ribothymidine diphosphate
thermal death point
thoracic duct pressure
thymidine diphosphate
tryptophan-deaminase-positive (microorganism)

Tdp torsade des pointes [Fr. (twisted toes)]

TdR thymidine (thymine-2-desoxyriboside); also T

TDS temperature, depth, salinity
total dissolved solids

tds to be taken three times a day [L. *ter die sumendum*]

TDT tentative discharge tomorrow
terminal deoxynucleotidyl transferase; also TdT
thermal death time
tone decay test
tumor doubling time

TdT terminal deoxynucleotidyl transferase; also TDT

TDWB touch down weight-bearing

TDX therapeutic drug monitoring (instrument)

TDZ thymus-dependent zone (of lymph node)

TE echo-time
folic Teply and Elvehjem (medium)
tennis elbow
test ear
tetanus; also Te, TET, tet
tetracycline; also T, TC, Tc, TCN, TCNE, TETCYC
threshold energy
thromboembolism
thymus epithelium
thyrotoxic exophthalmos
time estimation
tissue-equivalent
tooth extracted
total estrogen
Toxoplasma encephalitis
trace element
tracheoesophageal; also TO
transepithelial elimination (terminated)

treadmill exercise
trial and error; also T&E

T&E testing and evaluation
training and experience
trial and error; also TE

Te tellurium
tetanic (contraction)
tetanus; also TE, TET, tet

te effective halflife; also teff

TEA temporal external artery
tetraethylammonium
thermal energy analyzer
thromboendarterectomy
total-elbow arthroplasty
transient emboligenic aortoarteritis
transversely excited atmospheric (pressure)
triethanolamine; also TREA

TE$_A$ total error goal

TEAB tetraethylammonium bromide

TEAC tetraethylammonium chloride

TEAE triethylaminoethyl

TEAM Training in Expanded Auxiliary
Management

TEB tris-ethylenediaminetetraacetate borate

TEBG, TeBG testosterone-estradiol-binding
globulin

TEC total electron content
total eosinophil count
total exchange capacity (of a resin)
transient erythroblastopenia of childhood

T&EC Trauma and Emergency Center

TECA technetium albumin (study)

Tech technician
technologist

tech technical
technique

TECV traumatic epiphyseal coxa vara

TED Tasks of Emotional Development
threshold erythema dose
thromboembolic disease (hose, stockings)
tracheoesophageal dysraphism
tris-ethylenediaminetetraacetate dithiothreitol
(buffer)

TEDD total end-diastolic diameter

TEDP tetraethyl dithionopyrophosphate

TEE thermal effect of exercise
transesophageal echocardiography
tyrosine ethyl ester

TEEM tanned erythrocyte electrophoretic
mobility

TEF thermal effect of food
tracheoesophageal fistula
trunk extension-flexion (unit)

teff effective halflife; also te

TEFS transmural electrical field stimulation

TEG thromboelastogram

TEGDMA tetraethylene glycol dimethacrylate

TEI transesophageal imaging

TEIB triethyleneiminobenzo quinone

TEL telemetry; also tele
tetraethyl lead

tele telemetry; also TEL

TEM transmission electron microscope
transmission electron microscopy
transverse electromagnetic
triethylenemelamine

TEMED tetramethylethylenediamine

TEMP, temp temperature; also T, T°, *t*, TPR
temple
temporal; also t
temporary; also T

temp dext to the right temple [L. *tempori
dextro*]

temp sinist to the left temple [L. *tempori
sinistro*]

TEN tension (intraocular pressure); also T
total enteral nutrition
total epidermal necrolysis
total excretory nitrogen
toxic epidermal necrolysis
toxic epidermal necrosis

tenac tenaculum

TENS transcutaneous electrical nerve
stimulation
transcutaneous electrical nerve stimulator

TEP thromboendophlebectomy
tracheoesophageal puncture
tubal ectopic pregnancy

TEPA triethylenephosphoramide (aphoxide);
also APO

TEPG triethyl phosphine gold

TEPP tetraethyl pyrophosphate
triethylenepyrophosphate

TEQU test equivocal (possible low titer)

TER total elbow replacement
total endoplasmic reticulum
transcapillary escape rate

ter rub [L. *tere*]
terminal or end; also term, TRML, Trml
ternary

ter —cont'd
  tertiary; also T, t, tert, *tert*
  threefold [L. *ter*]
  three times [L. *ter*]; also t

Terb terbutaline; also TRB

term full term (infant)
  terminal; also t, ter, TRML, Trml

ter sim rub together [L. *tere simul*]

tert, *tert* tertiary; also T, t, ter

TES tetradecyl sulfate, ethanol, saline
  thymic epithelial supernatant
  toxic epidemic syndrome
  transcutaneous electrical stimulation
  transmural electrical stimulation
  treatment of emergent symptoms
  trimethylaminoethanesulfonic acid

TESD total end-systolic diameter

TESPA triethylenethiophosphoramide; also
  Thio-T, thiotepa, Thio-TEPA, thio-TEPA,
  TSPA, TTPA

TESS treatment-emergent symptom scale

testos testosterone; also T

TET tetanus; also TE, Te, tet
  tetralogy (of Fallot); also Tet
  tetroxoprim
  total exchangeable thyroxine
  transcranial electrostimulation therapy
  treadmill exercise test; also TMET
  triethyltryptamine

Tet tetralogy (of Fallot); also TET

tet tetanus; also TE, Te, TET

TETA test-estrin timed action
  triethylenetetramine

TETCYC tetracycline; also T, TC, Tc, TCN,
  TCNE, TE

TETD tetraethylthiuram disulfide (disulfiram)

TETRAC tetraiodothyroacetic acid; also TA$_4$

tet tox tetanus toxoid; also TT

TEV talipes equinovarus

TEWL transepidermal water loss; also TWl

TF tactile fremitus
  tail flick (reflex)
  temperature factor
  testicular feminization
  tetralogy of Fallot; also TOF
  thymol flocculation
  thymus factor
  thymus tolerance factor
  thymus transfer factor
  tissue-damaging factor; also TDF
  tissue factor
  to follow
  total flow
  transfer factor
  transferrin; also Tf, TFN
  transformation frequency
  transfrontal
  tube feeding
  tuberculin filtrate
  tubular fluid
  tuning fork

Tf transferrin; also TF, TFN

T$_f$ temperature, freezing

TFA total fatty acids
  total fibrinolytic activity
  transverse fascicular area
  trifluoracetic acid

TFB trifascicular block

TFd transfer factor, dialyzable

TFE polytetrafluoroethylene (Teflon)
  tetrafluoroethylene
  two-fraction fast exchange

TFEV timed force expiratory volume

TFF tube-fed food

Tf-Fe transferrin-bound iron

TFL tensor fascia lata

TFM testicular feminization male
  testicular feminization mutation
  total fluid movement
  trifluoromethlyl nitrophenol

Tfm testicular feminization (syndrome); also
  TSF

TFN total fecal nitrogen
  totally functional neutrophil
  transferrin; also TF, Tf

TFP treponemal false positive
  trifluoperazine; also TFZ

TF/P tubule fluid to plasma (ratio)

(TF/P) In tubule fluid to plasma inulin (ratio)

TFR total fertility rate
  total flow resistance

TFS testicular feminization syndrome
  tube-fed saline

TFT thrombus formation time
  thyroid function test
  tight filum terminale
  transfer factor test
  trifluorothymidine

TFZ trifluoperazine; also TFP

TG tendon graft

TFCC – Triangular
fibrocartilage complex

testosterone glucuronide
tetraglycine
theophylline-guaifenesin
thermogravimetry
thioglucose
thioglycollate (broth); also THIO
thioguanine; also Tg
thyroglobulin; also Tg, Thg
toxic goiter
transglutaminase; also Tgase
transmissible gastroenteritis (virus of swine);
also TGE
treated group
triacylglycerol; also TAG
trigeminal ganglion
trigeminal (neuralgia)
triglyceride; also TGL, TRIG, Trig, trig
tumor growth
type genus; also tg

Tg generation time; also GT
teragram
thioguanine; also TG
thyroglobulin; also TG, Thg

T$_g$ glass transition temperature

tg type genus; also TG

tG$_1$ time required to complete G$_1$ phase of cell
cycle

tG$_2$ time required to complete G$_2$ phase of cell
cycle

TGA taurocholate gelatin agar
thioglycolic acid
thyroglobulin antibody; also TgAb
total glycoalkaloids
transient global amnesia
transposition of the great arteries
tumor glycoprotein assay

TgAb thyroglobulin antibody; also TGA

TGAR total graft area rejected

Tgase transglutaminase; also TG

TGB thyroid-binding globulin

TGC time-gain compensation
time-gain compensator
time-varied gain control

TGD thermal green dye

TGE theoretical growth evaluation
transmissible gastroenteritis (virus of swine);
also TG
tryptone glucose extract (agar)

TGF T-cell growth factor
transforming growth factor
tubuloglomerular feedback
tumor growth factor

TGFA triglyceride fatty acid

TGG turkey gamma globulin

TGI tuberculin globulineuse (Behring's formula for tuberculin) [Fr. *globulineuse*
(globulinous)]

TGIF thank God it's Friday
tumor-growth inhibitory factor

TGL triglyceride; also TG, TRIG, Trig, trig
triglyceride lipase

TGN trans-Golgi network

TGP tobacco glycoprotein

TGR tenderness, guarding, rigidity (abdominal
exam)

T-group training group

TGS tincture of green soap
trichlorogalactosucrose
triglycine sulfate

TGT thromboplastin generation test
thromboplastin generation time
tolbutamide-glucagon test

TGV thoracic gas volume
transposition of the great vessels; also TOGV

TGXT thallium-graded exercise test

TGY tryptone glucose yeast (agar)

TGYA tryptone glucose yeast agar

TH tetrahydrocortisol; also THC
T helper (cell)
theophylline; also T, TL
thoracic; also T, Th, th, thor
thrill
thyrohyoid
thyroid hormone (thyroxine)
thyrotropic hormone (thyrotropin); also TTH
topical hypothermia
torcular herophili
total hysterectomy
tube holder
tyrosine hydroxylase

T&H type and hold

Th thenar
thigh
thigh amputation
thoracic; also T, TH, th, thor
thorax; also T, th, thor
thorium
throat

th thoracic; also T, TH, Th, thor
thorax; also T, Th, thor

THA tetrahydroaminoacridine (tacrine)
total hip arthroplasty
total hydroxyapatite

THA—cont'd
transient hemispheric attack
Treponema hemagglutination

ThA thoracic aorta

THAL thalamus

THAM tris(hydroxymethyl)aminomethane (tromethamine); also TRIS, Tris

THAN transient hyperammonemia of newborn

THARIES total hip arthroplasty with internal eccentric shells

THb total hemoglobin

THBP 7,8,9,10-tetrahydrobenzol[*a*]pyrene

THC tetrahydrocannabinol
tetrahydrocortisol; also TH
thiocarbanidin
transhepatic cholangiogram
transplantable hepatocellular carcinoma
Troisier-Hanot-Chauffard (syndrome)

Δ9THC delta-9-tetrahydrocannabinol

THCA trihydroxycoprostanoic acid

THCCRC tetrahydrocannabinol cross-reacting cannabinoids

TH-CULT throat culture; also TC

THD thioridazine
transverse heart diameter

Thd ribothymidine (thymidine); also T

THDOC tetrahydrodeoxycorticosterone

THE tetrahydrocortisone E
tonic hind limb extension
transhepatic embolization
tropical hypereosinophilia

theor theoretical
theory

ther therapeutic; also therap
therapy; also therap, Tx, T$_x$
thermometer; also therm

therap therapeutic; also ther
therapy; also ther, Tx, T$_x$

Ther Ex, ther ex therapeutic exercise

therm thermometer; also ther

THF tetrahydrocortisone F
tetrahydrofluorenone
tetrahydrofolate
tetrahydrofolic (acid)
tetrahydrofuran
thymic humoral factor

THFA tetrahydrofolic acid
tetrahydrofurfuryl alcohol

Thg thyroglobulin; also TG, Tg

THH telangiectasia hereditaria haemorrhagica

THI transient hypogammaglobulinemia of infancy
trihydroxyindole

THIO thioglycollate (broth); also TG

Thio-T triethylenethiophosphoramide; also TESPA, thiotepa, Thio-TEPA, thio-TEPA, TSPA, TTPA

thiotepa, Thio-TEPA, thio-TEPA triethylenethiophosphoramide; also TESPA, Thio-T, TSPA, TTPA

THIP tetrahydroisoxazolopyridinol

THIQ tetrahydroisoquinoline; also TIQ

THKAFO trunk-hip-knee-ankle-foot orthosis

THM total heme mass
trihalomethane

THO Thogoto orthomyxovirus
titrated water; also TH$_2$O

TH$_2$O titrated water; also THO

THOMAM trihydroxymethylaminomethane

THOR thoracentesis (fluid)

thor thoracic; also T, TH, Th, th
thorax; also T, Th, th

thou thousandth

THP take-home pack
tetrahydropapaveroline
tissue hydrostatic pressure
total hip replacement; also THR
total hydroxyproline
transhepatic portography
trihexyphenidyl

THPA tetrahydropteric acid

THPC tetra-bis(hydroxymethyl) phosphonium chloride

ThPP thiamine pyrophosphate; also TPP

tHPT tertiary hyperparathyroidism

THPV transhepatic portal vein

THQ tetroquinone

THR target heart rate
total hip replacement; also THP
training heart rate
transhepatic resistance

Thr threonine; also T

thr thyroid; also T
thyroidectomy; also TX

THR-CT thrombin control

THRF thyrotropic hormone-releasing factor

throm thrombosis; also thromb
thrombus; also T, thromb

thromb thrombosis; also throm
thrombus; also T, throm

THS tetrahydro-compound S
tetrahydrodeoxycortisol

THSC totipotent hematopoietic stem cell

THU tetrahydrouridine

THUG thyroid uptake gradient

THVO terminal hepatic vein obliteration

Thx thromboxane; also TBX, TX

Thy thymine; also T

thy thymectomy
thymus; also T
thymus (cell); also T

Thy-ALL acute lymphoblastic leukemia of
thymic phenotype

THz terahertz

TI inversion time
temporal integration
terminal ileum
thalassemia intermedia
therapeutic index
thoracic index
thymus independent
thyroxine iodine
threshold of intelligibility
tibia, complete (congenital absence of limb)
time information
time interval
tissue invasiveness
tonic immobility
total iron
translational inhibition
translational inhibitor
transverse diameter between ischia
transverse inlet
tricuspid incompetence
tricuspid insufficiency; also TCI
trunk index
tumor inducing
tumor induction

Ti titanium
tumor inducing (plasmid)

ti tibia, incomplete (congenital absence of
limb)

TIA transient ischemic attack
tumor-induced angiogenesis

TIAH totally implanted artificial heart

TIA-IR transient ischemic attack, incomplete
recovery

TIB total ischemic burden
tumor immunology bank

Tib, tib tibia

TIBC total iron-binding capacity

tib-fib tibia and fibula

TIBO tetrahydroimidazobenzodiazepinone

TIC ticarcillin
Toxicology Information Center
trypsin inhibitory capability
trypsin inhibitory capacity
tumor-inducing complex

tic diverticulum

TICCC time interval between cessation of contraception and conception

TID three times a day [L. *ter in die*]; also tdd,
tid
time interval difference
titrated initial dose

tid three times a day [L. *ter in die*]; also tdd,
TID

TIDA tuberoinfundibular dopamine
tuberoinfundibular dopaminergic (system)

TIE transient ischemic episode

TIF tumor-inducing factor
tumor-inhibiting factor

TIFB thrombin-increasing fibrinopeptide B

TIG, TIg tetanus immune globulin

TIH time interval histogram

TIL tumor-infiltrating lymphocyte

TIM transthoracic intracardiac monitoring
triose isomerase

TIMC tumor-induced marrow cytotoxicity

TIMI Thrombolysis in Myocardial Infarction
(study group)

TIMP tissue inhibitor of metalloproteinase

TIN three times a night [L. *ter in nocte*]; also
tin
tubulointerstitial nephropathy

tin three times a night [L. *ter in nocte*]; also
TIN

tinc tincture; also T, tinct, TR, Tr, tr

tinct tincture; also T, tinc, TR, Tr, tr

TIP thermal inactivation point
Toxicology Information Program
transient ischemic paroxysm
translation-inhibiting protein
tumor-inducing principle
tumor-inhibiting principle
tumor-insularis pancreatis

TIPPS tetraiodophenolphthalein sodium

TIQ tetrahydroisoquinoline; also THIQ

TIR terminal innervation ratio
total immunoreactive (insulin)

TIS tetracycline-induced steatosis
transdermal infusion system
trypsin-insoluble segment
tumor in situ

TISP total immunoreactive serum pepsinogen

TISS Therapeutic Intervention Scoring System

TIT *Treponema pallidum* immobilization test
triiodothyronine; also T_3, TITh, TRIT

TITh triiodothyronine; also T_3, TIT, TRIT

TIU trypsin-inhibiting unit

TIUP term intrauterine pregnancy

TIUV total intrauterine volume

TIV Tipula iridescent virus
trivalent inactivated influenza vaccine

TIVC thoracic inferior vena cava

TIW, tiw three times a week [L. *ter in* (three times a)]; also tiwk

tiwk three times a week [L. *ter in* (three times a)]; also TIW, tiw

TJ tendon jerk
terajoule
tight junction
triceps jerk
Troell-Junet (syndrome)

TJA total joint arthroplasty

TJN twin jet nebulizer

TJR total joint replacement

TK through the knee
thymidine kinase
tourniquet; also TQ, Tq
transketolase; also TRK
triose-kinase
Turner-Kieser (syndrome)

TKA total knee arthroplasty
transketolase activity

TKD thymidine kinase deficiency
tokodynamometer

TKE terminal knee extension

TKG tokodynagraph

TKLI tachykinin-like immunoreactivity

TKM thymidine kinase, mitochondrial
Tris/KCl/MgCl$_2$ (buffer)

TKNO to keep needle open

TKO to keep open (vein for IV)

TKP thermokeratoplasty

TKR total knee replacement

TKS thymidine kinase, soluble

TKVO to keep vein open

TL team leader
temporal lobe
terminal limen
theophylline; also T, TH
thermolabile
thermoluminescence
Thorndike-Lorge
threat to life
thymic lymphocyte
thymus-dependent lymphocyte; also TDL, T-L
thymus-derived lymphocyte
thymus leukemia (antigen)
thymus lymphoma
time lapse
time limited
tolerance level
total lipids
transverse line
trial leave
tubal ligation

T-L thymus-dependent lymphocyte; also TDL, TL

T/L terminal latency (electromyography)

Tl teraliter
thallium

TLA tissue lactase activity
translaryngeal aspiration
translumbar aortogram
transluminal angioplasty
trypsin-like amidase

TLAA T-lymphocyte-associated antigen

TLC tender loving care
thin-layer chromatography
total L-chain concentration
total lung capacity
total lung compliance
total lymphocyte count
triple-lumen catheter

^{201}TlCl radioactive thallium chloride

TLD thermoluminescent dosimeter
thermoluminescent dosimetry
thoracic lymphatic duct
transluminescent dosimeter
tumor lethal dose

T/LD$_{100}$ minimum lethal dose causing death or malformation of 100 percent of fetuses

TLE temporal lobe epilepsy
thin layer electrophoresis
total lipid extract

TLI thymidine labeling index
tonic labyrinthine inverted

total lymphoid irradiation
Totman's Loss Index
translaryngeal intubation
trypsin-like immunoactivity

TliSA1 T-lineage-specific activation antigen 1

TLMO truncated localized molecular orbital (method)

TLNB term living newborn

TLP transitional living program

TLQ total living quotient

TLR tonic labyrinthine reflex

TLS tumor lysis syndrome

TLSO thoracic lumbar sacral orthosis
thoracolumbar spinal orthosis
thoracolumbosacral spinal orthosis; also TLSSO

TLSSO thoracolumbosacral spinal orthosis; also TLSO

TLT tryptophan load test

TLV threshold limit value
total lung volume

TLW total lung water

TLX trophoblast-lymphocyte cross-reactivity

TM tectorial membrane
temperature by mouth
temporalis muscle
temporomandibular (joint)
teres major (muscle)
term milk
thalassemia major
Thayer-Martin (medium); also T-M
time and modifying
time-motion
tobramycin; also TOB
trabecular meshwork
trademark
Transcendental Meditation
transitional mucosa
transmediastinal
transmetatarsal
transport maximum; also Tm
transport mechanism
transport medium
transverse myelitis
trimester; also TRI
Tropical Medicine
tubular myelin
tumor; also T
tympanic membrane
tympanometric

TM trade mark

T&M type and cross-match; also TC, T&C, T&X, TXM

T-M Thayer-Martin (medium); also TM

Tm maximum tubular excretory capacity of the kidneys; also T_m
temperature, muscle
terameter
thulium
transport maximum; also TM
tumor-bearing mice

Tm² square terameter

Tm³ cubic terameter

T_m maximum tubular excretory capacity of the kidneys; also Tm
melting temperature
temperature midpoint (Kelvin)

tM time required to complete M phase of cell cycle

t_m, t_m temperature midpoint (Celsius)

TMA tetramethylammonium
thermomechanical analysis
thrombotic microangiopathy
thyroid microsomal antibody; also TMAb
trace mineral analysis
transmetatarsal amputation
trimethoxyamphetamine
trimethoxyphenyl aminopropane
trimethylamine
trimethylxanthine amphetamine

TMAb thyroid microsomal antibody; also TMA

TMAH trimethylphenylammonium hydroxide

TMAI trimethylphenylammonium iodide

TMAO trimethylamine oxide

TMAS Taylor Manifest Anxiety Scale

T-MAX time for maximum concentration; also T_{max}

T_{max} highest temperature
time of maximum concentration; also T-MAX

TMB tetramethyl benzidine
transient monocular blindness
trimethoxybenzoate
tris-maleate buffer

TMBA trimethoxybenzaldehyde
trimethylbenzanthracene

TMC transmural colitis
triamcinolone and terramycin capsule

TMCA trimethylcolchicinic acid

TMCS trimethylchlorosilane

TMD trimethadione; also TMO

TMDA tetramethyldiamine

TMDS, t-MDS therapy-related myelodysplasia

TME thermolysin-like metalleondopeptidase
total metabolizable energy
transmissible mink encephalopathy
transmural enteritis

TMET treadmill exercise test; also TET

TMF transformed mink fibroblast

TMG 3,3-tetramethyleneglutaric acid

TmG, TM$_G$, T$_{mg}$ maximal tubular reabsorption
of glucose

TMH tetramethylammonium hydroxide

TMI threatened myocardial infarction
transmandibular implant
transmural infarction

TMIC Toxic Materials Information Center

TMIF tumor-cell migration inhibition factor

TMIS Technicon Medical Information System

TMJ temporomandibular joint
temporomandibular joint (dysfunction)

TMJ-PDS temporomandibular joint–pain dysfunction syndrome

TMJS temporomandibular joint syndrome

TMK Tris/MgCl$_2$/KCl (buffer)

TML terminal motor latency
tetramethyl lead

TMM torn medial meniscus

Tmm McKay-Marg tension

TMNG toxic multinodular goiter

TMO trimethadione; also TMD

T-MOP thioguanine, methotrexate, Oncovin,
and prednisone

TMP thallium myocardial perfusion
thymidine monophosphate
thymine ribonucleoside-5′-phosphate
thymolphthalein
thymolphthalein monophosphate
transmembrane hydrostatic pressure
transmembrane potential
trimethoprim
trimethylpsoralen

T$_4$-MP T$_4$ by Murphy-Pattee

TM$_{PAH}$, T$_{mPAH}$ maximum tubular excretory
capacity of the kidneys for *para*-amino-
hippuric acid

TMPD tetramethyl-*para*-phenylenediamine

TMPDS temporomandibular pain and dysfunction syndrome

TMP-SMX trimethoprim-sulfamethoxazole;
also TMP-SMZ

TMP-SMZ trimethoprim-sulfamethoxazole;
also TMP-SMX

TMR tetramethylrhodamine
tissue maximal ratio
topical magnetic resonance
trainable mentally retarded

TMRI tetramethylrhodamine isothiocyanate;also TRMC

TMS tetramethylsilane
thallium myocardial scintigraphy
thread mate system
trimethylsilane
trimethylsilyl; also TMSi

TMSI trimethysilylimidazole

TMSi trimethylsilyl; also TMS

TMST treadmill stress test; also TST

TMT tarsometatarsal
Trail-Making Test (psychiatry)
treadmill test

TMTC too many to count

TMTD tetramethylthiuram disulfide (thiram)

TMTX trimetrexate

TMU tetramethylurea

TMV tobacco mosaic virus
tracheal mucous velocity

TMX tamoxifen; also T, TAM

TMZ temazepam
transformation zone

TN intraocular tension, normal; also Tn
talonavicular
team nursing
temperature normal
tiodazosin
total negatives
trigeminal nucleus
trochlear nucleus
true negative

T/N tar and nicotine

T&N tension and nervousness

T$_4$N normal serum thyroxine

Tn intraocular tension, normal; also TN
thoron
transposon

TNA total nutrient admixture

TNB term newborn
Tru-Cut needle biopsy

TNC turbid, no creamy (layer)

TNCA thionaphthenecarboxylic acid

TNCB trinitrochlorobenzene

TNCC trauma nursing core course

TND term normal delivery

TNEE titrated norepinephrine excretion

TNF trinitrofluorenone
true negative fraction
tumor necrosis factor

TNG toxic nodular goiter
trinitroglycerol (nitroglycerin)

Tng training; also trg, trng

tng tongue

TNH transient neonatal hyperammonemia

TNI total nodal irradiation

TNM thyroid node metastasis
tumor, node, metastasis (tumor staging)

TNMR tritium nuclear magnetic resonance

TNP total net positive
trinitrophenol

TNPM transient neonatal pustular melanosis

TNR tonic neck reflex
true negative rate

TNS total nuclear score
transcutaneous nerve stimulation; also TCNS
tumor necrosis serum

TNT triamcinolone and nystatin
2,4,6-trinitrotoluene

TNTC too numerous to count

TNV tobacco necrosis virus

TO no evidence of primary tumor
oral temperature; also T(O)
original tuberculin
target organ
telephone order
Theiler's Original (mouse encephalomyelitis
virus)
tincture of opium [L. *tinctura opii*]; also to
total obstruction
tracheoesophageal; also TE
transfer out
tubo-ovarian
turned on
turnover
Tyler's original (mice)

T(O) oral temperature; also TO

T&O tandem and ovoids
tubes and ovaries

TO₂ oxygen transport rate

to tincture of opium [L. *tinctura opii*]; also TO

TOA a tuberculin apparently corresponding to
Denys' bouillon filtré. [Ger. *Tuberculin
original alt*]
time of arrival
tubo-ovarian abscess

TOAP thioguanine, Oncovin, Ara-C (cytarabine), and prednisone

TOB tobramycin; also TM

TOBP tobramycin, peak

TobRV tobacco ringspot virus; also TRSV

TOBT tobramycin, trough

TOC test of cure
total organic carbon
tubo-ovarian complex

TOCE transcatheter oily chemoembolization

TOCO tocodynamometer

TOCP triorthocresyl phosphate

TOD tail on detector
tension of right eye [L. *oculus dexter* (right
eye)]
Time-Oriented Data (Bank)

TOE tracheo(o)esophageal

TOES toxic oil epidemic syndrome

TOF tetralogy of Fallot; also TF
time of flight (mass spectrometry)
total of four
tracheo(o)esophageal fistula

T of A transposition of the aorta

TOGV transposition of the great vessels; also
TGV

TOH throughout hospitalization
transient osteoporosis of hip

TOL trial of labor

tol tolerance
tolerated

tolb tolbutamide

TOM tomorrow
transcutaneous oxygen monitor; also TCOM

tomo tomogram
tomography

TON tonight; also tonoc

TONAR the oral-nasal acoustic ratio

tonoc tonight [to + L. *nocte* (night)]; also TON

TOP temporal, occipital, parietal
termination of pregnancy
tissue oncotic pressure

top topical; also T

TOPS Take Off Pounds Sensibly

TOPV trivalent oral polio vaccine

TORCH toxoplasmosis, rubella, cytomegalovirus, and herpes simplex (titer)

TORP total ossicular chain replacement prosthesis

torr Torecelli units (same as mm Hg)

TOS tension of left eye [L. *oculus sinister* (left eye)]
thoracic outlet syndrome

Tos tosyl (*p*-toluenesulfonyl); also Ts

TOT tincture of time
total operating time
transovarial transmission

TOTAL-C total cholesterol; also TC

TOTP triothotolyl phosphate

TOTPAR total pain relief

tot prot total protein; also TP, T PROT

TOV thrombosed oral varix
trial of void

TOWER testing, orientation, work, evaluation, rehabilitation

Tox toxicity; also T, tox

tox toxic
toxicity; also T, Tox
toxicology
toxoid

TOXGR toxic granulation (on differential)

TOXICON Toxicology Information Conversational On-Line Network

TOXLINE Toxicology Information On-Line

TOXO, Toxo toxoplasmosis

TP posterior tibial; also PT
tail pinch
target polynucleotide
temperature and pressure
temporal peak
temporoparietal
terminal phalanx
testosterone propionate
tetanus-pertussis
therapeutic pass
thiamphenicol
thickly padded
threshold potential
thrombocytopenic purpura
thrombophlebitis
thymic polypeptide
thymidine phosphorylase
thymus protein
tissue pressure
Todd's paralysis

toilet paper
total population
total positives
total protein; also Tot prot, T PROT
trailing pole
transforming principle
transition point; also T
transpyloric
transverse polarization
treating physician
treatment period
Treponema pallidum
triazolophthalazine
trigger point
trigonal prism (complexes)
triphosphate
true positive
tryptophan; also Tp, T_p, Trp, Try, Tryp, W
tryptophan pyrrolase
tube precipitin
tuberculin precipitation

TP5 thymopoietin pentapeptide

TP-6 trigonal prismatic

T&P temperature and pulse; also T+P
turn and position; also T+P

T+P temperature and pulse; also T&P
turn and position; also T&P

Tp tampon
tryptophan; also TP, T_p, Trp, Try, Tryp, W

T_p tryptophan; also TP, Tp, Trp, Try, Tryp, W

tp physical halflife(time)

TPA tannic acid, polyphosphomolybdic acid, and amido acid (staining technique)
12-*o*-tetradecanoylphorbol-13-acetate
thermal polarization analysis
thermoparticulate analysis
tissue plasminogen activator; also t-PA
tissue polypeptide antigen
total parenteral alimentation
total phobic anxiety
Treponema pallidum agglutination
tumor-derived polypeptide antigen

t-PA tissue plasminogen activator; also TPA

TPAG total protein and albumin to globulin ratio

TPAL term infants, premature infants, abortions, living children (obstetric history)

TPB tryptone phosphate broth

TPBF total pulmonary blood flow

TPBS three-phase (radionuclide) bone scanning

TPC telescoping plugged catheter
telopeptide-poor collagen
thromboplastic plasma component
time-to-pulse-height converter
total patient care
total plasma catecholamines
total plasma cholesterol
total proctocolectomy
treatment planning conference
Treponema pallidum complement
true partition coefficient

TPCC *Treponema pallidum* cryolysis complement fixation (test)

TPCF *Treponema pallidum* complement fixation (test)

TPCV total packed cell volume

TPD temporary partial disability
thiamine propyl disulfide
tropical pancreatic diabetes
tumor-producing dose

TPE therapeutic plasma exchange
total protective environment

TPEY tellurite polymyxin egg yolk (agar)

TPF thymus permeability factor
trained participating father
true positive fraction

TPG therapeutic play group
transmembrane potential gradient
transplacental gradient
tryptophan peptone glucose (broth)

TPGYT trypticase-peptone-glucose-yeast extract-trypsin (medium)

TPH thromboembolic pulmonary hypertension
trained participating husband
transplacental hemorrhage
tryptophan hydroxylase

TPHA *Treponema pallidum* hemagglutination (assay)

TPHOS triple phosphate (crystal)

TPI treponemal immobilization test (cardiolipin)
Treponema pallidum immobilization (test)
triose phosphate isomerase

TPIA *Treponema pallidum* immobilization immune adherence

TPL triphosphate of lime
tyrosine phenol-lyase

T plasty tympanoplasty

TPM temporary pacemaker
thrombophlebitis migrans
total particulate matter

total passive motion
triphenylmethane
trophopathia pedis myelodysplastica

TPMT thiopurine methyltransferase

TPN thalamic projection neuron
total parenteral nutrition
triphosphopyridine nucleotide (NADP)

TPN+ oxidized triphosphopyridine nucleotide (NADP+)

TPNH reduced triphosphopyridine nucleotide (NADPH)

TPO thrombopoietin
thyroid peroxidase
trial prescription order
tryptophan peroxidase

TPP tetraphenylporphyrin
thiamine pyrophosphate; also ThPP
transpulmonary pressure

TP&P time, place, and person

TPPase thiamine pyrophosphatase

TPPN total peripheral parenteral nutrition

TPPV trans pars plana vitrectomy

TPR temperature; also T, T°, *t*, TEMP, temp
temperature, pulse, and respiration
testosterone production rate
total peripheral resistance
total pulmonary resistance
true positive rate (probability)

TPRI total peripheral resistance index

T PROT total protein; also Tot prot, TP

TPS trypsin
tumor polysaccharide substance

TPS-7 trigonal prismatic square-faced monocapped

TPS-8 trigonal prismatic square-faced bicapped

TPS-9 trigonal prismatic square-faced tricapped

TPSE 2-(*p*-tritylphenyl)sulphonylethanol

TPST true positive stress test

TPT tetraphenyl tetrazolium
time to peak tension
total protein tuberculin
treadmill performance test
typhoid-paratyphoid (vaccine)

TPT-8 trigonal prismatic triangular-faced bicapped

TPTE 2-(*p*-tritylphenyl)thioethanol

TPTHS total parathyroid hormone secretion

TPTX thyroid-parathyroidectomy

TPTZ tripyridyltriazine

TPUR transperineal urethral resection

TPV tetanus-pertussis vaccine

TPVR total peripheral vascular resistance
total pulmonary vascular resistance

TQ Fagerstrom Tolerance Scale
time questionnaire
tocopherolquinone
tourniquet; also TK, Tq

Tq tourniquet; also TK, TQ

TR recovery time
rectal temperature; also T(R)
repetition time
residual tuberculin
tetrazolium reduction
therapeutic radiology
therapeutic recreation
timed release
tincture; also T, tinc, tinct, Tr, tr
to return
total repair
total resistance
total response; also R
trace; also T, Tr, tr
trachea; also trach
transfusion reaction
transplant recipient
treatment; also Tr, tr, treat, trt, TX, Tx T$_x$
tremor; also tr
tricuspid regurgitation
triradial
tuberculin R (new tuberculin) [Ger.
Tuberculin Rückstand]
tuberculin residue
tubular reabsorption
tumor registry
turbidity reducing
turnover rate

T(°R) absolute temperature on the Rankine
scale

T(R) rectal temperature; also TR

T&R tenderness and rebound

Tr tincture; also T, tinc, tinct, TR, tr
trace; also T, TR, tr
tragion
treatment; also TR, tr, treat, trt, TX, Tx, T$_x$

T$_r$ radiologic halflife(time)
retention time

tr tincture; also T, tinc, tinct, TR, Tr, tr
trace; also T, TR, Tr, tr
traction; also tract, TX, Tx, T$_x$, TXN, txt
treatment; also TR, Tr, treat, trt, TX, Tx, T$_x$

tremor; also TR

TRA therapeutic recreation associate
to run at
total renin activity
transaldolase; also TA
tumor-resistant antigen

tra transfer; also trf, TSR

TRAb thyrotrophin receptor antibody

trach trachea; also TR
tracheal
tracheostomy
tracheotomy

tract traction; also Tr, TX, Tx, T$_x$, TXN, txt

TRAJ timed repetitive ankle jerk

TRAM transverse rectus abdominis myocuta-
neous (breast reconstruction)
Treatment Rating Assessment Matrix
Treatment Response Assessment Method

TRAN transfusion

trans transference
transverse; also T

trans D transverse diameter; also TD

transm transmission
transmitted

transpl transplantation; also TX, Tx, T$_x$
transplanted; also TX

trans sect transverse section; also TS, T sect

transsex transsexual; also TS

TRAP tartrate-resistant leukocyte acid
phosphatase
thioguanine, rubidomycin, Ara-C, and
prednisone

TRAS transplant renal artery stenosis

trau trauma; also traum
traumatic; also traum

traum trauma; also trau
traumatic; also trau

TRB terbutaline; also Terb

TRBF total renal blood flow

TRC tanned red cell(s)
total renin concentration
total respiratory conductance
total ridge count

TRCA tanned red cell agglutination

TRCH tanned red cell hemagglutination

TRCHI tanned red cell hemagglutination
inhibition

TRCV total red cell volume

TRD tongue-retaining device
traction retinal detachment

TRE thymic reticuloepithelial
true radiation emission

TREA thoroughness, reliability, efficiency, analytic (ability)
triethanolamine; also TEA

treat treatment; also TR, Tr, tr, trt, TX, Tx, T$_x$

TREELS Time-resolved electron energy loss spectroscopy

TREES Time-resolved europium III excitation spectroscopy

Tren Trendelenburg (position); also TREND, TRND

TREND Trendelenburg (position); also Tren, TRND

TRF T-cell replacing factor
thyrotropin-releasing factor

trf transfer; also tra, TSR

TRFC total rosette-forming cell

TRG T-cell-rearranging gene

trg training; also Tng, trng

trng training; also Tng, trg

TRGI triglycerides incalculable

TRH tension-reducing hypothesis
thyroid-releasing hormone
thyroid-stimulating hormone-releasing hormone
thyrotropin-releasing hormone

TRH-ST thyrotropin-releasing hormone stimulation test

TRI tetrazolium reduction inhibition
Thyroid Research Institute
total response index
trifocal
trimester; also TM
tubuloreticular inclusion

tri tricentric

T$_3$RIA, T$_3$(RIA) triiodothyronine radio-immunoassay

T$_4$RIA, T$_4$(RIA) tetraiodothyronine (thyroxine) radioimmunoassay

TRIAC, Triac triiodothyroacetic acid

TRIC trachoma and inclusion conjunctivitis (group of organisms)

TRICB trichlorobiphenyl

TRICH, Trich trichinosis
Trichomonas

Trid, trid three days [L. *triduum*]

TRIG, Trig, trig triglyceride; also TG, TGL

TRIMIS Tri-Service Medical Information System

TRIS, Tris 2-amino-2-hydroxymethyl-propane-1,3-diol
tris (hydroxymethyl) aminomethane (tromethamine); also THAM

TRISS Trauma and Injury Severity Score

TRIT triiodothyronine; also T$_3$, TIT, TITh

Trit, trit triturate

TRITC tetrarhodamine isothiocyanate

TRK transketolase; also TK

TRMC tetramethylrhodamino isothiocyanate; also TMRI

TRML, Trml terminal; also t, ter, term

TRMS time-resolved mass spectrometry

tRNA transfer ribonucleic acid

TRND Trendelenburg (position); also Tren, TREND

TRNG tetracycline-resistant *Neisseria gonorrhoeae*

TRO tissue reflectance oximeter
to return to office

TROCA tangible reinforcement operant conditioning audiometry

TROCH, Troch lozenge [L. *trochiscus* (troche)]

Trop tropical

TRP Tactical Reproduction Pegboard
total refractory period
trichorhinophalangeal (syndrome)
tubular reabsorption of phosphorus

Trp tryptophan; also TP, Tp, T$_p$, Try, Tryp, W

TRPA tryptophan-rich prealbumin

TrPl treatment plan

TRPS trichorhinophalangeal syndrome

TRPT theoretical renal phosphorus threshold

TRR total respiratory resistance

TRS Therapeutic Recreation Specialist
total reducing sugars
tuberculosis record system
tubuloreticular structure

TrS traumatic surgery

TRSV tobacco ringspot virus; also TobRV

TRT thermoradiotherapy
total reading time

Trt Trityl (triphenylmethyl)

trt treatment; also TR, Tr, tr, treat, TX, Tx, T$_x$

TRU turbidimetry unit
turbidity-reducing unit

T₃RU triiodothyronine resin uptake (test)

TRUS transrectal ultrasound

TRUSP transrectal ultrasound of prostate

TRV tobacco rattle virus
Tupaia retrovirus

Try tryptophan (obsolete abbreviation, preferred: Trp); also TP, Tp, T_p, Trp, Tryp, W

Tryp tryptophan; also TP, Tp, T_p, Trp, Try, W

TRZ tartrazine
triazolam; also TZ

TS Tay-Sachs (disease)
temperature sensitive; also ts
temporal stem
terminal sensation
testosterone sulfate
test solution
thermostable
thiosporin
thoracic surgery
tissue space
tocopherol supplemented
toe sign
total solids (in urine)
Tourette's syndrome
toxic substance
toxic syndrome
tracheal sound
tracheal spiral
transitional sleep
transsexual; also transsex
transverse section; also trans sect, T sect
transverse sinus
Trauma Score
treadmill score
trichostasis spinulosa
tricuspid stenosis
triple strength
tropical sprue
trypticase soy (agar)
T suppressor (cell); also Ts
tuberous sclerosis
tubular sound
tumor specific
Turner's syndrome
type specific

T+S type and screen; also T&S

T/S thyroid to serum (iodide ratio)

T&S type and screen; also T+S

Ts skin temperature
tension by Schiøtz's tonometer
tosyl (*p*-toluenesulfonyl); also Tos
tosylate

T suppressor (cell); also TS

tS time required to complete S phase of cell cycle

ts teaspoon; also t, tsp
temperature sensitive; also TS

TSA technical surgical assistance
Test of Syntactic Ability
tissue-specific antigens
toluenesulfonic acid
Total Severity Assessment
total shoulder arthroplasty
total solute absorption
toxic shock antigen
trypticase-soy agar
tumor-specific antigen
tumor surface antigen
tumor susceptible antigen
type-specific antibody

T₄SA thyroxine-specific activity

TSAb thyroid-stimulating antibody

TSAP toxic shock-associated protein

Tsaph temperature in saphenous vein

TSAS total severity assessment score

TSAT tube slide agglutination test

TSB total serum bilirubin
trypticase soy broth
tryptone soy broth

TSBA total serum bile acids

TSBB transtracheal selective bronchial brushing

TSBC Time-Sample Behavioral Checklist

TSC technetium sulfur colloid
theophylline serum concentration
thiosemicarbazide
total static compliance
transverse spinal sclerosis

TSCA Toxic Substance Control Act

TSCS Tennessee Self-Concept Scale

TSD target to skin distance
Tay-Sachs disease
theory of signal detectability
transfer summary dictated

TSE testicular self-examination
total skin examination
trisodium edetate

TSEB total skin electron beam

T sect transverse section; also trans sect, TS

TSEM transmission scanning electron microscopy

T set tracheotomy set

TSF testicular feminization (syndrome); also Tfm
thrombopoiesis-stimulating factor
tissue-coding factor; also TCF
total systemic flow
triceps skinfold
T-suppressor factor

TSG Touraine-Solente-Golé (syndrome)
tumor-specific glycoprotein; also TSG(P)

TSG(P) tumor-specific glycoprotein; also TSG

TSH thyroid-stimulating hormone (thyrotropin)

TSH-RF thyroid-stimulating hormone-releasing factor

TSH-RH thyroid-stimulating hormone-releasing hormone

TSI thyroid-stimulating immunoglobulin; also TSIg
triple sugar iron (agar); also TSIA

TSIA total small intestinal allotransplantation
triple sugar iron agar; also TSI

TSIg thyroid-stimulating immunoglobulin; also TSI

TSL terminal sensory latency

TSM type-specific M protein

TSN tryptophan peptone sulfide neomycin (agar)

TSP thrombin-sensitive protein
total serum protein
total suspended particulate
tribasic sodium phosphate
trisodium phosphate
tropical spastic paraparesis

tsp teaspoon; also t, ts

TSPA triethylenethiophosphoramide; also TESPA, Thio-T, thiotepa, Thio-TEPA, thio-TEPA, TTPA

TSPAP total serum prostatic acid phosphatase

T-spica thumb spica (bandage)

T-spine, T/spine thoracic spine

TSPP tetrasodium pyrophosphate

TSR testosterone-sterilized (female) rat
theophylline-sustained release
thyroid to serum ratio
total shoulder replacement
total systemic resistance
transfer; also tra, trf
transient situational reaction

TSRBC trypsinized sheep red blood cell

TSS toxic shock syndrome

transcription start signal
tropical splenomegaly syndrome

TSSA tumor-specific cell surface antigen

TSSE toxic shock syndrome exoprotein
toxic shock syndrome exotoxin

TSSNM Technologists Section of the Society of Nuclear Medicine

TSST toxic shock syndrome toxin

TSSU (operating) theater sterile supply unit

TST tail suspension test
temporal scaling test
thromboplastin screening test
total sleep time
transcrotal testosterone
transition state theory
treadmill stress test; also TMST
tumor skin test

TSTA toxoplasmin skin test antigen
tumor-specific tissue antigen
tumor-specific transplantation antigen

TSU triple sugar urea (agar)

TSV total stomach volume

TSY trypticase soy yeast

TT tablet triturate
tactile tension
talking task
terminal transferase
tetanus toxin
tetanus toxoid; also tet tox
tetrathionate (broth)
tetrazol
thrombin time
thymol turbidity
tibial tubercle
tibial tuberosity
tilt table
tine test
token test
tooth treatment
total thyroxine; also TT-4, TT_4
total time
transferred to
transient tachypnea
transit time
transthoracic
transtracheal
tuberculin test
tuberculin tested
tube thoracostomy
tumor thrombus
turnover time
tyrosine transaminase

TT-3, TT$_3$ total triiodothyronine

TT-4, TT$_4$ total thyroxine; also TT

T/T trace of/trace of (different substances on tests)

T&T time and temperature
tobramycin and ticarcillin
touch and tone

TTA tetanus toxoid antibody
tetracyclic antidepressants; also TCA
timed therapeutic absence
total toe arthroplasty
transtracheal aspiration

TTAP threaded titanium acetabular prosthesis

TTBV total trabecular bone volume

TTC triphenyltetrazolium chloride (test)

TTD temporary total disability
tetraethylthiuram disulfide
tissue tolerance dose
total temporary disability
transient tic disorder
transverse thoracic diameter

TTFD thiamine tetrahydrofurfuryl disulfide

TTG tellurite, taurocholate, gelatin

TTGA tellurite, taurocholate, and gelatin agar

TTH thyrotropic hormone (thyrotropin); also TH
tritiated thymidine

TTI tension-time index
time-tension index
tissue thromboplastin inhibition (test)
transtracheal insufflation

TTIB tension-time index per beat

TTL training and test lung
transistor-transistor logic

TTLC true total lung capacity

TTM transtelephonic (electrocardiographic) monitoring

TTN transient tachypnea of newborn; also TTNB

TTNA transthoracic needle aspiration

TTNB transient tachypnea of newborn; also TTN
transthoracic needle aspiration biopsy

TTO to take out
transtracheal oxygen

TTOD tetanus toxoid outdated

TTOT transtracheal oxygen therapy

TTP Testicular Tumour Panel
thrombotic thrombocytopenic purpura

thymidine triphosphate
time to peak

TTPA triethylenethiophosphoramide; also TESPA, Thio-T, thiotepa, Thio-TEPA, thio-TEPA, TSPA

TTP-HUS thrombotic thrombocytopenic purpura–hemolytic uremic syndrome

TTR transthoracic resistance
triceps tendon reflex
type to token ratio

TTS tarsal tunnel syndrome
temporary threshold shift
through the skin
transdermal therapeutic system

TTT thymol turbidity test
tolbutamide tolerance test
total twitch time

TTTT test tube turbidity test

TTUTD tetanus toxoid up to date

TTV tracheal transport velocity
transfusion transmitted virus

TTVP temporary transvenous pacemaker

TTWB touch-toe weight-bearing

TTX tetrodotoxin; also TD

TU thiouracil
thiourea
thyroidal uptake
Todd unit(s)
toxic unit
toxoid unit
transmission unit
transurethral
tuberculin unit
turbidity unit

T$_3$U triiodothyronine uptake (test); also T$_3$UP

TUB tubouterine (junction)

tuberc tuberculosis; also T, TB, Tb, tb, TBC, Tbc, tbc
tuberculous; also T, TB, Tb, tb, TBC, Tbc, tbc

TUD total urethral discharge

TUDC tauroursodeoxycholate

TUDCA tauroursodeoxycholic acid

TUF total ultrafiltration

TUG total urinary gonadotropin

TUI transurethral incision

TUN total urinary nitrogen

T$_3$UP triiodothyronine uptake (test); also T$_3$U

TUPR transurethral prostatic resection

TUR transurethral resection

T₃UR triiodothyronine uptake ratio

TURB transurethral resection of bladder (tumor)

turb turbid
turbidity

TURBN transurethral resection of bladder neck

TURBT transurethral resection of bladder tumor

TURP transurethral prostatectomy
transurethral resection of prostate

TURV transurethral resection of valves

tus cough [L. *tussis*]

TUU transureteroureterostomy

TV talipes varus
temporary visit
tetrazolium violet
thoracic vertebra
tick-borne virus
tidal volume
total volume
toxic vertigo
transfer vesicle
transvenous
trial visit
Trichomonas vaginalis
Trichomonas vaginitis
tricuspid valve
trivalent
true vertebra
truncal vagotomy
tuberculin volutin
tubulovesicular

T/V touch/verbal

TVA truncal vagotomy plus antrectomy

TVC third-ventricle cyst
timed ventilatory capacity
timed vital capacity
total viable cells
total volume capacity
transvaginal cone
triple voiding cystogram
true vocal cord

TVD transmissible virus dementia
triple vessel disease

TVDALV triple vessel disease with abnormal left ventricle

TVF tactile vocal fremitus

TVG time-varied gain (control)

TVH total vaginal hysterectomy
turkey virus hepatitis

TVL tenth value layer (radiation)

TVP tensor veli palatini
textured vegetable protein
transvenous pacemaker
transvesicle prostatectomy
tricuspid valve prolapse
truncal vagotomy plus pyloroplasty

TVR total vascular resistance
total vibration reflex
tricuspid valve replacement

TVSC transvaginal sector scan

TVT transmissible venereal tumor
tunica vaginalis testis

TVU total volume of urine

TVUS transvaginal ultrasound

TW tap water
terminal web
test weight
Thibierge-Weissenbach (syndrome)
thymic weight
total body water; also TBW, TBWA

TWA time-weighted average

Twb wet bulb temperature

TWBC total white blood cells

TWD total white and differential (cell count)

TWE tap water enema
tepid water enema

TWETC tap water enema 'til clear

TWG total weight gain

TWHW toe walking and heel walking

TWIS treatment of emergent symptoms
write-in scale

TWiST time without symptoms of toxicity

TWL transepidermal water loss; also TEWL

TWN twin

TWR total wrist replacement

TWWD tap water wet dressing

TWZ triangular working zone

TX derivative of contagious tuberculin
thromboxane; also TBX, Thx
thyroidectomized
thyroidectomy; also thr
traction; also tr, tract, Tx, T$_x$, TXN, txt
transplant; also Tx, T$_x$, Txn
transplantation; also transpl, Tx, T$_x$
transplanted; also transpl
treatment; also TR, Tr, tr, treat, trt, Tx, T$_x$

T&X type and cross-match; also TC, T&C, T&M, TXM

Tx, T$_x$ therapy; also ther, therap
traction; also tr, tract, TX, TXN, txt
transfuse
transplant; also TX, Txn
transplantation; also transpl, TX
treatment; also TR, Tr, tr, treat, trt, TX
tympanostomy; also Tymp

TXA, TxA thromboxane A

TXA2, TXA$_2$ thromboxane A$_2$

TXB2, TXB$_2$ thromboxane B$_2$

TXM T-cell cross-match
type and cross-match; also TC, T&C, T&M,
T&X

TXN traction; also tr, tract, TX, Tx, T$_x$, txt

Txn transplant; also TX, Tx, T$_x$

txt traction; also tr, tract, TX, Tx, T$_x$, TXN

Ty thyroxine
type; also T
typhoid
tyrosine; also Tyr, Y

TYCO Tylenol with codeine

Tyl Tylenol
tyloma [Gr. tylōma (a callus)]

TYMP tympanogram

Tymp tympanic
tympanicity (auscultation of chest)
tympanium
tympanostomy; also Tx, T$_x$

TYMV turnip yellow mosaic virus

ty-neg tyrosinase-negative (oculocutaneous
albinism)

typ typical

TYR tyramine
tyrode

Tyr tyrosine; also Ty, Y

TyRIA thyroid radioimmunoassay

TZ transition zone
triazolam; also TRZ
zymoplastic tuberculin [Ger. *Tuberculin
zymoplastiche*]

U internal energy
International Unit (of enzyme activity)
kilurane (radioactivity unit)
Mann-Whitney rank sum statistic; also *U*
potential difference (in volts)
ulna; also uln
ulna, complete (congenital absence of limb)
ultralente (insulin)
uncertain
unerupted
unit
unknown; also *U*, UK, UNK, unk, unkn
upper
uracil; also URA, Ura
uranium
urethra; also UA, ureth
uridine; also Urd
uridylic acid; also UA
urinary (concentration)
urine; also UR, Ur, ur
urologist; also Urol
urology; also UR, URO, Urol
uvula
wave on electrocardiogram

U Mann-Whitney rank sum statistic; also U
unknown; also U, UK, UNK, unk, unkn

U100 100 units per millimeter

U/1 one fingerbreadth below umbilicus

1/U one fingerbreadth above umbilicus

U/3 upper third (of long bone)

u atomic mass unit
to be used [L. *utendus*]; also utend
ulna, incomplete (congenital absence of limb)
unified atomic mass unit

235U uranium 235, radioactive uranium;
halflife, 7.1 x 10^8 years

UA Ulex agglutinin
ultra-audible (sound)
ultrasonic arteriogram
umbilical artery
unaggregated
unauthorized absence
uncertain about
unit of analysis
unrelated children raised apart
unstable angina
upper airway
upper arm
urethra; also U, ureth

uric acid; also U/A, URC-A
uridylic acid; also U
urinalysis; also U/A, ur anal
urinary aldosterone
urine aliquot
urine analysis; also ur anal
urocanic acid
uronic acid
uterine aspiration

U/A uric acid; also UA, URC-A
urinalysis; also UA, ur anal
uterine activity

ua as far as, up to [L. *usque ad* (as far as)]

UAC umbilical artery catheter
underactive
upper airway congestion

UA/C uric acid to creatinine (ratio)

UAD upper airway disease

UAE unilateral absence of excretion

UAG uracil-adenine-guanine

UAI uterine activity integral

UAL up (out of bed) [up + L. *ad libidinem*
(as desired)]; also up ad lib
umbilical artery line

UA&M urinalysis and microscopy

U-AMY urinary amylase

UAN uric acid nitrogen

UAO upper airway obstruction

UAP unstable angina pectoris; also USAP

UAPF upon arrival patient found

UAR upper airway resistance

UAS upper abdominal surgery

UASA upper airway sleep apnea

UAT up (out of bed) as tolerated

UAU uterine activity unit

UAVC univentricular atrioventricular connection

UB ultimobranchial body
Unna's boot
urinary bladder

UBA undenatured bacterial antigen
universal beer agar

UBBC unsaturated vitamin B$_{12}$-binding
capacity

UBC University of British Columbia (brace)
unsaturated binding capacity

UBF unknown black female
uterine blood flow

UBG ultimobranchial gland(s)
urobilinogen; also UROB, UROBIL

UBI ultraviolet blood irradiation

UBIP ubiquitous immunopoietic polypeptide

UBL undifferentiated B-cell lymphoma

UBM unknown black male

UBO unidentified bright object

UBP ureteral back pressure

UBW usual body weight

UC ulcerative colitis
Uldall catheter
ultracentrifugal
umbilical cholesterol
umbilical cord
unchanged
unclassifiable
unconscious; also UCS, Ucs, ucs
unfixed cryostat
unit clerk
unit coordinator
unsatisfactory condition
untreated cell
urea clearance; also UCL
urethral catheterization
urinary catheter
urine concentrate
urine culture; also U/C, UCX
usual care
uterine contraction(s)

U/C urine culture; also UC, UCX

U&C urethral and cervical (cultures)
usual and customary

U$_{Ca}$V urinary calcium volume (excretion rate)

UCB unconjugated bilirubin; also UCBR

UCBC umbilical cord blood culture

UCBR unconjugated bilirubin; also UCB

UCC urgent care center

UCD urine collection device
usual childhood diseases; also UCHD

UCE urea cycle enzymopathy

UCG ultrasonic cardiogram
ultrasonic cardiography
urinary chorionic gonadotropin

UCHD usual childhood diseases; also UCD

UCHI usual childhood illnesses; also UCI

UCHS uncontrolled hemorrhagic shock

UCI urethral catheter in

urinary catheter in
usual childhood illnesses; also UCHI

UCL ulna collateral ligament
uncomfortable listening level
uncomfortable loudness level; also ULL
upper confidence limit
urea clearance; also UC

UCLA University of California at Los Angeles

UCLP unilateral cleft of lip and palate

UCO urethral catheter out
urinary catheter out

UCP urethral closure pressure
urinary coproporphyrin
urinary C-peptide

UCPP urethral closure pressure profile

UCPT urinary coproporphyrin test

UCR unconditioned reflex; also uncond ref,
UR
unconditioned response; also UR
usual, customary, and reasonable (fees)

UCRE urine creatinine

UCRP Universal Control Reference Plasma

UCS unconditioned stimulus; also UnCS,
unCS, UnS, US
unconscious; also UC, Ucs, ucs

Ucs, ucs unconscious; also UC, UCS

UCT unchanged conventional treatment

UCTD unclassifiable connective tissue disease
undifferentiated connective tissue disease

UCU urinary care unit

UCV ulcus cruris varicosum
uncontrolled variable

UCX urine culture; also UC, U/C

UD ulcerative dermatosis
ulcerogenic dose
ulnar deviation
underdeveloped
undesirable discharge
unipolar depression
unit dose
urethral discharge
uridine diphosphate; also UDP
uroporphyrinogen decarboxylase; also UROD
uterine distention
uterus delivery

ud as directed [L. *ut dictum*]; also ut dict

UDC ursodeoxycholate
usual diseases of childhood

UDCA ursodeoxycholic acid; also URSO

UDE undetermined etiology; also UE

UDN updraft nebulizer

UDO undetermined origin; also UO

UDP uridine diphosphate; also UD

UDPG uridine diphosphoglucose; also UDPGlc, UDP-glucose

UDPGA uridine diphosphoglucuronic acid; also UDP-GlcUA

UDPGal uridine diphosphogalactose; also UDP-galactose

UDP-galactose uridine diphosphogalactose; also UDPGal

UDPGlc uridine diphosphoglucose; also UDPG, UDP-glucose

UDP-GlcUA uridine diphosphoglucuronic acid; also UDPGA

UDP-glucose uridine diphosphoglucose; also UDPG, UDPGlc

UDP-glucuronate uridine diphosphoglucuronate

UDPGT uridine diphosphoglucyronyl transferase

UdR uracil deoxyriboside (deoxyuridine)

UDRP uridine diribose phosphate

UDS ultra-Doppler sonography
unscheduled deoxynucleic acid synthesis
unscheduled deoxyribonucleic acid synthesis

UDV under direct vision

UE uncertain etiology
under elbow
undetermined etiology; also UDE
uninvolved epidermis
upper esophagus
upper extremity; also U/E, u/ext

U/E upper extremity; also UE, u/ext

UEA upper extremity arterial

UEG unifocal eosinophilic granuloma

UEM universal electron microscope

UEMC unidentified endosteal marrow cell

UER unaided equalization reference

UES upper esophageal sphincter

UESP upper esophageal sphincter pressure

u/ext upper extremity; also UE, U/E

UF Ullrich-Feichtiger (syndrome)
ultrafilterable
ultrafiltrate
ultrafiltration
ultrafine
ultrasonic frequency
unflexed

universal feeder
unknown factor
until finished
urea formaldehyde

UFA unesterified fatty acids

UFC urinary free cortisol

UFD ultrasonic flow detector

UFE uniform food encoding

UFF unusual facial features

UFFI urea formaldehyde foam insulation

UFN until further notice

UFO unflagged order
unidentified foreign object

UFR ultrafiltration rate
urine filtration rate
uroflowmetry

uFSH urinary follicle-stimulating hormone

UFV unclassified fecal virus

UG until gone
urinary glucose
urogastrone
urogenital; also URO-GEN
uteroglobulin

UGA under general anesthesia

UGD urogenital diaphragm

UGDP University Group Diabetes Project

UGF unidentified growth factor

UGH unstable-type glycated hemoglobin
uveitis-glaucoma-hyphema (syndrome)

UGH+ uveitis-glaucoma-hyphema plus (vitreous hemorrhage, syndrome)

UGI upper gastrointestinal

UGIH upper gastrointestinal hemorrhage

UGIS upper gastrointestinal series

UGIT upper gastrointestinal tract

UGK urine glucose ketone

UGPP uridyl diphosphate glucose pryophosphorylase

UGS urogenital sinus

UH umbilical hernia
University Hospital
upper half

UHBI upper hemibody irradiation

UHC ultrahigh carbon

UHD unstable hemoglobin disease

UHDDS Uniform Hospital Discharge Data Set

UHF ultrahigh frequency
unrestricted Hartree-Fock

UHL universal hypertrichosis lanuginosa

UHMW ultrahigh molecular weight

UHR underlying heart rhythm

UHRC ulcerohemorrhagic rectocolitis

UHSC university health services clinic

UHT ultrahigh temperature

UHV ultrahigh vacuum
ultrahigh voltage

UI Ulcer Index
urinary incontinence
uroporphyrin isomerase

U/I unidentified; also UNID

UIBC unbound iron-binding capacity
unsaturated iron-binding capacity

UICC International Union Against Cancer
(Geneva, Switzerland) [Union International
Contre le Cancer]

UID once daily [L. *uno in die*]

UIF undegraded insulin factor

UIP usual interstitial pneumonia
usual interstitial pneumonitis

UIQ upper inner quadrant

UIS Utilization Information Service

UJT unijunction transistor

UK United Kingdom
unknown; also U, *U*, UNK, unk, unkn
urinary kallikrein; also UKa
urine potassium [L. *kalium* (potassium)]
urokinase

UKA unicompartmental knee arthroplasty

UKa urinary kallikrein; also UK

U$_k$V urinary potassium volume (excretion rate)
[L. *kalium* (potassium)]

UL unauthorized leave
Underwriters' Laboratories
undifferentiated lymphoma
upper limb
upper limit
upper lobe
utterance length

U&L upper and lower; also U/L

U/L units per liter; also U/l
upper and lower; also U&L

U/l units per liter; also U/L

ULA undedicated logic array

ULBW ultralow birth weight

ULL uncomfortable loudness level; also UCL

ULLE upper lid, left eye

ULN upper limits of normal; also U:N

uln ulna; also U
ulnar

ULPE upper lobe pulmonary edema

ULQ upper left quadrant

ULRE upper lid, right eye

ULT ultralow temperature

ult last [L. *ultimus*]
ultimate
ultimately

ult praes last prescribed [L. *ultimum praescriptum*]

ULV ultralow volume

ULYTES urine electrolytes

UM unmarried
upper motor (neuron)
uracil mustard
Utilization Management

UMA urinary muramidase activity

Umax maximal urinary osmolality

UMB umbilical; also umb
umbilicus; also umb

Umb umbelliferyl

umb umbilical; also UMB
umbilicus; also UMB

UMC unidimensional chromatography

U$_{Mg}$V urinary magnesium volume (excretion rate)

UMLS Unified Medical Language System

UMN upper motor neuron

UMNB upper motor neurogenic bladder

UMNL upper motor neuron lesion

UMP uridine 5′-monophosphate (uridylic acid)

UMPK uridine monophosphate kinase

UMS urethral manipulation syndrome

UMT unit of medical time

UN ulnar nerve
undernourished
unilateral neglect
urea nitrogen
urinary nitrogen

U:N upper limits of normal; also ULN

UNA urinary nitrogen appearance

UNa urinary sodium [L. *natrium* (sodium)]

U$_{Na}$ urinary concentration of sodium
[L. *natrium* (sodium)]

uncomp uncompensated

uncond unconditioned

uncond ref unconditioned reflex; also UCR, UR

uncor uncorrected; also uncorr

uncorr uncorrected; also uncor

UnCS, unCS unconditioned stimulus; also
UCS, UnS, US

unct smeared [L. *unctus*]

UNCV ulnar nerve conduction velocity

undet undetermined

UNE urinary norepinephrine

UNESCO United Nations Educational,
Scientific and Cultural Organization

Ung, ung ointment [L. *unguentum*]; also ungt

ungt ointment [L. *unguentum*]; also Ung, ung

U$_{NH4}^+$ urinary ammonium

UNICEF United Nations International
Children's Emergency Fund (now: United
Nations Children's Fund)

UNID unidentified; also U/I

unilat unilateral

univ universal
university

UNK, unk unknown; also U, *U*, UK, unkn

unkn unknown; also U, *U*, UK, UNK, unk

UNL upper normal limit

UNOS United Network of Organ Sharing

UNRRA United Nations Relief and
Rehabilitation Administration (defunct)

UNS, uns unsatisfactory; also unsat
unsymmetrical; also *uns-*, unsym, *unsym-*

UnS unconditioned stimulus; also UCS, UnCS,
unCS, US

uns- unsymmetrical; also UNS, uns, unsym,
unsym-

unsat unsatisfactory; also UNS, uns
unsaturated

unsym, *unsym-* unsymmetrical; also UNS,
uns, *uns-*

UNTS unilateral nevoid telangiectasia syndrome

UO under observation; also U/O, u/o
undetermined origin; also UDO
ureteral orifice
urinary output; also UOP

U/O, u/o under observation; also UO

UOP urinary output; also UO

UOQ upper outer quadrant

UOS units of service

UOsm, Uosm urinary osmolality

UOV unit of variance

UOZ upper outer zone (quadrant)

UP ulcerative proctitis
ultrahigh purity
unipolar
Unna-Pappenheim (stain)
upright posture
uretero-pelvic
uridine phosphorylase
uroporphyrin; also URO
uteroplacental

U/P urine to plasma (ratio)

up ad lib up (out of bed) [up + L. *ad libidinem*
(as desired)]; also UAL

UPC Universal Product Code
usual provider continuity

UPD urinary production (rate)

UPEP urine protein electrophoresis

UPF universal proximal femur (prosthesis)

UPG uroporphyrinogen; also URO

UPI uteroplacental insufficiency
uteroplacental ischemia

UPJ ureteropelvic junction

UPK uninvolved psoriatic keratinocyte

UPL unusual position of limbs

UPN unique patient number

UPOR usual place of residence

UPP urethral pressure profile
urethral pressure profilometry
uvulopalatoplasty

UPPP uvulopalatopharyngoplasty

UPPRA upright peripheral plasma renin
activity

UPS ultraviolet photoelectron spectroscopy
uninterruptible power supply
uroporphyrinogen synthase
uterine progesterone system

UPT uptake
urine pregnancy test

UQ ubiquinone
upper quadrant

UR unconditioned reflex; also UCR,
uncond ref
unconditioned response; also UCR
unrelated; also url
upper respiratory
urinal

UR—cont'd
urine; also U, Ur, ur
urology; also U, URO, Urol
utilization review

Ur, ur urinary
urine; also U, UR

URA upper respiratory allergy
uracil; also U, Ura

Ura uracil; also U, URA

ur anal urinalysis; also UA, U/A
urine analysis; also UA

URC upper rib cage
utilization review committee

URC-A uric acid; also UA, U/A

URC SP uric acid urine spot (test)

URD undifferentiated respiratory disease
unilateral renal disease
upper respiratory disease

Urd uridine; also U

UREA-S urea nitrogen urine spot (test)

URED unable to read (lab result)

ureth urethra; also U, UA

URF unidentified reading frame
uterine-relaxing factor

UR-FST urine-fasting

urg urgent

UR HR urine–number of hours for glucose tolerance

URI upper respiratory illness
upper respiratory infection

URIN random urine

URIS upper respiratory infections

url unrelated; also UR

UR&M urinalysis, routine and microscopic

URO urology; also U, UR, Urol
uroporphyrin; also UP
uroporphyrinogen; also UPG

UROB urobilinogen; also UBG, UROBIL

UROBIL urobilinogen; also UBG, UROB

UROD uroporphyrinogen decarboxylase; also UD

URO-GEN urogenital; also UG

URO-2H urobilinogen–2 hours

Urol urologist; also U
urology; also U, UR, URO

UROS uroporphyrinogen synthetase

URQ upper right quadrant

URS ultrasonic renal scanning

URSO ursodeoxycholic acid; also UDCA

URT upper respiratory tract

URTI upper respiratory tract illness
upper respiratory tract infection

UR-TIM urine-time

URVD unilateral renovascular disease

UR VOL urine volume

US ultrasonic
ultrasonography; also USG
ultrasound; also U/S, UTS, UTZ
unconditioned stimulus; also UCS, UnCS, unCS, UnS
unit secretary
upper segment
Usher's syndrome

U/S ultrasound; also US, UTS, UTZ

U1S uroporphyrinogen-1-synthase

USA unit services assistant

USACQ Universal Secure Affordable Medical Care with Choice & High Quality

USAEC United States Atomic Energy Commission

USAFH United States Air Force Hospital

USAFRHL United States Air Force Radiological Health Laboratory

USAH United States Army Hospital

USAHC United States Army Health Clinic

USAIDR United States Army Institute of Dental Research

USAMEDS United States Army Medical Service

USAN United States Adopted Names (Council)

USAP unstable angina pectoris; also UAP

USASI United States of America Standards Institute (now: ANSI, American National Standards Institute)

USB upper sternal border

USBS United States Bureau of Standards

USCVD unsterile controlled vaginal delivery

USD United States Dispensatory

USDA United States Department of Agriculture

USDHHS United States Department of Health and Human Services

USE ultrasonic echography (ultrasonography)

USFMG United States foreign medical graduates

USG ultrasonogram
ultrasonography; also US

USH usual state of health

USHL United States Hygienic Laboratory

USI urinary stress incontinence

USMG United States medical graduate

USMH United States Marine Hospital

USN ultrasonic nebulizer

USNH United States Naval Hospital

USNRP United States National Reference Preparation

USO unilateral salpingo-oophorectomy

USOGH usual state of good health

USP United States Pharmacopeia

USPC United States Pharmacopeial Convention

USPDI United States Pharmacopeia Drug Information

USPET Urokinase-Streptokinase Pulmonary Embolism Trial

USPHS United States Public Health Service

USR unheated serum reagin (test)

USS ultrasound scanning

ust burnt [L. *ustulatus*]

USUCVD unsterile uncontrolled vaginal delivery

USVB United States Veterans Bureau

USVH United States Veterans Hospital

USVMD urine specimen volume measuring device

USVMS urine specimen volume measuring system

USW ultrashortwave

UT Ullrich-Turner (syndrome)
Unna-Thost (syndrome)
unrelated children raised together
untested
untreated
urinary tract
urticaria

Ut uterus; also ut

uT unbound testosterone

ut uterus; also Ut

U$_{TA}$ urinary titratable acidity

UTBG unbound thyroxin-binding globulin

UTD up to date

ut dict as directed [L. *ut dictum*]; also ud

UTDR unexpected or toxic drug reaction

utend to be used [L. *utendus*]; also u

utend mor sol to be used in the usual manner [L. *utendus more solito*]

UTF usual throat flora

UTI urinary tract infection
urinary trypsin inhibitor

uti to make use of [L. *uti, utor*]; also uto

UTLD Utah Test of Language Development

UTO unable to obtain
upper tibial osteotomy

uto to make use of [L. *utor, uti*]; also uti

UTP unilateral tension pneumothorax
uridine triphosphate

UTPA uterine plasminogen tissue activator

UTS Ullrich-Turner syndrome
ulnar tunnel syndrome
ultimate tensile strength
ultrasound; also US, U/S, UTZ

ut supr as above [L. *ut supra*]

UTZ ultrasound; also US, U/S, UTS

UU urinary urea
urine urobilinogen

UUN urine urea nitrogen

UUO unilateral ureteral occlusion

UUP urine uroporphyrin

U UREA urinary concentration of urea

UV ultraviolet; also uv
umbilical vein; also uv
ureterovesical
urine volume

U$_v$ Uppsala virus

uv ultraviolet; also UV
umbilical vein; also UV

UVA ultraviolet A (ultraviolet radiation, long wavelength)
ureterovesical angle

UVB ultraviolet B (ultraviolet radiation, midrange wavelength)

UVC ultraviolet C (ultraviolet radiation, short wavelength)
umbilical venous catheter
urgent visit center

UVEB unifocal ventricular ectopic beat

UVER ultraviolet-enhanced reactivation

UVI ultraviolet irradiation

UVJ ureterovesical junction

UVL ultraviolet light
umbilical venous line

UVP ultraviolet photometry

UVR ultraviolet radiation
UW unilateral weakness
Urbach-Wiethe (syndrome)
U/WB unit of whole blood
UWF unknown white female
UWL unstirred water layer
UWM unknown white male
unwed mother
UX uranium X (protactinium)
ux wife [L. *uxor*]
UYP upper yield point

V

V coefficient of variation
electrical potential (in volts)
gas volume
logical binary relation that is true if any argument is true and false otherwise
luminous efficiency
minute volume (of air or blood)
potential energy (joules)
unipolar chest lead
vaccinated
vaccine; also vac
vagina; also VAG, Vag, vag
vaginal; also VAG, Vag, vag
valine (one-letter notation); also VAL, Val
valve; also val
vanadium (element)
variable; also Var, var
variation; also Var, var
varnish
vector; also vect
vegetarian
vegetation
vein; also v
velocity; also v, v, vel, veloc
venous; also v
ventilation; also VE, Ve, VENT, vent
ventral; also VENT, vent
ventricle; also ventric
ventricular (fibrillation)
venule
verbal (comprehension factor)
vertebral; also vert
vertex; also VE, VTX, Vtx, Vx
vertex sharp transient (electroencephalography)
Vibrio species; also *V*
violet
viral; also Vir
virulence; also VI, Vi
virus; also v, Vir
vision; also *V*, vis, vsn
visual acuity; also *V*, VA, Va
visual capacity; also VC
voice
volt(s); also v
voltage; also *V, v,*
volume; also q, V, vol
vomiting

V *Vibrio* species; also V
vision; also V, vis, vsn
visual acuity; also V, VA, Va

voltage; also V, v
volume; also q, V, vol

$\dot{V}$ gas volume per unit of time (gas flow) (frequently used with subscripts indicating location and chemical species)
ventilation (frequently with subscript)

V_1–V_6 precordial chest leads (electrocardiogram)

v rate of reaction catalyzed by an enzyme
see [L. *vide*]; also vid
specific volume
vein; also V
velocity; also V, v, vel, veloc
venous; also V
versus; also VS, vs
very
virus; also V, Vir
vitamin; also VIT, Vit, vit
volt(s); also V

v. A vitamin A (vitamin A_1, retinol)

v. A_1 vitamin A_1 (retinol)

v. A_2 vitamin A_2 (dehydroretinol)

v. B_1 vitamin B_1 (thiamine)

v. B_2 vitamin B_2 (riboflavin)

v. B_3 vitamin B_3 (niacinamide, pantothenic acid)

v. B_4 vitamin B_4 (adenine)

v. B_5 vitamin B_5 (niacinamide, pantothenic acid)

v. B_6 vitamin B_6 (pyridoxine hydrochloride)

v. B_8 vitamin B_8 (adenylic acid)

v. B_{10} and B_{11} vitamins B_{10} and B_{11} (compounds allied to folic acid reported to be necessary for feathering and growth in chicks)

v. B_{12} vitamin B_{12} (cyanocobalamin)

v. B_{12a} vitamin B_{12a} (hydroxocobalamin)

v. B_{12b} vitamin B_{12b} (aquocobalamin)

v. B_{12c} vitamin B_{12c} (nitrosocobalamin)

v. B_{14} vitamin B_{14} (compound isolated from urine; said to check the reproduction of cancer cells and to act as an anti-pernicious anemia factor)

v. B_{15} vitamin B_{15} (pangamic acid)

v. B_{17} vitamin B_{17} (misleading term applied to amygdalin)

v. Bc vitamin Bc (folic acid)

v. Bc conjugate   vitamin Bc conjugate (pteroylhexaglutamylglutamic acid)

v. B$_T$ vitamin B$_T$ (carnitine)

v. B$_x$ vitamin B$_x$ (*para*-aminobenzoic acid)

v. C   vitamin C (ascorbic acid)

v. D$_1$ vitamin D$_1$ (1:1 molecular compound of lumisterol and vitamin D$_2$)

v. D$_2$ vitamin D$_2$ (ergocalciferol)

v. D$_3$ vitamin D$_3$ (cholecalciferol)

v. D$_4$ vitamin D$_4$ (22,23-dihydroergocalciferol)

v. E   vitamin E (alpha-tocopherol); also VE

v. F   vitamin F (name given to the fatty acids, linoleic, linolenic, and arachidonic acids)

v. G   vitamin G (riboflavin [vitamin B$_2$])

v. H   vitamin H (biotin)

v. H′   vitamin H′ (*para*-aminobenzoic acid)

v. J   vitamin J (apparently necessary for development in guinea pigs)

v. K$_1$ vitamin K$_1$ (phytonadione)

v. K$_2$ vitamins K$_2$ (menaquinones)

v. K$_3$ vitamin K$_3$ (menadione)

v. L$_1$ vitamin L$_1$ (*ortho*-aminobenzoic acid)

v. L$_2$ vitamin L$_2$ (necessary for lactation in rats; found in yeast)

v. M   vitamin M (folic acid [vitamin Bc])

v. P complex   vitamin P complex (bioflavonoids)

v. PP   vitamin PP (niacinamide [vitamin B$_5$])

v. R   vitamin R (necessary for proper development of chicks)

v. S   vitamin S (necessary for proper development of chicks)

v. T   vitamin T (tegotin)

v. U   vitamin U (methylmethioninesulfonium chloride)

v. V   vitamin V (in the development of chicks)

v. X   vitamin X (former name for vitamin P)

v   velocity; also V, v, vel, veloc
voltage; also V, *V*

v-, *v*-   vicinal (adjacent) isomer

v̄   as a subscript, refers to mixed venous blood

+v   positive vertical divergence; also +VD

VA   alveolar ventilation; also V$_A$, Va
vacuum aspiration
valeric acid
valproic acid; also VPA
vancomycin
vasodilator agent

ventricular arrest
ventricular arrhythmia
ventriculoatrial; also V-A
ventroanterior
vertebral artery
Veterans Administration
Vinyl acetate
viral antigen
visual activity
visual acuity; also V, *V*, Va
visual aid
visual axis
visual discriminatory acuity; also VDA
volcanic ash
volt-ampere; also Va, va
volume, alveolar
volume averaging

V$_A$ alveolar ventilation; also VA, Va

V/A   variety; also Var, var
volt per ampere

V-A   ventriculoatrial; also VA

V&A   vagotomy and antrectomy

Va   alveolar ventilation; also VA, V$_A$
arterial gas volume
visual acuity; also V, *V*, VA
volt-ampere; also VA, va

va   volt-ampere; also VA, Va

VAB   vincristine, actinomycin D, and bleomycin

VAB-6   vinblastine, actinomycin D, bleomycin, cisplatin, and cyclophosphamide

VABCD   vinblastine, Adriamycin, bleomycin sulfate, CCNU (lomustine), and dacarbazine

VABP   ventroarterial bypass pumping

VAC   vascular anticoagulant
ventriculoarterial connection
ventriculoatrial condition
ventriculoatrial conduction
vincristine, actinomycin D, and cyclophosphamide
vincristine, Adriamycin, and cyclophosphamide
virus capsid antigen

vac   vaccine; also V
vacuum

vacc   vaccination

VACTERL   vertebral abnormalities, anal atresia, cardiac abnormalities, tracheoesophageal fistula and/or esophageal atresia, renal agenesis and dysplasia, and limb (defects)

VAD vascular (venous) access device
ventricular assist device
vincristine, Adriamycin, and dexamethasone
virus-adjusting diluent
vitamin A deficiency

VADA vincristine, Adriamycin, dexamethasone, and actinomycin D

V_A**eff** effective alveolar ventilation

VAER visual auditory evoked response

VAFAC vincristine, Adriamycin, fluorouracil, Amethopterin, and cyclophosphamide

VAG, Vag, vag vagina; also V
vaginal; also V

VAG HYST vaginal hysterectomy; also VH

VAH vertebral ankylosing hyperostosis
Veterans Administration Hospital
virilizing adrenal hyperplasia

VAHS virus-associated hemophagocytic syndrome

VAIN vaginal intraepithelial neoplasia; also VIN

VAKT visual, association, kinesthetic, tactile (reading)

VAL, Val valine; also V

val valve; also V

VALE visual acuity, left eye

VALG Veterans Administration Lung Cancer Study Group

VAM ventricular arrhythmia monitor
Vepesid, Adriamycin, and methotrexate

VAMC Veterans Administration Medical Center

VAMP vincristine, actinomycin, methotrexate, and prednisone
vincristine, Amethopterin, and prednisone
vincristine, Amethopterin, mercaptopurine, and prednisone

VAMS Visual Analogue Mood Scale

VAN ventricular aneurysmectomy

VANCO/P vancomycin–peak

VANCO/T vancomycin–trough

V and T volume and tension (of pulse); also V&T

VAP variant angina pectoris
venous access port
vincristine, Adriamycin, and prednisone
vincristine, Adriamycin, and procarbazine
vincristine, asparaginase, and prednisone

vap vapor

$\dot{V}A/\dot{Q}, \dot{V}a/\dot{Q}$ ventilation-perfusion quotient ratio; also V_A/Q_C, $\dot{V}/\dot{Q}$, VQR

V_A/Q_C ventilation-perfusion quotient ratio; also $\dot{V}A/\dot{Q}, \dot{V}a/\dot{Q}, \dot{V}/\dot{Q}$, VQR

VAR variant; also Var, var
visual auditory range

Var, var variable; also V
variant; also VAR
variation; also V
variety; also V/A

VARE visual acuity, right eye

VAS vascular; also VASC, vasc
vasectomy; also vas
vesicle attachment site
Visual Analogue Scale (pain)

vas vasectomy; also VAS

VASAG Veterans Administration Surgical Adjuvant Cancer Chemotherapy Study Group

VASC vascular; also VAS, vasc
Verbal Auditory Screen for Children
Visual-Auditory Screen Test for Children

vasc vascular; also VAS, VASC

vasodil vasodilation; also VD
vasodilator; also VD

VAS RAD vascular radiology

vas vit glass vessel [L. *vas vitreum*]; also vas vitr

vas vitr glass vessel [L. *vas vitreum*]; also vas vit

VAT atrial synchronous ventricular (pacemaker code)
variable antigen type
ventricular activation time
ventricular pacing, atrial sensing, triggered mode (pacemaker)
Veterinary Aptitude/Admission Test
visual action time
visual apperception test
vocational apperception test

VATER vertebral defects, imperforate anus, tracheoesophageal fistula with esophageal atresia, radial and renal dysplasia

VATH vinblastine, Adriamycin, thiotepa, and Halotestin

VATs variable antigen, surface

VAV Vepesid (etoposide), Adriamycin, and vincristine

VB vagina bulbi
valence bond

VB—cont'd
Van Buren (catheter)
venous blood
ventricular bradycardia
ventrobasal
veronal buffer
viable birth
vinblastine; also VBL, Vbl
vinblastine and bleomycin
virus buffer
voided bladder

VB$_1$ first voided bladder specimen

VB$_2$ second midstream bladder specimen

VB$_3$ third midstream bladder specimen

VBAC vaginal birth after cesarean

VBAIN vertebrobasilar artery insufficiency

VBAP vincristine, BCNU (carmustine), Adriamycin, and prednisone

VBC vinblastine, bleomycin, and cisplatin

VBD veronal-buffered diluent

VBG vagotomy and Billroth gastroenterostomy
venoaortocoronary artery bypass graft
venous blood gas
veronal-buffered serum with gelatin
vertical-banded gastroplasty

VBI vertebrobasilar insufficiency
vertebrobasilar ischemia

VBL vinblastine; also VB, Vbl

Vbl vinblastine; also VB, VBL

VBM vinblastine, bleomycin, and methotrexate

VBMCP vincristine, BCNU (carmustine), melphalan, cyclophosphamide, and prednisone

VBOS veronal-buffered oxalated saline

VBP vinblastine, bleomycin, and Platinol

VBR ventricular-brain ratio

VBS veronal-buffered saline
vertebral-basilar artery system

VBS:FBS veronal-buffered saline:fetal bovine serum

VBT vertebral body tenderness

VC color vision
pulmonary capillary blood volume; also V$_c$
vascular change
vasoconstriction
vena cava
venous capacitance
venous capillary
ventilatory capacity
ventral column

ventricular contractions
Vepesid and carboplatin
verbal comprehension
vertebral canal
Veterinary Corps
videocassette
vincristine; also VCR, Vcr
vinyl chloride
vision, color
visual capacity; also V
visual cortex
vital capacity; also VIT CAP, vit cap
vocal cord(s)
volume, capillary
voluntary closing
vomiting center
vowel-consonant

V/C ventilation to circulation (ratio)

V&C vertical and centric (bite)

Vc pulmonary capillary gas volume

V$_c$ pulmonary capillary blood volume; also VC

VCA vancomycin, colistin, and anisomycin
viral capsid antigen

VCA-EB viral capsid antigen, Epstein-Barr

VCAP vincristine, cyclophosphamide, Adriamycin, and prednisone

VCC vasoconstrictor center
ventral cell column

VCCA velocity, common carotid artery

VCD vibrational circular dichroism

VCDQ verbal comprehension deviation quotient

VCE vagina, ectocervix, and endocervix (smear)

V$_{CE}$ velocity of contractile element

V$_{CF}$ velocity of circumferential fiber (shortening)

VCG vectorcardiogram
vectorcardiography
voiding cystogram

VCI volatile corrosion inhibitor

V-Cillin penicillin V

VCIU voluntary control of involuntary utterances

VCM vinyl chloride monomer

VCMP vincristine, cyclophosphamide, melphalan, and prednisone

VCN vancomycin, colistimethate, and nystatin (medium)
Vibrio cholerae neuraminidase

VCO, V$_{CO}$ carbon monoxide (endogenous production)

VCO$_2$, V$_{CO2}$ carbon dioxide output
volume, carbon dioxide elimination

VCP vincristine, cyclophosphamide, and prednisone

VCR vasoconstriction rate
vincristine; also VC, Vcr
vincristine sulfate
volume clearance rate
volume to concentration ratio

Vcr vincristine; also VC, VCR

VCS vasoconstrictor substance
vesicocervical space
Vocabulary Comprehension Scale

VCSA viral cell surface antigen

VCSF ventricular cerebrospinal fluid

VCT venous clotting time

VCTM viral-chlamydial transport medium

VCU videocystourethrogram
videocystourethrography
voiding cystourethrogram; also VCUG

VCUG vesicoureterogram
voiding cystourethrogram; also VCU

VCV vowel-consonant-vowel

VD vapor density
vascular disease
vasodilation; also vasodil
vasodilator; also vasodil
venereal disease
ventricular dilator
vertical deviation
vessel disease
video disk
viral diarrhea
voided
volume of distribution; also Vd

+VD positive vertical divergence; also +v

V&D vomiting and diarrhea

V$_D$ ventilation per minute of dead space
volume of dead air space; also Vd, VDS

Vd volume of dead air space; also V$_D$, VDS
volume of distribution; also VD

V$_d$ apparent volume of distribution (V area)

vd double vibrations

VDA venous digital angiogram
visual discriminatory acuity; also VA

V$_D$A ventilation of alveolar dead space
volume of alveolar dead space

VDAC vaginal delivery after cesarean

voltage-dependent anion-selective channel

V$_D$an ventilation of anatomic dead space
volume of anatomic dead space

VDBR volume of distribution of bilirubin

VDC vasodilator center

VDD atrial synchronous ventricular inhibited (pacemaker code)

VDDR vitamin D-dependent rickets

VDEL Venereal Disease Experimental Laboratory

VDEM vasodepressor material; also VDM

VDF ventricular diastolic fragmentation

VDG, VD-G venereal disease, gonorrhea

Vdg, vdg voiding

VDH valvular disease of the heart
vascular disease of the heart

VDL vasodepressor lipid
visual detection level

VDM vasodepressor material; also VDEM

V$_{DM}$ volume of mechanical dead space

VD or M venous distention or mass

VDP vinblastine, dacarbazine, and Platinol
vincristine, daunorubicin, and prednisone

VDR venous diameter ratio

V$_D$rb rebreathing ventilation

VDRL Venereal Disease Research Laboratories

VDRR vitamin D-resistant rickets

VDRS Verdun Depression Rating Scale

VDRT Venereal Disease Reference Test

VDS vasodilator substance
venereal disease, syphilis; also VD-S
vindesine
volume of dead air space; also V$_D$, Vd

VD-S venereal disease, syphilis; also VDS

Vd shunt dead space effect of Qs/Qt

VDT visual display terminal
visual distortion test

VDU visual display unit

VDV ventricular end-diastolic volume

VD/VT, V$_D$/V$_T$ dead-space gas volume to tidal gas volume (ratio)

V$_D$V$_T$ physiologic dead space in percent of tidal volume

VE vacuum extraction
vaginal examination
Venezuelan encephalitis
venous emptying
venous extension
ventilation; also V, Ve, VENT, vent

VE—cont'd
ventricular elasticity
ventricular escape
ventricular extrasystole
vertex; also V, VTX, Vtx, Vx
vesicular exanthema
viral encephalitis
visual efficiency
visual examination
vitamin E (alpha-tocopherol); also v. E
vocational evaluation
volumic ejection
voluntary effort

V_E environmental variance
respiratory minute volume (expired)
volume airflow per unit of time
volume of expired gas

Ve ventilation; also V, VE, VENT, vent

VEA ventricular ectopic activity
ventricular ectopic arrhythmia
viral envelope antigen

VEAD visually evoked afterdischarge

VEB ventricular ectopic beats
ventricular extra beats

VEC vecuronium

VECG vector electrocardiogram

VECP visually evoked cortical potential

vect vector; also V

VED ventricular ectopic depolarization
vital exhaustion and depression

VEDP ventricular end-diastolic pressure

VEE Venezuelan equine encephalitis
Venezuelan equine encephalomyelitis

V-EEG vigilance-controlled electroencephalogram

VEF ventricular ejection fraction
visually evoked field

V_{EH} extrahepatic distribution

vehic vehicle

vel or [L. *vel*]
velocity; also V, v, *v*, veloc

veloc velocity; also V, v, *v*, vel

VEM vasoexcitor material

V_{Emax} maximal flow per unit of time

VEMP vincristine, Endoxan, mercaptopurine,
and prednisone

VENT, vent ventilation; also V, VE, Ve
ventilator
ventral; also V
ventricular

vent fib ventricular fibrillation; also VF, Vfib

ventric ventricle; also V

VEP visual evoked potential

VER ventricular escape rhythm
veratridine
visual evoked response

vert vertebra
vertebral; also V
vertical

VES, ves bladder [L. *vesica*]
vesicular
vessel

vesica blister [L. *vesicula*]
vesicatorium [L. *vesicula*. (a blister)]

vesp evening [L. *vesper*]

ves ur urinary bladder [L. *vesica urinaria*]

VESV vesicular exanthema of swine virus

VET vestigial testis
veteran; also Vet

Vet veteran; also VET
veterinarian
veterinary

vet see also [L. *vide etiam*]

Vet Med veterinary medicine

VETS Veterans Adjustment Scale

Vet Sci veterinary science

VEWA Vocational Evaluation and Work
Adjustment

VF left leg electrode (electrocardiogram)
ventricular fibrillation; also vent fib, Vfib
ventricular fluid
ventricular flutter; also VFL
ventricular fusion
video frequency
vigil, fatiguing
visual field (field of vision); also Vf, vf
vitreous fluorophotometry; also VFP
vocal fremitus

Vf, vf visual field (field of vision); also VF

V_f variant frequency

VFA volatile fatty acid

Vfactor verbal comprehension factor

VFAM vincristine, fluorouracil, Adriamycin,
and mitomycin C

VFC ventricular function curve

VFD visual feedback display

VFDF very fast death factor

VFI visual field(s) intact; also VFIT

Vfib ventricular fibrillation; also vent fib, VF

VFIT visual field(s) intact; also VFI
VFL ventricular flutter; also VF
VFP ventricular filling pressure
ventricular fluid pressure
vitreous fluorophotometry; also VF
VFPN Volu-feed preemie nipple
VFR voiding flow rate
VFRN Volu-feed regular nipple
VFT venous filling time
ventricular fibrillation threshold
VG vein graft
ventilated group
ventricular gallop
very good
V&G vagotomy and gastroenterotomy
V_G genetic variance
VGH very good health
veterinary general hospital
VGP viral glycoprotein
VH vaginal hysterectomy; also VAG HYST
venous hematocrit
ventricular hypertrophy
veteran's hospital
viral hepatitis
vitreous hemorrhage
V_H hepatic distribution volume
variable domain of heavy chain immunoglobulin
VHD valvular heart disease
ventricular heart disease
viral hematodepressive disease
VHDL very high-density lipoprotein
VHF very high frequency
viral hemorrhagic fever
visual half-field
VHN Vickers hardness number
VHOC volatile halogenated organic compounds
VHSV viral hemorrhagic septicemia virus
VI vaginal irrigation
valgus index
variable interval
vastus intermedius
virgin [L. *virgo intacta* (untouched girl)]
virulence; also V, Vi
virulent; also Vi, vir
viscosity index
Visual Imagery
visual impairment
visual inspection

vitality index
volume index
V_I volume of inspired gas (per minute)
Vi virginium
virulence; also V, VI
virulent; also VI, vir
VIA virus-inactivating agent
virus infection-associated antigen
vib vibration
VIBS vocabulary, information, block design,
similarities (psychology)
VIC vasoinhibitory center
vehicle for initial crawling
Vepesid, ifosfamide, carboplatin, and mesna
visual communication (therapy)
voice intensity controller
VICA velocity internal carotid artery
VID vaginal intraepithelial dysplasia
video-densitometry
visible iris diameter
vid see [L. *vide*]; also v
VIF virus-induced interferon
VIG, VIg vaccinia immune globulin
vig vigorous
VIH violence-induced handicap
VIM ventral impaired medium (neuron)
video-intensification microscopy
VIN vaginal intraepithelial neoplasia;also
VAIN
vinbarbital
vulvar intraepithelial neoplasia
vin wine [L. *vinum*]
VIP vasoactive intestinal peptide
vasoactive intestinal polypeptide
vasoactive intracorporeal pharmacotherapy
vasoinhibitory peptide
venous impedance plethysmography
very important patient
very important person
vinblastine, ifosfamide, and Platinol
voluntary interruption of pregnancy
VIQ Verbal Intelligence Quotient
VIR virology
Vir viral; also V
virus; also V, v
vir green [L. *virdis*]
virulent; also VI, Vi
VIR AC viral antibody, acute
VIS vaginal irrigation smear
visible

VIS—cont'd
visual information storage
vocational interest schedule

vis vision; also V, *V*, vsn
visiting
visitor
visual

VISA ventriculus inhibited synchronously with the atrium

VISC vitreous infusion suction cutter

visc viscera
visceral
viscosity
viscous

VISI volar-flexed intercalated segment instability

VIT venom immunotherapy
vital; vit
vitamin; also v, Vit, vit

Vit vitamin; also v, VIT, vit

vit vital; also VIT
vitamin; also v, VIT, Vit
vitrectomy; also Vx
vitreous; also vitr
yolk [L. *vitellus*]; also vitel

VIT CAP vital capacity; also VC, vit cap

vit cap vital capacity; also VC, VIT CAP
vitamin capsule

vitel yolk [L. *vitellus*]; also vit

vit ov sol dissolved in egg yolk [L. *vitello ovi solutus*]; also vos

vitr glass [L. *vitrum*]
vitreous; also vit

vits vitamins

VI/VI may be heard with the stethoscope entirely off the chest (heart murmur)

viz that is, namely [L. *videlicet* (one can see, it is clear)]
visualized

VJ Vogel-Johnson (agar)

VK vervet (African green monkey) kidney (cell)
Vogt-Koyanagi (syndrome)

VKC vernal keratoconjunctivitis

VKH Vogt-Koyanagi-Harada (syndrome)

VL left arm electrode (electrocardiogram)
vastus lateralis
ventralis lateralis
ventrolateral
visceral leishmaniasis
vision, left eye; also VOS

V_L actual volume of lung
variable domain of light chain immunoglobulin

VLA vanillactic acid
very late antigen
virus-like agent

VLB vincaleukoblastine (vinblastine)

VLBR very low birth rate

VLBW very low birth weight

VLCD very low calorie diet

VLCFA very long chain fatty acid

VLD very low-density

VLDL very low density lipoprotein; also VLDLP

VLDLP very low-density lipoprotein; also VLDL

VLDL-TG very low-density lipoprotein triglyceride

VLDS Verbal Language Development Scale

V lead voltage lead

VLF very low frequency

VLG ventral nucleus of the lateral geniculate (body)

VLH ventrolateral nucleus of the hypothalamus

VLI vasopressin-like immunoreactivity

VLM visceral larval migrans

VLP ventriculolumbar perfusion
vincristine, L-asparaginase, and prednisone
virus-like particle

VLSI very large scale integration

VM vasomotor
vastus medialis
ventricular mass
ventricular muscle
ventromedial
Verner-Morrison (syndrome)
vestibular membrane
viomycin
viral myocarditis
voltmeter

V/m volts per meter

VM-26 teniposide

VMA vanillylmandelic acid (inaccurate name for vanilmandelic acid)
vanilmandelic acid

V-Mask Venturi mask

V_{max} maximum velocity (of an enzyme catalyzed reaction)
peak flow velocity (Doppler)

VMC vasomotor center
village malaria communicator
void metal composite
von Meyenburg's complex

VMCG vector magnetocardiogram

VMCP vincristine, melphalan, cyclophosphamide, and prednisone

VMD Doctor of Veterinary Medicine [L. *Veterinariae Medicinne Doctor*]

vMDV virulent Marek's disease virus

VMF vasomotor flushing
Vepesid (etoposide), methotrexate, and fluorouracil

VMH ventromedial hypothalamic (neuron, nuclei)

VMI visual motor integration

V-MI Volpe-Manhold Index

VMIT visual-motor integration test

VMN ventromedial nucleus

VMO vastus medialis oblique (muscle)

VMP variable major protein

VMR vasomotor rhinitis

VMS visual memory span

VMSC Vineland Measurement of Social Competence

VMST Visual-Motor Sequencing Test

VMT vasomotor tone
ventilatory muscle training
ventral mesencephalic tegmentum
ventromedial tegmentum

VN vesicle neck
vestibular nucleus
virus neutralization
virus-neutralizing
visceral nucleus
Visiting Nurse
visual naming
Vocational Nurse
vomeronasal

VNA Visiting Nurse Association

VNC vesicle neck contracture

VNDPT Visual Numerical Discrimination Pretest

VNE verbal nonemotional (stimuli)

VNO vomeronasal organ

VNR ventral nerve root
vitronectin receptor

VNS villonodular synovitis; also VS
Visiting Nursing Service

VNTR variable number of tandem repeats (genetics)

VO verbal order
volume (ventricular) overload

VO$_2$, V$_{O2}$ oxygen uptake
volume of oxygen consumption per unit of time

VOC volatile organic compounds
voltage-operated channel

voc vocational

vocab vocabulary

VOCTOR void on call to operating room

VOD venous occlusive disease
vision, right eye [L. *visio, oculus dextra*]; also VR

vol volar
volatile
volume; also q, V, *V*
volumetric
voluntary
volunteer

vol% volume percent

vol adm voluntary admission

volfr volume fraction

vol/vol volume per volume (ratio)

VOM volt-ohm-milliammeter
vomited; also vom

vom vomited; also VOM

VO$_2$max, V$_{O2}$max maximum oxygen consumption

VOO ventricular asynchronous (pacemaker code)

VOP venous occlusion plethysmography

VOPP veterinary, optometry, podiatry, pharmacy

VOR vestibulo-ocular reflex

VOS vision, left eye [L. *visio, oculus sinister*]; also VL

vos dissolved in egg yolk [L. *vitello ovi solutus*]; also vit ov sol

VOT Visual Organization Test
voice onset time

VOU vision, each eye [L. *visio, oculus uterque*]

voxel volume element

VP etoposide; also VP-16, Vp-16, VP-16-213
vapor pressure; also vp
variegate porphyria
Variot-Pironneau (syndrome)
vascular permeability
vasopressin

VP—cont'd
velopharyngeal
venipuncture
venous pressure; also Pv
venous volume plethysmography
ventricular pacing
ventricular pause
ventricular premature (beat); also Vp
ventriculoperitoneal (shunt)
vertex potential
vincristine and prednisone
vindesine and Platinol
vinylpyrroildone
viral protein
virus protein
Voges-Proskauer (medium, reaction, test)
voiding pressure (bladder)
volume-pressure
vulnerable period

V-P, V/P ventilation and perfusion; also V&P

V&P vagotomy and pyloroplasty
ventilation and perfusion; also V-P, V/P

Vp plasma volume
ventricular premature (beat); also VP

VP-16, Vp-16 etoposide; also VP, VP-16-213

VP-16-213 etoposide; also VP, VP-16, Vp-16

vp vapor pressure; also VP

VPA valproic acid; also VA

VP + A vincristine, prednisone, and asparaginase

VPB ventricular premature beat

VPC vapor-phase chromatography
ventricular premature complex
ventricular premature contraction
volume of packed cells
volume percent

VPCMF vincristine, prednisone, cyclophosphamide, methotrexate, and fluorouracil

VPCT ventricular premature contraction threshold

VPD ventricular premature depolarization

VPDF vegetable protein diet plus fiber

VPF vascular permeability factor

VPG velopharyngeal gap

VPI velopharyngeal insufficiency
ventral posterior inferior
virus structural protein

VPIR vapor-phase infrared (spectra)

VPL ventroposterolateral

VPM vascular permeability mediator
ventilator pressure manometer
ventroposteromedial

vpm vibrations per minute

VPO velopharyngeal opening

VPP viral porcine pneumonia

VPR volume-pressure response

VPRBC volume of packed red blood cells

VPRC volume of packed red cells

VPS valvular pulmonic stenosis
visual pleural space
Volume Performance Standards

vps vibrations per second

VPW ventral prostate weight

VQ ventilation-perfusion; also V/Q
voice quality

V/Q ventilation flow
ventilation-perfusion; also VQ

$\dot{V}/\dot{Q}$ ventilation-perfusion quotient ratio;
also $\dot{V}A/\dot{Q}$, $\dot{V}a/\dot{Q}$, V_A/Q_C, VQR

VQE Visa Qualifying Exam

VQR ventilation-perfusion quotient ratio;
also $\dot{V}A/\dot{Q}$, $\dot{V}a/\dot{Q}$, V_A/Q_C, $\dot{V}/\dot{Q}$

VQ scan ventilation quantitation imaging technique

VR right arm electrode (electrocardiogram)
valve replacement
variable rate
variable ratio
vascular resistance
venous reflux
venous return
ventilation rate
ventilation ratio
ventral root; also Vr, vr
ventricular rate
ventricular response
ventricular rhythm
verbal reprimand
vesicular rosette
vision, right eye; also VOD
visual reproduction
vital record
vocal resonance
vocational rehabilitation

Vr ventral root; also VR, vr
volume of relaxation

vr ventral root; also VR, Vr

VRA visual reinforcement audiometry
Vocational Rehabilitation Administration

VRBC volume of red blood cells

VRC venous renin concentration

VR CON viral antibody, convalescent

VRD ventricular radial dysplasia

VR&E vocational rehabilitation and education

V region variable region (of an antibody)

VRI viral respiratory infection

VRL ventral root, lumbar
Virus Reference Laboratory
Virus Reference Library

VRNA viral ribonucleic acid

VROM voluntary range of motion

VRP very reliable product (written on prescription)

VRR ventral root reflex

VRT variance of resident time
ventral root, thoracic
Visual Retention Test

VRV ventricular residual volume
viper retrovirus

VS vaccination scar
vaccine serotype
vagal stimulation
vasospasm
venesection; also Vs
ventral subiculum
ventricular sense
ventricular septum
verbal scale (IQ)
versus; also v, vs
vertically selective (visual cell)
very sensitive
vesicular sound
vesicular stomatitis
veterinary surgeon
villonodular synovitis; also VNS
visual storage
vital signs; also V/S, vs
Vogt-Spielmeyer (disease)
volumetric solution
voluntary sterilization

V/S vital signs; also VS, vs

V·s vibration-second; also vs, v-s
volt-second

v-s vibration-second; also V·s, vs

V x s volts by seconds

Vs venesection; also VS

vs against [L. *versus*]
see above [L. *vide supra*]
single vibration
to draw blood [L. *venae sectio* (cutting of vein)]

versus; also v, VS
vibration-second; also V·s, v-s
vital signs; also VS, V/S
voids

VSA variant-specific surface antigen

VsB, vsb drawing blood from a vessel in arm
[L. *venae sectio brachii*]

VSBE very short below-elbow (cast)

VSC voluntary surgical contraception

VSCC voltage-sensitive calcium channel

VSCS ventricular specialized conduction system

VSD ventricular septal defect
virtually safe dose

VSEPR valence shell electron pair repulsion

VSFP venous stop flow pressure

VSG variable surface glycoprotein

VSHD ventricular septal heart defect

VSL very serious list

VSM vascular smooth muscle

VSMS Vineland Social Maturity Scale

vsn vision; also V, *V*, vis

VSO vertical subcondylar oblique

VSOK vital signs okay (normal)

VSR venereal spirochetosis of rabbits
venous stasis retinopathy

VSS vital signs stable

VSULA vaccination scar, upper left arm

VSV vesicular stomatitis virus

VSW ventricular stroke work

VT tetrazolium violet (stain)
tidal volume; also V$_T$
total ventilation
vacuum tube
vacuum tuberculin
vasotocin
vasotonin
venous thrombosis
ventricular tachyarrhythmia
ventricular tachycardia; also V Tach, V-TACH, V tach
Vero cytotoxin

V$_T$ tidal volume; also VT

V$_t$ pulmonary parenchymal tissue volume

V&T volume and tension (of pulse); also V and T

VTA ventral tegmental area

V$_T$A alveolar tidal volume

VTach, V-TACH, V tach ventricular tachycardia; also VT

VTCS vinyltrichlorosilane

VTE venous thromboembolism
ventricular tachycardia event
vicarious trial and error

VTEC verotoxin-producing *Escherichia coli*

V-test Voluter test (radiology)

VTG volume thoracic gas

VTI volume thickness index

VTM mechanical tidal volume
variegated translocation mosaicism
virus transport medium

VTMoV virusoid of velvet tobacco mottle virus

VTR variable tandem repetition

VTS vesicular transport system

VTSRS Verdun Target Symptom Rating Scale

VTVM vacuum tube voltmeter

VTX, Vtx vertex; also V, VE, Vx

VU varicose ulcer
very urgent
volume unit

VUR vesicoureteral reflux
vesicoureteral regurgitation

VUV vacuum ultraviolet

VV vaccinia virus
varicose veins; also VVs
vesicovaginal (fistula); also V-V
viper venom
vulva and vagina; also V&V

V/V volume of solute per total volume of solution; also v/v

V-V vesicovaginal (fistula); also VV

V&V vulva and vagina; also VV

vv veins

v/v vice versa
volume of solute per total volume of solution; also V/V

VVC village voluntary collaborator

VVD vaginal vertex delivery
vascular volume of distribution

VVFR vesicovaginal fistula repair

VVI ventricular demand inhibited (pacemaker code)

V/VI very loud, may be heard with a stethoscope partly off the chest (heart murmur)

vvi vocal velocity index

vvMDV very virulent Marek's disease virus

VVOR visual vestibulo-ocular reflex

VVQ verbalizer-visualization questionnaire

VVS vesicovaginal space

VVs varicose veins; also VV

VVT ventricular demand triggered (pacemaker code)

VW vascular wall
vessel wall
von Willebrand's (disease, factor, syndrome); also vW

vW von Willebrand's (disease, factor, syndrome); also VW

v/w volume per weight

V wave vertex sharp transient

VWD ventral wall defect
von Willebrand's disease; also vWD, vWd

vWD, vWd von Willebrand's disease; also VWD

VWF velocity waveform
vibration-induced white finger
von Willebrand's factor; also vWF, vWf

vWF, vWf von Willebrand's factor; also VWF

VWFT variable-width forms tractor

VWM ventricular wall motion

vWS, vWs von Willebrand's syndrome

Vx vertex; also V, VE, VTX, Vtx
vitrectomy; also vit

VY veal yeast

V-Y shape of incisions in V-Y procedure (plasty)

VZ, V-Z varicella-zoster (virus)

VZIG, VZIg varicella-zoster immune globulin

VZL vinzolidine

VZV varicella-zoster virus

W

W   dominant spotting (mouse)
   energy (work)
   section modulus
   shape of surgical incisions (plasty)
   tryptophan (one-letter notation); also TP, Tp,
      T_p, Trp, Try, Tryp
   tungsten [Ger. *wolfram*]
   watch the finding
   water
   watt; also w
   Weber's (test)
   week; also w, WK, wk
   wehnelt (unit of roentgen ray penetrating
      ability)
   weight; also w, WT, wt
   well closed
   west
   wetting
   white; also w, Wh, wh, wt
   white cell; also WC
   whole (response)
   widow; also w, WID, wid
   widowed; also w, WID, wid
   widower; also w, WID, wid
   width
   wife; also w
   Wilcoxon rank sum statistic
   Wistar (rat); also WI
   with; also c̄, w, w/, w̄
   wolframium (tungsten)
   word fluency; also WF
   work; also *W*, WK, wk

185W   tungsten 185, radioactive tungsten;
      halflife, 75.8 days

W+   weakly positive; also WP

W   work; also W, WK, wk

w   velocity (m/s)
   watt; also W
   week; also W, WK, wk
   weight; also W, WT, wt
   white; also W, Wh, wh, wt
   widow; also W, WID, wid
   widowed; also W, WID, wid
   widower; also W, WID, wid
   wife; also W
   with; also c̄, W, w/, w̄

w/, w̄   with; also c̄, W, w

WA   Wellness Associates
   when awake

while awake; also wa
Widal-Abrami (syndrome)
wide awake; also W/A
Wiskott-Aldrich (syndrome)

W/A   watt per ampere
   wide awake; also WA

W or A   weakness or atrophy

wa   while awake; also WA

WAB   Western Aphasia Battery (Test)

WABRS   Ward Adjustment and Behavior
   Rating Scale

WABT   Western Aphasia Battery Test

WACE   weakly acidic cation-exchange (resin)

WACH   wedge adjustable cushioned heel (shoe)

WADAO   weak and dizzy all over

WAF   weakness, atrophy, and fasciculation
   white adult female

WAGR   Wilms tumor, aniridia, genitourinary
   abnormalities, and mental retardation (syndrome)

WAIS   Wechsler Adult Intelligence Scale

WAIS-R   Wechsler Adult Intelligence
   Scale–Revised

WAM   white adult male

WAP   wandering atrial pacemaker

WAR   whole abdominal radiotherapy

WARDT   Welfare of Animals Used for
   Research in Drugs and Therapy

Ward X   the morgue

WARF   warfarin

WAS   Ward Atmosphere Scale (psychology)
   weekly activity summary
   Wiskott-Aldrich syndrome

WASP   World Association of Societies of
   Pathology (Anatomic and Clinical)

Wass   Wassermann (reaction, test)

WAT   Word Association Test

WAXI   Wistar adult xiphisternum (chondrocyte)

WB   waist belt
   washable base
   washed bladder
   water bottle
   Wechsler-Bellevue (Scale)
   weight-bearing; also Wb
   well baby
   Western blot

WB—cont'd
wet bulb
whole blood; also QB, W Bld
whole-body
Willowbrook (virus)

Wb weber (coulomb)
weigh-bearing; also WB

WBA wax bean agglutinin
whole body activity

Wb/A webers per ampere

WBAPTT whole-blood activated partial thromboplastin time

WBAT weight bearing as tolerated

WBC weight bearing with crutches
well-baby clinic
white blood cell
white blood cell count

WBC/hpf white blood cells per high power field

WBC/lpf white blood cells per low power field

WBCT whole-blood clotting time

WBDS whole-body digital scanner

WBE whole-body extract

WBF whole-blood folate

WBGT wet bulb globe temperature

WBH whole-blood hematocrit
whole-body hyperthermia

WBI Ward behavior inventory
will be in

W Bld whole blood; also QB, WB

WBM whole boiled milk

Wb/m² webers per square meter

WBN wellborn nursery
wide band noise

WBPTT whole-blood partial thromboplastin time

WBQC wide-base quad cane

WBR whole-body radiation
whole-body retention

WBRS Ward Behavior Rating Scale

WBRT whole-blood recalcification time

WBS Wechsler-Bellevue Scale
whole-body scan
whole-body shower
withdrawal body shakes
wound-breaking strength

WBT wet bulb temperature

WBTF Waring Blender tube feeding

WBTT weight bearing to tolerance

WBUS weeks by ultrasound

WC ward clerk
ward confinement
water closet
Weber-Christian (syndrome)
wet compress
wheelchair; also W/C, wc, w/c, wh ch
white cell; also W
white cell casts
white cell count; also WCC
whole complement; also WC'
whooping cough
will call
word connection (list)
work capacity
writer's cramp

WC' whole complement; also WC

W/C wheelchair; also WC, wc, w/c, wh ch

wc, w/c wheelchair; also WC, W/C, wh ch

WCB will call back

WCC Walker carcinoma cell
well-child care
white cell count; also WC

WCD Weber-Christian disease

WCE work capacity evaluation

WCL Wenckebach's cycle length
whole-cell lysate
word connection list

WCOT wall coated open tubular

WCR Walthard cell rest

WCSG Western Cancer Study Group

WCST Wisconsin Card Sorting Test

WD wallerian degeneration
ward; also Wd, wd
warm and dry; also W/D, W&D
well-developed; also wd, w/d
well-differentiated
wet dressing
Whitney Damon (dextrose)
Wilson's disease
with disease
withdrawal dyskinesia
without dyskinesia
Wolman's disease
word; also Wd
wound; also wd, WND, wnd
wrist disarticulation

W/D warm and dry; also WD, W&D
withdrawal
withdrawn

W&D warm and dry; also WD, W/D

W→D wet to dry

Wd ward; also WD, wd
word; also WD

wd ward; also WD, Wd
well-developed; also WD, w/d
wound; also WD, WND, wnd
wounded

w/d well-developed; also WD, wd

W4D Worth Four-Dot (test)

WDCC well-developed collateral circulation

WDF white divorced female

WDHA watery diarrhea, hypokalemia,
achlorhydria (syndrome)
watery diarrhea with hypokalemic alkalosis

WDHH watery diarrhea, hypokalemia, and
hypochlorhydria

WDI warfarin dose index

WDLL well-differentiated lymphocytic
lymphoma

WDM white divorced male

WDS Watery diarrhea syndrome
wavelength-dispersive x-ray spectrometry
Web drug-delivery system
wet dog shakes (syndrome)
wounds; also wds

wds wounds; also WDS

WDWN well-developed, well-nourished

WE wage earner
wax ester
weekend; also W/E
western encephalitis
western encephalomyelitis
whiskey equivalent

W/E weekend; also WE

WEE western equine encephalitis
western equine encephalomyelitis

WEG water–ethylene glycol

WEP weekend pass

WEST work evaluation systems technology

WEUP willful exposure to unwanted pregnancy

WF Waterhouse-Friderichsen (syndrome)
Weil-Felix (reaction, test)
white female; also W/F, wf
Wistar-Furth (rat)
word fluency; also W

W/F, wf white female; also WF

WFE Williams' flexion exercises; also
Wms flex ex

WFI water for injection

WFL within functional limits

WF-O will follow in office

WFOT World Federation of Occupational
Therapists

WFR Weil-Felix reaction
wheal-and-flare reaction

WFSS Wolpe Fear Survey Schedule

WG water gauge
Wegener's granulomatosis
Wright-Giemsa (stain)

WGA wheat germ agglutinin

WH walking heel (cast)
well-healed
well-hydrated
Werdnig-Hoffmann (disease, syndrome)
whole homogenate
wound healing

Wh white; also W, w, wh, wt

wh whisper
whispered
white; also W, w, Wh, wt

w-h watt-hour; also whr

WHA warmed, humidified air
World Health Assembly

WHAP Women's Health and Abortion Project

wh ch wheelchair; also WC, W/C, wc, w/c
white child

WHD Werdnig-Hoffmann disease

WHHL Watanabe heritable hyperlipidemic
(rabbit)

WHML Wellcome Historical Medical Library

WHO World Health Organization (Geneva,
Switzerland)
World Health Organization (histologic classification of ovarian tumors)
wrist-hand orthosis

WHP, Whp, whp whirlpool; also WP, W/P

WHPB whirlpool bath; also WPB

WHR waist to hip circumference ratio

whr watt-hour; also w-h

WHRC World Health Research Center

WHS Werdnig-Hoffmann syndrome
Wolf-Hirschhorn syndrome

WHV woodchuck hepatitis virus

WHVP wedged hepatic venous pressure

WI walk-in (medicine, patient)
wash-in
water ingestion
waviness index
Wistar (rat); also W

W/I within

W&I work and interest

WIA walking imagined analgesia
wounded in action

WIC women, infants, and children

WID, wid widow; also W, w
widowed; also W, w
widower; also W, w

WIPI Word Intelligibility by Picture
Identification

WIQ Waring Intimacy Questionnaire

WIS Ward Initiation Scale
Wechsler Intelligence Scale

WISC Wechsler Intelligence Scale for Children

WISC-R Wechsler Intelligence Scale for
Children–Revised

WIST Whitaker Index of Schizophrenic
Thinking

WITT Wittenborn (Psychiatric Rating Scale)

W-J Woodcock-Johnson

WJPB Woodcock-Johnson Psychoeducational
Battery

WK week; also W, w, wk
Wernicke-Korsakoff (syndrome)
Wilson-Kimmelstiel (syndrome)
work; also W, *W*, wk

wk weak
week; also W, w, WK
work; also W, *W*, WK

WKD Wilson-Kimmelstiel disease

WKF well-known fact

W/kg watts per kilogram

WKS Wernicke-Korsakoff syndrome

wks weeks

WKY Wistar-Kyoto (rat)

WL waiting list
waterload (test)
wavelength; also wl, λ
weight loss
workload

wl wavelength; also WL, λ

WLE wide local excision

WLD Werner linear dichroism

WLF whole lymphocyte fraction

WLI weight-length index

WLM work-level month

WLS wet lung syndrome

WLT waterload test
whole-lung tomography

WM Waldenström's macroglobulinemia
wall motion
ward manager
warm, moist
Weill-Marchesani (syndrome)
Wernicke-Mann (syndrome)
wet mount
white male; also W/M, wm
whole milk; also wm
whole mount (microscopy); also wm
Wilson-Mikity (syndrome)
woman milk

W/M white male; also WM, wm

wm white male; also WM, W/M
whole milk; also WM
whole mount (microscopy); also WM

w/m² watts per square meter

WMA wall-motion abnormality
World Medical Association

WMC weight-matched control

WME Williams' medium E

WMF white married female
white middle-aged female

WMM white married male
white middle-aged male

WMP weight management program

WMR work metabolic rate
World Medical Relief

WMS wall-motion study
Wechsler Memory Scale

Wms flex Williams' flexion

Wms flex ex Williams' flexion exercises;
also WFE

WMX whirlpool, massage, and exercise

WN, wn, w/n well-nourished

WND, wnd wound; also WD, wd

WNE West Nile encephalitis

WNF well-nourished female

WNL within normal limits

WNLS weighted nonlinear least squares

WNM well-nourished male

WNV West Nile virus

WO wash-out
Weber-Osler (syndrome)
weeks old; also wo
without; also s, s̄, W/O, wo, w/o
written order

W/O water in oil (emulsion)
without; also s, s̄, WO, wo, w/o

w/o without; also s, s̄, WO, W/O, wo

wo weeks old; also WO
  without; also s, s̄, WO, W/O, w/o
WOB work of breathing
WOFL wound fluid
WOP without pain
WOR Weber-Osler-Rendu (disease)
WORM write once, read many
WOU women's outpatient unit
WOW, W/O/W water in oil in water
WOWS Weak Opiate Withdrawal Scale
WP water packed
  weakly positive; also W+
  wet pack; also WPk
  wettable powder
  whirlpool; also WHP, Whp, whp, W/P
  white pulp
  word processor
  working point
W/P water to powder (ratio)
  whirlpool; also WHP, Whp, whp, WP
WPB whirlpool bath; also WHPB
WPCU weighted patient care unit
WPFM Wright peak flowmeter
WPk Ward pack
  wet pack; also WP
WPN white mucosa with punctation
WPPSI Wechsler Preschool and Primary Scale
  of Intelligence
WPRS Wittenborn Psychiatric Rating Scale
WPSI Wittenborn Psychiatric Symptoms
  Inventory
WPT marbled pure tone
WPW Wolff-Parkinson-White (syndrome)
WR washroom
  Wassermann reaction; also Wr
  water retention
  weakly reactive
  whole response
  wiping reaction
  work rate
  wrist; also Wr, wr
W/R with respect (to)
Wr Wassermann reaction; also WR
  wrist; also WR, wr
wr wrist; also WR, Wr
Wr^a Wright antigen
WRAMC Walter Reed Army Medical Center
WRAT Wide Range Achievement Test
WRBC washed red blood cells

WRC washed red cells
  water-retention coefficient
WRE whole ragweed extract
WRK Woodward's reagent K (*N*-ethyl-5-
  phenylisoxazolium-3′-sulphonate)
WRMT Woodcock Reading Mastery Test
WRST Wilcoxon rank sum test
WRVP wedged renal vein pressure
WS Wardenburg syndrome
  ward secretary
  Warthin-Starry (stain)
  water soluble; also ws
  water swallow
  watt-seconds; also W·s, ws, w-s
  Werner syndrome
  Westphal-Strümpell (syndrome)
  West's syndrome
  wet swallow
  whole response plus white space
  Wilder's silver (stain)
  Williams' syndrome
  work simplification
W&S wound and skin
W·s watt-seconds; also WS, ws, w-s
ws water soluble; also WS
  watt-seconds; also WS, W·s, w-s
w-s watt-seconds; also WS, W·s, ws
WSA water-soluble antibiotic
WSB wheat soy blend
WSD water seal drainage
WSepF white separated female
WSepM white separated male
WSF white single female
WSL Wesselsbron (virus)
WSM white single male
WSP wearable speech processor
WSR Weisenburg-Sicard-Robineau
  (syndrome)
  Westergren sedimentation rate
W/sr watts per steradian
WSS weight sum of squares
WT walking tank
  wall thickness
  water temperature
  weight; also W, w, wt
  wild type (cells, strain)
  Wilms' tumor
  wisdom teeth
  work therapy

wt weight; also W, w, WT
  white; also W, w, Wh, wh

WTD wet tail disease

WTE whole time equivalent

WTF weight transferral frequency

wt/vol weight per volume

wt/wt weight ratio (weight per weight)

W/U, w/u workup

WV walking ventilation
  whispered voice

W/V, w/v weight of solute per volume of solution

W$_v$ variable dominant spotting (mouse)

WV-MBC walking ventilation to maximal
  breathing capacity (ratio)

WW Weight Watchers
  wet weight

W/W, w/w weight of solute per weight of total
  solution

WWAC walk with aid of cane

WWidF white widowed female

WWidM white widowed male

WWK Wilson-Westphal-Konoyalor (syndrome)

WWTP wastewater treatment plant

WX wound of exit

WxB wax bite

WxP wax pattern

WY women years

WY/NRT Weidel Yes/No Reliability Test

WZa wide zone alpha (hemolysis)

X

Ξ XI, UPPER CASE, fourteenth letter of the Greek alphabet

ξ xi, lower case, fourteenth letter of the Greek alphabet

X abscissa (horizontal axis of rectangular coordinate system); also x, x
androgenic (zone)
break
chromosome X
cross
cross-bite
crossed with
cross-match; also XM, X-mat, X-match
cross-section; also XS
except; also X, x, x̄
exophoria distance; also x
exposure
extra
female sex chromosome
homeopathic symbol for the decimal scale of potencies
ionization exposure rate
Kienböck's unit (of x-ray exposure)
magnification
multiplied by; also x
no times
reactance (electric current); also X
removal of
respirations (anesthesia chart)
start of anesthesia
times
translocation between two X chromosomes
transverse; also xvse
unknown quantity
xanthine; also Xan
xanthosine; also Xao
xerophthalmia
X-unit; also XU, Xu

X reactance (electric current); also X
Xenopsylla species

X̄, x̄ average for all X's
except; also X,x
mean (average)
sample mean

X+ xyphoid plus (number of fingerbreadths)

X′ exophoria, near viewing; also x′

|x| absolute value of X

x abscissa (horizontal axis of rectangular coordinate system); also X, x
axis of cylindrical lens
except; also X,X̄,x̄

exophoria distance; also X
mole fraction
multiplied by; also X
roentgen (rays)

x abscissa (horizontal axis of rectangular coordinate system); also X, x

x′ exophoria, near viewing; also X′

XA xanthurenic acid

X-A xylene-alcohol (mixture)

Xa chiasma

Xaa unknown amino acid

Xan xanthine; also X

XANES x-ray absorption near-edge structure

XANT xanthochromic

Xanth xanthomatosis

Xao xanthosine; also X

XBT xylose breath test

XC, Xc excretory cystogram
excretory cystography

Xc medical decision level

XCCE extracapsular cataract extraction

XD times daily
X-linked dominant

X&D examination and diagnosis

XDH xanthine dehydrogenase

XDP xanthine diphosphate
xeroderma pigmentosum; also XP

XDR transducer

Xe xenon

XeCT xenon-enhanced computed tomography

X-ed crossed

XEF excess ejection fraction

XES x-ray energy spectrometer
x-ray energy spectrometry

XF xerophthalmic fundus

Xfmr transformer

Xgᵃ antigen in the Xg blood group system

XGP xanthogranulomatous pyelonephritis; also XPN

XH extra high

XIP x-ray in plaster

XKO not knocked out

XL excess lactate
extra large
xylose-lysine (agar base)

X-LA X-linked agammaglobulinemia

XLD xylose-lysine-deoxycholate (agar)

X-leg cross leg

XLH X-linked hypophosphatemia

XLI X-linked ichthyosis

XLJR X-linked juvenile retinoschisis

XLMR X-linked mental retardation

XLP X-linked lymphoproliferative (syndrome)

XLR X-linked recessive

XM cross-match; also X, X-mat, X-match

X_m magnetic susceptibility

X-mat, X-match cross-match; also X, XM

XMM xeromammography

XMP xanthine monophosphate (xanthosine-5'-phosphate)

XN night blindness

Xn Christian

XO gonadal dysgenesis of Turner type
presence of only one sex chromosome
xanthine oxidase

XOAN X-linked (Nettleship) ocular albinism

XOM extraocular movement

XOP x-ray out of plaster

XOR exclusive operating room

XP xeroderma pigmentosum; also XDP

Xp short arm of chromosome X

Xp- deletion of short arm of chromosome X

XPA xeroderma pigmentosum, group A

XPC xeroderma pigmentosum, group C

XPN xanthogranulomatous pyelonephritis; also XGP

X-Prep bowel evacuation prior to radiography

XPS x-ray photoemission spectroscopy

Xq long arm of chromosome X

Xq- deletion of long arm of chromosome X

XR X-linked recessive
x-ray

XRD x-ray diffraction

XRF x-ray fluorescence (spectrometry)

XRG Xonics radiography

XRT external radiation therapy
x-ray technician
x-ray therapy (radiotherapy)

XS corneal scar
cross-section; also X

excess
excessive
xiphisternum

XSA cross-sectional area
xenograph surface area

XS-LIM exceeds limits (of procedure)

XSLR crossed straight leg-raising (sign)

XSP xanthoma striatum palmare

XSPL extrasplanchnic (circulation)

XT, xT exotropia

X^2t chi-square test

X(T), x(T) intermittent exotropia

Xta chiasmata

Xtab cross-tabulating

XTE xeroderma, talipes, and enamel (defect)

XTM xanthoma tuberosum multiplex

XTP xanthosine triphosphate

XU excretory urogram
excretory urography
X-unit; also X, Xu

Xu X-unit; also X, XU

XULN times upper limit of normal

XUV extreme ultraviolet

xvse transverse; also X

XX double strength
normal female sex chromosome type

XX/XY sex karyotypes

XY normal male sex chromosome type

46,XX 46 chromosomes, 2 X chromosomes
(normal female)

46,XY 46 chromosomes, 1 X and 1 Y chromosomes (normal male)

47,XXY 47 chromosomes, 2 X and 1 Y chromosomes (Klinefelter's syndrome)

47,XY +21 47 chromosomes, male, additional chromosome 21 (Down syndrome, chromosome 21 trisomy)

47,XYY 47 chromosomes, 1 X and 2 Y chromosomes (XYY syndrome, supermale)

49,XXXXY 49 chromosomes, 4 X and 1 Y chromosomes (XXXXY syndrome)

XYL Xylocaine; also XYLO

Xyl xylose

XYLO Xylocaine; also XYL

Υ

Υ UPSILON, UPPER CASE, twentieth letter of the Greek alphabet

υ upsilon, lower case, twentieth letter of the Greek alphabet

ϒ UPSILON, UPPER CASE, twentieth letter of the Greek alphabet, variant

Y chromosome Y
  coordinate axis in plane
  male sex chromosome
  ordinate (vertical axis of rectangular coordinate system); also y, *y*
  tyrosine (one-letter notation); also Tyr, Ty
  year(s); also y, yr
  yellow; also Yel, yel
  young
  yttrium; also YT, yt

Y Yersinia species

y ordinate (vertical axis of rectangular coordinate system); also Y, *y*
  wave on phlebogram
  year(s); also Y, yr
  yield

y ordinate (vertical axis of rectangular coordinate system); also Y, y

YA Yersinia arthritis

YAC yeast artificial chromosome

YACP young adult chronic patient

YADH yeast alcohol dehydrogenase

YAG yttrium aluminum garnet
  yttrium-argon-garnet (laser)

Y/B yellow/blue

Yb ytterbium

YBT Yerkes-Bridges Test (psychology)

YCB yeast carbon base

YCT Yvon's coefficient test

yd yard(s)

yd^2 square yard(s)

yd^3 cubic yard(s)

YE yeast extract
  yellow enzyme

YEH$_2$ reduced yellow enzyme

YEI *Yersinia enterocolitica* infection

Yel, yel yellow; also Y

YET youth effectiveness training

YF yellow fever

YFI yellow fever immunization

YHMD yellow hyaline membrane disease

YHT Young-Helmholtz theory

YJV yellow jacket venom

Yk York (antibody)

YLC youngest living child

YLF yttrium lithium fluoride

YLS years of life saved

YM yeast and mold (medium)

YMA yeast morphology agar

YMM yeast minimal medium

YMT Yaba monkey tumor

Y/N yes/no

YNB yeast nitrogen base

YNS yellow nail syndrome

YO, Y/O, yo, y/o years old

YOB year of birth

YORA younger-onset rheumatoid arthritis

YP yeast phase
  yield point
  yield pressure

YPA yeast, peptone, and adenine sulfate

YPLL years of potential life lost (before age 65)

yr year(s); also Y, *y*

YRD Yangtze River disease

YS yellow spot (on retina); also ys
  yolk sac; also ys
  Yoshida's sarcoma

ys yellow spot (on retina); also YS
  yolk sac; also YS

YSC yolk sac carcinoma

YST yeast (cells)
  yolk sac tumor

YT, yt yttrium; also Y

YTD year to date

YVS yellow vernix syndrome

Z

Z ZETA, UPPER CASE, sixth letter of the Greek alphabet

ζ zeta, lower case, sixth letter of the Greek alphabet

Z 5-amino-4-imidazolecarboxamide riboside-atomic number symbol; also Z, z
benzyloxycarbonyl (carbobenzoxy) contraction [Ger. *Zuckung* (spasm, twich, jerk)]
impedance; also Z
ionic charge number
no effect
point formed by line perpendicular to nasion-menton line through anterior nasal spine
proton number
section modulus
shape of surgical incision (-plasty)
standardized deviate
standard score; also z
symbol for glutamine (Gln) or glutamic acid (Glu) (one-letter notation to denote uncertainty between the two); also Glx
Z disk (band or line that separates sarcomeres) [Ger. *Zwischenscheibe* (intermediate disk)]; also z
zero
zone

Z atomic number symbol; also Z, z
impedance; also Z

Z′, Z″ increasing degrees of contraction [Ger. *Zuckung* (spasm, twich, jerk)]

z algebraic unknown of space coordinate
atomic number symbol; also Z, Z
axis of three-dimensional rectangular coordinate system
catalytic amount
standardized device
standard normal deviate
Z disk (band or line that separates sarcomeres) [Ger. *Zwischenscheibe* (intermediate disk)]; also Z

z charge
standard score; also Z

ZAH Zerewitinov active H atom

ZAP zymosan-activated plasma (rabbit)

ZAPF zinc adequate pair-fed

ZAS zymosan-activated autologous serum

ZB zebra body

ZC zona compacta

ZCP zinc chloride poisoning

ZD zero defects; also Z/D
zero discharge
zinc deficient

Z/D zero defects; also ZD

Z-DNA form of deoxyribonucleic acid

ZDP 5-amino-4-imidazolecarboxamide riboside diphosphate

ZDDP zinc dialkyldithiophosphate

ZDO zero differential overlap (method)

ZDS zinc depletion syndrome

ZDV zidovudine

ZE, Z-E Zollinger-Ellison (syndrome)

ZEC Zinsser-Engman-Cole (syndrome)

ZEEP zero end-expiratory pressure

ZES Zollinger-Ellison syndrome

Z-ESR zeta erythrocyte sedimentation ratio

ZF zero frequency
zona fasciculata

ZFY zinc finger Y

ZG zona glomerulosa

ZGM zinc glycinate marker

Z/G zoster immune globulin (vaccine); also ZIG, ZIg

ZHC Zajdela hepatoma cell

ZI zona incerta

ZI^a isotope with atomic number Z and atomic weight A

ZIG, ZIg zoster immune globulin (vaccine); also Z/G

ZIM zimelidine

ZIO zinc iodide and osmium

ZIP zoster immune plasma

ZK Zuelzer-Kaplan (syndrome[s])

Zm zygomaxillare

ZMA zinc meta-arsenite

ZMC zygomatic
zygormaxillary complex

ZMP 5-amino-4-imidazolecarboxamide riboside monophosphate

ZN Ziehl-Neelsen (method, stain)

Zn between [Ger. *zwischen*]
zinc

Zn fl zinc flocculation (test)

ZnOE zinc oxide and eugenol (white zinc);
also ZOE

ZNG zinc gluconate

ZNP zinc pyrithione; also ZPT

ZNS Ziehl-Neelsen stain

ZO Ziehen-Oppenheim (disease)
Zuelzer-Ogden (syndrome)

Zo$_2$ microliters of oxygen taken up per hour by
10^8 spermatozoa

ZOE zinc oxide and eugenol (white zinc); also
ZnOE

Zool zoological
zoology

ZPA zone of polarizing activity

ZPC zero point of charge
zopiclone

ZPG zero population growth

ZPLS Zimmerman Preschool Language Scale

ZPO zinc peroxide

ZPP zinc protoporphyrin

ZPT zinc pyrithione; also ZNP

ZR zona reticularis

Zr zirconium

^{95}Zr zirconium 95, radioactive zirconium;
halflife, 65 days

ZSB zero stool since birth

ZSO zinc suboptimal

ZSR zeta sedimentation ratio

ZT Ziehen's test

ZTN zinc tannate of naloxone

ZTP 5-amino-4-imidazolecarboxamide riboside
triphosphate

ZTS zymosan-treated serum

Z-TSP zephiran-trisodium phosphate

ZTT zinc turbidity test

Zy zygion

ZyC zymosan-complement reagent

Zylo Zyloprim

Zz ginger [L. *zingiber*]

Z.Z.'Z." increasing degrees of contraction [Ger.
Zuckung (spasm, twich, jerk)]

Prefixes & Suffixes

Introduction

This section contains the prefixes and suffixes used in medical nomenclature. Where applicable, the notation gives the language of origin, an English translation of the root term, and a brief definition of the prefix or suffix. Terms originating from Latin and Greek are indicated by L. and Gr., respectively. Other language origins are not abbreviated. Unlike abbreviations and symbols, prefixes and suffixes generally have a single accepted meaning or a set of closely related meanings. There are some exceptions. Most of these result from the development of the same term from more than one word in a language or from more than one language. These are indicated in the text of the particular descriptions.

There are some considerations about the development of terms in modern medical nomenclature from Latin and Greek. The classical Latin alphabet consists of 23 letters. The J, U, and W were added during medieval times to give the 26 letters of the modern alphabet used in English. The letter J may appear in the Latin roots given here even though this is not proper in classical Latin. Medical terminology developed from tl more modern form of Latin, hence some medical abbreviations, prefixes, and suffixes reflec this.

The process of transliterating Greek into English is a fairly smooth one. Dr. Steven Sheeley, whose work is acknowledged in the front matter of this book, gives two explanatory notes that relate to the development of prefixes and suffixes. First, Greek does not contain the letter H. Many words that begin with R or a vowel have aspirated first syllables indicated by a "rough" breathing mark. While this H sound would normally be transliterated by placing the H before the vowel or R (ie, hr), English spelling of Greek words tends to reverse that order (ie, rh as in rheumatism). A second note concerns the transliteration of the Greek letter upsilon (υ). Where this letter would be transliterated with a U, it shows up consistently in English spelling as a Y (i.e. hyper rather than huper).

Prefixes

a-	1. [Gr. *alpha* (privative or negative), usually "an-" before a vowel]. Signifying want or absence.
	2. [L. *a* (privative or negative, from, away from), usually "an-" before a vowel]. Signifying separation or away from.
ab-	[L. *ab* (from, away from)]. Signifying from, away from, or off.
abdomin-	[L. *abdomen* (belly)]. Denoting relationship to the abdomen.
abdomino-	[L. *abdomen* (belly)]. Denoting relationship to the abdomen.
acantho-	[Gr. *akantha* (thorn or prickle)]. Denoting relationship to a sharp spine or thorn, or meaning spiny or thorny.
acaro-	[Gr. *akari*, L. *acarus* (mite)]. Denoting relationship to mites.
acet-	1. Chemical prefix denoting the two-carbon fragment of acetic acid (eg, acetyl or aceto- compounds).
	2. Chemical prefix denoting replacement of an H atom by the acetyl radical, as in acetoacetic acid.
aceto-	Chemical prefix denoting replacement of an H atom by the acetyl radical, as in acetoacetic acid.
acou-	[Gr. *akouein* (to hear)]. Denoting relationship to hearing.
acro-	[Gr. *akron* (extremity)]. Meaning extremity, tip, end, peak, or topmost.
actino-	[Gr. *aktis*, *aktinos* (ray, beam)]. Meaning a ray, as of light, or any structure with radiating parts, or pertaining to some form of radiation.
acu-	[L. *acus* (needle)]. Denoting relationship to a needle.
ad-	[L. *ad* (to)]. Denoting increase, adherence, motion toward, nearness, addition to, or intensification.
aden-	[Gr. *adēn*, *adenos* (gland)]. Denoting relationship to a gland or glands.
adeno-	[Gr. *adēn*, *adenos* (gland)]. Denoting relationship to a gland or glands.
adip-	[L. *adeps*, *adipis* (fat)]. Relating to fat.
adipo-	[L. *adeps*, *adipis* (fat)]. Relating to fat.
adren-	[L. *ad* (toward, near) + *ren* (kidney)]. Relating to the adrenal gland.
adrenal-	[L. *ad* (toward, near) + *ren* (kidney)]. Relating to the adrenal gland.
adreno-	[L. *ad* (toward, near) + *ren* (kidney)]. Relating to the adrenal gland.
aer-	[Gr. *aēr* (air or gas)]. Denoting relationship to air or gas.
aero-	[Gr. *aēr* (air or gas)]. Denoting relationship to air or gas.
alge-	[Gr. *algos* (pain)]. Relating to pain.
algesi-	[Gr. *algos* (pain)]. Relating to pain.
algo-	[Gr. *algos* (pain)]. Relating to pain.
allelo-	[Gr. *allēlōn* (to one another)]. Denoting relationship to another.
allo-	[Gr. *allos* (other)]. Meaning "other" or differing from the normal or usual, or referring to another.
alveolo-	[L. *alveolus* (trough, hollow sac, cavity)]. Denoting relationship to an alveolus or to the alveolar process.
ambi-	[L. *ambo* (both)]. Meaning on all (both) sides.
ambly-	[Gr. *amblys* (dull)]. Denoting dullness.
ambo-	[L. *ambo* (both)]. Meaning on all (both) sides.
amido-	Chemical prefix denoting the amide radical, $R-CO-NH-$ or $R-SO_2-NH-$, etc.

amino-	Chemical prefix denoting a compound containing the radical group -NH$_2$.
ammonio-	Chemical prefix meaning ammoniated.
amnio-	[Gr. *amnion* (a bowl)]. Relating to the amnion.
amphi-	[Gr. *amphi* (two-sided, on both sides)]. Meaning on both sides, around, surrounding, double.
ampho-	[Gr. *amphō* (both)]. Meaning on both sides, surrounding, double.
amygdalo-	[Gr. *amygdalē* (almond)].

        1. Denoting relationship to an almond-shaped structure.

        2. Denoting relationship to the tonsil.

amyl-	[Gr. *amylon* (starch)]. Indicating starch or polysaccharide nature or origin.
amylo-	[Gr. *amylon* (starch)]. Indicating starch or polysaccharide nature or origin.
an-	[Gr. *alpha* (privative or negative), form of "a-" used before vowels]. Signifying not, without.
ana-	[Gr. *ana* (up, back, again)]. Meaning up, toward, backward, apart.
andr-	[Gr. *anēr, andros* (male, man)].

        1. Relating to man.

        2. Pertaining to the male of the species.

andro-	[Gr. *anēr, andros* (male, man)].

        1. Relating to man.

        2. Pertaining to the male of the species.

anemo-	[Gr. *anemos* (wind)]. Denoting relationship to wind.
angi-	[Gr. *angeion* (vessel)]. Relating to blood or lymph vessels.
angio-	[Gr. *angeion* (vessel)]. Relating to blood or lymph vessels.
anhydro-	[Gr. *an* (negative) + *hydōr* (water)]. Chemical prefix denoting the removal of water.
aniso-	[Gr. *anisos* (unequal)]. Denoting unequal or dissimilar.
ankylo-	[Gr. *ankylē* (the bend of the arm, hence bent or crooked; also noose or loop)]. Meaning bent, or in the form of a noose or loop.
anomalo-	[Gr. *anōmalos* (irregular), *anōmalia* (irregularity, unevenness); from *an* (negative) + *homalos* (even)]. Meaning irregular or uneven.
ant-	[Gr. *anti* (against)].

        1. Signifying against or opposing.

        2. Denoting curative (relative to symptoms and diseases).

ante-	[L. *ante* (before)]. Signifying before in time or place.
antero-	[L. *anterior* (before)]. Denoting anterior or before.
anthraco-	[Gr. *anthrax* (coal)].

        1. Denoting relationship to coal.

        2. Denoting relationship to a carbuncle.

        3. Denoting relationship to carbon dioxide.

anthropo-	[Gr. *anthrōpŏs* (man)]. Signifying human, or denoting some relationship to man.
anti-	[Gr. *anti* (against)].

        1. Signifying against or opposing.

        2. Denoting curative (relative to symptoms and diseases).

antro-	[L. *antrum,* from Gr. *antron* (a cave)]. Denoting relationship to any antrum (any nearly closed cavity).
ap-	[Gr. *apo* (from)]. Implying separation or derivation from.
apico-	[L. *apex* (summit or tip)]. Relating to any apex.
apo-	[Gr. *apo* (from)]. Implying separation or derivation from.
appendico-	[L. *appendix* (appendage)]. Relating, usually, to the vermiform appendix.

arch-   [Gr. *archē* (origin, beginning)].
    1. Meaning primitive or ancestral.
    2. Meaning first or chief.

arche-   [Gr. *archē* (origin, beginning)].
    1. Meaning primitive or ancestral.
    2. Meaning first or chief.

archi-   [Gr. *archē* (origin, beginning)].
    1. Meaning primitive or ancestral.
    2. Meaning first or chief.

archo-   [Gr. *archos* (rectum), from *archē* (origin, beginning. The rectum was considered the first part of the bowel)].
    1. Meaning primitive or ancestral.
    2. Meaning first or chief.
    3. Denoting relationship to the rectum or anus.

arrheno-   [Gr. *arrhēn* (male)]. Meaning male.

arseno-   Chemical prefix indicating the chemical group –As:As–.

arteri-   [L. *arteria,* from Gr. *artēria* (artery)]. Denoting relationship to an artery or arteries.

arterio-   [L. *arteria,* from Gr. *artēria* (artery)]. Denoting relationship to an artery or arteries.

arteriolo-   [L. *arteriola* (arteriole)]. Relating to arterioles.

arth-   [Gr. *arthron* (joint)]. Denoting relationship to a joint, or articulation, of the skeleton.

arthr-   [Gr. *arthron* (joint)]. Denoting relationship to a joint, or articulation, of the skeleton.

arthro-   [Gr. *arthron* (joint)]. Denoting relationship to a joint, or articulation, of the skeleton.

aryl-   Chemical prefix indicating a radical belonging to the aromatic series.

astro-   [Gr. *astron* (star)]. Denoting some relation to a star, as star-shaped.

atelo-   [Gr. *atelēs* (incomplete), from *a-* (privation) + *telos* (end or fulfillment)]. Meaning incomplete or imperfect.

athero-   [Gr. *athērē* (gruel)]. Relating to the deposit of gruel-like, soft, pasty materials, for example, material in arteries.

atlanto-   [Gr. *Atlas* (in Greek mythology a Titan who supported the earth on his shoulders)]. Relating to the skeletal atlas.

atlo-   [Gr. *Atlas* (in Greek mythology a Titan who supported the earth on his shoulders)]. Relating to the skeletal atlas.

atmo-   [Gr. *atmos* (vapor or steam)]. Denoting steam or vapor, or derived by action of same.

atreto-   [Gr. *atrētos* (not perforated)]. Denoting lack of normal opening; closed.

atrio-   [L. *atrium* (entrance hall)]. Relating to the atrium.

atto-   [Danish. *atten* (eighteen)]. Denoting one-quintillionth (10^{-18}).

audio-   [L. *audio* (to hear)]. Relating to hearing.

aut-   [Gr. *autos* (self)]. Denoting relationship to self or same.

auto-   [Gr. *autos* (self)]. Denoting relationship to self or same.

aux-   [Gr. *auxanō* (to increase)]. Denoting relation to increase, eg, in size, intensity, speed.

auxano-   [Gr. *auxanō* (to increase)]. Denoting relation to increase, eg, in size, intensity, speed.

auxo-   [Gr. *auxanō* (to increase)]. Denoting relation to increase, eg, in size, intensity, speed.

axio-   [L. *axis*, Gr. *axōn* (axle)]. Denoting relationship to an axis. In dentistry, used in special reference to the long axis of a tooth.

azo-   Chemical prefix denoting the presence in a molecule of the group –N=N–; the prefix "diazo-" is also used.

balan-   [Gr. *balanos* (acorn, glans)]. Relating to the glans penis or the glans clitoridis.

balano-   [Gr. *balanos* (acorn, glans)]. Relating to the glans penis or the glans clitoridis.

baro-   [Gr. *baros* (weight)]. Denoting relationship to weight or pressure.

bary-   [Gr. *barys* (heavy)]. Meaning heavy or difficult.

baryto-   Chemical prefix indicating the presence of barium in a mineral.

basi-   [Gr. *basis* (base, that on which one stands)]. Indicating relationship to a base or foundation.

basio-   [Gr. *basis* (base, that on which one stands)]. Indicating relationship to a base or foundation.

batho-   [Gr. *bathys* (deep), *bathos* (depth)]. Meaning deep or relating to depth.

bathy-   [Gr. *bathys* (deep), *bathos* (depth)]. Meaning deep or relating to depth.

benz-   Chemical prefix denoting association with benzene.

bi-   [L. *bi* (twice, double, two)]. Meaning twice or double.

bicro-   1. pico- [Italian *piccolo* (small)]. Used in the metric system to denote one-trillionth (10^{-12}).
             2. Meaning small.

bili-   [L. *bilis* (bile)]. Relating to bile.

bio-   [Gr. *bios* (life)]. Denoting relationship to life.

bis-   [L. *bis* (two, twice)]. Signifying two or twice. Used in chemistry to denote the presence of two complex groups in one molecule.

blasto-   [Gr. *blastos* (germ, sprout or shoot)]. Pertaining to the process of budding by cells or tissue.

blenn-   [Gr. *blennos* (mucous)]. Denoting relationship to mucous.

blenno-   [Gr. *blennos* (mucous)]. Denoting relationship to mucous.

blephar-   [Gr. *blepharon* (eyelid), *blephrais* (eyelash)]. Denoting relationship to the eyelid or eyelash.

blepharo-   [Gr. *blepharon* (eyelid), *blephrais* (eyelash)]. Denoting relationship to the eyelid or eyelash.

brachy-   [Gr. *brachys* (short)]. Meaning short.

brady-   [Gr. *bradys* (slow)]. Meaning slow.

brenz-   German prefix meaning burnt.

brepho-   [Gr. *brephos* (embryo or newborn infant)].
             1. Denoting relationship to the embryo or fetus.
             2. Denoting relationship to the newborn infant.

brevi-   [L. *brevis* (short)]. Meaning short.

bronch-   [Gr. *bronchos* (windpipe)]. Denoting bronchus, and, in ancient usage, the trachea.

bronchi-   [Gr. *bronchos* (windpipe)]. Denoting bronchus, and, in ancient usage, the trachea.

bronchiolo-   [Mod. L. *bronchiolus* (windpipe)]. Relating to the bronchiolus.

broncho-   [Gr. *bronchos* (windpipe)]. Denoting bronchus, and, in ancient usage, the trachea.

bucco-   [L. *bucca* (cheek)]. Denoting relationship to the cheek.

bufa-   Denoting origin from toads. Used in trivial and systematic names of a large number of toxic substances (genins), isolated from plants and animals, containing the bufanolide structure.

bufo   Denoting origin from toads. Used in trivial and systematic names of a large number of toxic substances (genins), isolated from plants and animals, containing the bufanolide structure.

butyr-   [L. *butyrum* (butter)]. Denoting relationship to butter.

cac-   [Gr. *kakos* (bad)]. Meaning bad or ill.

caci-   [Gr. *kakos* (bad)]. Meaning bad or ill.

caco-   [Gr. *kakos* (bad)]. Meaning bad or ill.

cantho-   [Gr. *kanthos* (curve or bend)]. Denoting relationship to the canthus (the corner of the eye).

carb-   Chemical prefix indicating the attachment of a group containing a carbon atom.

carba-   Chemical prefix indicating the attachment of a group containing a carbon atom.

carbo-   Chemical prefix indicating the attachment of a group containing a carbon atom.

carboxy-   Chemical prefix indicating the addition of CO or CO_2.

cardi-   [Gr. *kardia* (heart)]. Relating to the heart.

cardia-   [Gr. *kardia* (heart)]. Relating to the heart.

cardio-   [Gr. *kardia* (heart)]. Relating to the heart.

cario-   Relating to caries.

caryo-   [Gr. *karyon* (nucleus, or nut)]. Denoting relationship to a nucleus.

cata-   [Gr. *kata* (down)]. Meaning down, lower, under, against, very.

cec-   [L. *caecum* (cecum)]. Relating to the cecum.

ceco-   [L. *caecum* (cecum)]. Relating to the cecum.

celio-   [Gr. *koilia* (belly)]. Denoting relationship to the abdomen.

celo-   1. [Gr. *koilōma* (hollow [celom])]. Relating to the celom.
                2. [Gr. *kēlē* (hernia)]. Meaning hernia or relationship to a tumor or swelling.
                3. [Gr. *koilia* (belly)]. Relating to abdomen.

ceno-   1. [Gr. *kainos* (new, fresh)]. Meaning new.
                2. [Gr. *kenos* (empty)]. Meaning empty.
                3. [Gr. *koinos* (shared in common)]. Denoting relationship to a common feature or characteristic.

centi-   [L. *centrum* (one hundred)].
                1. Denoting relationship to 100.
                2. Used in the metric system to indicate one-hundredth (10^{-2}).

centro-   [Gr. *kentron* (center)]. Relating to a center.

cephal-   [Gr. *kephalē* (head)]. Denoting relationship to the head.

cephalo-   [Gr. *kephalē* (head)]. Denoting relationship to the head.

cerebello- [L. *cerebellum* (brain)]. Relating to the cerebellum.

cerebr-   [L. *cerebrum* (brain)]. Relating to the cerebrum.

cerebri-   [L. *cerebrum* (brain)]. Relating to the cerebrum.

cerebro-   [L. *cerebrum* (brain)]. Relating to the cerebrum.

cervico-   [L. *cervix* (neck)]. Relating to a cervix, or neck, in any sense.

cheil-   [Gr. *cheilos* (lip, an edge)].
                1. Relating to the lips.
                2. Relating to an edge or brim.

cheilo-   [Gr. *cheilos* (lip, an edge)].
                1. Relating to the lips.
                2. Relating to an edge or brim.

cheir-   [Gr. *cheir* (hand)]. Denoting relationship to the hand.

cheiro-   [Gr. *cheir* (hand)]. Denoting relationship to the hand.

chem-   [Gr. *chēmeia* (alchemy)]. Relating to chemistry or a chemical.

chemo-   [Gr. *chēmeia* (alchemy)]. Relating to chemistry or a chemical.

chil-   [Gr. *cheilos* (lip, an edge)].
                1. Relating to the lips.
                2. Relating to an edge or brim.

chilo-   [Gr. *cheilos* (lip, an edge)].
                1. Relating to the lips.
                2. Relating to an edge or brim.

chir-	[Gr. *cheir* (hand)]. Denoting relationship to the hand.
chiro-	[Gr. *cheir* (hand)]. Denoting relationship to the hand.
chlor-	[Gr. *chlōros* (green)]. 1. Denoting green. 2. Denoting association with chlorine.
chloro-	[Gr. *chlōros* (green)]. 1. Denoting green. 2. Denoting association with chlorine.
chol-	[Gr. *cholē* (bile)]. Denoting relationship to bile.
chole-	[Gr. *cholē* (bile)]. Denoting relationship to bile.
choledoch-	[Gr. *cholēdochos* (containing bile), from *cholē* (bile) + *dechomai* (to receive)]. Relating to the ductus choledochus (the common bile duct).
choledocho-	[Gr. *cholēdochos* (containing bile), from *cholē* (bile) + *dechomai* (to receive)]. Relating to the ductus choledochus (the common bile duct).
cholo-	[Gr. *cholē* (bile)]. Denoting relationship to bile.
chondr-	[Gr. *chondros* (cartilage)]. Meaning or denoting relationship to cartilage or cartilaginous substance.
chondri-	[Gr. *chondrion*, diminutive of *chondros* (groats [coarsely ground grain], grit, gristle, cartilage)]. 1. Meaning or relating to granular or gritty. 2. Meaning or relating to cartilage or cartilaginous substance.
chondrio-	[Gr. *chondrion,* diminutive of *chondros* (groats [coarsely ground grain], grit, gristle, cartilage)]. 1. Meaning or relating to granular or gritty. 2. Meaning or relating to cartilage or cartilaginous substance.
chondro-	[Gr. *chondros* (cartilage)]. Meaning or denoting relationship to cartilage or cartilaginous substance.
chord-	[Gr. *chordē* (cord)]. Denoting relationship to a cord.
chordo-	[Gr. *chordē* (cord)]. Denoting relationship to a cord.
choreo-	[L. *chorea* (a dance in a ring), from Gr. *choreia* (a dance)]. Relating to chorea.
chorio-	[Gr. *chorion* (membrane)]. Relating to any membrane, but especially that which encloses the fetus.
chorioid-	[Gr. *choroeidēs*, a false reading for *chorioeidēs* (like a membrane)]. Relating to the choroid.
chorioido-	[Gr. *choroeidēs*, a false reading for *chorioeidēs* (like a membrane)]. Relating to the choroid.
choroid-	[Gr. *choroeidēs*, a false reading for *chorioeidēs* (like a membrane)]. Relating to the choroid.
choroido-	[Gr. *choroeidēs*, a false reading for *chorioeidēs* (like a membrane)]. Relating to the choroid.
chrom-	[Gr. *chrōma* (color)]. Denoting relationship to color.
chromat-	[Gr. *chrōma* (color)]. Denoting relationship to color.
chromato-	[Gr. *chrōma, chrōmatos* (color)]. Denoting relationship to color.
chromo-	[Gr. *chrōma* (color)]. Denoting relationship to color.
chrono-	[Gr. *chronos* (time)]. Relating to time.
chrys-	[Gr. *chrysos* (gold)]. Denoting relationship to gold.
chryso-	[Gr. *chrysos* (gold)]. Denoting relationship to gold.
chylo-	[L. *chylus*, Gr. *chylos* (juice, chyle)]. Relating to chyle.
cin-	[Gr. *kineō,* future *kinēsō* (to move)]. Denoting movement.

cine- [Gr. *kineō*, future *kinēsō* (to move)]. Denoting movement.

circum- [L. *circum* (around, about)]. Denoting a circular movement, or a position surrounding the part indicated by the word to which it is joined.

cirso- [Gr. *kirsos* (varix)]. Denoting relationship to a varix.

cis- [L. *cis* (on the near side of)].
1. Meaning on this side, on the near side.
2. Used in genetics to denote the location of two or more genes on the same chromosome of a homologous pair.
3. In organic chemistry, denotes a form of isomerism in which similar functional groups are attached on the same side of the plane that includes two adjacent, fixed carbon atoms.
4. Opposite of "trans-".

cleid- [Gr. *kleis* (that which serves for closing; the collar bone [clavicle], so called because it locks the breast and neck together)].
1. Denoting relationship to the clavicle.
2. Denoting relationship to something barred.

cleido- [Gr. *kleis* (that which serves for closing; the collar bone [clavicle], so called because it locks the breast and neck together)].
1. Denoting relationship to the clavicle.
2. Denoting relationship to something barred.

co- [From L. preposition *con* (with). Corresponds to Greek "syn-".]. Meaning with. A form of "con-" that appears as "co-" before a vowel and as "com-" before p, b, or m.

cocto- [L. *coctus* (boiled)]. Indicating boiled or modified by heat.

coel- [Gr. *koilia* (cavity)]. Denoting relationship to a cavity or space. Sometimes spelled "cel-".

cole- [Gr. *koleos* (sheath)].
1. Denoting relationship to the vagina.
2. Denoting relationship to a sheath.

coleo- [Gr. *koleos* (sheath)].
1. Denoting relationship to the vagina.
2. Denoting relationship to a sheath.

colo- [Gr. *kolon* (colon)]. Relating to the colon.

colp- [Gr. *kolpos* (any fold or hollow; specifically, bosom-like hollow [vagina])]. Denoting relationship to the vagina.

colpo- [Gr. *kolpos* (any fold or hollow; specifically, bosom-like hollow [vagina])]. Denoting relationship to the vagina.

com- [From L. preposition *con* (with). Corresponds to Greek "syn-".]. Meaning with. A form of "con-" that appears as "com-" before p, b, or m, and as "co-" before a vowel.

con- [From L. preposition *con* (with). Corresponds to Greek "syn-".]. Meaning with. Appears as "com-" before p, b, or m, and as "co-" before a vowel.

contra- [L. *contra* (opposite, against)]. Signifying opposed, against.

copro- [Gr. *kopros* (dung)]. Relating to the feces.

cord- [Gr. *chordē* (cord)]. Denoting relationship to a cord.

core- [Gr. *korē* (pupil)]. Relating to the pupil of the eye.

coreo- [Gr. *korē* (pupil)]. Relating to the pupil of the eye.

coro- [Gr. *korē* (pupil)]. Relating to the pupil of the eye.

costo- [L., Gr. *costa* (rib)]. Relating to the ribs.

counter- [L. *countra* (against)]. Meaning opposite, opposed, against.

crani- [L. *cranium*, from Gr. *kranion* (skull)]. Denoting relationship to the cranium.

cranio- [L. *cranium*, from Gr. *kranion* (skull)]. Denoting relationship to the cranium.

cry- [Gr. *kryos* (cold)]. Relating to cold.

crymo- [Gr. *krymos* (cold, frost)]. Relating to cold.

cryo- [Gr. *kryos* (cold)]. Relating to cold.

crypt- [Gr. *kryptos* (hidden, concealed)].
    1. Relating to a crypt.
    2. Meaning hidden, obscure.
    3. Meaning without apparent cause.

crypto- [Gr. *kryptos* (hidden, concealed)].
    1. Relating to a crypt.
    2. Meaning hidden, obscure.
    3. Meaning without apparent cause.

cyan- [Gr. *kyanos* (blue)].
    1. Meaning blue.
    2. Chemical prefix frequently used in naming compounds that contain the cyanide group, CN, as part of the molecule.

cyano- [Gr. *kyanos* (blue)].
    1. Meaning blue.
    2. Chemical prefix frequently used in naming compounds that contain the cyanide group, CN, as part of the molecule.

cycl- [Gr. *kyklos* (circle)].
    1. Relating to a circle or cycle.
    2. Denoting association with the ciliary body of the eye.
    3. Chemical prefix indicating a continuous molecule, without end, or the formation of such a structure between two parts of a molecule.

cyclo- [Gr. *kyklos* (circle)].
    1. Relating to a circle or cycle.
    2. Denoting association with the ciliary body of the eye.
    3. Chemical prefix indicating a continuous molecule, without end, or the formation of such a structure between two parts of a molecule.

cymbo- [L. *cymba*, from Gr. *kymbē* (boat)]. Meaning boat-shaped.

cyn- [Gr. *kyōn* (dog)]. Meaning dog-like, or denoting relationship to a dog.

cyno- [Gr. *kyōn* (dog)]. Meaning dog-like, or denoting relationship to a dog.

cyst- [Gr. *kystis* (sac or bladder)].
    1. Relating to the urinary bladder.
    2. Relating to the cystic duct.
    3. Denoting a cyst or sac.

cysti- [Gr. *kystis* (sac or bladder)].
    1. Relating to the urinary bladder.
    2. Relating to the cystic duct.
    3. Denoting a cyst or sac.

cystido- [Gr. *kystis, kystides* (sac or bladder)].
    1. Relating to the urinary bladder.
    2. Relating to the cystic duct.
    3. Denoting a cyst or sac.

cysto- [Gr. *kystis, kystides* (sac or bladder)].
    1. Relating to the urinary bladder.
    2. Relating to the cystic duct.
    3. Denoting a cyst or sac.

cyt- [Gr. *kytos* (hollow vessel; anything that contains or covers)]. Meaning or denoting relationship to a cell.

cyto-   [Gr. *kytos* (hollow vessel; anything that contains or covers)]. Meaning or denoting relationship to a cell.

D-
1. Chemical prefix, printed as a small capital letter, indicating a chemical compound to be sterically related to δ-glyceraldehyde, the basis of stereochemical nomenclature.
2. In carbohydrate nomenclature, refers to the configurational family of the highest numbered asymmetric carbon atom.
3. In amino acid nomenclature, refers to the configurational family of the lowest numbered asymmetric carbon atom.
4. Opposed to L-.

D$_g$-   Chemical prefix used to emphasize that the rules of carbohydrate nomenclature are being employed. The subscript refers to the standard substance glyceraldehyde. Opposed to L$_g$-.

D$_s$-   Chemical prefix used in amino acid nomenclature to avoid possible confusion with carbohydrate nomenclature. The subscript refers to the standard substance serine. Opposed to L$_s$-.

d-   Chemical prefix (for "dextro-"), printed as a lower case italicized letter, indicating a chemical compound to be dextrorotatory. Opposed to *l-* ("levo-").

dacry-   [Gr. *dakryon* (tear)]. Relating to tears, or to the lacrimal sac or duct.

dacryo-   [Gr. *dakryon* (tear)]. Relating to tears, or to the lacrimal sac or duct.

dactyl-   [Gr. *daktylos* (finger)]. Relating to the fingers, and sometimes to the toes.

dactylo-   [Gr. *daktylos* (finger)]. Relating to the fingers, and sometimes to the toes.

de-   [L. *de* (from, away)].
1. Often carrying a privation or negative sense.
2. Denoting away from or cessation, and is frequently intensive.

deca-   [Gr. *deka* (ten)]. Used in the metric system to signify ten (10^1).

deci-   [L. *decimus* (tenth)]. Used in the metric system to signify one-tenth (10^{-1}).

dehydro-   Chemical prefix used in the names of those compounds that differ from other and more familiar compounds in the absence of two hydrogen atoms.

deka-   [Gr. *deka* (ten)]. Used in the metric system to signify ten. (10^1)

demi-   [L. *dimidius* (half), from *di-*(apart) + *medius* (middle)]. Denoting one-half.

dent-   [L. *dens* (tooth)]. Denoting relationship to a tooth or the teeth.

denta-   [L. *dens* (tooth)]. Denoting relationship to a tooth or the teeth.

denti-   [L. *dens* (tooth)]. Denoting relationship to a tooth or the teeth.

dentia-   [L. *dens* (tooth)]. Denoting relationship to a tooth or the teeth.

dento-   [L. *dens* (tooth)]. Denoting relationship to a tooth or the teeth.

deoxy-   Newer prefix indicating less oxygen than the reference material. Used in chemical names of substances containing carbohydrate moieties to indicate replacement of an –OH by an H. The spelling "desoxy-" is retained in some instances, and is official in the United States Pharmacopeia.

der-   [Gr. *derē* (neck)]. Denoting relationship to the neck.

derm-   [Gr. *derma, dermatos* (skin)]. Signifying relationship to the skin.

derma-   [Gr. *derma, dermatos* (skin)]. Signifying relationship to the skin.

dermat-   [Gr. *derma, dermatos* (skin)]. Signifying relationship to the skin.

dermato-   [Gr. *derma, dermatos* (skin)]. Signifying relationship to the skin.

dermo-   [Gr. *derma, dermatos* (skin)]. Signifying relationship to the skin.

des-   [L. *de* (from, away)].
1. Often carrying a privative or negative sense.
2. Denoting away from or cessation.

desm-   [Gr. *desmos* (band)].
                1. Meaning fibrous connection.
                2. Denoting relationship to a band or ligament.

desmo-   [Gr. *desmos* (band)].
                1. Meaning fibrous connection.
                2. Denoting relationship to a band or ligament.

desoxy-   Older prefix indicating less oxygen, used in chemical names of substances containing carbohydrate moieties to indicate replacement of an –OH by an H. The spelling "desoxy-" is official in the United States Pharmacopeia, but is generally replaced by "deoxy-".

deut-   [Gr. *deuteros* (second)]. Meaning two, or second (in a series).

deuterio-   Indicating "containing deuterium."

deutero-   [Gr. *deuteros* (second)]. Meaning two, or second (in a series).

deuto-   [Gr. *deuteros* (second)]. Meaning two, or second (in a series).

dextro-   [L. *dexter* (right)].
                1. Meaning right, toward or on the right side.
                2. Chemical prefix meaning dextrorotatory for which the symbol "+" is frequently substituted.
                3. Opposed to "levo-".

di-   [Gr. *dis* (two, twice, double)]. Denoting two, twice.

dia-   [Gr. *dia* (through)].
                1. Meaning across or apart.
                2. Meaning through, throughout, completely, or between.

diamido-   Chemical prefix indicating the possession of two amido groups.

diazo-   [Gr. *di-* (two) + French *azote* (nitrogen)]. Chemical prefix denoting a compound containing the $-N=N-$ or $N\equiv N-$ group.

didym-   [Gr. *didymos* (twin)]. Denoting relationship to the didymus (testis).

didymo-   [Gr. *didymos* (twin)]. Denoting relationship to the didymus (testis).

dihydro-   Chemical prefix indicating the addition of two hydrogen atoms.

dihydroxy-   Chemical prefix denoting the addition of two hydroxyl (OH) groups.

diiodo-   Chemical prefix indicating two atoms of iodine.

diplo-   [Gr. *diplous* (double)]. Meaning double, two-fold, twin, or twice.

dis-   [L. *dis-* (asunder, apart, in two)]. Meaning separation, taking apart, sundering in two.

disc-   [Gr. *diskos* (disk)]. Indicating relation or similarity to a disk.

disco-   [Gr. *diskos* (disk)]. Indicating relation or similarity to a disk.

DL-   Chemical prefix denoting that the substance consists of equal quantities of two enantiomorphs, one of which corresponds in configuration to D-glyceraldehyde, the other to L-glyceraldehyde.

dl-   Chemical prefix denoting that the substance consists of equal quantities of the dextrorotatory and levorotatory enantiomorphs, such as is produced by chemical synthesis without resolution or by the process of racemization.

dolicho-   [Gr. *dolichos* (long)]. Meaning long.

dorsi-   [L. *dorsum* (back)]. Denoting relationship to the back (posterior) aspect of an anatomic part or structure, or to the back of the body.

dorso-   [L. *dorsum* (back)]. Denoting relationship to the back (posterior) aspect of an anatomic part or structure, or to the back of the body.

dromo-   [Gr. *dromos* (a course)].
                1. Denoting relationship to conduction.
                2. Denoting running.

duodeno-	[Medieval L. *duodenum,* from L. *duodeni* (twelve)]. Relating to the duodenum (about 11 inches or 12 finger-breadths in length).
dynamo-	[Gr. *dynamis* (force, power)]. Relating to force, energy, power, or strength.
dys-	[Gr. *dys-* (bad, unlucky, difficult)]. Conveying the idea of bad, difficult, or painful. Opposite of "eu-".
ec-	[Gr. *ek* (from out of, from)]. Meaning out of, away from.
echin-	[Gr. *echinos* (hedgehog, sea urchin)]. Meaning prickly or spiny.
echino-	[Gr. *echinos* (hedgehog, sea urchin)]. Meaning prickly or spiny.
ect-	[Gr. *ektos* (outside)]. Denoting outer, on the outside.
ecto-	[Gr. *ektos* (outside)]. Denoting outer, on the outside.
eka-	[Sanscrit "one" or "first"]. Chemical prefix added to the name of a known chemical element as a provisional designation of the unknown element that should occur next in the same group in the periodic system.
electro-	[Gr *ēlektron* (amber [electricity])]. Denoting relationship to electric or electricity.
eleo-	[Gr. *elaion* (olive oil)]. Relating to oil.
elytro-	[Gr. *elytron* (sheath [vagina])].
	1. Denoting relationship to the vagina.
	2. Denoting relationship to a sheath.
em-	[Gr. *en* (in)]. Meaning in; a form of "en-" that appears as "em-" before b, p, or m.
embry-	[Gr. *embryon* (embryo)]. Relating to the embryo.
embryo-	[Gr. *embryon* (embryo)]. Relating to the embryo.
en-	[Gr. *en* (in)]. Meaning in; appears as "em-" before b, p, or m.
encephal-	[Gr. *enkephalos* (brain)]. Indicating the brain or some relationship to the brain.
encephalo-	[Gr. *enkephalos* (brain)]. Indicating the brain or some relationship to the brain.
end-	[Gr. *endon* (within)]. Indicating within, inner, absorbing, or containing.
endo-	[Gr. *endon* (within)]. Indicating within, inner, absorbing, or containing.
ent-	[Gr. *entos* (within)]. Meaning inner or within.
enter-	[Gr. *enteron* (intestine)]. Relating to the intestines.
entero-	[Gr. *enteron* (intestine)]. Relating to the intestines.
ento-	[Gr. *entos* (within)]. Meaning inner or within.
entomo-	[Gr. *entomon* (insect)]. Denoting relationship to an insect, or to insects.
epi-	[Gr. *epi* (on, upon, against)]. Meaning upon, following, or subsequent to.
epiplo-	[Gr. *epiploon* (omentum)]. Relating to the omentum.
episio-	[Gr. *epision* (the region of the pubes)]. Denoting relationship to the vulva.
epithelio-	[L. *epithelium,* from Gr. *epi* (on) and thēlē (nipple)]. Denoting relationship to the epithelium.
ergo-	[Gr. *ergon* (work)]. Denoting relationship to work.
eroto-	[Gr. *erōs* (love)]. Denoting relationship to love or sexual desire.
erythro-	[Gr. *erythros* (red)]. Meaning red, or relationship to red.
eso-	[Gr. *esō* (inward)]. Meaning within.
ethmo-	[Gr. *ēthmos* (sieve)]. Meaning ethmoid or relating to the ethmoid bone.
etio-	[Gr. *aitia* (cause)].
	1. Meaning cause.
	2. Chemical prefix used to indicate replacement of the C-17 side chain by H.
eu-	[Gr. *eu* (well)]. Meaning good, well, easily; opposite of *dys-*.
eury-	[Gr. *eurys* (wide)]. Meaning wide or broad.
ex-	[L. and Gr. *ex* (from out of, from)]. Denoting out of, from, away from, or outside; sometimes used to denote completely.

exa-	Prefix used in the metric system to signify quintillion (10^{18}).
exo-	[Gr. *exō* (outside)]. Meaning exterior, external, outward, or outside.
extra-	[L. *extra, exter* (outside, beyond, in addition)]. Meaning beyond, outside of, or in addition.
facio-	[L. *facies* (face)]. Denoting relationship to the face.
fascio-	[L. *fascia* (a band or fillet)]. Relating to a fascia.
femto-	[Danish *femten* (fifteen)]. Used in the metric system to signify one-quadrillionth (10^{-15}) of any unit.
ferri-	[L. *ferrum* (iron)]. Chemical prefix designating the presence in a compound of a ferric ion (Fe^{+++}).
ferro-	[L. *ferrum* (iron)]. Chemical prefix designating the presence of metallic iron or of the divalent ion Fe^{++} in a compound.
fibr-	[L. *fibra* (fiber)]. Denoting relationship to fibers.
fibro-	[L. *fibra* (fiber)]. Denoting relationship to fibers.
fluo-	[L. *fluo, fluere* (to flow)]. Denoting flow.
fructo-	[L. *fructus* (fruit)]. Prefix to the suffixes -furanose, -pyranose, -syl, -side, -san, etc, indicating the fructose configuration.
fructosyl-	Chemical prefix indicating fructose in –C–R– (not –C–O–R–) linkage through its carbon-2 (R usually C).
galact-	[Gr. *gala, galaktos* (milk)]. Denoting relationship to milk.
galacta-	[Gr. *gala, galaktos* (milk)]. Denoting relationship to milk.
galacto-	[Gr. *gala, galaktos* (milk)]. Denoting relationship to milk.
galvano-	[Named for Italian discoverer of galvanic current, Luigi Galvani]. Meaning electrical, denoting primarily direct current.
gam-	[Gr. *gamos* (marriage)]. Denoting relationship to marriage or sexual union.
gameto-	[Gr. *gametēs* (husband), *gametē* (wife)]. Relating to a gamete.
gamo-	[Gr. *gamos* (marriage)]. Denoting relationship to marriage or sexual union.
gangli-	[Gr. *ganglion* (knot)]. Denoting relationship to a ganglion.
ganglio-	[Gr. *ganglion* (knot)]. Denoting relationship to a ganglion.
gastr-	[Gr. *gastēr, gastr-* (stomach)]. Denoting relationship to the stomach or abdomen.
gastro-	[Gr. *gastēr, gastr-* (stomach)]. Denoting relationship to the stomach or abdomen.
gem-	[L. shortened form of *geminus* (twin)]. Chemical prefix denoting twin substitutions on a single atom.
gen-	[Gr. *gennaō* (birth)]. Meaning producing or coming to be.
genito-	[L. *genitalis* (belonging to birth)]. Denoting relationship to the organs of reproduction.
geno-	[Gr. *gennaō* (to produce)]. Denoting relationship to reproduction or to sex.
geny-	[Gr. *genys* (jaw)]. Denoting relationship to the jaw.
geo-	[Gr. *gē* (earth)]. Relating to the earth or to soil.
ger-	[Gr. *gēras* (old age), Gr. *gerōn* (old man)]. Relating to old age or the aged.
gerat-	[Gr. *gēras* (old age)]. Relating to old age or the aged.
gero-	[Gr. *gerōn* (old man)]. Relating to old age or the aged.
geront-	[Gr. *gerōn* (old man)]. Relating to old age or the aged.
geronto-	[Gr. *gerōn* (old man)]. Relating to old age or the aged.
giga-	[Gr. *gigas* (giant, mighty)]. Prefix used in the metric system to signify one billion (10^9).
giganto-	[Gr. *gigas, gigantos* (giant, huge)]. Meaning huge or gigantic size.
gingivo-	[L. *gingiva* (gum)]. Relating to the gingiva (gum).
glio-	[Gr. *glia* (glue)]. Denoting relationship to a gluey substance, specifically to the neuroglia.

gloss-	[Gr. *glōssa* (tongue)]. Relating to the tongue.
glosso-	[Gr. *glōssa* (tongue)]. Relating to the tongue.
gluco-	[Gr. *gleukos* (sweetness)]. Denoting relationship to glucose.
glyco-	[Gr. *glykys* (sweet)]. Denoting relationship to sugars in general.
gnath-	[Gr. *gnathos* (jaw)]. Relating to the jaw.
gnatho-	[Gr. *gnathos* (jaw)]. Relating to the jaw.

gon-	1. [Gr. *gonē* (seed)].
	  a. Denoting relationship to seed.
	  b. Denoting relationship to semen.
	2. [Gr. *gony* (knee)]. Denoting relationship to the knee.

gonad-	[Modern L. *gonas,* from Gr. *gonē* (seed)]. Relating to the gonads.
gonado-	[Modern L. *gonas,* from Gr. *gonē* (seed)]. Relating to the gonads.
gonio-	[Gr. *gōnia* (angle)]. Denoting relationship to an angle.

gono-	[Gr. *gonē* (seed)].
	  1. Denoting relationship to seed.
	  2. Denoting relationship to the semen.

gony-	[Gr. *gony* (knee)]. Denoting relationship to the knee.
granulo-	[L. *granulum* (granule)]. Meaning granular, or denoting relationship to granules.
grapho-	[Gr. *graphō* (to write), *graphein* (to record)]. Denoting a writing, or description.
gymno-	[Gr. *gymnos* (naked)]. Meaning naked or denoting relationship to nakedness.
gyn-	[Gr. *gynē, gynaikos* (woman)]. Denoting relationship to woman or the female sex.
gyne-	[Gr. *gynē, gynaikos* (woman)]. Denoting relationship to woman or the female sex.
gyneco-	[Gr. *gynē, gynaikos* (woman)]. Denoting relationship to woman or the female sex.
gyno-	[Gr. *gynē, gynaikos* (woman)]. Denoting relationship to woman or the female sex.

gyro-	[Gr. *gyros* (ring or circle)].
	  1. Meaning round.
	  2. Denoting relationship to a gyrus.

haem-	[Gr. *haima, haimatos* (blood)]. Denoting relationship to blood.
haemo-	[Gr. *haima, haimatos* (blood)]. Denoting relationship to blood.
halo-	[Gr. *halas* (salt)]. Denoting relationship to a salt.
hamarto-	[Gr. *hamartia* (defect, sin)]. Denoting relationship to a defect.
haplo-	[Gr. *haploos* (single, simple)]. Meaning single or simple.
hapt-	[Gr. *haptein* (to touch, seize upon, or hold fast)]. Denoting relationship to touch or seizure.
hapte-	[Gr. *haptein* (to touch, seize upon, or hold fast)]. Denoting relationship to touch or seizure.
hapto-	[Gr. *haptein* (to touch, seize upon, or hold fast)]. Denoting relationship to touch or seizure.
hecto-	[Gr. *hekaton* (one hundred)]. Used in the metric system to signify one hundred (10^2).

helico-	[Gr. *helix* (coil)].
	  1. Denoting relationship to a coil.
	  2. Denoting relationship to a snail.

helio-	[Gr. *hēlios* (sun)]. Denoting relationship to the sun.

helo-	[Gr. *hēlos* (nail, corn, or callus)].
	  1. Denoting relationship to a nail.
	  2. Denoting relationship to a wart or callus.

hem-	[Gr. *haima, haimatos* (blood)]. Denoting relationship to blood.
hema-	[Gr. *haima, haimatos* (blood)]. Denoting relationship to blood.

hemangio- [Gr. *haima* (blood) + *angeion* (vessel)]. Relating to the blood vessels.

hemat- [Gr. *haima*, *haimatos* (blood)]. Denoting relationship to blood.

hemata- [Gr. *haima*, *haimatos* (blood)]. Denoting relationship to blood.

hemato- [Gr. *haima*, *haimatos* (blood)]. Denoting relationship to blood.

hemi- [Gr. *hēmi-* (half). Corresponds to Latin "semi-".]. Signifying one-half.

hemo- [Gr. *haima*, *haimatos* (blood)]. Denoting relationship to blood.

hepat- [Gr. *hēpar*, *hēpat-* (liver)]. Denoting relationship to the liver.

hepatico- [Gr. *hēpar*, *hēpat-* (liver)]. Denoting relationship to the liver.

hepato- [Gr. *hēpar*, *hēpat-* (liver)]. Denoting relationship to the liver.

hept- [Gr. *hepta* (seven)]. Denoting seven.

hepta- [Gr. *hepta* (seven)]. Denoting seven.

heredo- [L. *heres* (an heir)]. Denoting heredity.

hernio- [L. *hernia* (rupture)]. Relating to hernia.

heter- [Gr. *heteros* (other)]. Meaning other or different, or denoting relationship to another.

hetero- [Gr. *heteros* (other)]. Meaning other or different, or denoting relationship to another.

hex- [Gr. *hex* (six)]. Denoting six.

hexa- [Gr. *hex* (six)]. Denoting six.

hidro- [Gr. *hidrōs* (sweat)]. Denoting relationship to sweat or a sweat gland.

hier- [Gr. *hieron* (sacred, or sacrum)].
  1. Denoting relationship to the sacrum.
  2. Denoting relationship to religion.

hiero- [Gr. *hieron* (sacred, or sacrum)].
  1. Denoting relationship to the sacrum.
  2. Denoting relationship to religion.

hippo- [Gr. *hippos* (horse)]. Denoting relationship to a horse.

hist- [Gr. *histos* (web, tissue)]. Denoting relationship to tissue.

histio- [Gr. *histion*, diminutive of *histos* (web, tissue)]. Relating to tissue.

histo- [Gr. *histos* (web, tissue)]. Denoting relationship to tissue.

hol- [Gr. *holos* (whole, entire, complete)]. Denoting entirety or relationship to a whole.

holo- [Gr. *holos* (whole, entire, complete)]. Denoting entirety or relationship to a whole.

homeo- [Gr. *homoios* (like, unchanging)]. Meaning the same, alike, or a constant unchanging state.

homo- [Gr. *homos* (the same)]. Meaning the same or alike.

homoeo- [Gr. *homoios* (like, unchanging)]. Meaning the same, alike, or a constant unchanging state.

homoio- [Gr. *homoios* (like, unchanging)]. Meaning the same, alike, or a constant unchanging state.

hyal- [Gr. *hyalos* (glass)]. Denoting resemblance to glass.

hyalo- [Gr. *hyalos* (glass)]. Denoting resemblance to glass.

hydr- [Gr. *hydōr* (water)]. Denoting association with water or hydrogen.

hydro- [Gr. *hydōr* (water)]. Denoting association with water or hydrogen.

hydroxy- Chemical prefix indicating addition or substitution of the –OH group to or in the compound whose name follows.

hygro- [Gr. *hygros* (moist)]. Meaning moist or denoting relationship to moisture.

hyl- [Gr. *hylē* (matter)]. Denoting relationship to matter.

hyle- [Gr. *hylē* (matter)]. Denoting relationship to matter.

hylo- [Gr. *hylē* (matter)]. Denoting relationship to matter.

hyp-   [Gr. *hypo* (under); variation of "hypo-" often used before a vowel, equivalent to Latin "sub-".].
1. Denoting a location beneath something else.
2. Denoting a diminution or deficiency.
3. Denoting the lowest, or least rich in oxygen, of a series of chemical compounds.

hyper-   [Gr. *hyper* (above, over), equivalent to Latin "super-".]. Denoting excessive, above the normal, or beyond.

hypno-   [Gr. *hypnos* (sleep)].
1. Relating to sleep.
2. Relating to hypnosis.

hypo-   [Gr. *hypo* (under); equivalent to Latin "sub-".].
1. Denoting a location beneath something else.
2. Denoting a diminution or deficiency.
3. Denoting the lowest, or least rich in oxygen, of a series of chemical compounds.

hypsi-   [Gr. *hypsi* (high)]. Meaning high, or denoting relationship to height.

hypso-   [Gr. *hýpsos* (height)]. Denoting relationship to height.

hyster-   1. [Gr. *hystera* (uterus)].
a. Denoting the uterus.
b. Denoting hysteria.
2. [Gr. *hysteros* (later)]. Meaning late or following.

hystero-   1. [Gr. *hystera* (uterus)].
a. Denoting the uterus.
b. Denoting hysteria.
2. [Gr. *hysteros* (later)]. Meaning late or following.

iatro-   [Gr. *iatros* (physician)]. Denoting relationship to physicians or medicine.

ichthyo-   [Gr. *ichthys* (fish)]. Denoting relationship to fish.

ideo-   [Gr. *idea* (form, notion)]. Pertaining to ideas or ideation.

idio-   [Gr. *idios* (one's own)]. Meaning private, distinctive, peculiar to or relationship to self.

ileo-   [L. *ileum*, Gr. *eileō* (to roll up, twist)]. Denoting relationship to the ileum.

ilio-   [L. *ilium* (groin, flank)]. Denoting relationship to the ilium or flank.

im-   Chemical prefix indicating the bivalent group >NH.

imido-   Chemical prefix denoting a compound containing an imide group (=NH attached to one or two carbons), attached to an acid radical.

imino-   Chemical prefix denoting a compound containing an imide group (=NH attached to one or two carbons), attached to a non-acid radical.

in-   1. [L. *in* (in, on, into, to), *in-* (negative particle, un-, not)].
a. Conveying a sense of negation.
b. Denoting in, within, inside.
c. Denoting an intensive action.
2. [Gr. *is, inos* (fiber)]. Denoting fibrous tissue or fibrin. Appears as "im-" before b, p, or m.

increto-   [L. *in* (within) + *secernere* (to separate)]. Pertaining to internal secretion.

infra-   [L. *infra* (underneath, below)]. Meaning situated, formed, or occurring below or beneath the part denoted by the word to which it is joined.

inio-   [Gr. *inion* (occiput)]. Denoting relationship to the occiput.

ino-   [Gr. *is, inos* (fiber)]. Obsolete combining form relating to fiber, or meaning fibrous. In most terms it is replaced by "fibro-".

inter-   [L. *inter* (between)]. Conveying the meaning of between, among.

intra-	[L. *intra* (on the inside, within; during)]. Meaning situated, found, or occurring within the element indicated by the word to which it is joined.
intro-	[L. *intro* (into, within)]. Meaning into or within.
irid-	[Gr. *iris*, *iridos* (rainbow)]. 1. Relating to the iris of the eye. 2. Relating to a colored circle.
irido-	[Gr. *iris*, *iridos* (rainbow)]. 1. Relating to the iris of the eye. 2. Relating to a colored circle.
ischio-	[Gr. *ischion* (hip-joint, haunch [ischium])]. Relating to the ischium or the hip.
ischo-	[Gr. *ischein* (to suppress)]. Meaning suppressed, or denoting relationship to suppression.
iso-	[Gr. *isos* (equal)]. Meaning equal, like, or the same.
jejuno-	[L. *jejunum* (empty)]. Denoting relationship to the jejunum.
kal-	[L. *kalium* (potassium)]. Relating to potassium. Sometimes the combining form "kalio" is used, but this is improper.
kali-	[L. *kalium* (potassium)]. Relating to potassium. Sometimes the combining form "kalio-" is used, but this is improper.
kalio-	[L. *kalium* (potassium)]. Relating to potassium.
kat-	[Gr. *kata* (down)]. Meaning down or against.
kata-	[Gr. *kata* (down)]. Meaning down or against.
karyo-	[Gr. *karyon* (nut, nucleus)]. Denoting relationship to a nucleus.
keno-	[Gr. *kenos* (empty)]. Signifying empty.
kerat-	[Gr. *keras* (horn, cornea)]. 1. Denoting the cornea. 2. Denoting horny tissue or cells.
kerato-	[Gr. *keras* (horn, cornea)]. 1. Denoting the cornea. 2. Denoting horny tissue or cells.
keto-	In chemistry, used with reference to any compound containing a ketone group (–CCOC–).
kilo-	[Gr. *chilioi* (one thousand)]. Prefix used in the metric system to signify one thousand (10^3).
kin-	[Gr. *kinēsis* (movement)]. Denoting movement or relationship to movement.
kine-	[Gr. *kinēsis* (movement)]. Denoting movement or relationship to movement.
kinesio-	[Gr. *kinēsis* (movement)]. Denoting movement or relationship to movement.
kineto-	[Gr. *kinēteos* (moving, movable)]. Meaning moveable or relating to motion.
kino-	[Gr. *kinein* (to move)]. Denoting relationship to movement.
klepto-	[Gr. *kleptein* (to steal)]. Denoting relationship to theft or stealing.
koilo-	[Gr. *koilos* (hollow)]. Meaning hollow or concave.
krymo-	[Gr. *krymos*, *kryos* (cold)]. Denoting cold.
kryo-	[Gr. *krymos*, *kryos* (cold)]. Denoting cold.
kysth-	[Gr. *kysthos* (vagina)]. Denoting or relating to the vagina.
kystho-	[Gr. *kysthos* (vagina)]. Denoting or relating to the vagina.
kyto-	[Gr. *kytos* (a hollow, a receptacle)]. Denoting or relating to a cell.
L-	1. Chemical prefix, printed as a small capital letter, specifying that the substance corresponds in configuration to the standard substance L-glyceraldehyde. 2. In carbohydrate nomenclature, refers to the configurational family of the highest numbered asymmetric carbon atom.

3. In amino acid nomenclature, under rules adopted in 1947, refers to the configurational family of the lowest numbered asymmetric carbon atom.

4. Opposed to D-.

L_g- Chemical prefix occasionally used to emphasize that the rules of carbohydrate nomenclature are being employed. The subscript refers to the standard substance glyceraldehyde. Opposed to D_g-.

L_s- Chemical prefix used in amino acid nomenclature to avoid possible confusion with carbohydrate nomenclature. The subscript refers to the standard substance serine. Opposed to D_s-.

labio- [L. *labium* (lip)]. Denoting relationship to the lips, especially of the mouth.

lacri- [L. *lacrima* (tear)]. Pertaining to the tears.

lact- [L. *lac, lactis* (milk)]. Denoting relationship to milk.

lacto- [L. *lac, lactis* (milk)]. Denoting relationship to milk.

lalo- [Gr. *lalein* (to babble or speak)]. Denoting relationship to speech or babbling.

laparo- [Gr. *lapara* (flank, loins)]. Denoting relationship to the loins or flank, or, less properly, the abdomen in general.

laryng- [Gr. *larynx* (larynx)]. Relating to the larynx.

laryngo- [Gr. *larynx* (larynx)]. Relating to the larynx.

latero- [L. *latus* (side)]. Denoting relationship to the side; on the side (position).

lecitho- [Gr. *lekithos* (yolk)]. Denoting relationship to the yolk of an egg or ovum.

leio- [Gr. *leios* (smooth)]. Meaning smooth.

lepto- [Gr. *leptos* (slender)]. Meaning light, slender, thin, or frail.

leuc- [Gr. *leukos* (white)]. Meaning white.

leuco- [Gr. *leukos* (white)]. Meaning white.

leuk- [Gr. *leukos* (white)]. Meaning white.

leuko- [Gr. *leukos* (white)]. Meaning white.

levo- [L. *laevus* (left)].

1. Denoting left, toward the left or on the left.

2. Chemical prefix meaning levorotatory for which the symbol "-" is frequently substituted.

3. Opposed to dextro-.

lien- [L. *lien* (spleen)]. Obsolete prefix relating to the spleen. The preferred prefix is "splen".

lieno- [L. *lien* (spleen)]. Obsolete prefix relating to the spleen. The preferred prefix is "spleno".

lip- [Gr. *lipos* (fat)]. Denoting relationship to fat, or lipid.

lipo- [Gr. *lipos* (fat)]. Denoting relationship to fat, or lipid.

lith- [Gr. *lithos* (stone)]. Relating to a stone or calculus, or to calcification.

litho- [Gr. *lithos* (stone)]. Relating to a stone or calculus, or to calcification.

logo- [Gr. *logos* (word)]. Denoting relationship to words or speech.

lymph- [L. *lympha* (water [especially clear spring or river water], lymph)]. Relating to lymph.

lympho- [L. *lympha* (water [especially clear spring or river water], lymph)]. Relating to lymph.

lyo- [Gr. *lyein* (to dissolve)]. Meaning dissolved.

lyso- [Gr. *lysis* (dissolution)]. Indicating lysis or dissolution.

lysso- [Gr. *lyssa* (frenzy)]. Denoting relationship to rabies or hydrophobia.

macr- [Gr. *makros* (large, long)]. Meaning large or abnormal size or length.

macro- [Gr. *makros* (large, long)]. Meaning large or abnormal size or length.

malaco- [Gr. *malakos* (soft)]. Meaning a condition of abnormal softness.

mammo-	[L. *mamma*, Gr. *mammē* (the mother's breast)]. Denoting relationship to the breast (mammary gland).
mast-	[Gr. *mastos* (breast)]. Denoting relationship to the breast.
masto-	[Gr. *mastos* (breast)]. Denoting relationship to the breast.
mechano-	[Gr. *mēchanē* (machine)]. Meaning mechanical or denoting relationship to a machine.
meco-	[Gr. *mēkos* (length)]. Indicating length.

mega-	[Gr. *megas* (big, great)].
	    1. Meaning large, oversize.
	    2. Used in the metric system to signify one million (10^6).

megal-	[Gr. *megas* (large), *megaleios* (magnificent)]. Meaning large.
megalo-	[Gr. *megas* (large), *megaleios* (magnificent)]. Meaning large.
meio-	[Gr. *meioun* (to make smaller, to lessen)]. Signifying decrease in size or number.
mel-	1. [Gr. *melos* (limb)]. Indicating limb. 2. [Gr. *mēlon* (cheek)]. Indicating cheek. 3. [L. *mel*, *mellis* (honey), Gr. *meli*, *melitos* (honey)]. Relating to honey.

melan-	[Gr. *melas*, *melan-* (black)].
	    1. Meaning black or extreme darkness of hue.
	    2. Denoting relation to melanin.

melano-	[Gr. *melas*, *melan-* (black)].
	    1. Meaning black or extreme darkness of hue.
	    2. Denoting relation to melanin.

meli-	[Gr. *meli* (honey)]. Meaning sweet, or denoting relationship to honey.
melo-	1. [Gr. *melos* (limb)]. Indicating limb. 2. [Gr. *mēlon* (cheek)]. Indicating cheek. 3. [L. *mel*, *mellis* (honey), Gr. *meli*, *melitos* (honey)]. Relating to honey.

mening-	[Gr. *mēninx* (membrane)].
	    1. Denoting any membrane.
	    2. Specifically, denoting relationship to the membranes covering the brain and/or spinal column.

meningo-	[Gr. *mēninx* (membrane)].
	    1. Denoting any membrane.
	    2. Specifically, denoting relationship to the membranes covering the brain and/or spinal column.

meno-	[Gr. *mēn* (month), *mēniaia* (the menses)]. Denoting relationship to the menses.
mercapto-	Chemical prefix indicating the presence of a thiol group (-SH).
mere-	[Gr. *mēros* (part)]. Meaning part or one of a series of similar parts.
mero-	[Gr. *mēros* (part)]. Meaning part or one of a series of similar parts.
mes-	[Gr. *mesos* (middle)]. Meaning middle, or mean.
meso-	[Gr. *mesos* (middle)]. Meaning middle, or mean.

meta-	[Gr. *meta* (after, between, over)].
	    1. In chemistry, a prefix denoting that a compound is formed by two substitutions in the benzene ring arranged unsymmetrically, ie, 1st & 3rd, 2nd & 4th. Abbreviated "*m-*".
	    2. Prefix in many words denoting a change, transformation, or occurrence behind or after something else in the series.
	    3. Meaning after or next; corresponds to Latin "post-".

methoxy-	Chemical prefix denoting addition of a methoxyl group (CH_3O-).
metopo-	[Gr. *metōpon* (forehead)]. Denoting relationship to the forehead.
metr-	[Gr. *mētra* (uterus)]. Denoting relationship to the uterus.

metra- [Gr. *mētra* (uterus)]. Denoting relationship to the uterus.

metro- [Gr. *mētra* (uterus)]. Denoting relationship to the uterus.

micr- [Gr. *mikros* (small)].
1. Denoting smallness.
2. When prefixed to a term denoting a unit of any kind, it denotes the one-millionth (10^{-6}) of such unit.
3. Applied to words denoting chemical examination, methods, etc, means that minimal quantities of the substance to be examined are used.
4. A combining form meaning microscope.

micro- [Gr. *mikros* (small)].
1. Denoting smallness.
2. When prefixed to a term denoting a unit of any kind, denotes one-millionth (10^{-6}) of such unit.
3. Applied to words denoting chemical examination, methods, etc, means that minimal quantities of the substance to be examined are used.
4. A combining form meaning microscope.

micromicro- Prefix (symbol $\mu\mu$) sometimes used to signify one-trillionth (10^{-12}); preferred term is "pico-".

milli- [L. *mille* (one thousand)]. Prefix used in the metric system to signify one-thousandth (10^{-3}).

millimicro- Prefix sometimes used to signify one-billionth (10^{-9}); the preferred prefix is "nano-".

mio- [Gr. *meiōn* (less)]. Indicating less.

miso- [Gr. *misein* (to hate)]. Meaning hatred of.

mito- [Gr. *mitos* (thread)]. Meaning thread-like, or denoting relationship to a thread.

mogi- [Gr. *mogis* (with difficulty)]. Meaning difficult or with difficulty.

mon- [Gr. *monos* (single)]. Denoting the participation or involvement of a single element or part.

mono- [Gr. *monos* (single). Equivalent to Latin "uni-".]. Denoting the participation or involvement of a single element or part.

morpho- [Gr. *morphē* (form)]. Denoting relationship to form.

multi- [L. *multus* (much, many)]. Denoting many or much; properly joined only to words of Latin derivation.

muci- [L. *mucus* (the clear, viscous secretion of the mucous membranes)]. Denoting relationship to mucus, or to mucin.

mucin- [L. *mucus* (the clear, viscous secretion of the mucous membranes)]. Denoting relationship to mucus, or to mucin.

mucino- [L. *mucus* (the clear, viscous secretion of the mucous membranes)]. Denoting relationship to mucus, or to mucin.

muco- [L. *mucus* (the clear, viscous secretion of the mucous membranes)]. Denoting relationship to mucus, or to a mucous membrane.

multi- [L. *multus* (many, much). Corresponds to the Greek "poly-".]. Signifying many or much. Correctly joined only to words of Latin derivation.

my- [Gr. *mys* (muscle)]. Relating to muscle.

myc- [Gr. *mykēs* (fungus)]. Relating to fungus.

mycet- [Gr. *mykēs* (fungus)]. Relating to fungus.

myceto- [Gr. *mykēs* (fungus)]. Relating to fungus.

myco- [Gr. *mykēs* (fungus)]. Relating to fungus.

myel- [Gr. *myelos* (marrow)].
1. Denoting relationship to the bone marrow.
2. Denoting relationship to the spinal cord.

myelo- [Gr. *myelos* (marrow)].
    1. Denoting relationship to the bone marrow.
    2. Denoting relationship to the spinal cord.

myo- [Gr. *mys* (muscle)]. Relating to muscle.

myria- [Gr. *myrios* (numberless)]. Meaning a great number.

myringo- [L. *myringa* (drum membrane)]. Denoting relationship to the membrana tympani.

myx- [Gr. *myxa* (mucus)]. Relating to mucus.

myxo- [Gr. *myxa* (mucus)]. Relating to mucus.

nano- [Gr. *nānos* (dwarf)].
    1. Used in the metric system to signify one-billionth (10^{-9}) of any unit.
    2. Designating small size.

narco- [Gr. *narkoun* (to benumb, deaden), *narkē* (numbness)]. Relating to stupor.

naso- [L. *nasus* (nose)]. Relating to the nose.

necr- [Gr. *nekros* (dead, corpse)]. Denoting relationship to death or a corpse.

necro- [Gr. *nekros* (dead, corpse)]. Denoting relationship to death or a corpse.

nemato- [Gr. *nēma* (thread)].
    1. Denoting relationship to a thread-like structure.
    2. Denoting relationship to a nematode.

neo- [Gr. *neos* (new)]. Meaning new or recent.

neph- [Gr. *nephros* (kidney)]. Relating to the kidney.

nephelo- [Gr. *nephelē* (cloud or mist)]. Indicating relationship to cloudiness or mistiness.

nephr- [Gr. *nephros* (kidney)]. Relating to the kidney.

nephro- [Gr. *nephros* (kidney)]. Relating to the kidney.

neur- [Gr. *neuron* (nerve)]. Denoting relationship to a nerve or nerves, or to the nervous system.

neuro- [Gr. *neuron* (nerve)]. Denoting relationship to a nerve or nerves, or to the nervous system.

nitrilo- Chemical prefix indicating the presence of a cyanide group ($-C\equiv N$).

nitro- Chemical prefix denoting the presence of the group $-NO_2$.

nitroso- Chemical prefix denoting a compound containing the univalent atom group $-N=O$; Nitrosyl.

noci- [L. *nocere* (to injure)].
    1. Signifying relationship to injury.
    2. Denoting relationship to a noxious or deleterious agent or influence.

nomo- [Gr. *nomos* (law)]. Denoting relationship to usage or law.

nor-   1. Chemical prefix denoting the elimination of one methylene group from a chain, the highest permissible locant being used.
    2. Chemical prefix denoting the contraction of a (steroid) ring by one CH_2 unit, the locant being the capital letter identifying the ring. Elimination of two methylene groups is denoted by the prefix "dinor-", three groups by "trinor-", etc.
    3. Chemical prefix denoting "normal" (ie, unbranched chain of carbon atoms as opposed to branched) in aliphatic compounds.
    4. Chemical prefix indicating a parent compound (no longer limited to nitrogenous compounds).

normo- [L. *norma* (rule)]. Meaning conforming to the rule; normal or usual.

noso- [Gr. *nosos* (disease)]. Relating to disease.

noto- [Gr. *nōton* (back)]. Relating to the back.

nycto- [Gr. *nyx* (night)]. Denoting relationship to night or darkness.

nympho-   [L. *nympha*, from Gr. *nymphē* (bride)]. Denoting relationship to the nymphae or labia minora.

oari-   [L. *ovarium* (ovary)]. Denoting relationship to an ovary.

ob-   [L. *ob* (against)]. Indicating against, in front of.

octa-   [L. *octo*, Gr. *oktō* (eight)]. Meaning eight.

oculo-   [L. *oculus* (eye)]. Denoting relationship to the eye.

odont-   [Gr. *odous, odont-* (tooth)]. Denoting a tooth or teeth. Properly used only in words formed from Greek roots.

odonto-   [Gr. *odous, odont-* (tooth)]. Denoting a tooth or teeth. Properly used only in words formed from Greek roots.

odyn-   [Gr. *odynē* (pain)]. Meaning pain.

odyno-   [Gr. *odynē* (pain)]. Meaning pain.

oleo-   [L. *oleum* (oil)]. Relating to oil.

olig-   [Gr. *oligos* (few, little)].
                  1. Meaning "a few" or "a little".
                  2. In chemistry, used in contrast to "poly-" in describing polymers; eg, oligosaccharide.

oligo-   [Gr. *oligos* (few, little)].
                  1. Meaning "a few" or "a little".
                  2. In chemistry, used in contrast to "poly-" in describing polymers; e.g. oligosaccharide.

omo-   [Gr. *ōmos* (shoulder)]. Indicating relationship to the shoulder.

omphalo-   [Gr. *omphalos* (the navel)]. Denoting relationship to the umbilicus.

oncho-   [Gr. *onkos* (bulk, mass)]. Meaning a tumor or relationship to a tumor, swelling, or mass.

onco-   [Gr. *onkos* (bulk, mass)]. Meaning a tumor or relationship to a tumor, swelling, or mass.

oneiro-   [Gr. *oneiros* (dream)]. Denoting relationship to a dream.

onych-   [Gr. *onyx* (nail)]. Denoting relationship to a nail or nails.

onycho-   [Gr. *onyx* (nail)]. Denoting relationship to a nail or nails.

onyx-   [Gr. *onyx* (nail)]. Denoting relationship to a nail or nails.

oo-   [Gr. *ōon* (egg)]. Denoting relationship to an egg or ovum.

oophor-   [Gr. *ōophoros* (egg-bearing), from *ōon* (egg) + *phoros* (bearing)]. Denoting relationship to the ovary.

oophoro-   [Gr. *ōophoros* (egg-bearing), from *ōon* (egg) + *phoros* (bearing)]. Denoting relationship to the ovary.

oothec-   [Modern L. *ootheca* (ovary), from Gr. *ōon* (egg) + *thēkē* (case)]. Denoting relationship to the ovary.

ootheco-   [Modern L. *ootheca* (ovary), from Gr. *ōon* (egg) + *thēkē* (case)]. Denoting relationship to the ovary.

ophthalm-   [Gr. *ophthalmos* (eye)]. Denoting relationship to the eye.

ophthalmo-   [Gr. *ophthalmos* (eye)]. Denoting relationship to the eye.

opistho-   [Gr. *opisthen* (behind, at the back)]. Meaning backward or denoting relationship to the back.

opo-   [Gr. *ops, op-* (face, eye)]. Relating to the face or eye.

opto-   [Gr. *optos* (seen)]. Meaning visible, or denoting relationship to vision or sight.

orchi-   [Gr. *orchis* (testis)]. Denoting relationship to the testes.

orchid-   [Gr. *orchis* (testis)]. Denoting relationship to the testes.

orchido-   [Gr. *orchis* (testis)]. Denoting relationship to the testes.

orchio-   [Gr. *orchis* (testis)]. Denoting relationship to the testes.

organo-   [Gr. *organon* (organ)]. Denoting relationship to an organ.

oro-   1. [L. *os, oris* (mouth)]. Denoting relationship to the mouth.
     2. [Gr. *oros* (whey, or the watery part of the blood)]. Denoting relationship to serum.

orrho-   [Gr. *orrhos* (serum)]. Relating to serum.

ortho-   [Gr. *orthos* (correct, straight)].
     1. Meaning straight, normal, or in proper order.
     2. In chemistry, denoting that a compound has two substitutions on adjacent carbon atoms in a benzene ring. Abbreviated "*o-*".

osche-   [Gr. *osche* (scrotum)]. Denoting relationship to the scrotum.

oscheo-   [Gr. *oscheon* (scrotum)]. Denoting relationship to the scrotum.

oscillo-   [L. *oscillare* (to swing)]. Denoting relationship to a backward and forward motion, or oscillation.

osmo-   1. [Gr. *ōsmos* (impulse)]. Relating to an impulse or osmosis.
     2. [Gr. *osmē* (smell)]. Relating to smell or odors.

osphresio-   [Gr. *osphrēsis* (smell)]. Denoting relationship to odors.

ossi-   [L. *os* (bone)]. Denoting bone.

ost-   [Gr. *osteon* (bone)]. Relating to bone.

oste-   [Gr. *osteon* (bone)]. Relating to bone.

osteo-   [Gr. *osteon* (bone)]. Relating to bone.

ot-   [Gr. *ous, ōtos* (ear)]. Relating to the ear.

oto-   [Gr. *ous, ōtos* (ear)]. Relating to the ear.

ovario-   [L. *ovarium* (ovary)]. Denoting relationship to the ovary.

ovi-   [L. *ovum* (egg)]. Relating to an egg or ova.

ovo-   [L. *ovum* (egg)]. Relating to an egg or ova.

oxa-   Term inserted in the name of organic compounds to signify the presence or addition of oxygen atom(s).

oxo-   Denoting the addition of oxygen, eg, oxotestosterone.

oxy-   [Gr. *oxys* (keen)].
     1. Denoting sharp, pointed.
     2. Denoting acid.
     3. Denoting acute.
     4. Denoting shrill.
     5. Denoting quick [incorrectly used for "ocy-", from Gr. *okys* (swift)], as in oxytocia.
     6. In chemistry, denoting the presence of oxygen in the substance whose name follows (oxybiotin).

pachy-   [Gr. *pachys* (thick)]. Signifying thick; correctly applied only to words from Greek roots.

palato-   [L. *palatum* (palate)]. Relating to the palate.

paleo-   [Gr. *palaios* (old)]. Meaning old.

pali-   [Gr. *palin* (backward, again)]. Meaning again, frequently denoting pathologic condition.

palin-   [Gr. *palin* (backward, again)]. Meaning again, frequently denoting pathologic condition.

pan-   [Gr. *pas, pan* (all)]. Implying all or entire.

pancreat-   [Gr. *pankreas* (pancreas [the sweetbread])]. Relating to the pancreas.

pancreatico-   [Gr. *pankreas* (pancreas [the sweetbread])]. Relating to the pancreas.

pancreato-   [Gr. *pankreas* (pancreas [the sweetbread])]. Relating to the pancreas.

pancreo-   [Gr. *pankreas* (pancreas [the sweetbread])]. Relating to the pancreas.

pant-   [Gr. *pas, pantos* (all)]. Implying all or entire.

panto-   [Gr. *pas, pantos* (all)]. Implying all or entire.

para-   [Gr. *para* (alongside of, near)].
1. Denoting a departure from the normal.
2. Referring to an involvement of two like parts (a pair), as the two lower extremities.
3. In chemistry, a compound formed by two substitutions in the benzene ring, arranged symmetrically, ie, linked to opposite carbon atoms in the ring. Abbreviated "*p-*".

parieto-   [L. *paries,* pl. *parietes* (wall)]. Meaning parietal; denoting relationship to any wall or paries.

path-   [Gr. *pathos* (suffering, disease)]. Relating to disease.

patho-   [Gr. *pathos* (suffering, disease)]. Relating to disease.

pedia-   [Gr. *pais, paidos* (child)]. Signifying relationship to a child.

pedo-   1. [Gr. *pais, paidos* (child)]. Signifying relationship to a child.
2. [L. *pes, pedis* (foot)]. Denoting relationship to a foot.

pelo-   [Gr. *pēlos* (mud)]. Indicating relationship to mud.

pelvi-   [L. *pelvis,* from Gr. *pellis* (bowl)]. Denoting relationship to the pelvis.

pent-   [Gr. *pente* (five)]. Meaning five.

penta-   [Gr. *pente* (five)]. Meaning five.

per-   [L. *per* (through)].
1. Meaning throughout (in space and time)
2. Meaning completely or extremely, carrying an idea of intensity.
3. In chemistry, denoting either
    a. More or most, with respect to the amount of a given element or radical contained in a compound.
    b. Degree of substitution for hydrogen.

peri-   [Gr. *peri* (around)]. Denoting the idea of around or about.

pero-   [Gr. *pēros* (maimed)]. Meaning maimed or deformed.

peroxi-   Chemical prefix denoting the presence of an extra oxygen atom, as in peroxides.

peroxy-   Chemical prefix denoting the presence of an extra oxygen atom, as in peroxides.

perthio-   Chemical prefix denoting substitution of sulfur for every oxygen atom in a compound, as perthiocarbonic acid (H_2CS_3).

petalo-   [Gr. *petalon* (leaf)]. Denoting relationship to a leaf.

phaco-   [Gr. *phakos* (lentil, or anything shaped like a lentil; a spot on the body, a freckle)].
1. Meaning lens-shaped, or relating to a lens.
2. Denotes "mother-spot" (as in phacomatosis).

phako-   [Gr. *phakos* (lentil, or anything shaped like a lentil; a spot on the body, a freckle)].
1. Meaning lens-shaped, or relating to a lens.
2. Denotes "mother-spot" (as in phacomatosis).

phago-   [Gr. *phagein* (to eat)]. Relating to eating or devouring.

phallo-   [Gr. *phallos* (penis)]. Denoting relationship to the penis.

pharmaco-   [Gr. *pharmakon* (medicine)]. Signifying relationship to a drug or medicine.

pharyng-   [Gr. *pharynx, pharyng-* (throat)]. Denoting relationship to the pahrynx.

pharyngo-   [Gr. *pharynx, pharyng-* (throat)]. Denoting relationship to the pahrynx.

phen-   [Gr. *phainō* (to appear, show forth)].
1. Referring to appearance.
2. Denoting a derivation from benzene.

pheo-
1. [Gr. *phaios* (dusky)]. Meaning dusky, gray, or dun.
2. Prefix denoting the same substituents on a phorbin or phorbide (porphyrin) residue as are present in chlorophyll, excluding any ester residues and magnesium.

phleb-   [Gr. *phleps, phlebos* (vein)]. Denoting relationship to a vein or veins.

phlebo-   [Gr. *phleps, phlebos* (vein)]. Denoting relationship to a vein or veins.

phlogo-   [Gr. *phlogōsis* (inflammation)]. Denoting relationship to inflammation.

phon-   [Gr. *phōnē* (sound)]. Denoting relationship to sound.

phono-   [Gr. *phōnē* (sound)]. Denoting relationship to sound.

phos-   [Gr. *phōs* (light)]. Denoting light.

phot-   [Gr. *phōs, phōt-* (light)]. Relating to light.

photo-   [Gr. *phōs, phōt-* (light)]. Relating to light.

phren-   [Gr. *phrēn* (the mind, heart, seat of emotions, diaphragm)].
1. Denoting relationship to the diaphragm.
2. Denoting relationship to the mind.

phreno-   [Gr. *phrēn* (the mind, heart, seat of emotions, diaphragm)].
1. Denoting relationship to the diaphragm.
2. Denoting relationship to the mind.

phyco-   [Gr. *phykos* (seaweed)]. Denoting relationship to seaweed.

phyllo-   [Gr. *phyllon* (leaf)]. Denoting relationship to leaves.

physio-   [Gr. *physis* (nature)]. Denoting relationship to physiology or nature.

physo-   [Gr. *physaō* (to inflate, distend), *physa* (air)].
1. Denoting a tendency to swell or inflate.
2. Relating to air or gas.

phyto-   [Gr. *phyton* (a plant)]. Denoting relationship to plants.

pico-   [Italian *piccolo* (small)].
1. Meaning small.
2. Prefix used in the metric system to denote one-trillionth (10^{-12}).

picro-   [Gr. *pikros* (bitter)]. Meaning bitter.

pilo-   [L. *pilus* (hair)]. Meaning resembling or composed of hair, or denoting relationship to hair.

pimelo-   [Gr. *pimelē* (fat)]. Denoting relationship to fat.

pio-   [Gr. *pion* (fat)]. Denoting relationship to fat.

pipsyl-   *p*-iodophenyl sulfonyl-, the radical of pipsyl chloride used to combine with NH_2 groups of amino acids and proteins.

plasmo-   [Gr. *plasma* (anything formed)]. Denoting relationship to plasma, or to the substance of a cell.

platy-   [Gr. *platys* (flat, broad)]. Conveying the idea of width or flatness.

pleio-   [Gr. *pleiōn* (more)]. Meaning more.

pleo-   [Gr. *pleiōn* (more)]. Meaning more.

pleur-   [Gr. *pleura* (rib, side)]. Denoting relationship to the rib, side, or pleura.

pleuro-   [Gr. *pleura* (rib, side)]. Denoting relationship to the rib, side, or pleura.

pluri-   [L. *plus, plur-* (more)]. Meaning several, or more.

pneo-   [Gr. *pnein* (to breath)]. Indicating relationship to breath or respiration.

pneum-   [Gr. *pneuma, pneumatos* (air, breath)]. Indicating relationship to air or gas, or to breathing.

pneuma-   [Gr. *pneuma, pneumatos* (air, breath)]. Indicating relationship to air or gas, or to breathing.

pneumat- [Gr. *pneuma, pneumatos* (air, breath)]. Indicating relationship to air or gas, or to breathing.

pneumato- [Gr. *pneuma, pneumatos* (air, breath)]. Indicating relationship to air or gas, or to breathing.

pneumo- [Gr. *pneumōn* (lung)]. Indicating relationship to the lung or lungs.

pneumon- [Gr. *pneumōn* (lung)]. Indicating relationship to the lung or lungs.

pneumono- [Gr. *pneumōn* (lung)]. Indicating relationship to the lung or lungs.

pod- [Gr. *pous, podos* (foot)]. Meaning foot or foot-shaped, or relating to the foot.

podo- [Gr. *pous, podos* (foot)]. Meaning foot or foot-shaped, or relating to the foot.

poikilo- [Gr. *poikilos* (varied)]. Meaning irregular or varied.

polio- [Gr. *polios* (gray)]. Denoting relationship to the gray matter of the nervous system.

poly- [Gr. *polys* (much, many)].
  1. Denoting many or much, correctly used only with words formed from Greek roots; corresponding to the Latin "multi-".
  2. In chemistry, a prefix meaning "polymer of", as in polypeptide.

pono- [Gr. *ponos* (hard work, bodily exertion, or distress; consequences of toil, suffering, or pain)]. Denoting relationship to hard work or pain.

post- [L. *post* (after). Corresponds to Greek "meta-"]. Prefix to words derived from Latin roots, denoting after, behind, or posterior.

postero- [L. *posterus* (behind)]. Denoting the posterior part or position.

prae- [L. *prae* (before)]. Prefix to words from Latin origins, denoting anterior or before (in space or time).

pre- [L. *prae* (before)]. Prefix to words from Latin origins, denoting anterior or before (in space or time).

presby- [Gr. *presbys* (old)]. Meaning old, or denoting relationship to old age.

pro- [L. and Gr. *pro* (before)].
  1. Denoting before or forward.
  2. In chemistry, a prefix indicating "precursor of".

proct- [Gr. *prōktos* (anus)]. Signifying relationship to the anus, or, more frequently, the rectum.

procto- [Gr. *prōktos* (anus)]. Signifying relationship to the anus, or, more frequently, the rectum.

propionyl- Chemical prefix for the radical of propionic acid (CH_3CH_2CO-).

propyl- Chemical prefix for the radical of propyl alcohol or propane ($CH_3CH_2CH_2-$).

proso- [Gr. *prosō* (forward)]. Meaning forward or anterior.

prosopo- [Gr. *prosōpon* (face)]. Denoting relationship to the face.

prostat- [L. *prostata*, from Gr. *prostatēs* (one standing before)]. Relating to the prostate gland.

prostato- [L. *prostata*, from Gr. *prostatēs* (one standing before)]. Relating to the prostate gland.

prot- [Gr. *prōtos* (first)]. Prefix in words derived from Greek roots, denoting first, the first in a series, or the highest in rank.

proto- [Gr. *prōtos* (first)]. Prefix in words derived from Greek roots, denoting first, the first in a series, or the highest in rank.

psammo- [Gr. *psammos* (sand)]. Signifying relationship to sand or to sand-like material.

pseud- [Gr. *pseudēs* (false)]. Signifying false or spurious; denoting a resemblance, often deceptive.

pseudo- [Gr. *pseudēs* (false)]. Signifying false or spurious; denoting a resemblance, often deceptive. Before a vowel it is often contracted to "pseud".

psych- [Gr. *psychē* (soul, mind)]. Relating to the mind or psyche.

psycho-	[Gr. *psychē* (soul, mind)]. Relating to the mind or psyche.
psychro-	[Gr. *psychros* (cold)]. Relating to cold.
ptyal-	[Gr. *ptyalon* (saliva)]. Denoting relationship to saliva or the salivary glands.
ptyalo-	[Gr. *ptyalon* (saliva)]. Denoting relationship to saliva or the salivary glands.
pulmo-	[L. *pulmo* (the organ of respiration)]. Denoting relationship to the lungs.
pulmono-	[L. *pulmo* (the organ of respiration)]. Denoting relationship to the lungs.
pupillo-	[L. *pupilla* (pupil)]. Denoting relationship to the pupil of the eye.
pyel-	[Gr. *pyelos* (trough, pelvis)]. Relating to the renal pelvis.
pyelo-	[Gr. *pyelos* (trough, pelvis)]. Relating to the renal pelvis.
pygo-	[Gr. *pygē* (rump)]. Signifying relationship to the buttocks.
pykno-	[Gr. *pyknos* (thick, frequent)]. Meaning thick, compact, or frequent.
pyle-	[Gr. *pylē* (gate)]. Denoting relationship to the portal vein.
pyloro-	[Gr. *pylōros*, from *pylē* (gate) + *ouros* (guard)]. Denoting relationship to the pylorus.
pyo-	[Gr. *pyon* (pus)]. Denoting suppuration or an accumulation of pus.
pyreto-	[Gr. *pyretos* (fever)]. Denoting relationship to fever.
pyro-	[Gr. *pyr* (fire)]. 1. Denoting fire or heat. 2. In chemistry, denotes prepared by heating.
quadri-	[L. *quattuor* (four)]. Meaning four or four-fold.
rachi-	[Gr. *rhachis* (spine)]. Relating to the spine.
rachio-	[Gr. *rhachis* (spine)]. Relating to the spine.
radio-	[L. *radius* (ray)]. 1. Relating to radiation; in medicine, denoting chiefly "x-ray". 2. Denoting the radioactive isotope of the element to which it is prefixed.
re-	[L. *re, red* (again, back, contrary)]. Meaning again, backward, or contrary to.
recto-	[L. *rectus* (straight)]. Relating to the rectum.
reno-	[L. *ren* (kidney)]. Relating to the kidney.
retro-	[L. *retro* (back, backward, behind)]. Prefix in words from Latin roots, denoting backward or located behind.
rhabdo-	[Gr. *rhabdos* (rod)]. Meaning rod-shaped or denoting relationship to a rod.
rheo-	[Gr. *rheos* (current, flow)]. 1. Indicating blood flow. 2. Indicating electrical current.
rhin-	[Gr. *rhis, rhin-* (nose)]. Relating to the nose or a nose-like structure.
rhino-	[Gr. *rhis, rhin-* (nose)]. Relating to the nose or a nose-like structure.
rhizo-	[Gr. *rhiza* (root)]. Relating to a root.
rhodo-	[Gr. *rhodon* (rose)]. Meaning red.
saccharo-	[L. *saccharum*, from Gr. *sakcharon* (sugar)]. Denoting relationship to sugar.
sacr-	[L. *sacrum* (sacred)]. Relating to the sacrum.
sacro-	[L. *sacrum* (sacred)]. Relating to the sacrum.
salping-	[Gr. *salpinx* (trumpet, tube)]. Denoting relationship to a tube, specifically the Fallopian or Eustachian tube.
salpingo-	[Gr. *salpinx* (trumpet, tube)]. Denoting relationship to a tube, specifically the Fallopian or Eustachian tube.
sangui-	[L. *sanguis* (blood)]. Denoting relationship to blood.
sapro-	[Gr. *sapros* (rotten)]. Meaning rotten, or denoting relationship to decay or decaying material.

sarco-	[Gr. *sarx, sarkos* (flesh)]. 1. Denoting muscular substance. 2. Denoting a resemblance to flesh.
scato-	[Gr. *skōr, skatos* (dung)]. Denoting relationship to feces.
schisto-	[Gr. *schistos,* from *shizein* (split)]. Denoting split or cleft.
schiz-	[Gr. *schizō* (to split or cleave)]. Denoting split, cleft, or division.
schizo-	[Gr. *schizō* (to split or cleave)]. Denoting split, cleft, or division.
scirrho-	[Gr. *skirrhos* (hard)]. Meaning hard, or denoting relationship to hard.
scler-	[Gr. *sklēros* (hard)]. 1. Meaning hard. 2. Denoting relationship to the sclera.
sclero-	[Gr. *sklēros* (hard)]. 1. Meaning hard. 2. Denoting relationship to the sclera.
scole-	[Gr. *skōlēx* (worm)]. Denoting relationship to a worm.
scoleco-	[Gr. *skōlēx* (worm)]. Denoting relationship to a worm.
scolio-	[Gr. *skolios* (twisted)]. Meaning twisted or crooked.
scoto-	[Gr. *skotos* (darkness)]. Denoting relationship to darkness.
semi-	[L. *semis* (half); corresponding to the Greek prefix *hemi-*.]. Prefix used with words from Latin origins, denoting one-half.
semio-	[Gr. *sēmeion* (sign)]. 1. Relating to signs or symbols in language. 2. Denoting signs or symbols relating to the body.
sero-	[L. *serum* (whey)]. 1. Relating to serum. 2. Denoting a watery consistency.
sesqui-	[L. *sesqui* (one and one-half, one-half more)]. Denoting 1 and 1/2. At one time, used in chemistry to indicate a ratio of 3 to 2 between the two parts of a compound. Presently used only for sesquihydrates, ie, compounds crystallizing with 1.5 molecules of water.
sial-	[Gr. *sialon* (saliva)]. Relating to saliva or the salivary glands.
sialo-	[Gr. *sialon* (saliva)]. Relating to saliva or the salivary glands.
sidero-	[Gr. *sidēros* (iron)]. Relating to iron.
sinistro-	[L. *sinister* (left)]. Meaning left, or signifying relationship to the left side.
sito-	[Gr. *sitos* (food, corn, or grain)]. Denoting relationship to food.
skia-	[Gr. *skia* (shadow)]. Denoting reference to shadows, especially of internal structures as produced by roentgen rays.
sodio-	Chemical prefix denoting a compound containing sodium, as sodiotartrate (a tartrate of some element also containing sodium).
somat-	[Gr. *sōma* (body)]. Denoting relationship to the body.
somatico-	[Gr. *sōma* (body)]. Denoting relationship to the body.
somato-	[Gr. *sōma* (body)]. Denoting relationship to the body.
somni-	[L. *somnus* (sleep)]. Denoting relationship to sleep.
spano-	[Gr. *spanios* (scarce)]. Meaning scarce or scanty.
spasmo-	[L. *spasmus,* Gr. *spasmos* (spasm)]. Indicating relationship to a spasm.
sperma-	[Gr. *sperma* (seed)]. Relating to sperm or spermatozoa.
spermato-	[Gr. *sperma* (seed)]. Relating to sperm or spermatozoa.
spermio-	[Gr. *sperma* (seed)]. Relating to sperm or spermatozoa.
spermo-	[Gr. *sperma* (seed)]. Relating to sperm or spermatozoa.

spheno- [Gr. *sphēn* (wedge)].
    1. Meaning wedge or wedge-shaped.
    2. Relating to the sphenoid bone.

spher- [Gr. *sphaira* (ball or globe)]. Meaning round, or denoting relationship to a sphere.

sphero- [Gr. *sphaira* (ball or globe)]. Meaning round, or denoting relationship to a sphere.

sphygm- [Gr. *sphygmos* (pulse)]. Denoting relationship to the pulse.

sphygmo- [Gr. *sphygmos* (pulse)]. Denoting relationship to the pulse.

splanch- [Gr. *splanchnon, splanchnos* (viscus)]. Relating to the viscera or to the splanchnic nerve.

splanchno- [Gr. *splanchnon, splanchnos* (viscus)]. Relating to the viscera or to the splanchnic nerve.

splen- [Gr. *splēn* (spleen)]. Relating to the spleen.

spleno- [Gr. *splēn* (spleen)]. Relating to the spleen.

spodo- [Gr. *spodos* (ashes)]. Relating to waste materials.

spondyl- [Gr. *spondylos* (vertebra)]. Relating to the vertebrae or spinal column.

spondylo- [Gr. *spondylos* (vertebra)]. Relating to the vertebrae or spinal column.

spongio- [L., Gr. *spongia* (sponge)]. Meaning like a sponge, or signifying relationship to a sponge.

spor- [Gr. *sporos* (seed)]. Denoting relationship to a seed or spore.

sporo- [Gr. *sporos* (seed)]. Denoting relationship to a seed or spore.

staphyl- [Gr. *staphylē* (bunch of grapes [or the uvula when swollen, thus resembling a bunch of grapes])].
    1. Denoting the uvula.
    2. Denoting any process, organ, or mass resembling a bunch of grapes.

staphylo- [Gr. *staphylē* (bunch of grapes [or the uvula when swollen, thus resembling a bunch of grapes])].
    1. Denoting the uvula.
    2. Denoting any process, organ, or mass resembling a bunch of grapes.

stearo- [Gr. *stear, steatos* (tallow, fat)]. Relating to fat.

steato- [Gr. *stear, steatos* (tallow, fat)]. Relating to fat.

steno- [Gr. *stenos* (narrow)]. Denoting narrowness or constriction.

sterco- [L. *stercus* (dung)]. Denoting relationship to feces.

stereo- [Gr. *stereos* (solid)].
    1. Denoting a solid, or a solid condition or state.
    2. Denoting spatial qualities, three-dimensionality.

sterno- [Gr. *sternon* (sternum)]. Relating to the sternum.

steth- [Gr. *stēthos* (chest)]. Relating to the chest.

stetho- [Gr. *stēthos* (chest)]. Relating to the chest.

stheno- [Gr. *sthenos* (strength)]. Denoting relationship to strength.

stom- [Gr. *stoma* (mouth)]. Denoting the mouth.

stoma- [Gr. *stoma* (mouth)]. Denoting the mouth.

stomat- [Gr. *stoma*, pl. *stomas* or *stomata* (mouth)]. Denoting the mouth.

stomato- [Gr. *stoma*, pl. *stomas* or *stomata* (mouth)]. Relating to the mouth.

streph- [Gr. *strephein* (to twist)]. Meaning twisted.

strepho- [Gr. *strephein* (to twist)]. Meaning twisted.

strepto- [Gr. *streptos* (curved, twisted)].
    1. Meaning curved or twisted.
    2. Denoting relationship to streptococcus.

stylo-   [Gr. *stylos* (pillar, post), L. *stilus* (stake, pole)]. Denoting resemblance to a stake or pole, hence, relating to a styloid process; specifically, the styloid process of the temporal bone.

sub-   [L. *sub* (under); corresponds to the Greek "hypo-".]. Prefix to words formed from Latin roots.
1. Denoting beneath, under, near, almost, or moderately.
2. Denoting less than the normal or typical.
3. Denoting inferior.

sulf-   Chemical prefix denoting that the compound to the name of which it is attached contains a sulfur atom. This spelling (rather than "sulph-") is preferred by the American Chemical Society and has been adopted by the United States Pharmacopeia and National Formulary.

sulfo-   Chemical prefix denoting that the compound to the name of which it is attached contains a sulfur atom. This spelling (rather than "sulpho-") is preferred by the American Chemical Society and has been adopted by the United States Pharmacopeia and National Formulary.

sulph-   Prefix denoting that the compound to the name of which it is attached contains a sulfur atom. The preferred spelling is "sulf-".

sulpho-   Prefix denoting that the compound to the name of which it is attached contains a sulfur atom. The preferred spelling is "sulfo-".

super-   [L. *super* (above, beyond); corresponds to the Greek "hyper-".]. Prefix to words from Latin roots signifying in excess, above, superior, or in the upper part of.

supra-   [L. *supra* (above)]. Denoting a position above the part indicated by the word to which it is joined.

sympath-   [Gr. *sympathētikos*, from *sympatheō* (to feel with)]. Relating to the sympathetic (autonomic) nervous system.

sympatheto-   [Gr. *sympathētikos*, from *sympatheō* (to feel with)]. Relating to the sympathetic (autonomic) nervous system.

sympathico-   [Gr. *sympathētikos*, from *sympatheō* (to feel with)]. Relating to the sympathetic (autonomic) nervous system.

sympatho-   [Gr. *sympathētikos*, from *sympatheō* (to feel with)]. Relating to the sympathetic (autonomic) nervous system.

syn-   [Gr. *syn* (together, with); corresponds to Latin "con-".]. Prefix to words of Greek origin indicating together, with, or joined. It appears as "sym-" before b, p, ph, or m.

syndesmo-   [Gr. *syndesmos* (band or ligament)]. Denoting relationship to connective tissue, particularly the ligaments.

syringo-   [Gr. *syrinx* (pipe, tube, fistula)]. Denoting relationship to a tube or fistula.

tacho-   [Gr. *tachos* (speed)]. Denoting relationship to speed.

tachy-   [Gr. *tachys* (quick, swift, rapid)]. Meaning rapid or swift.

tarso-   [Gr. *tarsos* (a broad, flat surface)].
1. Denoting relationship to the edge of the eyelid.
2. Denoting relationship to the instep of the foot.

tauto-   [Gr. *tauto* (the same)]. Meaning the same.

tel-   [Gr. *tēle* (distant, end)]. Denoting distance, end, or other end.

tele-   [Gr. *tēle* (distant, end)]. Denoting distance, end, or other end.

telo-   [Gr. *telos* (end)]. Denoting distance, end, or other end.

teno-   [Gr. *tenōn, tenontos* (tendon)]. Denoting relationship to a tendon.

tenonto-   [Gr. *tenōn, tenontos* (tendon)]. Denoting relationship to a tendon.

ter-   [L. *ter* (thrice)]. Meaning three, three-fold.

tera-	[Gr. *teras* (monster)]. 1. Prefix used in the metric system to denote one trillion (10^{12}). 2. Relating to a teras, or monster.
terato-	[Gr. *teras, teratos* (monster)]. Denoting relationship to a monster.
tetra-	[Gr. *tetra* (four)]. Prefix to words from Greek origins, meaning four.
tetrahydro-	Chemical prefix denoting the attachment of four hydrogen atoms.
therm-	[Gr. *thermē* (heat), *thermos* (warm or hot)]. Relating to heat.
thermo-	[Gr. *thermē* (heat), *thermos* (warm or hot)]. Relating to heat.
thia-	Chemical prefix indicating the replacement of carbon for sulfur in a ring or chain.
thio-	[Gr. *theion* (sulfur)]. Chemical prefix denoting that sulfur has replaced oxygen in the compound to the name of which it is attached.
thioxo-	Chemical prefix indicating =S in a thioketone.
thorac-	[Gr. *thōrax, thōrakos* (chest)]. Denoting relationship to the chest.
thoraco-	[Gr. *thōrax, thōrakos* (chest)]. Denoting relationship to the chest.
thromb-	[Gr. *thrombos* (clot)]. Denoting or relating to blood clot.
thrombo-	[Gr. *thrombos* (clot)]. Denoting or relating to blood clot.
thymo-	1. [Gr. *thymos* (the mind or heart as the seat of strong feelings or passion)]. Denoting relationship to the mind, soul, or emotions. 2. [Gr. *thymos* (thymus)]. Relating to the thymus.
thyr-	[Gr. *thyreos* (shield)]. Relating to the thyroid gland.
thyreo-	[Gr. *thyreos* (shield)]. Relating to the thyroid gland.
thyro-	[Gr. *thyreos* (shield)]. Relating to the thyroid gland.
toco-	[Gr. *tokos* (birth)]. Relating to childbirth or labor.
toko-	[Gr. *tokos* (birth)]. Relating to childbirth or labor.
tomo-	[Gr. *tomē* (a cutting)]. Denoting relationship to a cutting or a designated layer, as might be achieved by cutting or slicing.
tono-	[Gr. *tonos* (tension)]. Denoting relationship to tone or tension.
topo-	[Gr. *topos* (place)]. Meaning place.
toxico-	[Gr. *toxikon* (poison)]. Denoting relationship to poison.
toxo-	[L. *toxinum*, Gr. *toxikon* (poison)]. Denoting relationship to poison or a toxin.
trache-	[Gr. *tracheia* (windpipe, trachea)]. Denoting the trachea.
trachel-	[Gr. *trachēlos* (neck)]. Denoting relationship to the neck or a neck-like structure.
trachelo-	[Gr. *trachēlos* (neck)]. Denoting relationship to the neck or a neck-like structure.
tracheo-	[Gr. *tracheia* (windpipe, trachea)]. Relating to the trachea.
trans-	[L. *trans* (across, through)]. 1. Meaning across, through, or beyond. 2. In genetics, denoting the location of two genes on opposite chromosomes of a homologous pair. 3. In organic chemistry, a form of isomerism in which the atoms attached to two carbon atoms, joined by double bonds, are located on opposite sides of the molecule. 4. In biochemistry, a prefix to group name in an enzyme name, or a reaction denoting transfer of that group from one compound to another. 5. Opposite of "cis-".
traumato-	[Gr. *trauma, traumatos* (wound)]. Denoting relationship to trauma, a wound, or an injury.
tri-	[L. and Gr. *tri* (three)]. Denoting three.

tricho-	[Gr. *thrix, trichos,* (hair)]. Relating to the hair or denoting a hair-like structure.
tris-	Chemical prefix indicating three of the substituents that follow.
troph-	[Gr. *trophē* (nourishment)]. Relating to food or nutrition.
tropho-	[Gr. *trophē* (nourishment)]. Relating to food or nutrition.
tubo-	[L. *tubus* (a pipe, tube)]. Relating to a tube or tubes.
typhlo-	1. [Gr. *typhlon* (cecum)]. Relating to the cecum. 2. [Gr. *typhlos* (blind)]. Relating to blindness
tyro-	[Gr. *tyros* (cheese)]. Denoting relationship to cheese.
ule-	1. [Gr. *oulē* (scar)]. Denoting relationship to a scar. 2. [Gr. *oulon* (gum)]. Denoting relationship to the gingivae (gums).
ulo-	1. [Gr. *oulē* (scar)]. Denoting relationship to a scar. 2. [Gr. *oulon* (gum)]. Denoting relationship to the gingivae (gums).
ultra-	[L. *ultra* (beyond)]. Denoting excess, exaggeration, or beyond.
uni-	[L. *unus* (one). Equivalent to the Greek "mono-".]. Denoting one, single, or not paired.
ur-	[Gr. *ouron* (urine)]. Relating to urine, the urinary tract, or urination.
uranisco-	[Gr. *ouraniskos* (roof of the mouth)]. Denoting relationship to the palate.
urano-	[Gr. *ouranos* (sky vault, roof of the mouth)]. 1. Relating to the palate. 2. Sometimes relating to the sky or heaven.
ure-	[Gr. *ouron* (urine)]. Relating to urea or urine.
urea-	[Gr. *ouron* (urine)]. Relating to urea or urine.
ureo-	[Gr. *ouron* (urine)]. Relating to urea or urine.
uretero-	[Gr. *ourētēr* (urinary canal)]. Relating to the ureter.
urethr-	[Gr. *ourēthra* (urethra)]. Relating to the urethra.
urethro-	[Gr. *ourēthra* (urethra)]. Relating to the urethra.
uri-	[Gr. *ouron* (urine)]. Relating to uric acid.
uric-	[Gr. *ouron* (urine)]. Relating to uric acid.
urico-	[Gr. *ouron* (urine)]. Relating to uric acid.
urin-	[Gr. *ouron* (urine)]. Relating to urine.
urino-	[Gr. *ouron* (urine)]. Relating to urine.
uro-	[Gr. *ouron* (urine)]. Relating to urine, the urinary tract, or urination.
urono-	[Gr. *ouron* (urine)]. Relating to urine, the urinary tract, or urination.
vago-	Relating to the vagus nerve.
varico-	[L. *varix* (dilated vein)]. 1. Relating to a varix or varicosity. 2. Meaning twisted and swollen.
vas-	[L. *vas* (vessel)]. Relating to a vessel or duct.
vasculo-	[L. *vasculum* (small vessel)]. Relating to the blood vessels.
vaso-	[L. *vas* (vessel)]. Relating to a vessel or duct.
vene-	1. [L. *vena* (vein)]. Relating to the veins. 2. [L. *venenum* (poison)]. Relating to venom.
veni-	[L. *vena* (vein)]. Relating to the veins.
veno-	[L. *vena* (vein)]. Relating to the veins.

ventr- [L. *venter* (belly)].
  1. Relating to the abdomen.
  2. Relating to the front of the body.

ventri- [L. *venter* (belly)].
  1. Relating to the abdomen.
  2. Relating to the front of the body.

ventro- [L. *venter* (belly)].
  1. Relating to the abdomen.
  2. Relating to the front of the body.

vertebro- [L. *vertebra*, from *vertere* (to turn)]. Denoting relationship to a vertebra or the vertebral column.

vesic- [L. *vesica* (bladder), *vesicula* (blister, vesicle)].
  1. Denoting a bladder.
  2. Denoting a blister.

vesica- [L. *vesica* (bladder), *vesicula* (blister, vesicle)].
  1. Denoting a bladder.
  2. Denoting a blister.

vesico- [L. *vesica* (bladder), *vesicula* (blister, vesicle)].
  1. Denoting relationship to the bladder.
  2. Denoting relationship to a blister.

viscero- [L. *viscus*, pl. *viscera* (organs of the body)]. Denoting relationship to the organs (viscera) of the body.

xanth- [Gr. *xanthos* (yellow)]. Meaning yellow or yellowish.

xantho- [Gr. *xanthos* (yellow)]. Meaning yellow or yellowish.

xeno- [Gr. *xenos* (strange, foreign)].
  1. Meaning strange.
  2. Denoting relationhsip to a foreign material.

xero- [Gr. *xēros* (dry)]. Meaning dry, or denoting relationship to dryness.

xiphi- [Gr. *xiphos* (sword)]. Denoting relationship to the xiphoid process.

xipho- [Gr. *xiphos* (sword)]. Denoting relationship to the xiphoid process.

xylo- [Gr. *xylon* (wood)]. Denoting relationship to wood.

zoo- [Gr. *zōon* (animal)]. Denoting relationship to an animal or animal life.

zyg- [Gr. *zygon* (yoke)]. Meaning yolked or joined, or relationship to a junction.

zygo- [Gr. *zygon* (yoke)]. Meaning yolked or joined, or relationship to a junction.

zym- [Gr. *zymē* (leaven, ferment)].
  1. Relating to fermentation.
  2. Relating to enzymes.

zymo- [Gr. *zymē* (leaven, ferment)].
  1. Relating to fermentation.
  2. Relating to enzymes.

Suffixes

-ad	[L. *ad* (to)]. Denoting toward or in the direction of the part indicated by the main portion of the word.
-agogue	[Gr. *agōgos* (leading, inducing)]. Indicating a promoter or stimulant of.
-agra	[Gr. *agra* (booty, a hunting, a draught of fishes, etc, hence a seizure)]. Meaning sudden onslaught of acute pain.
-algia	[Gr. *algos* (pain) + *-ia* (state or condition)]. Meaning pain or a painful condition.
-ase	Denoting an enzyme; suffixed to the name of the substance (substrate) upon which the enzyme acts.
-asis	[Gr.] Meaning state or condition.
-ate	Suffix forming a participial noun, as the object of the process indicated by the root to which it is affixed: eg, "injectate", something injected.
-blast	[Gr. *blastos* (offspring, germ)]. Indicating an immature precursor cell of the type indicated by the main word.
-cele	1. [Gr. *kēlē* (tumor, hernia)]. Denoting a swelling or hernia of the part signified by the main word. 2. [Gr. *koilia* (cavity)]. Signifying a relationship to a cavity.
-cleisis	[Gr. *kleisis* (a closing)]. Meaning closure.
-coele	[Gr. *koilia* (cavity)]. Denoting relationship to a space or cavity. Sometimes spelled "-cele".
-conid	Denoting the cusp of a tooth in the lower jaw.
-cyte	[Gr. *kytos* (hollow vessel; anything that contains or covers)]. Denoting a cell, the type of which is designated by the root to which it is attached.
-d	Indicating a deuterium-containing compound. Printed in lower case italics. Subscripts (d_2, d_3, etc.) indicate the number of such atoms.
-didymus	[Gr. *didymos* (twin, double, two-fold)]. Denoting a conjoined twin.
-diene	Used in chemistry to denote an unsaturated hydrocarbon containing two double bonds.
-dymus	1. [Gr. *-dymus* (fold)]. Indicates "-fold", as didymus (two-fold), tetradymus (four-fold), etc. 2. [Gr. *didymos* (twin)]. Occasionally used shortened form for "-didymus", denoting a conjoined twin.
-ectomize	[Gr. *ektomē* (excision) + *-izein* (to render)]. 1. Denoting deprivation by excision, as in adrenalectomize, etc. 2. By extension, used in terms to designate destruction or deprivation by other methods as well.
-ectomy	[Gr. *ektomē* (excision)]. 1. Indicating excision of the structure or organ designated by the root to which it is attached, eg, tonsillectomy. 2. By extension, used in terms to designate destruction or deprivation by other methods as well.
-emia	[Gr. *haima* (blood)]. Relating to blood.
-ene	Applied to a chemical name indicating the presence of a carbon-carbon double bond.
-esis	[Gr.] Meaning state or condition.
-facient	[L. *facio* (to make)]. Meaning one who, or that which, brings about.
-fugal	1. [L. *fugare* (to put to flight)]. Implying banishment, or driving away. 2. [L. *fugere* (to flee from)]. Implying traveling away from.
-fuge	[L. *fuga* (flight)]. Meaning flight or that which causes flight.

-gen	[Gr. *genos* (birth), *gennan* (to produce)]. 1. Meaning producing or coming to be. 2. In chemistry, indicating "precursor of".
-genic	[Gr. *gennan* (to produce)]. Meaning producing, or productive of.
-genin	Denoting the basic steroid unit of a toxic substance.
-gram	[Gr. *gramma* (that which is written, a mark)]. Denoting recording of many sorts.
-graph	[Gr. *graphō* (to write)]. Designating the instrument that makes the recording.
-graphy	[Gr. *graphō, graphein* (to write)]. Denoting a writing, recording, or description.
-ia	[Gr. *-ia* (denoting action or an abstract)]. Meaning state or condition; used in the formation of the names of many diseases.
-iasis	[Gr. *-iasis* (condition or state)]. Meaning a process or the condition resulting therefrom, particularly a morbid condition.
-ic	In chemistry, denoting that the element to the name of which it is attached is in combination in one of its higher valencies.
-ics	Denoting science, practice, or treatment.

-id	1. [Gr. *-eidos* (form, shape)].
	   a. Having the shape of, or resembling.
	   b. Indicating a state of sensitivity of the skin in which a part remote from the primary lesion reacts ("-id reaction") to substances of the pathogen, giving rise to a secondary inflammatory lesion. The lesion manifesting the reaction is designated by the use of "-id" as a suffix.
	2. [Gr. *-idios*, (one's own), diminutive ending]. Indicating a small or young specimen, eg, spermatid.

-ide	1. Denoting a binary chemical compound; formerly denoted by the qualification "-ureted", as in hydrogen sulfide or sulfureted hydrogen. 2. As a suffix to a sugar name, indicating substitution for the H of the hemiacetal OH (eg, glycoside).
-ine	1. Indicating an alkaloid. 2. Indicating an organic base. 3. Indicating a halogen.
-ism	[Gr. *-izō* + *-mos*]. 1. Meaning state, condition, or fact of being. 2. Meaning the process or result of an action.

-ite	[Gr. *-itēs* (fem. *-itis*)].
	   1. Denoting "of the nature of" or resembling the object to the name of which it is added.
	   2. In chemistry, denoting a salt of an acid whose name has the suffix "-ous".
	   3. In comparative anatomy, denoting an essential portion of the part of the name to which it is attached.

-ites	[Gr. *itēs* or *-itēs*, a masculine termination agreeing with *hydrōps* (dropsy)]. Indicating dropsy of the part indicated by the word stem to which it is attached.
-itis	[Gr. *-itis*, a feminine adjectival termination agreeing with Greek *nosos* (disease)]. Denoting inflammation of the part indicated by the word stem to which it is attached.
-ize	[Gr. *-izē* (causal idea, to make something take place)]. Denoting subjection to the specific action or treatment indicated by the stem to which it is attached.
-legia	[L. *legere* (to read)]. Relating to reading.
-lepsis	Denoting seizure.
-lepsy	Denoting seizure.
-lexis	[Gr. *-les-*, from *legein, lexai* (to speak)]. Relating to speech.

-lexy	[Gr. *-les-*, from *legein*, *lexai* (to speak)]. Relating to speech.
-logia	1. [Gr. *logos* (word, reason, discourse, treatise)]. Expressing in a general way the study of the subject noted in the main portion of the word, or a treatise on the same. 2. [Gr. *legō* (to collect)]. Signifying collecting or picking.
-logy	[Gr. *logos* (word, reason, discourse, treatise)]. Meaning the science or study of, or a treatise on, the subject designated by the stem to which it is attached.
-mania	[Gr. *mania* (frenzy)]. Referring to an abnormal love for, or morbid impulse toward, some specific object, place, or action.
-megaly	[Gr. *megas*, *megal-* (large)]. Meaning large.
-mer	Suffix attached to a prefix such as mono-, di-, tri-, poly, etc, to indicate the smallest unit of a repeating structure, eg, monomer.
-mere	[Gr. *mēros* (part)]. Indicating one of a series of similar parts, eg, blastomere.

-meter	[Gr. *metron* (measure)].
	     1. Designating relationship to measurement.
	     2. Denoting an instrument used in measurement.

-metry	[Gr. *metrein* (to measure)]. Meaning the act of measuring, or the measurement of, the object measured being indicated by the word stem to which it is attached.
-morph	[Gr. *morphē* (form, shape)]. Denoting relationship to form or shape.
-morphous	[Gr. morphē (form, shape)]. Indicating the manner of shape or form.
-odes	[Gr. *eidos* (form, resemblance)]. Meaning having the form of or like.
-odynia	[Gr. *odynē* (pain)]. Denoting pain.
-ogen	Often mistakenly construed as a combining form. However, the "o" is actually the final letter of a preceding combining form. Same as "-gen".
-oid	[Gr. *-o*, the stem vowel of the preceding word + *eidos* (form, appearance)]. Denoting resemblance to that which is indicated by the preceding element. Properly added only to words formed from Greek roots.
-ol	Denoting that a substance is an alcohol or phenol.
-ology	[Gr. *logos* (discourse, treatise)]. English suffix expressing in a general way the study of the subject noted in the body of the word, or a treatise on the same.
-oma	[Gr. *ōma* (tumor)]. Meaning a tumor or neoplasm. Properly added only to words derived from Greek roots.
-one	In chemistry, indicating quinquevalent nitrogen.
-onium	Indicating a positively charged compound ion, as ammonium (NH_4^+).
-opia	[Gr. *ōps* (eye). Meaning, or relating, to vision.
-ose	1. In chemistry, usually indicating a carbohydrate. 2. [L. -osus]. Appended to some Latin roots, signifying the more common form "-ous", denoting that the element to the name of which it is attached is in one of its lower valencies.

-osis	[Gr.]
	     1. Meaning a process, condition, or state, usually abnormal or diseased.
	     2. Denoting any production or increase (physiologic or pathologic), properly added only to words formed from Greek roots.
	     3. An invasion, and increase within the organism, of parasites.

-otomy	Denoting surgical incision.
-ous	Denoting that the element to the name of which it is attached is in one of its lower valencies, eg, phosphorus acid (H_3PO_3)
-pagus	[Gr. *pagos* (something fixed), from *pēgnymi* (to fasten together)]. Denoting conjoined twins, the first element of the word denoting the point of attachment, eg, craniopagus.
-pathy	[Gr. *pathos* (disease)]. Denoting a morbid condition, or disease.

-penia	[Gr. *penia* (poverty)]. Denoting deficiency.
-petal	[L. *petere* (to seek)]. Meaning directed or moving toward, the point of reference being indicated by the word stem to which it is attached.
-pexy	[Gr. *pēxis* (a fixing in place)]. Meaning fixation, usually surgical.
-phage	[Gr. *phagein* (to eat)]. Meaning eating or devouring.
-phagia	[Gr. *phagein* (to eat)]. Meaning eating or devouring.
-phagy	[Gr. *phagein* (to eat)]. Meaning eating or devouring.
-philia	[Gr. *philein* (to love, regard with affection)]. Denoting abnormal or notable fondness or attraction for.
-phrenia	[Gr. *phrēn* (the diaphragm, heart, seat of emotions, mind)].
	1. Denoting relationship to the diaphragm.
	2. Denoting relationship to the mind.
-plasia	[Gr. *plassō* (to form)]. Meaning formation.
-plast	[Gr. *plastos* (formed)]. Denoting any primitive living cell.
-plasty	[Gr. *plastos* (formed, shaped), *plassein* (to form, mold, or shape)]. Meaning molding or shaping or the result thereof, eg, of a surgical procedure.
-plegia	[Gr. *plēgē* (a blow, stroke)]. Meaning paralysis, or a stroke.
-ploid	[Gr. *-plo* (-fold) + *-ides* (in form)]. Meaning multiple in form.
	1. As an adjective, denoting condition in regard to degree of multiplication of chromosome sets in the karyotype.
	2. As a noun, denoting an individual or cell having chromosome sets of the particular degree of multiplication in the karyotype indicated by the root to which it is attached.
-ploidy	[Gr. *-plo* (-fold) + *-ides* (in form)]. Denoting the state of a cell nucleus with respect to the number of genomes it contains.
-poiesis	[Gr. *poiēsis* (a making)]. Meaning production.
-posia	[Gr. *posis* (drinking)]. Denoting relationship to drinking, or to intake of fluids.
-ptosis	[Gr. *ptōsis* (a falling)]. Denoting a falling or downward displacement of an organ.
-rhage	[Gr. *rhēgnymi* (to burst forth or erupt)]. Meaning a breaking or bursting forth, a profuse flow, as a hemorrhage.
-rhagia	[Gr. *rhēgnymi* (to burst forth or erupt)]. Denoting discharge from a burst vessel; usually denoting bleeding from a part.
-rhaphy	[Gr. *rhaphē* (seam)]. Meaning junction by a seam or suture.
-rhea	[Gr. *rhoia* (flux, flow), *rhein* (to flow, run or gush)]. Meaning a flowing.
-rrhage	[Gr. *rhēgnymi* (to burst forth or erupt)]. Denoting excessive or unusual discharge.
-rrhagia	[Gr. *rhēgnymi* (to burst forth or erupt)]. Denoting excessive or unusual discharge.
-rrhaphy	In surgery, indicating suturing, often denoting a fresh or recent laceration or wound.
-rrhea	[Gr. *rhoia* (flux, flow)]. Denoting flow or discharge.
-scope	[Gr. *skopeō* (to examine), *skopein* (to view or examine)]. Generally indicating an instrument for viewing, but also includes other methods of examination.
-scopy	[Gr. *skopein* (to examine)]. Meaning the act of examining.
-sis	Meaning state or condition.
-stomy	[Gr. *stoma* (mouth), *stomoun* (to provide with an opening)]. Denoting artificial or surgical creation of an artificial opening into a hollow organ, or a new opening between two such structures.
-thioic acid	Chemical suffix denoting the radical $-C(S)OH$ or $C(O)SH$.
-thione	Chemical suffix denoting the radical $=C=S$, the sulfur analogue of a ketone.

-thymia [Gr. *thymos* (the mind or heart as the seat of strong feelings or passion) + -*ia* (state or condition)]. Denoting relationship to the mind, soul, or emotions.

-tome [Gr. *tomos, tomē* (cutting, a cutting)].
  1. Denoting a cutting instrument, the first portion of the word usually indicating the part to be cut.
  2. A segment

-tomy [Gr. *tomē* (incision)]. Denoting a cutting operation or incision.

-trichia [Gr. *thrix, trich-* (hair)]. Denoting condition or type of hair.

-triene In chemistry, indicating the presence of three double bonds.

-trophic [Gr. *trophimos* (nourishing)]. Denoting relationship to nutrition.

-trophin [Gr. *trophimos* (nourishing)]. Denoting relationship to nutrition.

-trophy [Gr. *trophē* (nourishment)]. Relating to food or nutrition.

-tropic [Gr. *tropē, tropikos* (turn, turning)]. Denoting turning toward, changing, or tending to turn or change.

-uretic [Gr. *ourētikos* (relating to the urine)]. Denoting relationship to urine.

-uria [Gr. *ouron* (urine) + -*ia* (state or condition)]. Denoting a characteristic or constituent of the urine, indicated by the stem to which it is attached.

-yl [Gr. *hylē* (matter or substance)]. In chemistry, signifying that the substance is a radical, eg, phenyl.

-ylene 1. Chemical suffix denoting a bivalent hydrocarbon radical (eg, methylene, $-CH_2-$)
  2. In chemistry, denoting a double bond (eg, ethylene, $CH_2=CH_2$).

Symbols

Introduction

Symbols are letters, figures, or other marks used to indicate a specific thing within a specific setting. Many symbols consist only of ordinary letters (eg, chemical symbols). These are difficult to distinguish from abbreviations and are included in the Abbreviations and Acronyms section of this book. Symbols that are composed of characters other than simple letters are presented here.

   The symbols are arranged by their general shape or construction into the following groups: angles, arrows, boxes and circles, checks and radicals, dots, equalities and equivalents, numbers, pluses and minuses, primes, triangles, and weights and measures. The last is a miscellaneous group that contains all the symbols that do not readily fit into any of the other groups. If a proper name or term for a symbol is known, it is shaded and placed first at each entry. The meanings are then arranged alphabetically under this.

Angles

<	left single guillemet	∧	above
	caused by		diastolic blood pressure (anesthesia records)
	derived from		
	less than		elevated
	less severe than		enlarged
	produced by		improved
	proximal		increased
	right ear-bone conduction threshold		logical and
	smaller than		superior (position)
≮	not less than		upper
≤, ⩽	less than or equal to	∨	below
≲	less than or equivalent to		decreased
≨	neither less than nor equal to		deficiency
≪	left double guillemet		deficit
	much less than		depressed
⋘	left triple guillemet		deteriorated
	much much less than		diminished
>	right single guillemet		down
	causes		inferior (position)
	demonstrates		logical or
	derived from		lower
	distal		systolic blood pressure (anesthesia records)
	followed by	⊻	logical exclusive or
	greater than	∀	for all
	indicates	∠	angle
	larger than		flexion
	leads to		flexor
	left ear-bone conduction threshold	∠ᴇ	angle E
	more severe than		angle of entry
	produces	∠ˣ	angle X
	radiates to, radiating to		angle of exit
	results in	∡	measured angle
	reveals	∢	spherical angle
	shows	∟	right angle
	to	⌐	right angle
	toward		right lower quadrant
	worse than	⌐	right upper quadrant
	yields	¬	left upper quadrant
≯	not greater than	¬	logical not
≥, ⩾	greater than or equal to	⌐	left lower quadrant
≳	greater than or equivalent to	⊤	top
≩	neither greater than nor equal to	⊥	bottom
≫	right double guillemet		
	much greater than		
⋙	right triple guillemet		
	much much greater than		

Arrows

→ right single arrow
approaches limit of
causes to
demonstrates
direction of flow or reaction
distal
due to
followed by
indicates
is due to
leads to
no change
produces
progressing
radiating to
results in
reveals
shows, showed
to
to the right
toward
transfer to
vector
yields

→
← left single arrow
caused by
derived from
direction of flow or reaction
is due to
produced by
proximal
resulting from
secondary to
to the left

⇆,⇌ reversible chemical reaction
⇒ right double arrow
implies

⇐ left double arrow
implied by

↔ left and right arrow
stable
to and from
unchanging

↑ up arrow
above
alive
elevated
elevation
enlarged
gas

greater than
high
improved
increase, increased, increases
more than
rising
superior (position)
up, upper

⇑ up
↓ down arrow
below
dead
decrease, decreased
deficiency
deficit
depressed, depression
deteriorated, deteriorating
diminished
diminution
down
falling
inferior (position)
less than
low, lower, lowered
normal plantar reflex
precipitate, precipitates
restricted

↑C increase due to chemical interference
during assay
↓C decrease due to chemical interference
during assay
↑g increasing
rising
↓g decreasing
diminishing
falling
lowering

↑ICP increased intracranial pressure
↑V increase due to "in vivo" effect (lab)
↓V decrease due to "in vivo" effect (lab)
↑↑ extensor
extensor response, Babinski sign (neurologic examination)
positive babinski
testes undescended

↓↓ bilaterally descended
both down
flexor
plantar response, Babinski sign (neurologic examination)
testes descended

↑↓	reversible reaction up and down	↘	southeast arrow decreasing
↕	up-and-down arrow	↖	northwest arrow
↗	northeast arrow	↙	southwest arrow
	deviated displaced increasing		

Boxes & Circles

◯	circle empty respirations (anesthesia record) living female normal female right ear-air conduction threshold	⊕	plus positive present
●	affected female deceased female pulse rate (anesthesia record)	⊖	absent minus negative
◯◯	male	Ⓐ	circle A axilla (temperature)
⊙	circle dot start of operation (anesthesia record) carrier of sex-linked recessive	ⓐx	axilla (temperature)
	abortion or stillbirth, sex unspecified	Ⓒ	copyright confidential (patient may be unaware)
⊖	normal	Ⓗ ⓗ	circle H hypodermic, hypodermically
⊘	death empty set no none	ⓘM	intramuscular, intramuscularly
		ⓘV	intravenous, intravenously
♀	female female sex	Ⓛ	circle L left
♂	male male sex	Ⓜ	circle M murmur
		ⓜ	by mouth mouth (temperature) murmur

√⌐(m)	factitial murmur
(o)	circle O by mouth oral, orally
(R)	circle R rectal, rectally rectum (temperature) registered trademark right
(X)	circle X end of anesthesia (anesthesia 　　record) end of operation
♀	standing
⊶	recumbent
⚲	sitting
□	left ear-masked air conduction 　　threshold living male normal male
■	affected male deceased male
■◕	heterozygotes for autosomal 　　recessive
■●	proband or propositus
□♀	individual died without leaving 　　offspring
□⊤○	no issue

[3] (2)	number of children of sex indicated
⧄ ⊘	death male, death female
[□] [○]	adopted male, adopted female
□—○	mating
□=○	consanguinity
□⊤○	illegitimacy
I □⊤○ II □ ○	parents and offspring, in 　　generations
⌂	dizygotic twins
◬	monozygotic twins
⊞	examined professionally–normal 　　for trait
⊟	not examined–dubiously reported 　　to have trait
⊟	not examined–reliability reported to 　　have trait

Checks & Radicals

✓	check		✓g	checking
	flexion		✓ing	checking
	observe for		✓qs	voided quantity sufficient
	urine		√	radical
	voided			root
✓.	voided and bowels moved			square root
✓c̄	check with		²√	square root
✓d	checked		³√	cube root
	observed			

Dots

...	no data (in a given category)		∴	therefore
:	colon		::	four dots
	is to			as (in ratios)
	ratio			equality between ratios
;	semicolon			identical
.·	because			proportion
	since			proportional to

Equalities & Equivalents

~	tilde		≒	falling dots equals
	about			image
	approximate, approximately			nearly equal to
	proportionate to		≓	rising dots equals
	similar			reverse image
.~	approximate		÷	approximately equal to
+̇	not similar		≐	approaches
≃	similar or equal		⊥	quilateral
	approximately equal		△	equiangular
≠	not similar or equal		≟	questioned equality
≈	approximately equal			not equal, not equal to
	nearly equal to			unequal
≉	not approximately equal		≡	identical
≅	approximately			identical with
	approximately equals		≢	not identical
	congruent to			not identical with
≇	not congruent		≍	asymptotically equivalent
=	equal		≭	not asymptotically equivalent
	equal to		⇌	equivalent to
≠	does not equal, not equal to			isomorphic
			≵	not equivalent to
				not isomorphic

Numbers

0   zero
completely absent (pulse)
may indicate neuropathy
(reflexes)
no muscular contraction
(muscle strength)
no response (reflexes)

0/0   zero on either side

1   barely detectable flicker or
trace of contraction
(muscle strength)

1+   one plus
low normal (reflexes)
markedly impaired (pulse)
slight reaction or slight
trace (lab tests)
somewhat diminished (reflexes)

+1   markedly impaired (pulse)

1×   once
one time

1°   first degree
one hour
primary

$\bar{1}$, **etc.**   bowel movement (numeral indicates number of movements in a given period)

¹/₆ or I/VI   may not be heard in all positions, heard only after listener has "tuned in" (heart murmur)

2   active movement of the body part with gravity eliminated (muscle strength)

2+   two plus
average (reflexes)
moderately impaired (pulse)
normal (reflexes)
noticeable reaction or trace (lab tests)

+2   moderately impaired (pulse)

2×, ×2   twice
two times

2 × 2   gauze dressing, folded 2″ × 2″

2°   secondary
second degree
two hours

2d   second

2ndry   secondary

2/6 or II/VI   quiet, but heard immediately upon placing the stethoscope on the chest (heart murmur)

3   active movement against gravity (muscle strength)

3+   three plus
moderate reaction (lab tests)
more brisk than average (reflexes)
possibly, but not necessarily, indicative of disease (reflexes)
slightly impaired (pulse)

+3   slightly impaired (pulse)

3×, ×3   three times

3°   tertiary
third degree

3/6 or III/VI   moderately loud (heart murmur)

4   active movement against gravity and some resistance (muscle strength)

4+   four plus
hyperactive or very brisk (reflexes)
large amount (lab tests)
may indicate disease (reflexes)
normal (pulse)
often associated with clonus (reflexes)
pronounced reaction (lab tests)

+4   normal (pulse)

4 × 4   gauze dressing, folded 4″ × 4″

4/6 or IV/VI   loud (heart murmur)

5   active movement against full resistance without evident fatigue (normal) (muscle strength)

5/6 or V/VI   very loud, may be heard with a stethoscope partly off the chest (heart murmur)

6/6 or VI/VI   may be heard with the stethoscope entirely off the chest (heart murmur)

24°   24 hours

606   arsphenamine

914   neoarsphenamine

Plus & Minus

+ plus, one plus
acid reaction
add, added to
and
convex lens
excess
increased
less than 50% inhibition of hemolysis
(Wassermann)
low normal (reflexes)
markedly impaired (pulse)
mild (severity)
plus (slightly more than stated
amount)
positive
present
slight reaction or slight trace (lab tests)
sluggish (reflexes)
somewhat diminished (reflexes)

∔ dot plus
direct sum

(+) significant
uncommon or uncertain mode of
inheritance

(+)ive positive

+ to ++ slight pain

++ two plus
average (reflexes)
50% inhibition of hemolysis
(Wassermann)
moderate (pain, severity)
moderately impaired (pulse)
normally active (reflexes)
noticeable reaction or trace (lab tests)

+++ three plus
increased reflexes
75% inhibition of hemolysis
(Wassermann)
moderate amount
moderate reaction (lab tests)
moderately hyperactive (reflexes)
moderately severe (pain, severity)
more brisk than average (reflexes)
slightly impaired (pulse)

++++ four plus
complete inhibition of hemolysis
(Wassermann)
large amount (lab tests)
markedly hyperactive (reflexes)
markedly severe (pain, severity)
normal (pulse)
pronounced reaction (lab tests)
very brisk (reflexes)

++/+ 2 plus on the right, 1 plus on the left

± to + minimal pain

± plus or minus
doubtful
equivocal (reflexes, qualitative tests)
flicker (reflexes)
indefinite
more or less
no definite cause
not definite
positive or negative
possibly significant
questionable
suggestive
variable
very slight (reaction, severity, trace)
with or without

(±) possibly significant

∓ minus or plus

− minus
absent
alkaline reaction
concave lens
decreased
deficiency, deficient
diminished
negative
none
subtract
without

(-) insignificant

‡ double dagger
moderate (severity)
normally active (reflexes)

Primes

′   prime
- foot, feet
- minutes (1/60 of an hour or degree of angle)
- primary accent
- univalent

″   double prime
- bivalent
- ditto

″ (cont'd)
- inch
- seconds (1/60 of a minute of time or minute of angle)
- secondary accent

‴   triple prime
- line (1/12 inch)
- trivalent

Triangles

Δ   delta
- anion gap
- centrad prism
- change
- delta gap
- heat
- increment
- occipital triangle
- prism diopter
- right ear-masked air conduction threshold
- temperature (anesthesia records)

Δ+   time interval

ΔA   change in absorbance

ΔDb   difference in decibels

ΔH, H's Δ   Hesselbach's triangle

ΔP   change in intraocular pressure

ΔPh   change in pH

Δ scan   delta scan (computed tomography scan)

Δt   time interval

$\underline{\Delta}$ underscored triangle
- defined as

$\underset{\triangledown}{\underline{\underline{\Delta}}}$ corresponds to

∇   nabla

Weights & Measures
(Medication Orders/Prescriptions)

℥̇   one

℥̈   two

℥⃛   three

Ʒ   drachm (dram)

Ʒfl, fƷ   fluid drachm (fluid dram)

Ʒ   dram

Ʒfl, fƷ   fluid dram

♍   minim

℥   ounce

℥ss   half-ounce (tablespoon, approximately 15 ml)

℥fl, f℥   fluid ounce

 Э   scruple

Ʒ, flƷ, Ʒf   teaspoon (fluid dram, approximately 5 ml)

Miscellaneous

❤	heart
&	ampersand
	and
@	at
(	left parenthesis
)	right parenthesis
[	left bracket
	right ear-masked bone conduction threshold
]	right bracket
	left ear-masked bone conduction threshold
{	left brace
}	right brace
^	caret
¦	broken vertical bar
¶	paragraph sign
§	section sign
!	exclamation point
	factorial product
"	double quote
'	single quote
#	number/pound
	fracture
	gauge
	has been done
	has been given
	number
	pound(s)
	weight
*	asterisk
	birth
	multiplication
	not verified
	presumed
	supposed
?	question mark
	doubtful
	equivocal (reflexes)
	flicker (reflexes)
	not tested (severity)
	possible
	questionable
	question of
	suggested
	suggestive (severity)
	unknown

№	number (No.)
℞	prescription (Rx)
	recipe
	take
SM	servicemark
TM	trademark
®	registered trademark
©	copyright
%	percent
‰	per thousand
÷	division
	divided by
×	multiply
	times
†	dagger
	dead
	death
	deceased
	died
◊	lozenge
	sex unknown
	sex unspecified
∝	alpha particle
	proportional
/	virgule, slash
	and
	divided by
	either meaning
	extension
	extensor
	fraction
	of
	per
	to
	with
\	backslash
|	absolute value
	divides
∤	does not divide
|x|	absolute value of x
∥	parallel bars
	parallel
∦	not parallel
∈	element
	member
∋	such that

∃ there exists

∄ there never exists

∞ indefinitely more
infinite
infinity

° degree
hour (1/24 of a solar day)
measure of angle ($^1/_{360}$ of a circle)
severity (burns, wounds)
temperature
time (hour)

∫ integral

∏ product

∐ coproduct

•• combined with

∩ intersection

∪ union

⊎ U plus
multiset union

⊂ proper subset

⊆ reflex subset (contained in or equals)

⊄ subset but does not equal

⊃ proper superset

⊇ reflex superset (contains or equals)

⊉ superset but does not equal

∂ partial derivative

≺ precedes

≼ precedes or equals

⋠ neither procedes nor equals

≻ follows

⊁ does not follow

≽ follows or equals

⋡ neither follows nor equals

ⴵ between (quantic)

ℂ hollow C
complex number

𝕀 hollow I
integer

ℕ hollow N
natural number

ℝ hollow R
real number

ℰ script E
electromotive force

e script e
error

ℱ script F
fourier transform

ℒ script L
laplace transform

ℓ script l
liter

Greek Alphabet

	CAPITAL LETTERS	SMALL LETTERS	ENGLISH TRANSLATION
Alpha	A	α	A
Beta	B	β	B
	B (medial or terminal)	Ϭ (medial or terminal)	B
Gamma	Γ	γ	G
Delta	Δ	δ	D
Epsilon	E	ϵ	E
		ε (variant)	E
Zeta	Z	ζ	Z
Eta	H	η	Ē
Theta	Θ	θ	TH
		ϑ (variant)	TH
Iota	I	ι	TH
Kappa	K	κ	K, C (Latin)
		$\varkappa$ (variant)	K, C (Latin)
Lambda	Λ	λ	L
MU	M	μ	M
Nu	N	ν	N
Xi	Ξ	ξ	X
Omicron	O	o	O
Pi	Π	π	P
		ϖ (variant)	P
Rho	P	ρ	R, RH
		ϱ (variant)	R, RH
Sigma	Σ	σ	S
	Σ (terminal)	Ϛ (terminal)	S
		ς (variant)	S
Tau	T	τ	T
Upsilon	Y	υ	Y
	ϒ (variant)		Y
Phi	Φ	ϕ	PH
		φ (variant)	PH
Chi	X	χ	CH
Psi	Ψ	ψ	PS
Omega	Ω	ω	Ō
		Z (variant)	Ō

Greek Letters & Symbols

A ALPHA, UPPER CASE, 1st letter
α alpha, lower case, 1st letter
alpha particle
angular acceleration
constituent of alpha plasma protein
fraction
first in a series or group
heavy chain of immunoglobulin A
is proportional to
optical rotation (chemistry)
probability of type I error (statistics)
significance level
solubility coefficient (Bunsen's)
α_1AC alpha$_1$-anti-chymotrypsin
α-GLUC alpha-glucosidase
α-KG alpha-ketoglutarate
α-LP alpha-lipoprotein
α_2M alpha$_2$-macroglobulin
α_1PI human alpha$_1$ proteinase inhibitor

B BETA, UPPER CASE, 2nd letter
B BETA, UPPER CASE, medial or
terminal, 2nd letter
β beta, lower case, 2nd letter
anomer of carbohydrate
beta chain of hemoglobin
buffer capacity
carbon separated from carboxyl by one
other carbon in aliphatic compounds
constituent of beta plasma protein
fraction
probability of type II error (statistics)
second in a series or group
substituent group of steroid that projects above plane of ring
1-β power of statistical test
β_2**m** beta$_2$-microglobulin
β-**BuTX** beta-bungarotoxin
β beta, lower case, medial or terminal,
2nd letter

Γ GAMMA, UPPER CASE, 3rd letter
γ gamma, lower case, 3rd letter
10^{-4} gauss
carbon separated from the carboxyl
group by two other carbon atoms

constituent of gamma protein plasma
fraction
done
gamma chain of fetal hemoglobin
heavy chain of immunoglobulin G
microgram (former symbol, now μg)
photon (gamma ray)
plasma protein (globulin)
third in a series or group
γ-**Abu** gamma-aminobutyric acid
γ-**BHC** gamma-benzene hexachloride (lindane)
γG immunoglobulin G
γGT gamma-glutamyltranspeptidase
γ-**HCD** gamma-heavy chain disease

Δ DELTA, UPPER CASE, 4th letter
absence of heat in a reaction
change in a component of a physical
system
delta gap
diagnosis
difference (mathematics)
double bond
increment
Δ9 THC delta-9-tetrahydrocannabinol
Δ**EF** ejection fraction response
δ delta, lower case, 4th letter
fourth in a series or group
heavy chain of immunoglobulin D
delta chain of hemoglobin
thickness in a biological system, as of
a layer of fluid
δ-**ALA** delta-aminolevulinic acid

E EPSILON, UPPER CASE, 5th letter
ε epsilon, lower case, 5th letter
chain of hemoglobin
dielectric constant
fifth in a series or group
heavy chain of immunoglobulin E
molar absorption coefficient
molar absorptivity
molar extinction coefficient
permittivity
specific absorptivity
ε-**Acp** ε-aminocaproic acid
ε epsilon, lower case, variant, 5th letter

Z	ZETA, UPPER CASE, 6th letter		micro- (10^{-6})
ζ	zeta, lower case, 6th letter		micrometer (micron)
			mutation rate
H	ETA, UPPER CASE, 7th letter		permeability
η	eta, lower case, 7th letter		population mean (statistics)
	absolute viscosity	$\mu_\circ$	permeability of vacuum
	apparent (or dynamic) velocity	μA	microampere
		μb	microbar; also μbar
Θ	THETA, UPPER CASE, 8th letter	μ_β	Bohr's magneton
	thermodynamic temperature	μbar	microbar; also μb
θ	theta, lower case, 8th letter	μC	microcoulomb; also μcoul
	angular coordinate variable	μc	microcurie; also μCi
	customary temperature	μch	microcurie-hour; also μC-hr, μCi-hr
	latent trait (statistics)	μC-hr	microcurie-hour; also μch, μCi-hr
	temperature interval	μCi	microcurie; also μc
ϑ	theta, lower case, variant, 8th letter	μCi-hr	microcurie-hour; also μch, μC-hr
		μcoul	microcoulomb; also μC
I	IOTA, UPPER CASE, 9th letter	μ Eq	microequivalent
ι	iota, lower case, 9th letter	$\mu F, \mu f$	microfarad
		μg	microgram; also mcg
K	KAPPA, UPPER CASE, 10th letter	$\mu\gamma$	microgamma
κ	kappa, lower case, 10th letter	μGy	microgray
	magnetic susceptibility	μH	microhenry
	one of two types of immunoglobulin light chains	μHg	micrometer of mercury; also μmHg
ϰ	kappa, lower case, variant, 10th letter	μin	microinch
		μIU	one-millionth International Unit
Λ	LAMBDA, UPPER CASE, 11th letter	μkat	microkatal
λ	lambda, lower case, 11th letter	$\mu L, \mu l$	microliter
	craniometric point	μM	micromolar
	decay constant	μm	micrometer; also μ
	homosexuality		micromilli-
	junction of lambdoid and sagittal sutures (craniotomy)	μmg	micromilligram (nanogram)
	mean free path	μMhg	micrometer of mercury; also μHg
	microliter (now μl)	μmm	micromillimeter (nanometer)
	one of two forms of immunoglobulin light chains	$\mu m\mu$	meson
	thermal conductivity	μmol/L	micromolar
	wavelength	$\mu\Omega$	microhm
		μOsm	micro-osmolar
M	MU, UPPER CASE, 12th letter	$\mu R, \mu r$	microroentgen
μ	mu, lower case, 12th letter	μ/ρ	mass attenuation coefficient
	chemical potential	μs	microsecond; also μsec
	dynamic viscosity	μsec	microsecond; also μs
	electrophoretic mobility	μU	microunit
	heavy chain of immunoglobulin M	$\mu V, \mu v$	microvolt
	linear attenuation coefficient	$\mu W, \mu w$	microwatt
	magnetic moment	$\mu\mu$	micromicro- (10^{-12}, replaced by pico)
	mass absorption coefficient		micromicron
	mean		

$\mu\mu C$	micromicrocurie (picocurie); also $\mu\mu Ci$
$\mu\mu Ci$	micromicrocurie (picocurie); also $\mu\mu C$
$\mu\mu F$	micromicrofarad (picofarad)
$\mu\mu g$	micromicrogram (picogram)
N	NU, UPPER CASE, 13th letter
ν	nu, lower case, 13th letter
	frequency
	kinematic viscosity
	neutrino
	number of degrees of freedom
Ξ	XI, UPPER CASE, 14th letter
ξ	xi, lower case, 14th letter
O	OMICRON, UPPER CASE, 15th letter
o	omicron, lower case, 15th letter
Π	PI, UPPER CASE, 16th letter
	product of a sequence (math)
π	pi, lower case, 16th letter
	3.1416 (3.1415926536), ratio of the circumference of a circle to its diameter
	osmotic pressure
ϖ	pi, lower case, variant, 16th letter
P	RHO, UPPER CASE, 17th letter
ρ	rho, lower case, 17th letter
	correlation coefficient
	electrical resistivity
	electric charge density
	mass density
	population correlation coefficient
	reactivity
ϱ	rho, lower case, variant, 17th letter
Σ	SIGMA, UPPER CASE, 18th letter
	foaminess
	sigmoid
	sigmoidoscopy
	sum
	summation of all quantities following the symbol
	syphilis
Σ	SIGMA, UPPER CASE, terminal, 18th letter

σ	sigma, lower case, 18th letter
	conductivity
	cross-section
	millisecond (0.001 seconds)
	population standard deviation
	Stefan-Boltzmann constant
	stress
	surface tension
	type of molecular bond
	wavenumber
σ^2	population variance
$\sigma_{diff.}$	standard error of difference between scores
$\sigma_{est.}$	standard error of estimate
$\sigma_{meas.}$	standard error of measurement
ς	sigma, lower case, terminal, 18th letter
s	sigma, lower case, variant, 18th letter
T	TAU, UPPER CASE, 19th letter
τ	tau, lower case, 19th letter
	life (lifetime of radioactive isotopes)
	mean life
	relaxation time
	shear stress
	spectral transmittance
	torque
	transmission coefficient
$\tau^1/_2$	halflife (of radioactive isotopes)
Υ	UPSILON, UPPER CASE, 20th letter
Υ	UPSILON, UPPER CASE, variant, 20th letter
υ	upsilon, lower case, 20th letter
Φ	PHI, UPPER CASE, 21st letter
ϕ	phi, lower case, 21st letter
	ability continuum
	file
	magnetic flux
	osmotic coefficient
	phi coefficient (statistics)
φ	phi, lower case, variant, 21st letter
	none
X	CHI, UPPER CASE, 22nd letter
χ	chi, lower case, 22nd letter
χ^2	chi-square (distribution test)
χ_e	electric susceptibility
χ_m	magnetic susceptibility

Ψ PSI, UPPER CASE, 23rd letter
psychiatry

ψ psi, lower case, 23rd letter
pseudo
pseudouridine
wave function

Ω OMEGA, UPPER CASE,
24th letter
ohm

ω omega, lower case, 24th letter
angular frequency
angular velocity
carbon atom farthest from principal
functioning group

ϖ omega, lower case, variant, 24th letter

Appendix

Addendum

This addendum includes the abbreviations and acronyms discovered after this book went to press. The major portion of these entries relate to the expanding industry of Managed Health Care. Some of these entries are not enclued in the main list, while others are additional meanings of entries already listed.

5+2 cytarabine and daunorubicin

7+3 ARA-C and daunorubicin

AAPCC adjusted average per capita cost

AAPHO American Association of Physician-Hospital Organizations

AAPI American Accreditation Program, Inc.

AAPPO American Association of Preferred Provider Organizations

A/B Mods apnea/bradycardia moderate stimulation

AC assist control

ACDs anticonvulsant drugs

ACR adjusted community rating

ACSW Academy of Certified Social Workers

AD alternating days

ADA Americans with Disabilities Act

ADSU ambulatory diagnostic surgery unit

AFHHA American Federation of Home Health Agencies

AHCA American Health Care Association

AHP Accountable Health Partnership
Accountable Health Plan

AHS American Health Security Act (of 1993)

ALK-IOS alkaline phosphatase isoenzymes

2 alt every other day

AMCP Academy of Managed Care Pharmacy

AMCRA American Managed Care and Review Association

AMPRA American Medical Peer Review Association

AMR alternating motor rate

AN Associate Nurse

AOB assignment of benefits

AOD Assistant Officer of the Day

APG ambulatory patient group

APN Advanced Practice Nurse

APR average payment rate

APVR aortic pulmonary valve replacement

ARA-AC fazarabine

arr arrive

ASHRM American Society for Healthcare Risk Management

ASO administrative services only (contract)

ASR age/sex rates

ASS assessment

AT activity therapist

ATSO₄ atropine sulfate

AUD COMP auditory compensation

AVGs ambulatory visit groups

AVOC avocation

A waves atrial contraction waves

AWDW assault with a deadly weapon

AWP average wholesale price

BACT bacteria; also Bact, bact

BAERs brain-stem auditory evoked responses

BBS bilateral breath sounds

B cat *Branhamella catarrhalis*

BC/BE board certified/board eligible

BF breast-feed

BFM black female, married

B frag *Bacillus fragilis*

BIG 6 SMA 6 (analysis of 6 serum chemical components)

BLR blood flow rate

BMTT bilateral myringotomy with tympanic tubes

BPLA blood pressure, left arm; also BP lar

BPRA blood pressure, right arm; also BP rar

BSW Bachelor of Social Work

BVRT Benton Visual Retention Test

CAM Catchment Area Management (Project)

CAP capitation (a type of risk sharing reimbursement); also cap
carcinoma of the prostate; also cap

cap capitation (a type of risk sharing reimbursement); also CAP
carcinoma of the prostate; also CAP

CASP Child Analytic Study Program

CBP chronic benign pain

CCC-A Certificate of Clinical Competence in Audiology

CCC-SP Certificate of Clinical Competence in Speech-Language Pathology

CCN community care network

CCP coordinated care plan

CCRC continuing care retirement community (program)

CDP Child Development Program

CEC Council for Exceptional Children

CEO chief executive officer

CFS Child and Family Service

CH chronic

CHAP Child Health Associate Practitioner

CH₃-CCNU methylchloroethylcyclohexyl-nitrosourea (semustine); also MCCNU, MeCCNU, MeCcnu, methyl-CCNU

CHIP iproplatin

CHMIS Community Health Managed Information System

CIB Carnation Instant Breakfast

CLO close

CM case management
case manager

CMSA Case Management Society of America

CMT cutis marmorata telangiectasia

CO court order

C/O, c/o under care of

COA Certificate of Authority

COC Certificate of Coverage

COCCIDIO coccidioidomycosis

CODO codocytes

COI Certificate of Insurance

Coke Coca-Cola
cocaine

CONTU contusions; also cont

Co-Pay copayment

COPE cyclophosphamide, Oncovin, Platinol, and etoposide

CP Certified Paramedic
convenience package

C&P complete and pushing

CPA conditioned play audiometry

CPI-MCS consumer price index–medical care services

CPL criminal procedure law

CPP chronic pelvic pain

CPT-4 Physician's Current Procedural Terminology, 4th Edition

CQI continuous quality improvement

CRC community rating by class

CRI CHAMPUS reform initiative

CRM+ cross-reacting material positive

CRNI Certified Registered Nurse Intravenous

CS IV clinical stage four

CT cytarabine and thioguanine

CTA catamenia [Gr. *katamēnia* (menses)]

CTD cumulative trauma disorder

CTZ Co-Trimoxazole (sulfamethoxazole and trimethoprim)

CVI carboplatin, Vepesid, ifosfamide, and mesna uroprotection

C/W crutch walking; also CW, cw

CWW clinic without walls

Cx culture; also cult, CX
cylinder axis; also CX

CZN chlorzotocin

ΔOD 450 deviation of optical density at 450

D50 50% dextrose injection

DAG dianhydrogalactitol

DARP drug abuse reporting program

DC dual choice

DCI duplicate coverage inquiry

DCP vitamin D, calcium, and phosphorus (tablets)

DCYS Department of Children and Youth Services

D₅E₇₅ 5% dextrose and electrolyte #75

DFACS Department of Family and Children Services

DFW Dexide face wash

DHA docosahexaenoic acid

DHR Department of Human Resources

DHS Department of Human Services

DMO Dental Maintenance Organization

DNP do not publish

D5 1/2 NS dextrose 5% in 1/2 normal (0.45%) saline

DOB dangle out of bed

DOS date of service

DPR drug price review

DPT Driver Performance Test

DSM drink skim milk

DSM III *Diagnostic and Statistical Manual of Mental Disorders*, 3rd edition

DTD # dispense the given number of doses [L. *detur talis dosis* (let such a dose be given)]

DUM drug utilization management

DVR Division of Vocational Rehabilitation

5DW 5% dextrose in water

EAP Employee Assistance Program

EAPA Employee Assistance Professionals Association

EAS external anal sphincter

EASNA Employee Assistance Society of North America

EBAB equal breath sounds bilaterally

EBIS Employee Benefits Information System

EBR Employee Benefits Representative

EBRI Employee Benefits Research Institute

ECHO/NV echocardiography/radionuclide ventriculography

EDAX energy-dispersing analysis of X-rays

EDF elongation, derotation, and flexion

EDI electronic data interchange

EFM electronic fetal monitor

EKO echoencephalogram

EMO exclusive multiple option

ENC encourage

EOB explanation of benefits

E of I evidence of insurability

EOG Ethrane, oxygen, and gas (nitrous oxide)

EPC erosive prepyloric changes

ERISA Employee Retirement Income Security Act

ESD Emergency Services Department

Ext mon external monitor

FAAP Fellow of the American Academy of Pediatrics

FAA SOL formalin, acetic, and alcohol solution

FAB digoxin immune Fab (Digibind)

FACAG Fellow of the American College of Angiology

FACAL Fellow of the American College of Allergists

FACAN Fellow of the American College of Anesthesiologists

FACAS Fellow of the American College of Abdominal Surgeons

FACCPC Fellow of the American College of Clinical Pharmacology and Chemotherapy

FACEM Fellow of the American College of Emergency Medicine

FACEP Fellow of the American College of Emergency Physicians

FACGE Fellow of the American College of Gastroenterology

FACLM Fellow of the American College of Legal Medicine

FACN Fellow of the American College of Nutrition

FACNP Fellow of the American College of Neuropsychopharmacology

FACPRM Fellow of the American College of Preventive Medicine

FAS Financial Accounting Standards

FASHP Fellow of the American Society of Hospital Pharmacists

FDGS, Fdgs feedings

Fee Max fee maximum

FEF$_{25-75}$ forced expiratory flow during the middle half of the forced vital capacity

FEF$_{x-y}$ forced expiratory flow between two designated volume points in the forced vital capacity

FPP faculty practice plan

FQHMO federally qualified health maintenance organization

FR Father (priest)

FSALT Fletcher suite after loading tandem

F to N finger-to-nose; also FN, F-N, F➞N, FTN

F wave fibrillatory wave
flutter wave

GALI-PUT galactose-1-phosphate uridyltransferase; also GALT

Ga scan gallium scan

GDP gross domestic product

GNP gross national product

G$_4$P$_{3104}$ (example) gravida, para (subscripts represent number of occurrences: [L. *gravida* (pregnant)], 4 pregnancies; [L. *partus* (birth)], 3 went to term, 1 premature, no abortions or miscarriages, 4 living children)

GPWW group practice without walls

GRASS gradient recalled acquisition in a steady state

GRTT Graduate Respiratory Therapist Technician

H *Haemophilis* species; also *H*

3H high, hot, and a helluva lot; also HHH

HAM-A Hamilton Anxiety (Scale); HAMA

1 HB first-degree heart block; also HB1°

2 HB second-degree heart block; also HB2°

3 HB third-degree heart block; also HB3°

HCCP health care payment plan

HCP health care plan

HCPCS HCFA (Health Care Financing Administration) Common Procedural Coding System

HCQI Health Care Quality Improvement Act (of 1986)

HEC Health Education Center

HEDIS Health Plan Employer Data & Information Set

hep cap heparin cap

HFA health facility administrator

H flu *Haemophilus influenzae*; also HIF

HHH high, hot, and a helluva lot; also 3H

HHTC high-humidity trach collar

HHTM high-humidity trach mask

HI horizontal integration

HIAA Health Insurance Association of America

HIF *Haemophilus influenzae*; also H flu

HIN health insurance network

HIO Health Insuring Organization

HIPC health insurance purchasing cooperative

HISB Health Insurance Standards Board

HM human semisynthetic insulin

HOI Health Outcomes Institute

HONDA hypertensive, obese, Negro, diabetic, arthritic

HPA hospital-physician alliance

HPNS Healthcare Provider Networks Section (of the American Hospital Association)

HSA Health Services Agreement

HSB Health Standards Board

HT hyperthermia

HUS husband; also H, husb

Hx hospitalization; also H, Hosp, hosp, HX

hypopit hypopituitarism

I incisal

I₂ iodine

i Roman numeral one; also I

IAF industry adjustment factor

ICCU intermediate coronary care unit

ICD 9 CM International Classification of Diseases, 9th Revision - Clinical Modification

ICMA Individual Case Management Association

ID ifosfamide, doxorubicin, and mesna uroprotection

IDI Interpersonal Dependency Inventory

IDS integrated delivery system

IFEBP International Foundation of Employee Benefit Plans

IMVP-16 ifosfamide, mesna uroprotection, methotrexate, and VP-16 (etoposide)

Inc Spir incentive spirometer; also IS

INFC infected; also INF, inf, infect infection; also INF, inf, infect, infx

INTERP interpretation

Int mon internal monitor

intol intolerance

intub intubation

I/S instruct/supervise

ISHA International Subacute Healthcare Association

IS10S 10% invert sugar in saline

IS10W 10% invert sugar in water

IVA Intervir-A

IVSS intravenous Soluset

IWT impacted wisdom teeth

J jejunostomy (tube)

JLP juvenile laryngeal papillomatosis

JOMAC judgement, orientation, memory, affect, and cognition

JPA Joint Powers Authority

K₃ menadione (vitamin K₃)

KD Keto-Diastix

KTU kidney transplant unit

LAQ long arc quad

LCAH life care at home

LCM large case management

LD longdwell

LDR labor, delivery, and recovery

LL2 limb lead 2

LNCs lymph node cells

LOB line of business

LOT Licensed Occupational Therapist

LR left-right

LR1A labor room 1A
LS low salt
L5-S1 lumbar fifth vertebra to sacral first vertebra
LT laboratory technician
LTB$_4$ leukotriene B$_4$
LTC$_4$ leukotriene C$_4$
L&W living and well
LYM lymphocyte; also L, LY, lym, lymph
MAEEW moves all extremities equally well
MAP maximum allowable payment
MAT manual arts therapy
MaxLOS maximum length of stay
MC monocomponent (highly purified pork insulin)
McB pt McBurney's point
MCM medical care management
MCP managed care plan
MCTC metrizamide computed tomographic cisternogram
MDA methylenedioxyamphetamine
MDI methylenedioxyindenes
MDTM multidisciplinary team meeting
MEFR mid expiratory flow rate
MEL B melarsoprol
MEN (II) multiple endocrine neoplasia, type II
MERP medical expense reimbursement plan
MET multiple employer trust
MEWA Multiple Employer Welfare Association
MF *Malassezia furfur*
mg/kg/d milligrams per kilogram per day
mg/kg/hr milligrams per kilogram per hour
MGMA Medical Group Management Association
MHA Mental Health Assistant
MHCA Managed Health Care Association
MH/SA mental health/substance abuse
MHSS Military Health Service System
MIG Medicare-insured group
MIP Managed Indemnity Plan
MLP mid-level practitioner
MLR medical loss ratio
multiple logistic regression
MM member months
MMI 1-methylimidazole-2-thiol (methimazole)

MOB maintenance of benefits plan
MOR Monthly Operating Report
MPP Minimum Premium Plan
MPQ McGill Pain Questionnaire
MRDD mental retardation and development disabilities
MRE manual resistance exercise
MRSE methicillin-resistant *Staphylococcus epidermidis*
MSA metropolitan statistical area
MSO Management Services Organization
MSO$_4$ morphine sulfate
MTRS Licensed Master Therapeutic Recreation Specialist
MVV mixed vespid venom
NA Negro adult
NAEBA National Association of Employee Benefit Administrators
NAF Negro adult female
NAIC National Association of Insurance Commissioners
NAMCP National Association of Managed Care Physicians
NBCFH National Business Coalition Forum on Health
NBHH newborn helpful hints
NC Negro child
NCI nursing care institution
NCPA National Center for Policy Analysis
NCQA National Committee for Quality Assurance
NF Negro female
NGRI not quilty by reason of insanity
NHB National Health Board
NHLA National Health Lawyers Association
NLR net loss ratio
NM Negro male
NMHCC National Managed Health Care Congress
NonPar non-participatory provider
NSAIDS non-steroidal anti-inflammatory drugs
$^1/_2$ NSS $^1/_2$ normal saline solution (0.45% sodium chloride)
NSST-TWCS nonspecific ST-T wave changes
NZ enzyme
OA Overeaters Anonymous
OCC occlusal

OCCM open-chest cardiac massage

OD Officer of the Day

OHI oral hygiene instructions

OHMO Office of Health Maintenance Organization

OHS occupational health service

OJ, oj orthoplast jacket

OLTx orthotopic liver transplantation; also OLT, Olt

7-OMEN menogaril

OMH organic marine hydrocolloid

OMSB Outcomes Management Standards Board

OOA out-of-area (services)

OON out-of-network (services)

OPHCOO Office of Prepaid Health Care Operations and Oversight

OPL other party liability

OPM Office of Personnel Management

OROS osmotic release oral system

OSC organized system of care

OSCR on-site concurrent review

OSHA Occupational Safety and Health Act

OV ovary
ovum

OXZ oxazepam

PA paranoid

PACH pipers to after coming head

PAGA premature, appropriate for gestational age

PAROM passive assistive range of motion

PBMNC peripheral blood mononuclear cell; also PBMC, PMNC

PCLR paid claims loss ratio

PCP primary care person
primary care practitioner

PCPM per contract per month

PCR physician contingency reserve

PCV procarbazine, CCNU (lomustine), and vincristine

P₁E₁ pilocarpine 1%, epinephrine 1% (ophthalmic solution)

PEGG Parent Education and Guidance Group

peri perineum

Peri care perineum care

PERRRLA pupils equal, round, regular, react to light and accommodation

PFL Platinol, fluorouracil and leucovorin calcium

PFW pHisoHex face wash

PG paged in hospital

PGP paternal grandparent

PHA arterial pH

PHAR, phar pharmacist

PHCO Physician-Hospital-Community Organization

PHL Philadelphia (chromosome)

PLI professional liability insurance

PMPM per member per month

PNC prenatal course
Psychiatric Nurse Clinician

PNS practical nursing student

P of I proof of illness

POHA preoperative holding area

POLY polychromic erythrocytes

POP point-of-service plan

PP partial upper and lower dentures

PPI-H Producer Price Index–Hospital

PREMIE premature infant; also PI, preemie

prev prevent

prog prognathism

PRSs positive rolandic spikes

PS patient status
plastic surgeon
serum from pregnant women

PSAO Patient Services Administration Organization

PSC pediatric symptom checklist

PTB-SC-SP patellar tendon bearing–supracondylar–suprapatellar

PTMPY per thousand members per year

PWI pediatric walk-in clinic

QIP Quality Improvement Program

QMB qualified Medicare beneficiary

QMRP qualified mental retardation professional

QRC Quality Review Committee

qs every shift [L. *quaque* (every)]

RAC right atrial catheter

R₂AN second year resident's admission notes

RAP radiologists, anesthesiologists, and pathologists

R&C reasonable and customary (charge)

RCF residential care facility

RCPT Registered Cardiopulmonary Technician

RCT Registered Care Technologist

R↓E right lower extremity; also RLE, RLX

RED SUBS reducing substances

ref→ refer to

Reg block regional block (anesthesia)

Retro retrospective rate derivation

RFL request for information

RIMS Risk and Insurance Management Society

RMK #1 remark number 1

ROUL rouleaux

RPA Registered Physician's Assistant

R₂PN second year resident's progress notes

RPTA Registered Physical Therapist Assistant

rt ↑ ext right upper extremity; also RUE, RUX, R↑E

RTNM retreatment staging of cancer: tumor, nodes, and metastasis

RVF right ventricular function

RVS relative value of services

RWJF Robert Wood Johnson Foundation

SAD sugar and acetone determination

SAP Service Assessment Program

SBA stand-by assistant

SB-LM Stanford-Binet Intelligence Test–Form LM

SBOH State Board of Health

SBP small bowel phytobezoars

SCEMIA self-contained enzymatic membrane immunoassay

SCL - 90 symptom checklist–90 items

SCLs soft contact lenses

SCR seclusion room
standard class rate

SDB self destructive behavior

SDC sleep disorders center

SER-IV supination external rotation, type 4 fracture

SERs somatosensory evoked responses

S&F soft and flat

SHPM Society for Healthcare Planning & Marketing

SIC standard industry code

SIIA Self-Insurance Institute of America

Sin c̄ Fe Similac with iron [L. *cum* (with)]

SIW service intensity weights

SK SmithKline

SLMFVD sterile low midforceps vaginal delivery; also SLMFD

sl tr slight trace

SMAS superficial musculoaponeurotic system

SMI small volume infusion

SMILE safety, monitoring, intervention, length of stay, and evaluation

SNT suppan nail technique

SOBRA Sixth Omnibus Reconciliation Act

SPBA Society of Professional Benefit Administrators

SSEPs somatosensory evoked potentials

SSO second surgical opinion

SSSG similarly-sized subscriber group

STNM surgical-evaluation staging of cancer; tumor, nodes, and metastasis

STR stretcher

STT scaphoid, trapezium trapezoid

SUR Statistical Utilization Review

Surgi surgigator

S&WI skin and wound isolation

SWS student ward secretary

T₃/₄ ind triiodothyronine to thyroxine index

TC thioguanine and cytarabine

TEFRA Tax Equity and Fiscal Responsibility Act (of 1982)

TFTs thyroid function tests

TLA translumbar arteriogram

TPA third party administrator

TQM total quality management

TRM-SMX trimethoprim-sulfamethoxazole

TSRA tape surrounded Appli-rulers

TT tonometry
twitch tension

TU transrectal ultrasound

U/ at umbilicus

UB-92 Uniform Billing Code of 1992

UHP University Health Plan

umb ven umbilical vein

UNAC universal access

unacc unaccompanied

URAC Utilization Review Accreditation Commission

URO Utilization Review Organization

USA United States Army

USAF United States Air Force

USMC United States Marine Corp

USN United States Navy

+V positive vertical divergence; also +v, +VD

v. K$_4$ vitamin K$_4$ (menadiol diacetate)

VAERS vaccine adverse event reporting system

VAP vincristine, asparaginase, and prednisone

VCO centilator CPAP (continuous positive airway pressure) oxyhood

VIC Vepesid, ifosfamide, carboplatin, and mesna

VNAA Visiting Nurse Association of America

VP+A vincristine, prednisone, and asparaginase

VPDs ventricular premature depolarizations

VRC vocational rehabilitation counselor

VSI visual motor integration

WBGH Washington Business Group on Health

WDC weighed daily census

WDWN-BF well-developed, well–nourished black female

W+I work and interest

WPP Wechsler Preschool and Primary (Scale of Intelligence)

WTS whole tomography slice

X Xylocaine; also XYL, XYLO

X3 orientation to time, place, and person

X2d times two days

ZEBRA zero balanced reimbursement account

Amino Acid Notation

ABBREVIATION	NAME	ONE-LETTER NOTATION
Ala	Alanine	A
Arg	Arginine	R
Asn	Asparagine	N
Asp	Aspartic acid	D
Asx	Aasparagine or Aspartic acid	B
Cys	Cysteine	C
Gln	Glutamine	Q
Glu	Glutamic acid	E
Glx	Glutamin or Glutamic acid	Z
Gly	Glycine	G
His	Histidine	H
Ile	Isoleucine	I
Leu	Leucine	L
Lys	Lysine	K
Met	Methionine	M
Phe	Phenylalanine	F
Pro	Proline	P
Ser	Serine	S
Thr	Threonine	T
Trp	Tryptophan	W
Tyr	Tyrosine	Y
Val	Valine	V

Roman Numerals

The roman numeral system uses letters to represent numbers. It does not have a constant base system and hence makes calculations difficult or impossible. Roman numerals are used only to identify values and are used sporadically in writing. For example, in medicine roman numerals are used to indicate dosages of drugs and are written in apothecary units. Hence, one needs to understand roman numerals even though arabic numerals are much more common and useful.

Roman numerals are expressed as seven capital or lower case letters

ROMAN NUMERALS		ARABIC EQUIVALENT
Capital	**Lower**	
no roman numeral for 0		0
I	i	1
V	v	5
X	x	10
L	l	50
C	c	100
D	d	500
M	m	1000

A capital letter with a bar over it indicates 1000 times the simple letter.

$\bar{V}$	(5×1000)	5,000
$\bar{X}$	(10×1000)	10,000
$\bar{C}$	(100×1000)	100,000
$\bar{D}$	(500×1000)	500,000
$\bar{M}$	(1000×1000)	1,000,000

These letters are combined in specific ways to indicate the magnitude of a value. Following are some general rules for combining roman numerals.

1. When a numeral of lesser value follows one of greater value, add the two values.

$$V = 5 + 1 = 6$$
$$LX = 50 + 10 = 60$$
$$MDC = 1000 + 500 + 100 = 1600$$

2. When numerals of the same value are repeated in sequence, add the values.

$$XX = 10 + 10 = 20$$
$$iii = 1 + 1 + 1 = 3$$

3. When a numeral of lesser value precedes one of greater value, the value of the first is subtracted from the value of the second. The numerals V, L, and D are never used as a subtracted number.

$$IV = 5 - 1 = 4$$
$$XL = 50 - 10 = 40$$
$$XLV = 50 - 10 + 5 = 45 \text{ (not VL)}$$

4. When a number of lesser value is placed between two numerals of greater value, the numeral of lesser value is subtracted from the numeral following it.

$$XIV = 10 + 5 - 1 = 14$$
$$XXIX = 10 + 10 + 10 - 1 = 29$$

5. Numerals are never repeated more than three times in sequence.

$$XXX = 30$$
$$XL = 40 \text{ (not XXXX)}$$

6. Arrange the letters in order of decreasing value from left to right except for letters having values to be subtracted from the next letter.

$$MDCLXVI = 1666$$
$$MCM = 1900$$
$$MCMXLIV = 1944$$

EXAMPLES:

Arabic	Roman		Arabic	Roman
0			18	XVIII
1	I	i	19	XIX
2	II	ii	20	XX
3	III	iii	30	XXX
4	IV	iv	40	XL
5	V	v	50	L
6	VI	vi	60	LX
7	VII	vii	70	LXX
8	VIII	viii	80	LXXX
9	IX	ix	90	XC
10	X	x	100	C
11	XI	xi	1,000	M
12	XII	xii	5,000	$\bar{V}$
13	XIII	xiii	10,000	$\bar{X}$
14	XIV	xiv	100,000	$\bar{C}$
15	XV	xv	1,000,000	$\bar{M}$
16	XVI	xvi		
17	XVII	xvii		

Modified from: Campbell and Campbell, *Laboratory Mathematics: Medical and Biological Applications*, C.V. Mosby Co., 4th Edition.